AF681588

WITH THEM THROUGH HELL

Love drives me back to grope with them through hell.

Siegfried Sassoon, 'Banishment'

WITH THEM THROUGH HELL

New Zealand Medical Services in the First World War

ANNA ROGERS

MASSEY UNIVERSITY PRESS

CONTENTS

Part 3: Unexpected and Unsung

Part 4: Maimed and Mended

INTRODUCTION

> Whilst we honour our soldiers, let us not forget the medicos . . . There are no exceptions, wherever you go it is the same, just an unassuming attention to every need. Not in the limelight does such heroism shine, but the angels see it and take notice.
> — Chaplain Thomas Fielden Taylor, *Grey River Argus*, 17 February 1917

On the night of 11 August 1917, 24-year-old John Moloney of the New Zealand Rifle Brigade was digging a trench near the River Warnave in France when he and his companions were hit by a shell. 'Two poor lads working on either side of me were cut to ribbons. I could see their vertebrae. One whimpered and died. It was an awful scene, the cries of the wounded and dying sounded on all sides.' A 'melancholy procession' managed to reach the dressing station of medical officer Richard (Dicky) Barron.

> The lad on the stretcher in front of me . . . was wounded in the throat, he breathed with a heavy spluttering gurgle that got fainter and fainter . . . One fine big fellow sat propped up in a corner, his face ashen coloured. He had been badly smacked in the lungs, and there was foam at his mouth. He called gently 'Mother!' and his head dropped. He was gone . . . One little fellow had a left hand that looked like raw meat, it was mangled so. Dicky had a big shears and snipped off hunks of flesh. He whispered to me that the poor fellow couldn't feel it.[1]

There were many ways to be wounded or killed in the First World War. Bodies were pierced and mangled by the red-hot metal of shrapnel; limbs, hands and feet were torn or blown off; bones were shattered; tendons and arteries severed; faces mutilated beyond recognition. Men suffered brain injuries and deafness from the constant blast of shellfire. In close-quarter fighting there was the threat of stab wounds from bayonets or entrenching tools. Gas blinded and blistered and excoriated throats and lungs. The petroleum from flamethrowers caused appalling burns.[2] Added to terrible physical assaults were the high risk of infection and nerve damage, and the psychological effects of severe trauma. Although this was the first major conflict in which there were more combat deaths than fatalities caused by disease, serious sickness was widespread — dysentery, influenza, typhoid.

The thousands of men, wounded and ill, who were brought into regimental aid posts, dressing stations, casualty clearing stations and hospitals were cared for by another, less familiar fighting force, armed not with guns but with scalpels, bandages, drugs and compassion.[3] During the First World War, hundreds of New Zealand doctors, nurses, stretcher-bearers, orderlies and ambulance drivers, dentists, chiropodists, pharmacists, physiotherapists and chaplains carried out this vital work, often at great personal risk, as veterinarians also did for the horses, mules, donkeys and camels that provided essential military transport. Their extraordinary contribution has not always received the attention it deserves.

There is, of course, a central irony here. People trained to mend and heal were required to make hurt and ill soldiers and animals fit enough to fight again, so they could once more be wounded — or killed. There is an easy answer to this conundrum: to wage war a nation needs healthy troops, and the means of restoring them, without delay, to their place on the front line. This was certainly how New Zealand's military leaders, and its government, saw things, and the men themselves knew that unless they received a severe wound or were extremely sick, they would inevitably return to the front. One way of dealing with the ethical dilemma was to remove altogether the conflict between practising medicine and fulfilling military duty. 'We doctors simply go on healing the sick and patching up broken bodies . . . the enemy to us is not even an enemy but only part of our job of care. For a doctor there is no war, or at least there need be no war.'[4]

There is another paradox: war can stimulate significant medical advances. Many of the innovations born of the First World War are now second nature in military medicine: triage (ranking the urgency of casualties' condition to decide the order of treatment), debridement (the removal of unhealthy tissue from wounds to help healing), effective blood transfusions, the widespread use of X-rays, the vital importance of inoculation and vaccination, treatment of psychological war damage, life-altering maxillo-facial and oral surgery, and the role of physical therapy and rehabilitation in recovery. In the memorable words of medical historian Leo van Bergen, 'War was a colleague, war was a teacher. War was the doctor of doctors.' But, as he also notes, without improved medical care the terrible battles of the First World War would have been fought with far fewer men and would probably have ended before November 1918. It is worth remembering, too, the extraordinary advances, such as the discovery of penicillin, that have *not* been associated with war. As Bergen asks, 'Why don't we ever say: peace is good for medicine?'[5]

Because the sophisticated new weaponry of this war enabled attacks from a much greater distance, wounds and death were meted out far more impersonally and far more unpredictably: places of complete safety were rare. Slow, painful deaths were common, but most men died almost before they knew they had been hit.[6] The number of casualties in the First World War can never be certain — some 18 million were killed and 23 million wounded. Of New Zealand's 1.1 million inhabitants, almost 100,000 served overseas. Over 18,000 of them died during or soon after the conflict, and more than 40,000 were wounded or suffered from disease.

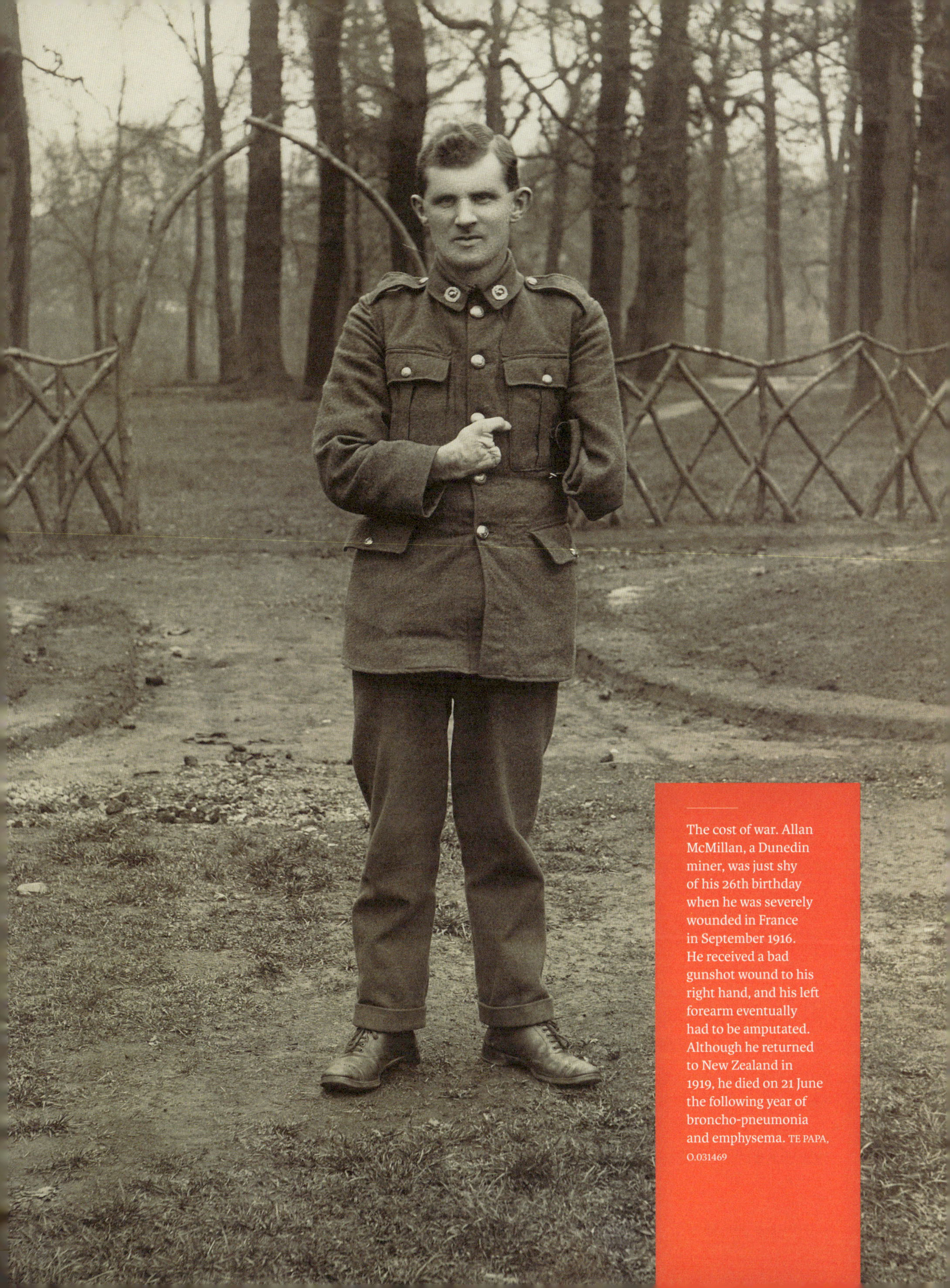

The cost of war. Allan McMillan, a Dunedin miner, was just shy of his 26th birthday when he was severely wounded in France in September 1916. He received a bad gunshot wound to his right hand, and his left forearm eventually had to be amputated. Although he returned to New Zealand in 1919, he died on 21 June the following year of broncho-pneumonia and emphysema. TE PAPA, O.031469

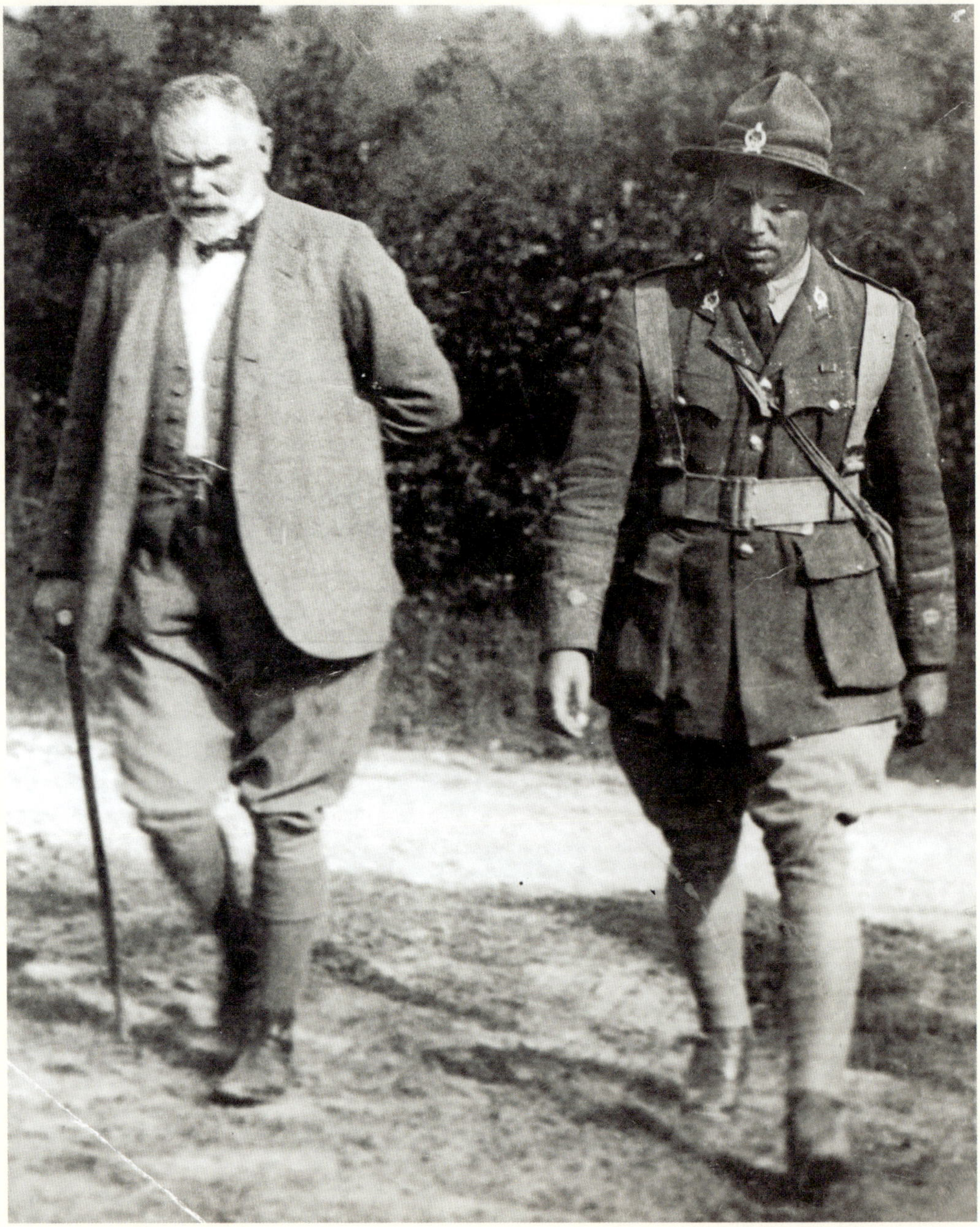

New Zealand's high commissioner to London, Sir Thomas Mackenzie (1853–1930), with Te Rangi Hīroa (Peter Buck) during a visit to New Zealand troops in France. Hīroa (1877?–1951), who was decorated for his work on Gallipoli, was the only Māori medical officer to serve in the war. Mackenzie was a kindly and sympathetic figure with a deep concern for the welfare of New Zealand soldiers overseas. His son, Clutha, was blinded on Gallipoli.
ALEXANDER TURNBULL LIBRARY, 1/2-037933-F

The New Zealand Medical Service in the Great War 1914–1918, written in 1924 by Andrew Carbery, a surgeon who was a serving officer, is a detailed and comprehensive account. Carbery was given an unenviable brief, especially when the principal technology available to him was a typewriter: one year to research his subject, six months to write it, and three to six months to see the book through the press. Particularly under these constraints, he did an admirable job — for a man of his time writing in an official military context only a few years after the war ended. Inevitably, there are omissions — the almost non-existent coverage of the nurses' role is the most glaring — and Carbery tends to gloss over or sidestep areas of controversy. There is, too, understandably, a strong imperial spirit, but the book is thorough and readable.

For that reason, and because it is written a century after the First World War ended, *With Them Through Hell* concentrates on telling the *story* of the men and women of New Zealand's medical services, where possible in their own words. Its scope goes beyond traditional military medicine to embrace others who fought to keep the men and animals of the war alive and healthy. For reasons of size, it focuses on those serving overseas.

It is very largely a Pākehā story. Only one Māori, Te Rangi Hīroa, also known as Peter Buck (Ngāti Mutunga), served as a medical officer in this war, with the mainly Māori Pioneer Battalion in the Middle East, Gallipoli and France. (Although not a front-line fighting unit, the battalion, which built roads, dug trenches and fulfilled other engineering and logistical duties, often found itself in perilous situations, working under fire.) He was twice mentioned in despatches and received the DSO. Māori served as stretcher-bearers, both officially and otherwise, and their pioneer role also made them invaluable in other ways. At Passchendaele, for example, they 'did yeoman service in bringing up planks and laying them crosswise to give a foothold' in the mud for the struggling stretcher-bearers.[7]

New Zealand's First World War medical story has much to say about the relationship with and attitudes towards the British. This was a period in which the regular newspaper headlines, 'New Zealanders at Home' and 'Our Boys in Britain', meant the same thing: Kiwis were serving the empire and Britain was home with a capital H. They certainly faced prejudice from some British doctors and nurses. The New Zealanders soon realised, however, that they were the equal of, if not often superior to, the Mother Country's military medics, and their reputation would grow as the war went on. The often-repeated idea that New Zealand discovered its nationhood in this war, particularly on Gallipoli, is clichéd and sweeping, but, like the troops, the men and women of the medical services certainly discovered that their skill, courage and devotion needed no imperial imprimatur.

The medical care for the men who fought in the New Zealand Expeditionary Force during the First World War went from head to toe, and from enlistment through often multiple experiences of sickness and wounding to their return home. Doctors (almost all male), nurses (and VADs — members of the Voluntary Aid Detachment), stretcher-bearers, orderlies and ambulance drivers were, of course, to the fore, but others played a significant part. Dentists looked after the soldiers' teeth, so they could chew their rations; chiropodists cared for their feet, so they could march; experts in massage (physiotherapy) encouraged wounded and disabled men towards recovery; pharmacists ensured they received the right drugs. There was skilled care, too, for the animals, from the New Zealand Veterinary Corps.

After a man was wounded on the battlefield, he moved along an evacuation chain that stretched from hasty, immediate front-line treatment to a casualty clearing station (CCS) to a stationary and/or a base hospital, and then, perhaps, to a cot on a hospital ship bound for Britain or home. New Zealand would send two stationary hospitals overseas during the war — despite their name, they moved about with the troops.[8] These served in Egypt and Salonika, and in France at Amiens, Hazebrouck and then Wisques. Wounded Kiwis were sent to British base hospitals in France and to New Zealand's three general hospitals in Britain, at Brockenhurst, Walton-on-Thames and Codford. The women of the New Zealand Army Nursing Service (NZANS) served in hospitals, in CCSs and on hospital ships. Although not allowed in the front line, they were often close to it. Untrained, but also essential, were VADs, who assisted with domestic and nursing work in hospitals and elsewhere, and the members of safe sex campaigner Ettie Rout's Volunteer Sisterhood.

Twenty-six medical officers (MOs), about a third of them from the volunteer New Zealand Medical Corps,[9] had accompanied the troops who fought in the 1899–1902 South African War. Each of the 10 contingents took at least one doctor, the larger ones two or more. They both acted as regimental medical officers (RMOs) and were posted to British military hospitals. But the imperial arrangements and equipment were poor. A hundred and thirty-nine New Zealand soldiers died of disease, usually typhoid, principally as a result of vestigial sanitation and ineffective treatment. Seventy-one were killed in action or died of wounds.[10] The treatment of the wounded and sick needed to be better in this war.

By 1914, what was now the New Zealand Medical Corps (NZMC) had been in existence for six years, but despite changes in the wake of the 1909 Defence Act, and regular camps at which field ambulance men practised such skills as 'stretcher drill, searching for wounded, the loading and unloading of ambulance waggons, and the placing of patients on and off stretchers',[11] the NZMC had problems. The various units were widely scattered, especially in rural areas, busy doctors had little time to devote to military work, the few officers were too far apart to easily share knowledge, and it was hard to make progress without a qualified, full-time Royal Army Medical Corps (RAMC) instructor. Despite the laudable enthusiasm and energy of the men themselves, 'New Zealand was not, from a medical point of view, prepared for war'.[12]

Sufficient medical personnel — four medical officers, two dental surgeons, 67 NCOs and men, plus six (later seven) nurses — were rapidly found for the Advance Party of the New Zealand Expeditionary Force that left in August 1914, in response to a request from Britain, to occupy the German colony of Samoa. The 48 officers who accompanied the Main Body of the NZEF when it departed for war in October were all volunteers with years of NZMC service behind them; some, like Christchurch surgeon Percival Fenwick, had served in South Africa. Almost all the 328 NCOs and other ranks were also corps men.[13] An outbreak of respiratory diseases, measles and cerebro-spinal meningitis at Trentham camp in the winter of 1915 killed 27 recruits and caused a nationwide scandal, laying horribly bare the faults of a 'loosely organized part time territorial medical service'.[14] Some sensible improvements were subsequently made.

Medical men throughout the country stepped up both to go overseas and to staff the training establishments at home. Until 6 October 1915, when Awapuni camp, at the racecourse outside Palmerston North, became the NZMC training centre, medical instruction at Trentham, amid the general preparation of hundreds of recruits, was 'haphazard'.[15] Ormond Burton, who would serve with the field ambulance, nevertheless found it 'interesting and very practical indeed. We had to look after the health of two thousand men and deal with incidental accidents. The doctors . . . were mainly young men who had recently qualified with a sprinkling of older men to stiffen them. Not a bad lot!'[16]

There were, however, complaints from doctors on Gallipoli about ill-prepared orderlies, and the first 20 who ended up at the New Zealand hospital in Cairo were not acceptable, in the view of commanding officer William Parkes. 'I regret that [they] are for the most part untrained,' he reported at the end of October 1915, 'and would strongly recommend that a proper course of instruction be given in Camp prior to embarkation and that a Medical Officer be detailed to continue instruction during the voyage.'[17] Not all the orderlies were below par. In May 1915 MO Thomas Ritchie felt compelled to 'say a word of praise' about his, a man named McCann. 'Although he had absolutely no knowledge of nursing or of drugs he has carried out my instructions to the letter . . . What he lacks in experience he makes up for in gentleness & application. He works night & day in the little hospital with another new chum from amongst the troops to help him.'[18]

General Alexander Godley, the General Officer Commanding the NZEF, had been concerned about the state of New Zealand's military medical services before Gallipoli. In February 1915 he was 'afraid that our men have not really got quite sufficient experience for managing a large number of casualties if we get them'. At the front he accepted the offered services of Englishman Colonel Neville Manders, a distinguished entomologist and military surgeon who would serve on the peninsula with the New Zealanders and Australians.[19] By April, wartime defence minister James Allen agreed that an experienced Royal Army Medical Corps officer was needed to head and instruct the NZMC at home,[20] and Colonel Robert Henderson arrived in New Zealand on 6 September 1915 to take up his duties as surgeon-general. Henderson made the establishment of the dedicated Awapuni camp one of his first initiatives.

For the 350 to 400 medical men training at Awapuni at any one time, the experience was not luxurious. Although amenities were added — lights, vegetable gardens and a 'shower bathroom' — the accommodation arrangements continued the bracing and money-saving pattern set when the camp had housed sick men sent from Trentham. 'There are,' the *Dominion* reported on 17 January 1916, 'neither tents nor hutments.'

> The officers and n.c.o.'s sleep on the balconies of the stewards' stand and secretary's offices, and the men have their quarters in the grandstand, sleeping in the upper part of it and taking their meals in the portion used as the public dining-room on race days . . . The end of the grandstand, which is exposed to the prevailing wind, is sheeted in with railway tarpaulins.

> The men have their beds on the broader of the ledges and place their gear in the seat above them. Everything is kept in ship-shape order and the quarters are comfortable and tidy.[21]

The camp was initially headed by the local military district commander, with Auckland doctor Major James Hardie Neil in charge of all the training, but by early 1916 Henderson had decided that an NZMC man should head the camp.

For everyone other than officers, the challenging programme comprised nine weeks of basic instruction at Awapuni, a month of practical hospital work at Featherston or Trentham, seven days of leave and then a final week back in camp. Norman Gray's practical experience was gained at Trentham. Because an NZMC man 'may have to act as a bearer, a nurse, a sanitary engineer, a water expert, a cook, a clerk, a storeman, or a driver, and these are only some of the positions', Gray and his companions took turns 'doing all the work of the place, nursing one week, on guard the next, sanitary work, cookhouse, dustmen, officers, orderlies'.[22] As well as ambulance drill with stretchers and wagons, there was 'field work reproducing as nearly as possible actual service conditions', along with lectures on everything from anatomy and physiology, wounds, fractures and bandaging to shock, fits, suffocation, 'choking, cold, foreign bodies in the eye and ear, drowning, poisoning, and so on'. The hospital work and nursing instruction included 'the use of surgical instruments, anaesthetics and antiseptics, the administration of medicines, surgical nursing, the treatment of infectious cases, observation of the sick'. Territorial officers gave lectures on such topics as discipline, military law, map-reading, judging distances and signalling. There was also drilling in infantry formations, to develop a 'soldierly spirit'.[23] It was little wonder, as the *New Zealand Herald* noted, that the men were 'busy from reveille — 5 a.m. — with short intervals for rest, until nightfall'.[24]

Those training at Awapuni could not choose their role in the NZMC; the authorities decided who went where. Some men who enlisted 'with an eye on a hospital ship' and missed out became 'very indignant'. They were, apparently, under the impression that such a post was a 'soft snap' but, said the *Dominion* sternly, and correctly, 'They are mistaken. It is very hard work.'[25] It was all relative, though. Front-line men like Gray would come to feel that some 'drafted to Stationary and Base Hospitals and Hosp. Ships . . . work all manner of "slinters" [tricks] to stay there for the duration' and 'should be given a chance to show their prowess at stretcher bearing and whizbang dodging . . . There is absolutely no comparison between the 2 kinds of work'.[26] Not all NZMC medics served overseas. Many were needed to staff the camps at home to ensure that the recruits were healthy and well cared for while training, and there were frequent calls throughout the war for more men, sometimes those not fit enough to return to the front, to do such work.

Awapuni-trained ambulance men sailed on the first charter of the hospital ship *Marama* in December 1915, and then left for overseas at regular intervals. As the *Dominion* reported in January 1917, 'every week fresh drafts have been going in to take the place of those who go on active service.'[27] The men continued to prepare while they waited to depart. Those embarking on the other hospital ship, the *Maheno*, in January 1917 travelled south to Christchurch to camp at the A & P showground at Addington, where they were 'revising their training with all kinds

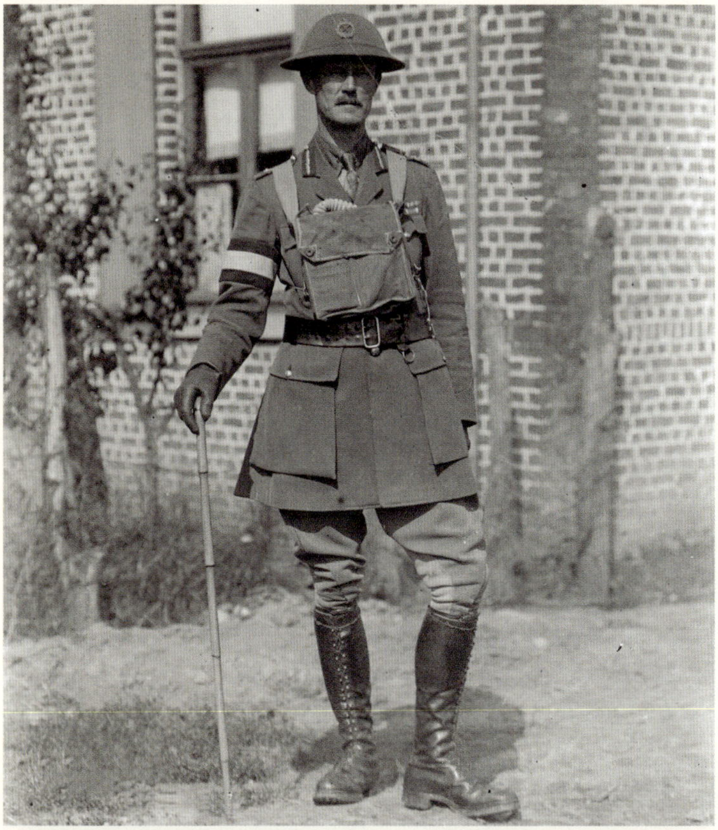

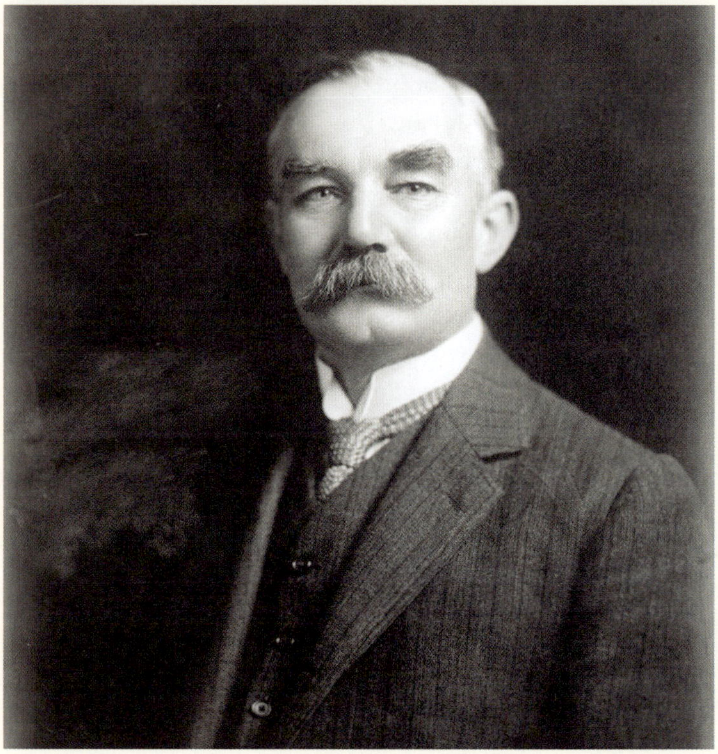

above A somewhat distant and formal figure who was not always liked or understood by the men he led and admired, British-born Alexander Godley (1867–1957) was General Officer Commanding the New Zealand Expeditionary Force throughout the war. ALEXANDER TURNBULL LIBRARY, 1/4-009477-G

below James Allen (1855–1942), who was knighted in 1917, held the challenging post of New Zealand defence minister from 1912 to 1919, and also acted as prime minister for lengthy periods while the country's joint leaders, William Massey and Joseph Ward, were overseas. He drew some criticism for his handling of the portfolio but was stoic and hard-working, especially in the face of his son John's death on Gallipoli in June 1915. ALEXANDER TURNBULL LIBRARY, 1/1-013396-G of ambulance work [and] being kept in condition by route marches'.[28] The learning continued during the voyages. When not on duty, the 25 NZMC other ranks going overseas with 500 Australian troops on HMS *Persia* in August 1915 practised stretcher drill and bandaging. 'All the Hospital work has fallen to our unit,' MO Ronald Orbell reported when the ship reached Suez, 'and I and my officers have taken every opportunity of teaching the men as much as possible of the ordinary hospital routine.'[29] Gray, on the *Tahiti*, considered 28 October 1915 'One of the best days so far, from our training standpoint' — lectures on the blood and circulatory system and the causes of disease were supplemented by 'signalling and stretcher drill'.[30]

Extra NZMC training was added in April 1917, when the Tauherenikau racecourse in Wairarapa became the venue for four weeks of practical instruction in military hospital and nursing work after a month of squad and stretcher training at Awapuni. At the racing club's expense, many alterations had been made, including converting the totalisator building into a 40-bed ward. The men also attended lectures and demonstrations, for which 'anatomical exhibits and specimens are provided'.[31]

New Zealand's medical profession was eager to serve. The nurses would have a much harder job convincing the authorities that they should go overseas — 550 would eventually do so — as would female doctors, but male doctors and surgeons were accepted without question. It is hard to put an exact figure on the number who served overseas with the NZMC. Carbery states that 385 of New Zealand's 700 or so registered doctors left the country, along with 3248 other ranks — recruits trained to work as orderlies and stretcher-bearers. But painstaking research by Pat Clarkson reveals a doctor/surgeon total nearer 430.[32] A number of New Zealand doctors also served with the RAMC, often because they were working in Britain and enrolled there when war broke out. The pay was better, too, in the British service.[33] Some later enlisted with the NZEF. Although the medical school at the University of Otago had opened in 1875, many of the older, more experienced doctors who served during the war were trained in Britain, particularly at the University of Edinburgh.[34]

Not everyone wanting to enlist was able to do so immediately. Initially, preference went to the waiting list of NZMC men — like Auckland surgeon Arthur Purchas, who had been with the volunteer force and then the territorials for 29 years when he enlisted on 26 August 1914[35] — as Thomas McKibbin from Hastings discovered when he tried to volunteer as a surgeon on 8 April 1915. He had been a territorial officer, but his membership had lapsed and the authorities regarded him as a civilian; he did not leave as an NZMC officer until mid-August. The Mother Country was calling too. In June 1915 the War Office requested an additional 100 New Zealand doctors, who would be 'temporary lieutenants of the R.A.M.C.' Those keen to apply were to do so via the inspector-general of hospitals or, if they were NZMC members, the director of medical services in Wellington.[36]

Some medical men, desperate to go but unable to get an NZMC place, headed overseas on their own initiative — and at their own expense. Louis Barnett took leave of absence from the chair of surgery at Otago University to sail for England in March 1915. From May to August, thanks to a temporary RAMC commission achieved with the help of New Zealand's high commissioner in London, Thomas (later Sir Thomas) Mackenzie, he was chief surgeon of the 1200-bed Imtarfa military hospital on Malta. 'I have got a splendid position at this great institution. I am busy from morning to night and am happy in the thought that I am doing something worth while.'[37] Barnett was then attached to the NZEF at Godley's request and in mid-1916 was appointed the force's consulting surgeon.

There were clearly some initial administrative problems. In a letter to the *Auckland Star* in July 1915, 'Sawbones' maintained that 'applicants who volunteered months ago have not yet received even the customary courtesy of an acknowledgment of their letters, much less any intimation as to whether they are, or will be, required . . . Only last week two junior resident medical officers left the local hospital for Australia, after waiting in vain for news for months.' The correspondent also believed that some doctors were '"wired" to proceed to Trentham at a few days' notice' and expected to wind up their affairs 'like the itinerant scissors-grinder his working outfit'.[38] There were also mistakes later in the war. NZMC Captain Edward Edie was serving in France in August 1918 when he felt obliged to write to the *Southland Times*, which had reported his calling up in the latest ballot (conscription had been introduced in 1916). 'For your benefit and also the benefit of others (including the Defence officials) I wish to state that I have now been sixteen months in France — all of that time (except a few weeks in hospital, the result of a wound) — I have spent as medical officer to a Battalion, which is not the softest of positions in this great game over here.'[39]

Speed in applying could be a factor too, even for NZMC members. The telegram Gore surgeon William McAra sent to his local MP expressing his willingness to serve overseas was forwarded to Allen on 12 August 1914; on the 16th he was told that he had 'delayed his application so long that when he applied, all the openings were filled and many wanting to take a chance of any vacancy that might occur'.[40] He did leave in December. One who moved swiftly was Major Charles Hand-Newton, 'who had only been a short time in practice' and had just been appointed to Christchurch Hospital as assistant surgeon. Two days after war was declared he and Dr Neil Guthrie went into camp at Addington; the next day they were transferred to Awapuni. Hand-Newton was appointed second in command of the Mounted Field Ambulance because he had been 'an active Territorial Medical Officer'. The other original MFA officers, all from Christchurch, were James Bell, Charles Hercus and Alexander Trotter, plus freshly graduated student doctors William Aitken, Donald Milne and Robert Withers. Their commander was South African War veteran Lieutenant-Colonel Charles Thomas from Timaru.[41]

The doctors who remained at home did their bit. On 10 August 1914 the *Nelson Evening Mail* reported that Wellington GPs would 'give free medical attendance to the wives and children of men who go to the front' and 'carry on the practices of doctors accompanying the troops'.[42] Reports like this, in the *New Zealand Herald* of 17 January 1916, became common. Alexander Grant, who had been acting superintendent of Auckland Hospital for 11 months in place of Charles Maguire, who was serving in Egypt, 'has received a commission as captain in the New Zealand Medical Corps . . . and will leave for the Awapuni camp to-morrow evening'.

He had 'been the recipient of several presentations': a silver spirit flask, an officer's kit-box, a travelling case and 'an enlarged photograph of themselves' from his returned soldier patients.[43] But the enthusiastic medical response, often by senior and highly trained men and women, left New Zealand badly short of medical professionals. In July 1917, the *Press* could report that 'in Christchurch alone, 23 out of 46 doctors in practice are either on service or have been'.[44]

The doctors who signed up had the requisite medical knowledge. Many, though, as NZEF officers, had to acquire military expertise, which included training and handling the men they would be commanding, ordering supplies and learning such unexpected skills as digging latrines. After Awapuni, they had a week's final leave before departing for duty. The pressure to keep the training cycle going was clear in an April 1916 letter from the camp commandant, Scottish-born Auckland surgeon Russell Tracey-Inglis. To get an extra two medical officers ready for the Twelfth Reinforcements, he would have to 'push on' with their training and cut their time by a week. Once they and others already chosen left, he would have only two men still in training, 'so that if you want officers trained to go with the Thirteenth Reinforcements I shall need them in camp at once'.[45]

William Barclay, who served on the second charter of the *Maheno*, certainly remembered a briefer experience. 'We had to get some military training so we went up to Awapuni [where they] tried to teach us to give instructions to squads. We were two weeks there and then back to Wellington to equip ourselves with a suitable uniform — Khaki serge and gabardine lighter uniform, riding breeches, spurs and sword [available from the barracks for £3], as we discovered to our consternation at the last moment.' Some returned their swords and got their money back.[46]

As the war went on, doctors and surgeons who had already served overseas or were home on leave shared their expertise as camp instructors. At the beginning of June 1916, the *Free Lance* reported that 'Doctor Arnold Izard — we beg his pardon, Captain Izard — has been spending his time ashore in the N.Z.M.C. Camp at Awapuni and instructing the "Linseed Lancers" (as they term themselves) in many things.' Izard was 'the most popular as well as the most practical officer in camp . . . the friendly little chats the Captain has with his own section during "smoko" or a "breather" are eagerly listened to by the boys, and [are] the proper way . . . to make soldiers aware of the dangers of the East [brothels] and the proper and manly way to meet or avoid these pitfalls.'[47] When No. 2 Field Ambulance was at Awapuni, it 'had the inestimable benefit of the services of Major A. A. Martin, who trained the men at the Palmerston North Public Hospital, and of Matron [Ada] Kilgour, of the Old Men's Home at Awapuni, under whose careful tuition they became remarkably efficient in ward duties and nursing'.[48] Returned doctors also often gave lectures about their experiences, to encourage recruitment and to inform and enthuse the public.

The medical men who left New Zealand with the Main Body included 21 Otago medical students in their final (fifth) year, who had responded with 'quite remarkable speed' when news of the outbreak of war was received. That very day, 5 August, they signed a letter stating their willingness 'if qualified, to place their services at the disposal of the New Zealand Government as Medical Officers for the Expeditionary Force'.[49] Among them was William Aitken. 'To meet the medical emergency,' he recalled many years later, the final exams were held in August rather than December, so 'I became qualified to practise medicine three months earlier than expected. At once I volunteered for service overseas and a week later a telegram came to say that I had been appointed a lieutenant in the N.Z. Mounted Field Ambulance which was being mobilised at Awapuni.' Aitken was on a train next morning.[50] Also eager to serve was a sizeable group of third-year students, whose first professional exams were brought forward; many who passed volunteered as stretcher-bearers. Others at various stages of their training would also enlist. Fourth-year student Thomas (Tom) Denniston, 'a very popular young fellow, of a most engaging disposition', was only 24 when he died of enteric fever (typhoid) on Malta after serving as a sergeant in the NZMC.[51]

Gallipoli was a brutal shock for these enthusiastic but inexperienced young men. John Russell of the 1st Battalion Wellington Infantry Regiment, who reached the peninsula in time for the horrors of Chunuk Bair, and did much to help the wounded, described 'an open-air operating theatre where . . . a very-severely wounded chap [was] being operated upon by an ex-Wanganui boy, Dr. Raymond Kitchen, for the removal of shell splinters from his middle area'. Twenty-one-year-old Kitchen, a first-year Otago student, would be mentioned in despatches for conspicuous gallantry at the Dardanelles. Later in the Gallipoli campaign, a number of the medical students who had left New Zealand in 1914 were sent home to complete their studies. Several returned to serve again.[52] Admirable though the students' patriotism had been, it was clear that proper preparation was required. Accordingly, a voluntary Officers' Training Corps was established at Otago University in mid-1916 to 'provide medical students in the Dominion with a standardised medico-military training' spread over four years.[53] Several of the students who went overseas in 1914 served with distinction. Aitken was awarded the Military Cross; both Kenneth MacCormick and Philip Jory received DSOs. After being mentioned in despatches for his work on Gallipoli, Aubrey Short won the MC in France.

Matters of age and experience caused problems when, in March 1915, all NZMC lieutenants who had sailed with the Main Body were promoted to captain, regardless of medical achievement. This meant that young, recently qualified men had the same rank as surgeons who may have held important hospital or university appointments.[54]

There was no question that male medics would be permitted to care for New Zealand's war casualties, but female nurses and doctors were another matter entirely. The New Zealand Medical Corps Nursing Reserve had been gazetted on 14 May 1908, and Janet Gillies, who had nursed in South Africa, became matron-in-chief. Her reserve, however, had no nurses and the authorities stonewalled her attempts at recruitment. Organisation was not her forte and living in Nelson made communication a problem. She faced, too, a determined and ambitious force in the redoubtable Hester Maclean, assistant inspector of hospitals in the Department of Hospitals and Charitable Aid, a vital force behind the New Zealand Trained Nurses' Association and the founding editor of the nursing journal *Kai Tiaki*. Close to the government, Maclean had power and influence, and knew how to use them.

In June 1910 a frustrated Gillies stepped down and Maclean stepped up, though she was not made matron-in-chief and asked to set up a New Zealand military nursing service until August 1911. Despite some progress, bureaucratic to-ing and fro-ing was still going on when war broke out. Since 'it would be likely a body of Nurses would . . . be sent with the troops', wrote an exasperated Maclean, would it not be sensible to ask for volunteers, sign up nurses and then deal with the red tape? The authorities disagreed. 'It is not intended to send any Nurses with the Expeditionary Force,' came the reply on 6 August, 'and you would be doing us a great favour by letting this be known among Nurses, as much time is spent in answering the numerous applications which are coming in.'[55]

But suddenly everything changed. On the morning of 7 August Maclean was asked to organise six nurses to travel to Samoa with the Advance Party, and by the next day she had approval to enrol women for the New Zealand Army Nursing Service. This did not, however, amount to a real beginning for the organisation: the authorities simply wanted replacements for the German nursing staff in Samoa.

Maclean and the government were deluged with impassioned requests from both nurses and untrained women burning to serve overseas. Mary Duff, for instance, had both a first aid certificate and 'a great deal of experience in nursing . . . I am most anxious to go, and do what I can for the brave fellows, who have to face so much danger and suffering.'[56] Allen remained unmoved. As he told Duff, 'we are not sending any nurses with the Main Expeditionary Force. I am grateful to you for the offer of your services, but under the circumstances you will see that they cannot be accepted.'[57] Allen was unwilling to budge: 'until the Mother Country asked us to provide nurses it would be almost a presumption to send them. It would look like interfering with the Imperial arrangements.' But pressure from other quarters, including a deputation from the New Zealand Trained Nurses' Association, and the realisation that more and more men were leaving to fight, finally propelled the defence minister into action. On 7 January 1915 the governor, Lord Liverpool, offered 50 nurses 'for service with British troops or with the French Red Cross if desired'.[58] London accepted, and by the end of January the decision was made; the nurses would, of course, be escorted overseas by Maclean. Later that year she could report that, although an amendment of the Defence Act was required, 'The New Zealand Army Nursing Service has at last been formed.'[59]

Liverpool had also asked Australia if New Zealand nurses could

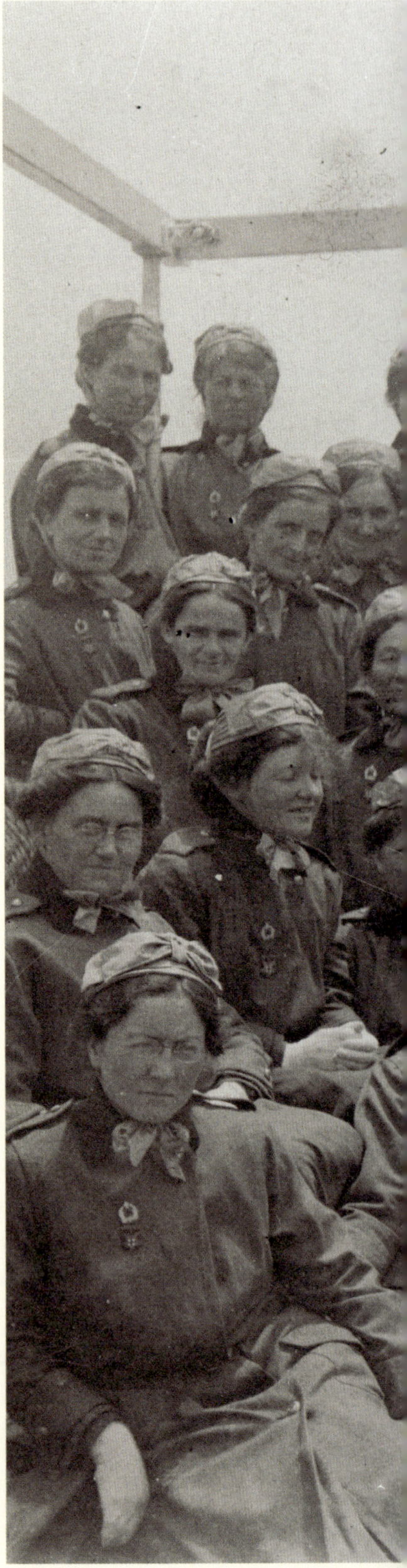

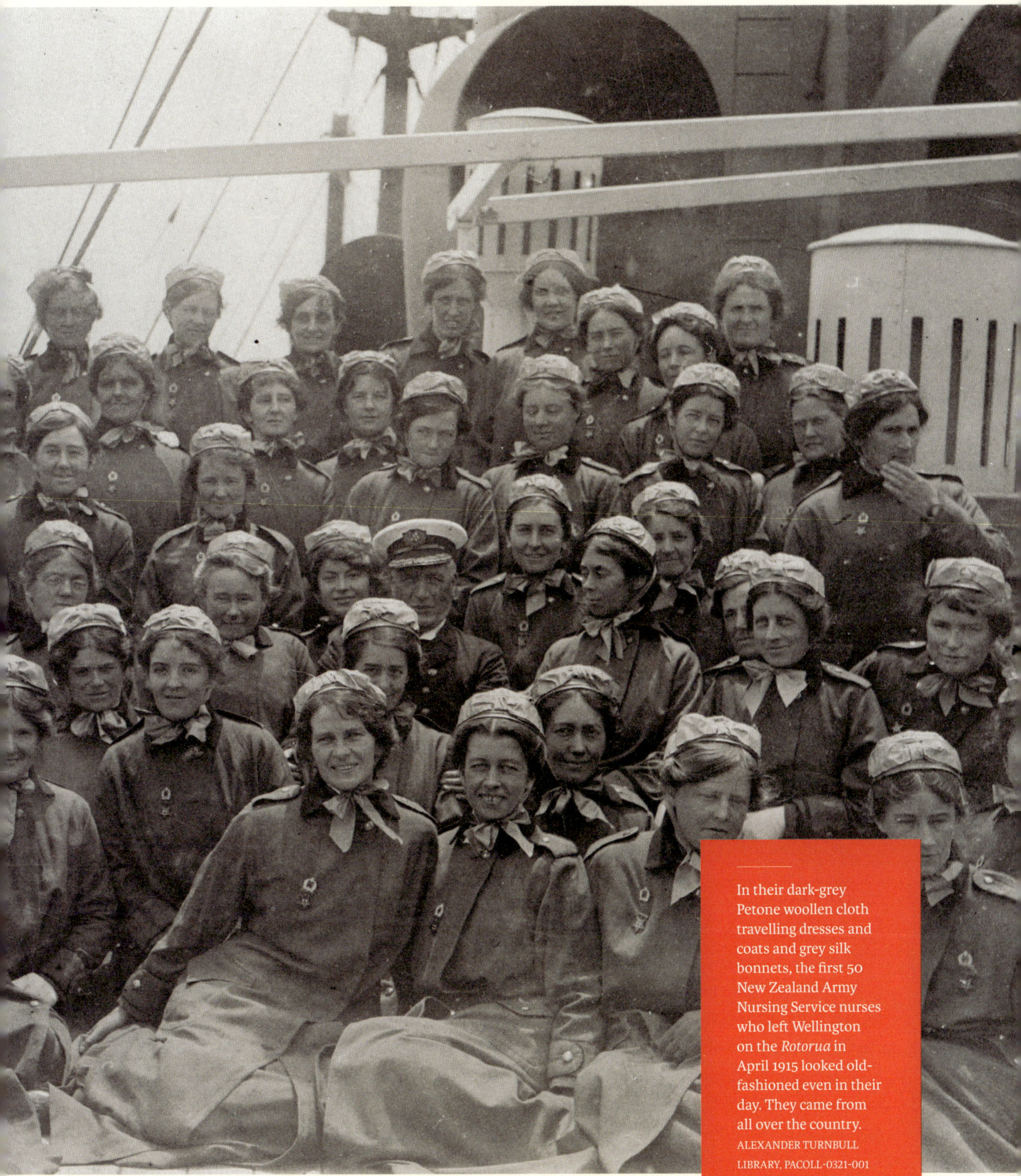

In their dark-grey Petone woollen cloth travelling dresses and coats and grey silk bonnets, the first 50 New Zealand Army Nursing Service nurses who left Wellington on the *Rotorua* in April 1915 looked old-fashioned even in their day. They came from all over the country.
ALEXANDER TURNBULL LIBRARY, PACOLL-0321-001

be considered for their overseas nursing contingent. On 25 March, Maclean received a cable requesting two sisters and 10 nurses to sail six days later, to join Australian nurses bound for Egypt. She hastily chose the required number from the reserve and volunteer lists, and the lucky dozen departed on 1 April 1915, a week before the first 50 left the capital.

All the women in the main NZANS group were Pākehā — no Māori nurses have been identified[60] — had at least six years of nursing experience and were single. Their average age was 27. All the women were farewelled by their own districts, with good wishes and helpful gifts. After reaching Wellington and organising their paybooks and uniforms, they received their badges at Parliament on 7 April. When she boarded the SS *Rotorua* the next morning, Mabel Crook from Palmerston North had with her 'Whisky Flask, Electric Torch, Hamper, Chocolate, books. Deck chair. Writing case in leather (officers style). Travelling Cabin Trunk. Suit case. Fountain pen. Hot water bag. Nail file. Woollen gloves, Muslin caps. Collars. Cuffs. Leather Purse bag (2). Gold Brooch. Gold chain. HRfs [handkerchiefs?]. Cushions (2). 2 blouses.' In warm Indian summer sunshine, the crowds on Wellington's Glasgow Wharf cheered as the *Rotorua* departed on the afternoon of 8 April. 'Had beautiful basket of flowers presented to me on board boat before leaving,' Crook wrote. 'Held strings of ribbon to those on wharf. Band played Tipperary, National Anthem & should old acquaintance . . . Many eyes held tears.'[61]

The nurse/orderly relationship was not always straightforward, as some NZMC men resented answering to women, but, like the patients, they more often appreciated the nurses' dedication and skill. While on night duty on the *Maheno* in Lottie Le Gallais' ward in 1915, orderly Guy Farrell wrote a letter to *Kai Tiaki* 'to draw your attention to the devoted and untiring work of our Sisters . . . one cannot fail to notice their splendid efforts to soothe the sick and wounded men . . . I shall never forget, the first few days on our initial trip to Anzac Bay . . . My poor Sister worked like a Trojan and it beats me how she kept up so long and with such frightful cases as we were getting.'[62]

Male prejudice was not absent, however. While travelling to war on the *Aparima* in 1917, Wilfred Smith told his wife, 'I have changed my opinion dear about having Nurses aboard Transports, it is only a farce because they don't do anything, but fool round with the Officers . . . and I really think that they do much more harm than good.'[63] As Claude Weston of the Wellington Infantry Battalion suggested, too, some wounded men, accustomed to being in command, could find it difficult 'to be controlled by the other sex . . . The sisters and nurses naturally like doing their work in their own way, and the soldiers have grown accustomed to insisting on everything being done as they ordain.'[64]

Gaining recognition of their rank and status proved difficult for the nurses. Despite a February 1916 directive that matrons, sisters and nurses held officer rank and were to be 'accorded the usual courtesy salute', this seldom happened,[65] and although many doctors showed respect and admiration, some foolish discrimination took place. Wellington nurse Edna Pengelly, travelling on the *Marama* from Egypt to England in June 1916, reported the putting up of a notice: '"Sisters are to have no communication with the officers on any account unless in the discharge of their duties." I suppose someone has been silly and so the whole crowd of us are to be treated in this fashion . . . There is a chalk line on the deck to divide the

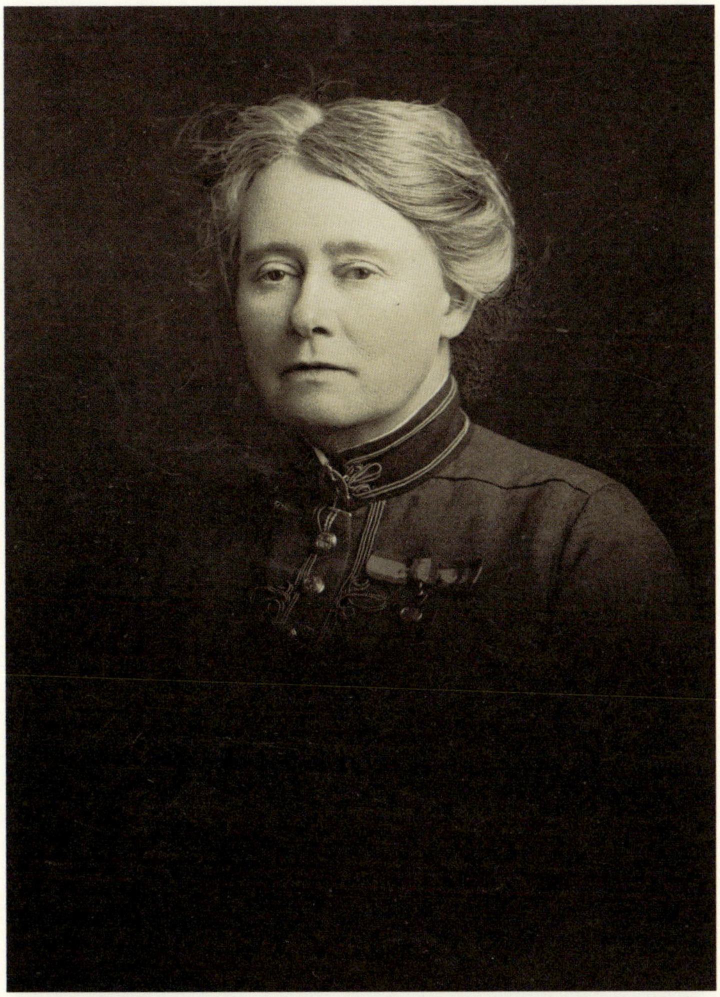

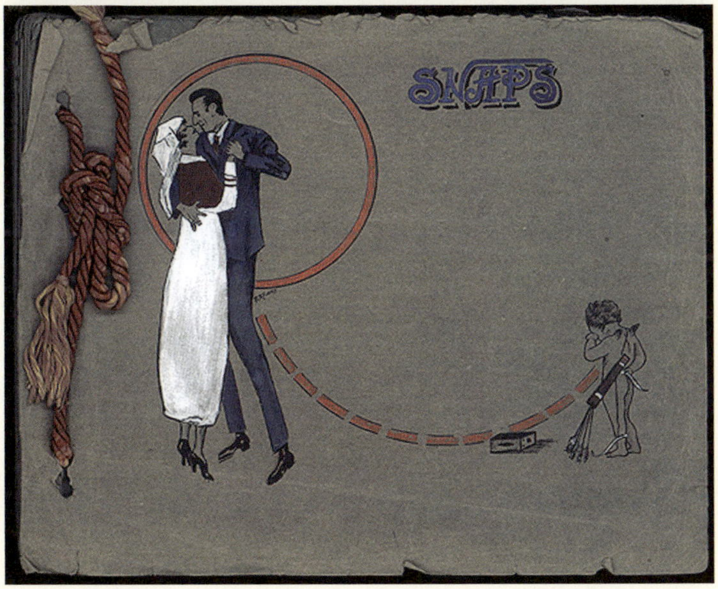

above Hester Maclean (1859–1932) was a woman of extraordinary energy. As well as being matron-in-chief of the New Zealand Army Nursing Service, which she fought to establish, she was assistant inspector of hospitals for the Department of Hospitals and Charitable Aid from 1906 to 1923 and a driving force in the New Zealand Trained Nurses' Association. In 1908 she founded the nursing journal *Kai Tiaki*, which she edited until her death. She defended the rights of nurses and their status as highly trained professionals. ALEXANDER TURNBULL LIBRARY, PACOLL-0785-1-106-02

below The nurses were almost universally admired by their patients, who often described them as angels. Images of improbably clean and pretty white-clad women, with equally immaculate patients, were often used on postcards and in recruiting material. Nurses were also the subject of poetry — 'When Peter dishes out the wings, he'll say in accents terse/Now stand aside, you soldiers! Step forward Angel Nurse!' — and, as this album cover shows, symbols of romance. NATIONAL ARMY MUSEUM, 1992.1156.2

men from the women.'[66] As she wrote later, 'It is a great pity, but it seems to me that the NZMC think that the sisters have no status at all . . . Clinical machines is what we are supposed to be — or ought to be, I suppose — to please them.'[67]

Like the doctors and men of the NZMC, nurses came and went from New Zealand, as new recruits joined up and were trained, or personnel were rested or returned to their pre-1914 civilian posts. Hester Maclean and Mabel Thurston, who was matron-in-chief for the NZEF in Britain, were constantly corresponding about nurses and their situations and placements.[68] While at No. 3 New Zealand General Hospital at Codford in July 1917, Pengelly noted, 'Miss Thurston has just asked for the names of the sisters who have not yet done service, either in Egypt or in France. I expect there will be a flutter soon, as some will be going and others returning.'[69]

Orderlies had an extensive range of duties, not all of them medical. It was they who 'carried the stretchers, who wheeled patients to the operating theatre, who set trays, dished out meals, and took on the less pleasant chores connected with bedpans'. They also washed and shaved men unable to care for themselves, and carried those whose legs had been amputated.[70] As Pengelly observed, they also had to deal with criticism from patients, though 'Orderlies are a genus quite distinct by themselves, and no doubt can put up with it all'.[71] Most of them had no medical background, save their pre-war training, and their suitability varied. In Weston's view, 'some should not have been allowed near a Hospital; there are others whose steady, sure hands seem to know instinctively how pain can be avoided and where ease lies'.[72]

Not everyone was happy to be in the NZMC. In January 1915 Walter Carruthers was hoping to soon 'be able to say that I am in the infantry . . . as there is a transfer going through'. He was particularly aggrieved at 'not even being a stretcher-bearer', but 'behind the firing line altogether'. He would not advise anyone to join the ambulance: 'There is no promotion out of the N.C.O. part of the business unless you are a qualified medical man.' In July he wrote, 'I don't want to go to England to look after wounded. That's a woman's or old man's job. I'm young and hefty and would much rather be in the thick.' Carruthers eventually got his wish, entering officer training early in 1918. He was killed in action on 29 September.[73]

Doctors often got good press, and the popular men featured frequently in letters and memoirs. Dentist Arthur Logan, the only non-doctor officer in No. 1 Field Ambulance during the first year in France, considered that 'a finer lot of mates to live with under any sort of circumstances, either grave or gay it would be very hard to find'.

> I believe that Army life to the average medical man is, except of course during those periods when active military operations are taking place, a relaxation and even a rest from the worries and trials of a busy medical practice. Consequently they can, as it were, let themselves go more and be more human than is expected of them in ordinary life.
>
> With one or two notable exceptions, I always found them most unassuming and friendly and, indeed, exceptionally good company.[74]

After MO William McAra was evacuated from Gallipoli with dysentery he was pleased to be visited in hospital by James Hardie Neil: 'Just same jolly old case as ever, only very thin.'[75] At one New Zealand hospital Sister Jeanne Sinclair heard many patients say of George Home, 'This Major is no good to me, he cures us too soon!'[76] The nurses, too, had their favourites. When wartime MO Mathew Holmes, who led the medical contingent to Samoa, died of influenza in 1918, *Kai Tiaki* remembered him as 'always . . . one with whom nurses were fellow-workers, to whom he accorded their just place in either hospital or private work'.[77]

There could, however, be discontent with — and even accusations of cowardice towards — the higher ranks of the medical service, though some of this may have stemmed from hearsay and gossip, or amounted to no more than traditional grousing about the top brass. On 8 May 1915, for example, when No. 1 Field Ambulance moved from Anzac Cove to Cape Helles on Gallipoli, John Thomson noted that 'Fanny (Capt. [Ernest] Boxer) is in charge, hence much messing about'. On the 14th he wrote: 'Also heard that Col. [Charles] Begg our O.C. got some shrapnel. There were no crocodile tears shed; the unpopularity he acquired in Egypt has not been lessened by his obvious disinclination to risk his own hide.'[78]

Godley, himself the subject of considerable, and not always merited, dislike, was very hard to please when it came to medical personnel. His wartime correspondence with Allen is full of impatient and often patronising complaints, particularly about those in top administrative positions and those he thought were insufficiently tough on malingerers. Although New Zealand's medical service had 'never been worse than anybody else's', he wrote in March 1916, 'of course, one would have liked to have had them much better'. Percival Fenwick, he considered, 'had neither the administrative ability nor the strength of character to cope with the situation' and 'William Parkes, I am afraid, is by no means a strong man, and I cannot find a strong one. But he is very sincere and painstaking and does on the whole very well.'[79] Godley had promoted Parkes to deputy director of medical services (DDMS) 'simply because I could not get anyone else', and would have preferred an RAMC man.[80] In August he told Allen, 'The Chaplains and the Doctors give us more trouble than anybody else. Begg is persistently tiresome.'[81]

But all these problems, whether of organisation, training, rank or personal unsuitability, were, finally, secondary to the enormous task that lay ahead of the men of the NZMC and the women of the NZANS as New Zealand went to war.

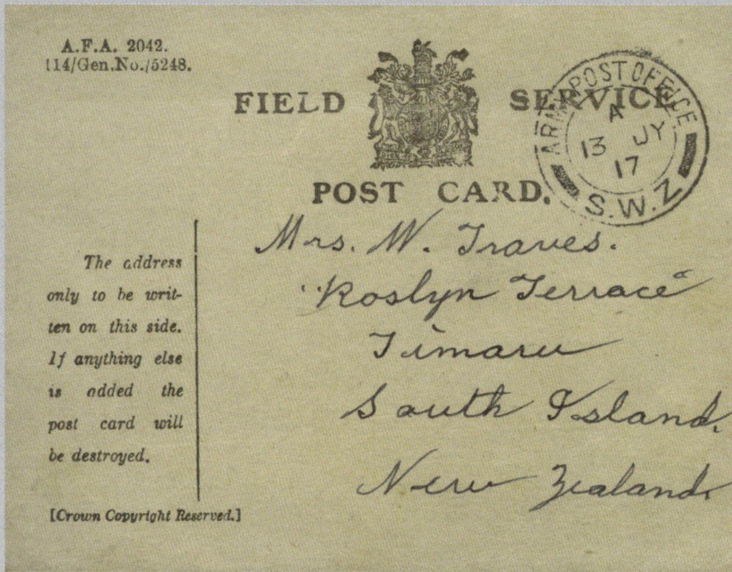
A.F.A. 2042.
114/Gen.No./5248.

FIELD SERVICE

POST CARD.

ARMY POST OFFICE A 13 JY 17 S.W.Z

The address only to be written on this side. If anything else is added the post card will be destroyed.

Mrs. W. Traves.
'Roslyn Terrace'
Timaru
South Island.
New Zealand.

[Crown Copyright Reserved.]

Soldiers could use a field service card with pre-printed sentences to send those at home a quick message of reassurance without having to worry about the censoring officer. Only a date and a signature were permitted to be added. Former ploughman George Traves from Timaru sent this one home after he received gunshot wounds to both arms in September 1917. SOUTH CANTERBURY MUSEUM, L2014/005.04

REGRET TO INFORM YOU

Informing distant loved ones when men were sick or wounded was a complex task, but the government was thorough in its response. When William Smallfield was admitted to a French hospital with trench fever in August 1917, his family received a telegram from defence minister James Allen and messages from Prime Minister William Massey and his coalition partner Joseph Ward on the same day. After Wilfred Smith died of wounds on 8 October 1917, his wife Ethel received cables from both Allen and, later, the governor-general, and a letter from Mackenzie.[82]

Sending the wrong message could cause undue alarm, as could the time lag involved with letters. Nurse Mary Grigor, who survived the sinking of the *Marquette* on 23 October 1915 (see Chapter 4), wrote from Alexandria on 10 November: 'New Zealand people will, I know, be worried until they hear from those they have over here. I cabled my father when I returned here, saying I was safe and well . . . nothing was mentioned in the Home papers about the Marquette, and he did not know I was on board, so . . . he must have wondered why I cabled. However, my letter to him will explain everything.'[83] When Len Coley was wounded and gassed at Messines, he was sent to No. 22 British General Hospital near Boulogne, where he soon discovered that he had been officially reported killed. 'I knew what that meant. I was out of bed like a shot. I found a doctor, explained and got him to cable my mother in New Zealand.'[84] When William McAra performed an appendectomy on Gallipoli in July 1915, 'Capt. tried to get me to agree that it was wise to cable as boy improving & so avoid frightening his people. Told him this was a mistake as boy not out of danger & would be great shock if first they knew was that he was dead.'[85]

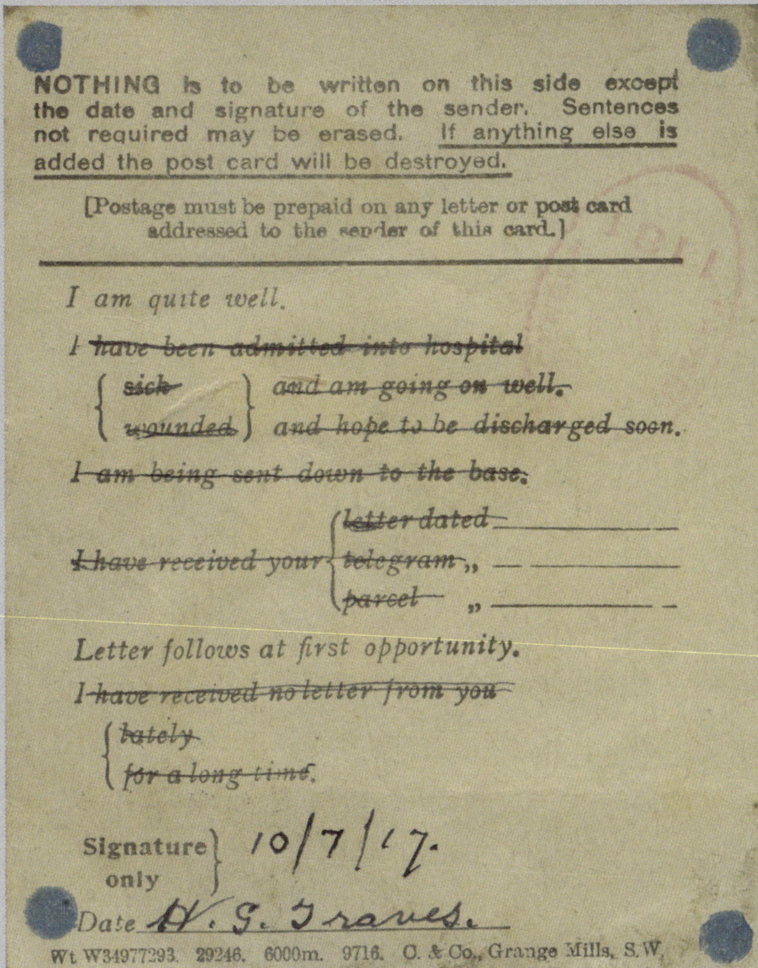

NOTHING is to be written on this side except the date and signature of the sender. Sentences not required may be erased. If anything else is added the post card will be destroyed.

[Postage must be prepaid on any letter or post card addressed to the sender of this card.]

I am quite well.

~~*I have been admitted into hospital*~~

~~*sick*~~ ~~*and am going on well.*~~

~~*wounded*~~ ~~*and hope to be discharged soon.*~~

~~*I am being sent down to the base.*~~

~~*I have received your*~~ ~~*letter dated*~~ ____
~~*telegram*~~ ,, ____
~~*parcel*~~ ,, ____

Letter follows at first opportunity.

~~*I have received no letter from you*~~
~~*lately*~~
~~*for a long time.*~~

Signature only } 10/7/17.

Date H. G. Traves.

Wt W34977293. 29246. 6000m. 9716. C. & Co., Grange Mills, S.W.

Because the official cabled information was, of necessity, basic, commanding officers, comrades, chaplains, and even busy doctors and nurses, also sent letters to relatives. 'I have been very busy writing,' padre Ronald Watson explained in December 1917. 'You have no idea what a difficult job it is. Still I want to do all I can, because the anxiety of relatives for all the news possible is pathetically great.'[86] When Frederick Welsh was killed on Gallipoli on 4 October 1915, two days before his twenty-first birthday, McAra wrote to his mother, Jessie, in Christchurch. The young man, ill with dysentery, was en route to a hospital ship when McAra and his ambulance men took him in for the night. Next morning, several patients were hit by Turkish shells, and 'your poor boy received a large piece of shell right into the lung. He did not suffer at all, but never rallied from the shock. He knew he was going, and smiled quite bravely at me as he told me that "he was not afraid".'[87] Such letters often blurred the truth, or lied, but Welsh did in fact die without trauma, as McAra noted in his diary: 'no pains — internal haemorrhage'.[88]

PART 1

Feeling the Heat

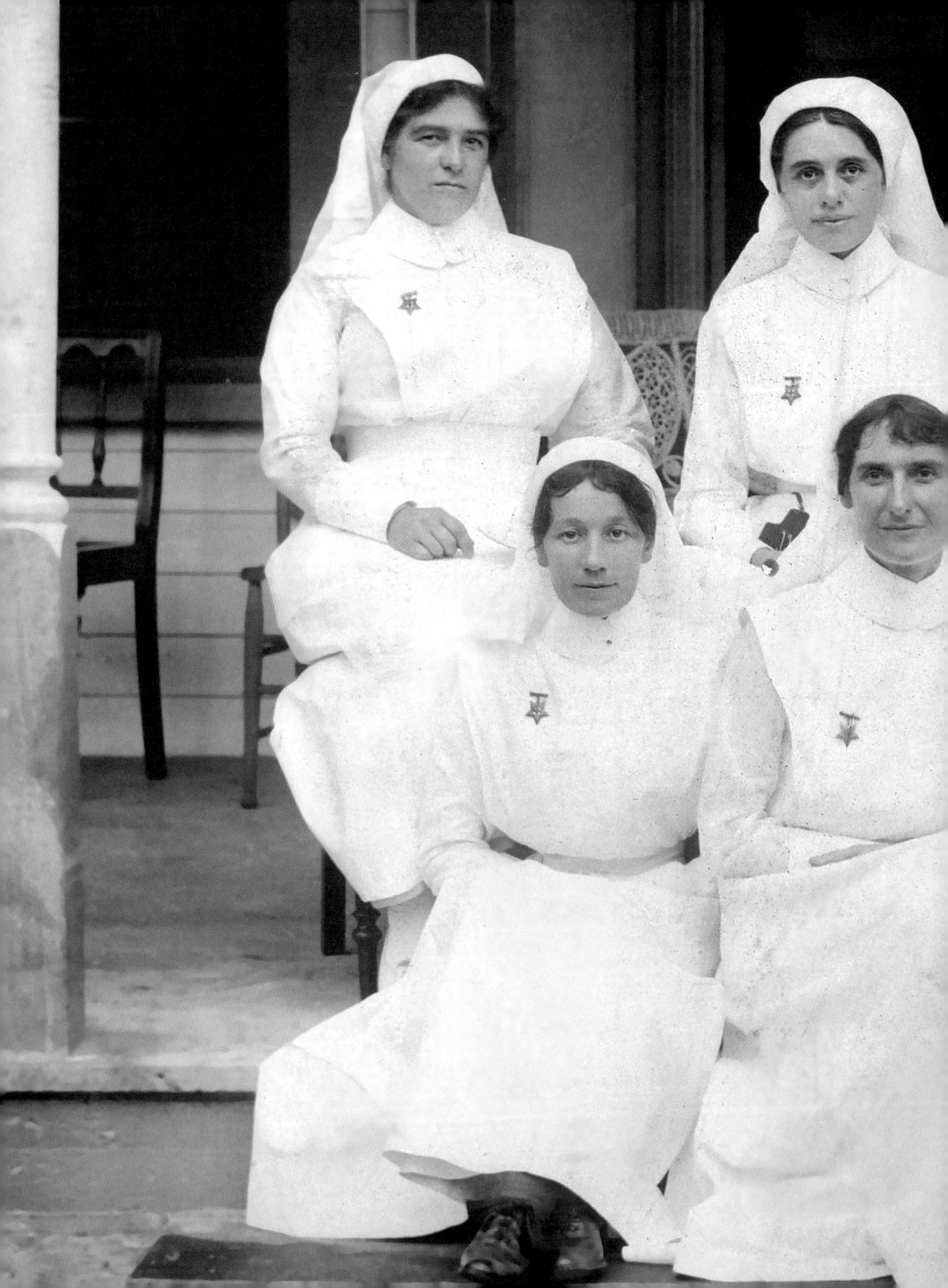

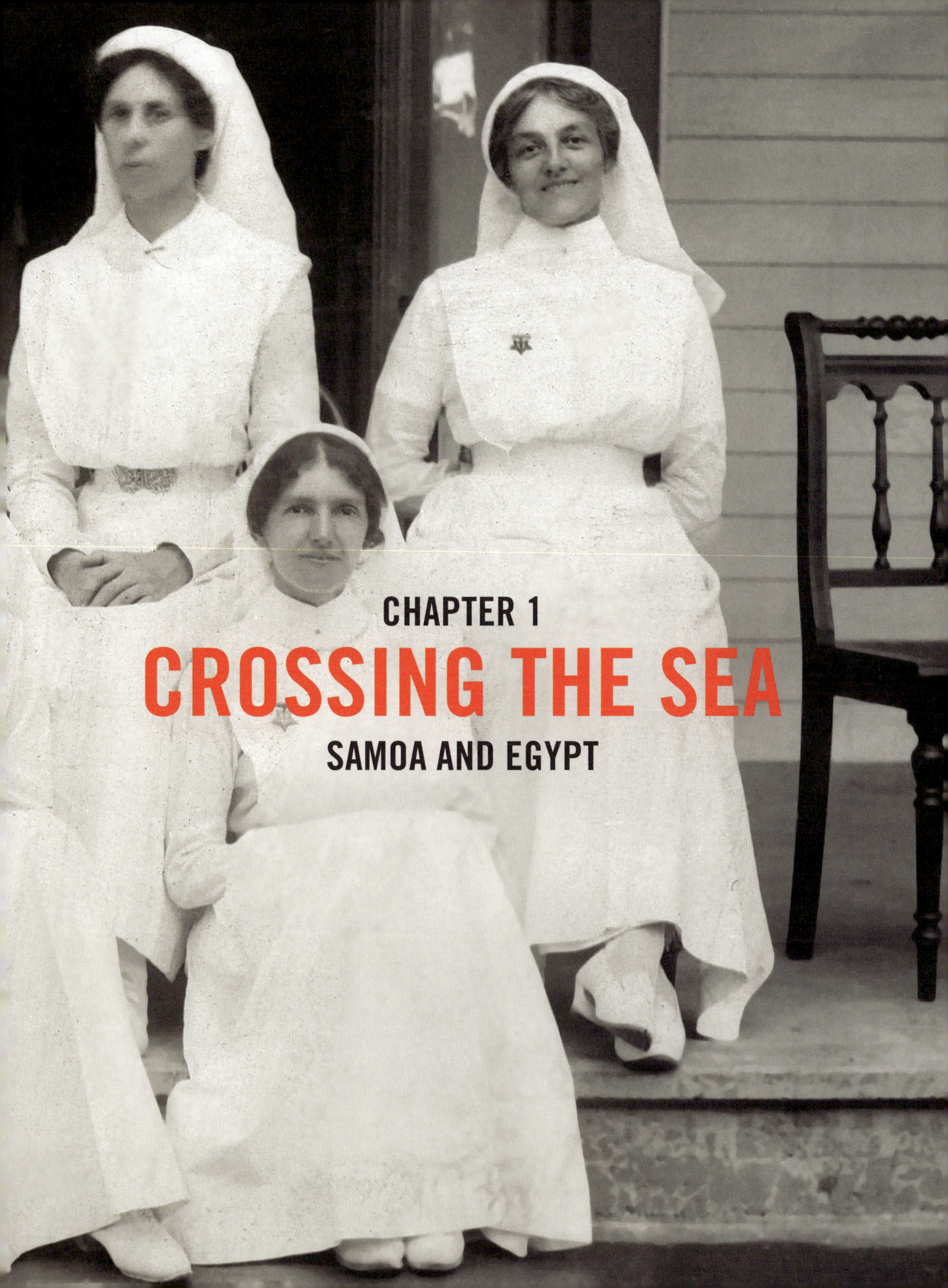

CHAPTER 1

CROSSING THE SEA

SAMOA AND EGYPT

previous pages
The first seven New Zealand nurses to serve overseas, photographed on the steps of the hospital at Apia in Samoa. Back row, from left: Ida Willis, Evelyn (Eva) Brooke, Bertha Nurse and Fanny Wilson. In the front row are Vida MacLean, Louise (Louie) McNie and Louise Brandon. ALEXANDER TURNBULL LIBRARY, 1/2-148862

On an enterprise of great and urgent Imperial necessity.

— *Evening Star*, 17 August 1914

It appears to have been a very poorly kept secret. Despite Godley insisting, on 10 August, that there was no truth in the rumour that a section of the Expeditionary Force was about to occupy German Samoa, and a request from James Allen for press silence, many felt, like the *Evening Star*, that it seemed 'a farce to try and make a mighty secret of the actual destination of the advance guard. Even the dogs seem to bark "Samoa."' The paper reported on 17 August that a 'compact force' had sailed out of Wellington on the *Monowai* and *Moeraki* two days before.[1]

Despite the shortcomings of the NZMC, the required medical component for the Samoan force, led by Major Mathew Holmes, was quickly assembled and equipped. This was mainly because the personnel were drawn from the No. 4 Field Ambulance based in the Wellington area. Telegrams sent out on 9 August brought more men than were needed to the capital the next day; NCOs were happy to join up as privates. With the staff went medical stores suitable for a small base hospital. The three doctors accompanying Holmes were Captain Alexander McKillop, who had been working at the Porirua mental hospital, distinguished surgeon Captain Duncan Stout, and Captain Kenneth Tapper from Wellington Hospital. Other doctors would later serve in Samoa.[2] The two dentists, with the rank of lieutenant, were Charles Ward and David Isaacs, both from Wellington. There was no preparation for the conditions they would encounter beyond the 'valuable advice and some literature dealing with . . . tropical diseases prevailing, also a small supply of necessary drugs' supplied by the chief medical officer in Fiji during a stopover in Suva.[3]

Hester Maclean had little time to select, notify and swear in her nurses, and have their uniforms made. For practical reasons, five came from the Wellington region; the sixth was Christchurch theatre sister Louise (Louie) McNie. The other women were Sisters Vida MacLean, formerly of Wanganui Hospital and now sub-matron of St Helen's Hospital in Wellington, Evelyn (Eva) Brooke and Fanny Wilson, both from Wellington Hospital, and Louise Brandon, also from the capital. The group was led by the appropriately named Wellington-based Sister

Bertha Nurse. The women's uniforms included two grey cotton frocks each, and a panama hat, since *Kai Tiaki*, too, had 'shrewdly surmised' that Samoa was the destination.[4] The nurses had supplies, the ingredients for invalid diets, a little bag each containing such items as surgical dressing instruments and a thermometer, canvas stretcher beds and bedding, and even deckchairs and cushions for the voyage.

On the morning of 12 August, the men marched down to the docks in steady rain while the nurses went by car. However, the two New Zealand transports did not sail until three days later. At Suva, a seventh nurse joined the group on 27 August. Ida Willis, who had worked in Australia and most recently in Wellington, was holidaying in Fiji when war was declared. Stranded, she was found by Holmes, who said she could join the other nurses if she was on board by 6.30 next morning. In 'something of a dream', she 'scarcely had time to realise that this was war'.[5] The journey to Samoa was not without its disruptions. Several men 'cracked up under the new life, and were marked for return to New Zealand', and the first anti-typhoid inoculation given en route 'brought to light the ubiquitous conscientious objectors', who were 'promptly tagged' to be sent home as soon as possible. When a private on the *Moeraki* developed acute appendicitis, the medical staff set up an improvised operating table in a cabin and performed their first wartime operation 'neatly and successfully'.[6]

Escorted by a convoy of warships, the two vessels reached Apia on 29 August. Samoa was taken without a struggle, the Union Jack soon flew above the post office, and the New Zealanders set about making the necessary medical arrangements. The public hospital, standing in 5 acres of pleasant grounds about a mile from the waterfront, was 'a large, airy bungalow building, the cool wards opening onto wide verandahs'. As Brandon explained to *Kai Tiaki* readers, 'The wards are well ventilated and plainly, but sensibly furnished, and white net mosquito curtains hang above each bed ready to tuck in when necessary.'[7] Nearby were two separate wards for Chinese and Samoan patients. The German medical staff still at the hospital included an eye specialist, whose clinic was always busy. A highly contagious eye disease spread chiefly by flies was endemic in Samoa; though easily treatable, it had blinded many locals.

The New Zealanders and the Germans rubbed along together until 11 September, when the German acting health officer announced that his entire staff had decided to stop work and would be leaving the hospital next morning. By this time many of the New Zealanders had

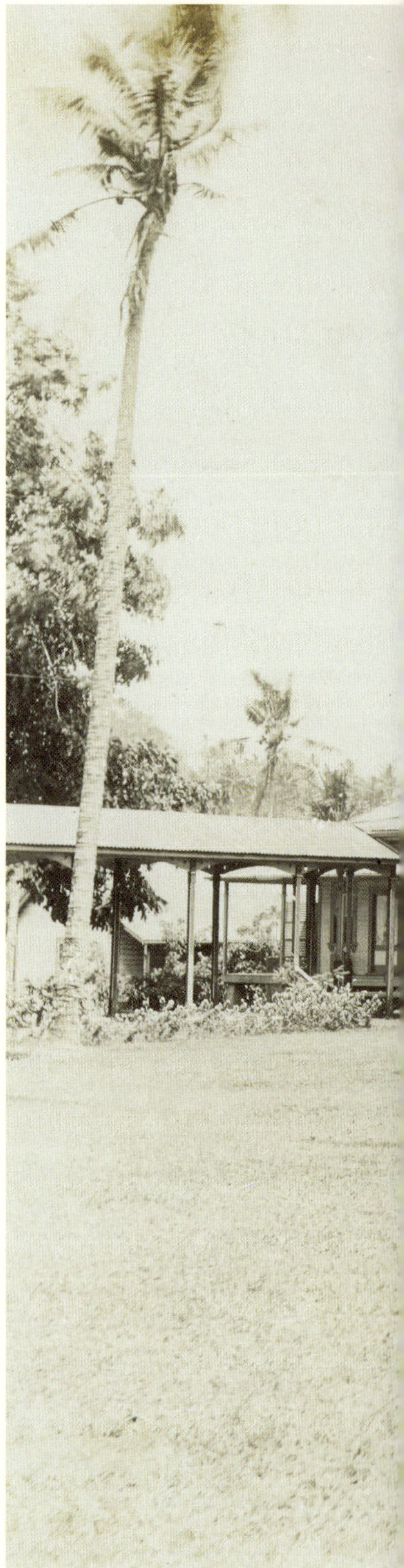

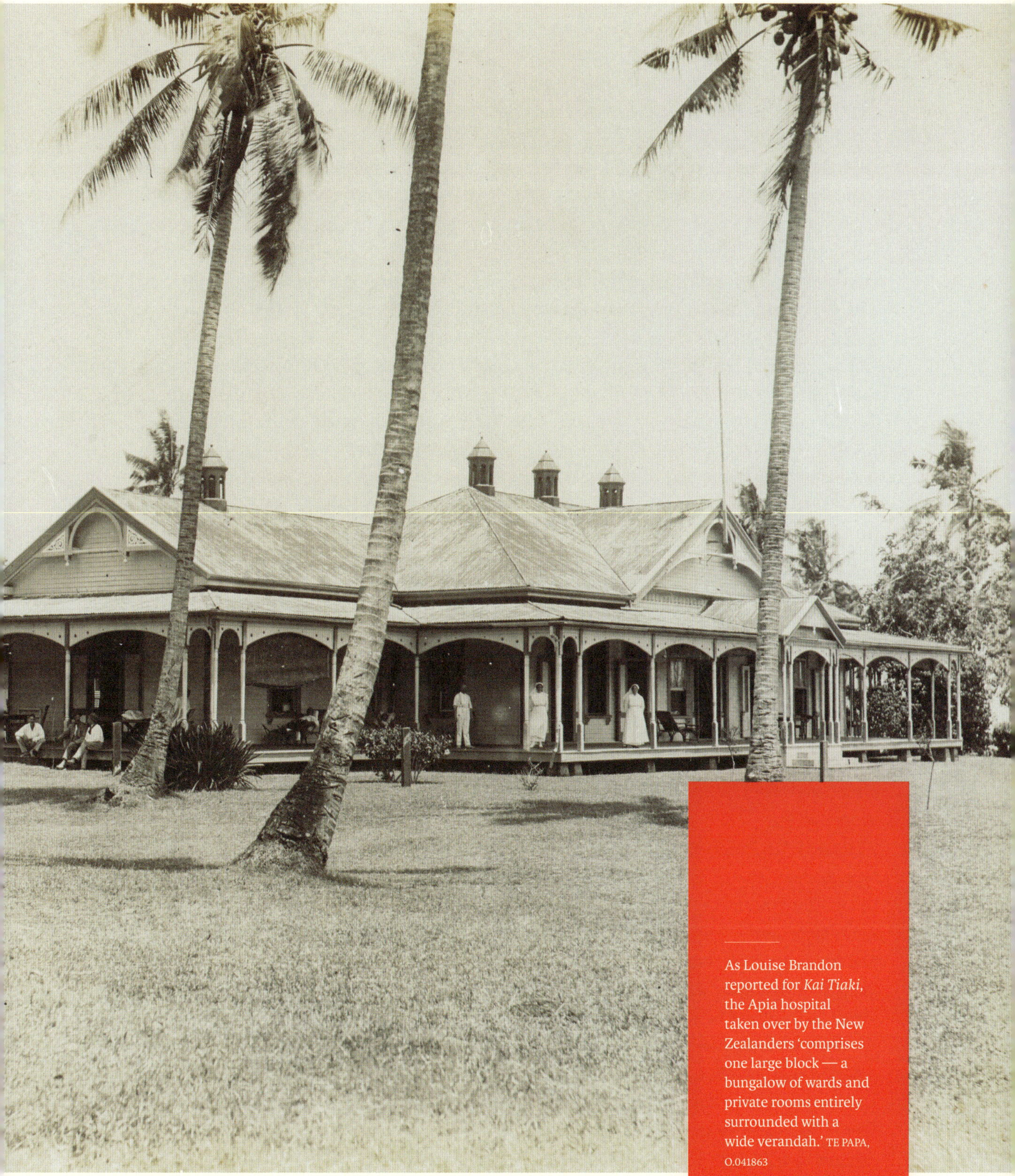

As Louise Brandon reported for *Kai Tiaki*, the Apia hospital taken over by the New Zealanders 'comprises one large block — a bungalow of wards and private rooms entirely surrounded with a wide verandah.' TE PAPA, O.041863

been infected by the prevailing eye disease, which meant the medical staff would have extra work caring for their own troops while covering all the local civil duties. Despite attempts to keep them, the Germans departed, taking with them the much-needed eye specialist. Ophthalmologist Henry Kendall left Auckland for Apia on 18 September; he replaced McKillop.

Even after discarding 'every possible article of apparel' and swapping their heavy, prickly woollen uniforms for singlets and shorts that became increasingly abbreviated, the troops soon began to suffer in the humid heat. The food was 'monotonous and inadequate'; initially there were no nets to repel the persistent mosquitoes (especially numerous as the rainy season approached); water had to be boiled; sunburn and sunstroke were common.[8] Another affliction was ear disease, probably caused by bathing in contaminated water. Then there were infected mosquito bites, boils and scratches that could quickly turn septic. An October outbreak of bacillary dysentery was treated with arrowroot supplied by the field ambulance. Dengue fever and dysentery also began to attack both the troops and the NZMC men. November brought the 'slight but nevertheless most unpleasant and irritating complaint known to the troops as Dhobie Itch (*Tinea cruris*)'.[9] While the men had received one typhoid inoculation on the voyage over, it was only when enteric fever, as typhoid was then known, threatened that a second required inoculation was hastily carried out. As sanitation and housing conditions were improved — the drainage system needed work — and the troops became more acclimatised, the sickness rate dropped.

Although the nurses were, as McNie reported, 'healthy and cheerful' while looking after their 25 to 30 patients, there were difficulties. The little operating theatre had 'some most up-to-date instruments', but a 'good many' necessary items were missing, perhaps removed by the Germans. 'However, with what we brought in the surgical panniers, we can manage to do anything required.' For the women, too, the climate was 'very trying'. 'I find that a light eight-hour duty really tries me more than did a heavy 12-hour one in Christchurch. It is so hot and steaming, one is never dry.' These conditions were bad for rheumatic or chest cases, who were sent back to New Zealand. But McNie thought Samoa 'certainly the most beautiful place I have seen. We never tire of exploring the roads and bush and finding fresh beauties every day.'[10]

Towards the end of November 1914, Holmes, with other staff officers, returned to New Zealand on the SS *Navua* to organise the Medical Corps that would accompany the Second Reinforcements bound for Egypt. He had been delighted by the 'keen enthusiasm of the Ambulance, and . . . the whole hearted manner in which they had carried out his commands'. The Samoa garrison was reduced in December, but it was not until 8 March 1915 that 'the long-looked-for radiogram arrived ordering the embarkation of 500 men for New Zealand'.[11] They were to be replaced by a relief force of men over the age limit for active service.

Sailing with the homeward-bound men were three of the nurses. On 11 November, having reported on their 'excellent work here', Holmes had asked that at least some of the seven women 'proceed to Europe'. Like the men, they were 'eager . . . to get nearer to the front'.[12] Hester Maclean also spoke up for them, and Vida MacLean, Bertha Nurse and Fanny Wilson reached New Zealand in time to join the first NZANS contingent that sailed from Wellington in

April 1915. The four remaining nurses also went on to serve overseas. Other NZANS members would work in Samoa during the occupation.

Not everyone entirely appreciated the NZMC's contribution in the Pacific. As one *Free Lance* reader pointed out, 'They are called non-combatants . . . and are dubbed "The Linseed Lancers" and "The Poultice Wallopers," but give them their dues. If they don't take a rifle and shoot an enemy they at least keep alive the men who are trained for that part of the game.' The paper doffed its hat to the medics: 'During the seven months' stay of about 1000 men in the tropical climate and pest-ridden camps of Samoa, not a single man was lost.' Venereal disease had not proved a problem either. 'You will be pleased to hear,' Allen told Godley, 'that not a single case of the disease which troubles you so much in Egypt has come back with the Samoans. This is highly gratifying.'[13]

When the 10 transports carrying the Main Body and First Reinforcements of the New Zealand Expeditionary Force left Wellington in October 1914, a much larger and more complex medical complement was organised. At its head, as assistant director of medical services (ADMS), was Colonel Thomas Will, who had been in charge of the country's military medical service before the war; his deputy was Christchurch's principal medical officer, surgeon Lieutenant-Colonel Percival Fenwick. Fenwick's Wellington counterpart, Lieutenant-Colonel Charles Begg, was in command of the field ambulance, while Lieutenant-Colonel Charles Thomas from Timaru headed the Mounted Field Ambulance.[14] Included was an 'X-Ray expert', Dunedin physician and surgeon Lieutenant-Colonel Ferdinand Batchelor, and 10 dental surgeons. With the medical staff went equipment: 1898 pattern medical panniers and light ambulance and GS (general service) wagons. (The latter transported medical, surgical and nursing equipment, tents and blankets. Their drivers came from the Army Service Corps.) The field ambulance (with their wagons, but without their horses and minus men attached to other units) travelled on the *Star of India*, while the Mounted Field Ambulance, with their horses and transport (minus 17 vehicles put on the *Athenic*), set sail in the *Maunganui*.[15]

The troopships were commercial vessels that had been chartered by the government and 'rapidly transformed . . . The main consideration was to pack as many men and horses on board as could reasonably be done.'[16] A medical officer was included among those who made recommendations about the alterations, and, according to Carbery, 'the sanitary appliances were satisfactory, there was one bath per 50 men'. But Cecil Malthus, on the *Athenic*, described how difficult it was to keep clothes clean — 'Washing is quite the horridest job we have on board. There is only one tub for 1500 men, cold water and poor soap' — and the super-efficient and scrupulous William Malone, commanding the Wellington Battalion, worried about hygiene standards.

On 3 November, while visiting his men in hospital on board the *Arawa*, he 'gave the orderly a talking to on the dirtiness and untidiness . . . I don't altogether understand [NZMC Captain George] Home. I am always discussing hygiene with him and he is classed as a sanitation expert and yet the dispensary and hospital are in my opinion disgraceful.'[17] The water was not solely for human use: each man was allowed only 3 gallons of fresh water a day as there were thirsty horses on all the ships. In one case, though, the water was 'absolutely black, so bad in fact that the Veterinary Officer would not allow it to be given to the horses'.[18]

Seasickness was a challenge that would affect most of the troops leaving New Zealand over the next four years. Sailing smoothly across Wellington Harbour was one thing, hitting the open ocean quite another, especially for the many men who had never been to sea. Only a few hardy souls were impervious to illness, and letters and diaries abound in often cryptic and teeth-gritting reports of vomiting and misery until the roll of the ship became familiar. 'The Tasman Sea was being very unkind,' William Taylor remembered, 'and many of the troops were sick. There was vomit everywhere so I went on deck to get a breath of fresh air. About a dozen of us were in pretty good shape so our O.C. rounded us up, and with brooms and water we descended into the hold and got busy. The stench was terrible. The chaps had used their dixies [mess tins] to contain what their stomachs couldn't.'[19] Rifleman Clifford Collingwood was so sick on the *Tofua* in November 1915 that he was hospitalised. He was soon feeling 'a lot better . . . and [we] are now getting cornflour and brandy'. The medical staff were not immune. On the *Willochra* in October 1916, Dr Thomas Watt, 'a grand little officer', was 'fearfully sick nearly all the way'.[20]

One of the most memorable aspects of the voyage, for all the wrong reasons, were the inoculations and vaccinations required, and particularly the two anti-typhoid injections that were usually given in either the top of the chest or the upper arm, 10 days apart.[21] Few did not suffer some kind of reaction. Private Peter Thompson, on the *Ruapehu*, did not find his first anti-typhoid injection painful, 'but the reaction affects one a little, and the fact of the men being relieved from all duties for 48 hours indicates that this is so'. Major Herbert Hart noted on 18 November: 'Commenced the inoculation of all ranks against typhoid fever . . . Some . . . had intense pains for an hour and nearly everyone becomes somewhat ill for a day.'[22] MO Alexander Trotter injected himself the second time ''cos I preferred my own technique. Considerable local tenderness but no constitutional reaction (felt pretty seedy after the first). Supply of vaccine considerably short even though bottle opened today is kept for tomorrow or the next day. Latterly have only been able to give half the correct dose which is a pity because it may not be so effective.'[23]

An otherwise peaceful voyage from Egypt to Marseilles in April 1916 was spoilt for Claude Weston by his second typhoid inoculation. 'The Medical Officer, in a genuine endeavour to save discomfort, injected the serum in what the Maories call my puku, with a result that neither he nor I anticipated. The slightest movement for five days was painfully punished.'[24] William Smallfield, who left with the Seventh Reinforcements, had suffered his first inoculation, in the left breast, while at Trentham. This left him 'feeling miserably sick', and the second dose a fortnight later brought 'another week's misery'. Then 'they very kindly filled our systems with another clever medical poison, and our arms are in an awful state'. At Featherston in November 1916, Stewart Callaghan saw some men 'go right out before they were touched at all and one fellow they had to hold up to the doctor while he stabbed him'.[25]

A number of men objected to inoculation, particularly on the *Ruapehu* after the 25 October death of dispenser Jack Gilchrist (see below), which was mistakenly attributed to the first anti-typhoid injections. Most of the more than 800 men on board refused to be injected again, 'asserting that they had not actually agreed to inoculation, but only vaccination as stated on the attestation form that each . . . had signed on enlistment'. (As historian Lea Doughty has pointed out, inoculation was considered dangerous because it used a live virus.) Although the attestation was a legally binding document, the 'imprecise wording' — 'Are you willing to be vaccinated or revaccinated?' — and the government's rather airy expectation of compliance caused problems. Clarity came only when the Military Service Act 1916, which brought in conscription, made vaccination or inoculation compulsory.[26]

There were problems on other ships. Malone, on the *Arawa*, was furious about the two dozen 'rotters' who objected. He blamed 'our stupid medical authorities in New Zealand [who] either didn't know of or forgot to provide for inoculation. I am not sure but that they thought that "vaccination" covered everything.' In a final effort at persuasion, Malone 'got Home to explain the matter and then made them understand that if they persisted, I . . . would try to get them sent back to New Zealand at once, as useless'.[27] There were refusals, too, on the *Hawke's Bay*.

Although the number of protesters was reduced — as Trooper Benjamin Colbran recorded on the *Hawke's Bay*, 'Some men objected & were told they would be classed as incapables and get no pay so they yielded' — there were still objectors after the convoy reached Egypt.[28] Godley, too, considered expulsion essential. Thirty-five men who 'persisted in their refusal' were put on the *Athenic* for return to New Zealand, along with some sick men, and discharged from the army. 'In this Country,' Godley told Allen, 'where everybody gets inoculated as a matter of course . . . I could not risk the health of the vast majority of the men, or an outbreak of enteric, by keeping those who refused [to] submit to reasonable precautions.' Allen, in return, assured the GOC that 'no man will leave here now without being inoculated or vaccinated, or without a positive assurance that he will submit to it on the voyage'.[29]

It was not always a needle that caused difficulties. Ambulance man Norman Gray, travelling on the *Tahiti* in October 1915, described the 'rather interesting' process of vaccination for smallpox. 'The men all bared their arms and filed past, 1st, 2 of the sisters one of whom washed the arm another dabbing it with ether, then to one Dr. who cut two series of small gashes with a knife . . . Then on to the 2nd. Dr. who applied the lymph [the material containing the virus]. Then onto one of our men who rubbed the lymph well over the cuts, and finally after letting the arm dry in the sun for a few minutes, on to 2 or 3 of our men who applied dressings.' The doctors on Gray's ship were careful, but he had heard of one who 'made marks the size of a ½ crown and the boat was tossing a bit as well'; the medical staff were still treating wounds on men's arms three months later.[30]

Landing at Alexandria did not mean an end to close encounters with needles. As the unnamed writer of 'Gossip from Egypt' reported for the *Dominion*, 'We are not without troubles . . . for there are already, two cases of smallpox, one of diphtheria, and four of scarlet fever, to say nothing of 28 cases of measles. Every member of the Force (with the exception of those who have been vaccinated within the last eighteen months) is to be vaccinated at once.'[31] In the view of Len Coley, the medical staff 'further justified their position with inoculation orgies.

I was in Egypt for seven and a half weeks and inoculated seven times. Their excuse was malaria, tetanus, smallpox — and goodness knows what the other ones were for unless they were to guard against dying from a natural death.'[32]

The doctors on the transports were not just seen as torturers. On the *Arawa*, George Home edited the shipboard newspaper, *The Arrower*. The senior MO on the *Orari*, Captain Henry McLean from Wellington, had 'a gruff, rough and ready way with him which made him the ideal regimental medical officer. The men loved him but it took a smart trooper to put one across the old Doc on sick parade.'[33] But reviews could vary. Eric Catchpole of the Auckland Mounted Rifles, on the *Star of India*, thought the doctors initially 'made light' of some 'very bad' cases of measles on board. 'One would think that the doctors here were out for a holiday; they don't seem to care what happens to the men in the least, and often keep a man who is hurt or ill waiting for hours before they will attend to him.'[34]

There were several major operations during the seven-week journey. For one, an 'acute abdominal surgery' successfully carried out by Charles Thomas, the *Maunganui* was 'hauled out of line and steamed head to swell to allow . . . the least possible movement of the ship'.[35] On the afternoon of 29 November, on the same vessel, Trotter performed a tonsillectomy under local anaesthetic.[36] Three NZMC men died before the convoy reached Colombo in Ceylon (Sri Lanka). On the evening of 25 October, 30-year-old dispenser and former Gore chemist Lance-Corporal Jack Gilchrist was found dead on the *Ruapehu*. The cause of death, according to Captain Cyril Baigent of the NZMC, was an overdose of morphine, taken to 'relieve the symptoms of ptomaine poisoning'. Gilchrist had been consuming 'large quantities of condensed milk; he left the tins opened & exposed to infection for over 24 hrs in the small & hot dispensary'. The night before he had been suffering from headaches, diarrhoea and vomiting. 'Empty tubes equivalent to 87.5 gms of Morphia [morphine] were found in his pockets.'[37] As Trooper William Pyle wrote on the 26th, when Gilchrist was buried, 'Poor chap, the war won't worry him anymore.' To Peter Thompson, Gilchrist was 'a thorough gentleman, and those who came under his jurisdiction were always ready to vouch for his care and attentiveness'.[38]

On 13 November, during the traditional celebrations for crossing the equator, 33-year-old Lieutenant Ernest Webb, one of the young Otago University doctors, dived into a shallow sail bath on the *Arawa* before anyone could stop him, and broke his neck. 'Of course he knew exactly what had happened to him, poor chap,' wrote Thomas.[39] Despite surgery at the military hospital in Colombo, he died on 18 November. Two days later, Trotter noted that Harold Lewis was 'desperately ill with pneumonia. Pulse all over the place, breathing embarrassed and face leaden in colour. Very little hope.' The 20-year-old, who was with the New Zealand Field Ambulance, died that day and was buried at sea the following morning. 'So it was that the N.Z.M.C. was the first unit of the Main Body to make sacrifice of lives in the great cause.'[40]

Once the New Zealanders reached Egypt on 3 December — their original final destination of France was altered after the Ottoman Empire entered the war — sick men were taken to the small No. 21 British Hospital at Ras-el-Tin, in former Egyptian Army barracks

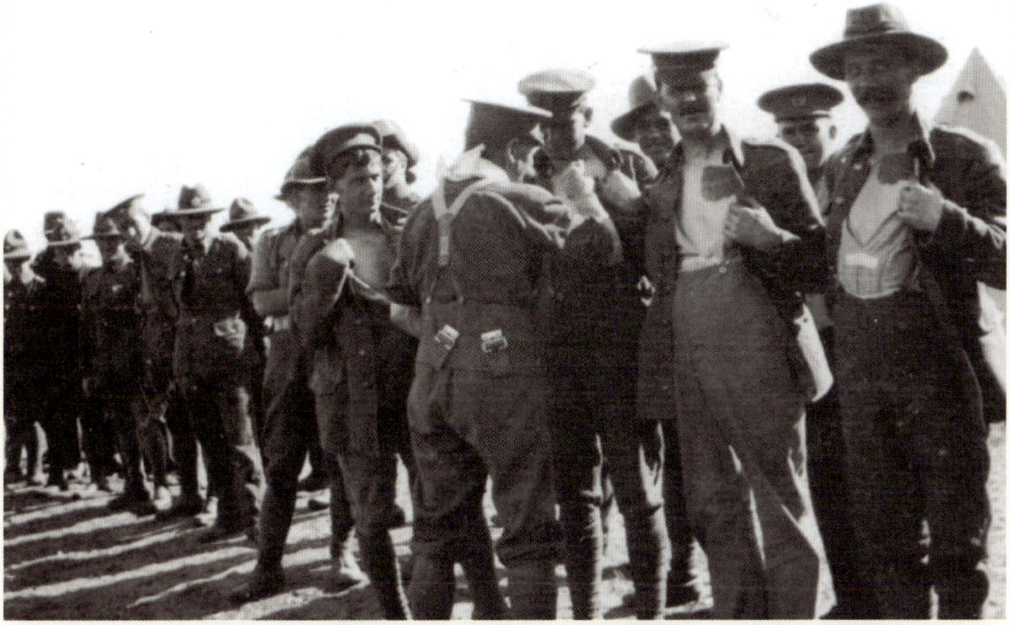

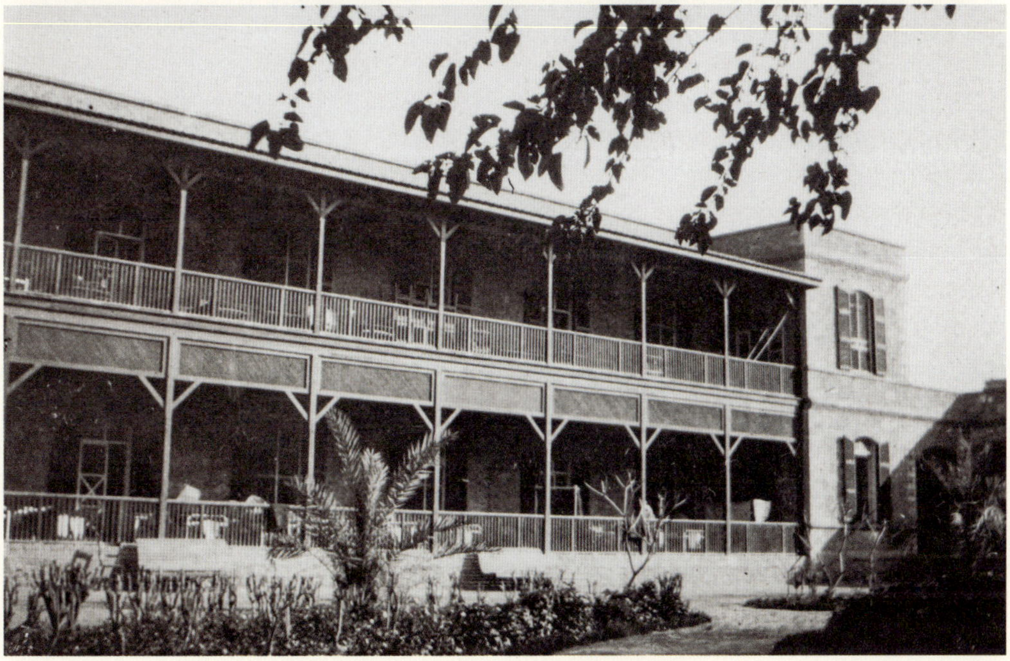

above In Egypt, a medical officer checks inoculation patches. Disease was a major enemy in this hot and unfamiliar climate. NATIONAL ARMY MUSEUM, 1991.587

below Originally the Egyptian Army Hospital, Pont de Koubbeh later became the New Zealand General Hospital. NELSON PROVINCIAL MUSEUM, A314.1, 300780 overlooking Alexandria's harbour. 'There are a good many sick with hen-flew-through-the-window [influenza] and measles,' wrote Catchpole on 22 December, 'and a few with minor injuries.'[41] Once the New Zealanders had established a camp at Zeitoun, near Cairo, the field ambulance set up a hospital capable of accommodating 200 patients, and the Egyptian Army Hospital at Pont de Koubbeh in nearby Abbassia was designated for the NZEF, whose patients at Ras-el-Tin were moved there. Some New Zealand ambulance men worked as orderlies at Pont de Koubbeh, which was run by an RAMC medical officer and had Australian nurses on its staff. 'Gossip from Egypt' was 'astonished at the extent of the hospital and how very comfortable and clean everything is'.[42]

When Benjamin Colbran contracted influenza on 14 December, he was sent to the camp hospital 'with 24 hours rations & blankets'. His day-long sleep on a stretcher was 'the most comfortable rest I had had since I left home'. Although he felt better the next day, he still had a headache. 'There are 15 of us in the hospital marquee today.' On the 16th, Colbran and four others were sent to Abbassia by ambulance wagon. 'It is a nice hospital & we get looked after well. We had stewed chicken & sago pudding for dinner.' The next day brought visits from 'several officers & chaplains'.[43] Godley turned up on the 19th. The GOC, who visited regularly, expected his commanders to look after their men in hospital, who should be provided with 'cigarettes, notepaper, newspapers, and other small luxuries, out of regimental funds'. Godley continued: 'I may have been unfortunate, but in the course of visits to the Egyptian Army Hospital, which I make fairly frequently, I have never yet seen a regimental officer there.'[44]

As well as participating in general training during the first three months of 1915, the medical men had plenty to occupy them: at New Year, there were more than 260 patients in the camp hospital suffering from various complaints and infectious diseases, some caused by the unfamiliar conditions. As early as 11 December Malone had recorded that although everyone was cheerful, he and Home were 'rather worried at our sick [in the Wellington Battalion] — over 130 reported this morning . . . We expected the change to send our numbers of sick up but it ought to have eased off by now.'[45] The carers were ailing, too, as Charles Begg noted on 3 January: 'the number of patients in the Field Ambulance lines is steadily increasing.' There had been 115 cases in a week, and on 7 January 40 orderlies were still at Pont de Koubbeh.

Begg was concerned, too, about the difficulties of training his medics when they were so scattered: some at Abbassia, others at the camp hospital's receiving, convalescent, venereal and infectious sections.[46] On 6 January, Walter Carruthers reported that 'I have been doing hospital work since Boxing Day morning and have been in the isolation camp attending scarlet fever cases since last Wednesday'. He felt, however, that 'there hasn't been a great deal of illness taking things all round'. A fortnight later, orderly Gordon Breen wrote that 'the work has just been ordinary routine which in my case is the Hospital, we now have 350 men in'.[47]

Dysentery, a crippling form of gastroenteritis that caused bloody diarrhoea, a fever and severe abdominal pain, was prevalent. On 14 February, when 12 of his men were hospitalised, Malone himself 'got an attack . . . Home says it is caused by swallowing fine sand'.[48] Gunner Norman Hassell of the New Zealand Field Artillery agreed: this 'sand-colic' was a 'cruel thing', causing agonising stomach pains. It did, however, last only a couple of days as the 'accumulated sand in the stomach [was] ultimately ejected by the bowels'. (Poor-quality water was also a likely culprit.) Hassell, who travelled to Egypt with the Fourth Reinforcements, spent only a few hours in Suez on 17 April 1915 before boarding a train for Cairo.

> Many of us were suffering from acute diarrhoea brought on by the unaccustomed heat and sand, and as the afflicted ones had to perform their functions somehow, the rest of the journey can perhaps be imagined! As far as we could ascertain there was not a single lavatory on the whole train, and so the unfortunate suffering ones were forced to go out on to the platforms and perch precariously on the couplings to obtain relief. Being still only a recruit and not hardened up to this sort of thing I felt very embarrassed over it at first, but soon discovered that there were hundreds of other men in even worse straits than myself.[49]

Dysentery would continue to plague later arrivals. Ambulance man Norman Gray used a popular remedy to treat his 'sharp attack' in November 1915: 'The cinnamon in the Otago kits is good.' In December, Rifleman Walter Widdowson explained that 'Dysentery usually lays a large number up for the first three weeks. I had three weeks in Pont de Koubbeh Hospital . . . but I am fit as the best of them now.' Gray, however, saw old friends at the hospital who had been suffering from dysentery for three months: 'They are wrecks and will take months to recover.'[50]

As the days lengthened, the heat was unlike anything the New Zealanders had ever encountered. As Cecil Malthus told his fiancée Hazel Watters, 'There is not an inch of shade all day, and the water in our bottles gets quite hot and worse than useless.' Peter Thompson described the torture of a forced march in the 'glare of the sun': 'discipline was strictly enforced and every man from the C.C. down was disallowed the priviledge of drinking water'. As men started 'simply dropping right and left', the ambulance wagons at the rear 'began to see signs of work, and this proved the case, for they were busy carting fatigued men to camp throughout the day'.[51] After arriving in Cairo late in May, the Fourth Reinforcements 'had to parade for inspection at 10 a.m. It was not fit for anyone to be out. Ten men dropped from the effect of the sun.' The worst affected was 'unconscious for a time and then delirious in hospital'.[52]

Challenging, too, was the sharp contrast between day and night temperatures. 'The days are invariably bright and warm . . . A soldier who discards his hat for a moment in the open learns at once that there is a risk of being sent into hospital with a raging headache.' But then came nights 'of almost Polar severity . . . and men who a few hours before were discarding their clothes bring out Balaclava caps, overcoats, scarves, and woollen gloves'. Trooper Frederick Foote and his companions rode all day until 8 p.m. in cotton shirts with the sleeves torn off. By 11 o'clock there were rugs on the horses' backs, the men had donned overcoats, 'and from then on till daylight we and our horses shiver as we ride through the night'.[53]

Such extreme changes of temperature caused sickness. Clifford Collingwood caught a severe chill while on guard duty on the night of 27/28 February 1916. A day later he was admitted to hospital with influenza and bronchitis, running a temperature of 103.4°F. By the evening he was delirious, 'seeing things and talking silly'. After 'two doses of whisky' he 'perspired heavily during the remainder of the night' and the fever broke. Still feeling 'very weak', he was discharged from hospital on 13 March. He managed a 15-mile route march on the 17th, 'but was ill on the return'.[54]

In Fred Hubbard's view, the fierce desert sun also had its advantages. 'My word you have no idea what a filthy hole Cairo is . . . The sun is the salvation of the place as it kills all germs and it is noticeable that when it rains and the sun is hidden there is immediately more sickness. At Hospital all washing water is just thrown on the sand outside the doors, and clothes laid in the sun for a couple of hours for all cases of measles, mumps, and scarlet [fever]. This is quite sufficient disinfection.' Everyone noticed the poor hygiene standards in Egypt compared with those at home. After riding through part of old Cairo shortly before Christmas, Herbert Hart took hours to rid himself of a smell that was 'worse than a bad public urinal'.[55]

Lice were another unwelcome novelty. In the words of Douglas Stark ('Starkie'), whose war experiences were fictionalised by Robin Hyde in *Passport to Hell*, they were 'really Egypt's oldest soldiers . . . These had been reared on soldiers' blood for a hundred generations, and liked it.'[56] Following the practice of the day, Foote and his mates were issued with cholera belts, 'heavy padded flannel, to wrap round over our kidneys and tie with tape. We were warned of dire consequences if we neglected to wear these.' Uncomfortable in the heat, they decided to go for a swim. After undressing, Foote 'felt a bit itchy [so] examined this flannel . . . and found it alive with lice. I remember . . . the feeling of horror as I threw the thing as far as I could, and never wore another as long as I was in the army . . . I never got rid of the lice either as long as I was on Active Service.'[57]

The first significant war casualties nursed by the men of the field ambulance were Ottoman Turks who were wounded when they tried to cross the Suez Canal at the beginning of February 1915. (One New Zealand soldier died of his wounds and another was slightly injured.) When two infantry battalions headed to Ismailia to help defend the canal, a section of the ambulance went with them. Between 3 and 5 February the NZMC cared for some 80 wounded Turkish prisoners, mostly at the advanced dressing station at the Cairo railway station. One man's severely wounded left hand had to be amputated. When Charles Thomas was there, there were 'two tables (operating) going hard all the afternoon . . . Most of the wounded I saw . . . were shot through the head from side to side.' One man had been blinded when a bullet grazed both his eyes.[58] This episode revealed that the regimental officers were short of medical stores and that the infantrymen had not been issued with enough of the field dressings they carried in their tunic or trouser pockets. The ambulance men at the canal also continued to treat the sick, sending them to Suez if necessary.

Training continued throughout March, with 'mimic battles, night marches and medical manoeuvres', which included 'six dusty horses hauling ambulance waggons through yielding sand' and 'casualties' laying themselves down 'in grateful ease beneath the waggon covers of improvised dressing stations'. As Adrian Delamore of the Auckland Infantry Battalion recalled, 'The idea was to test our ambulance and the doctors came along distributing tickets which entitled you to be [a] casuality, and lie in the shade for the rest of the day. There was great competition to be wounded.'[59] All too real was the death, on 17 March, of 19-year-old Private

Bethel (Beck) Simpson of the Wellington Infantry Battalion, who suffered heart failure after being given chloroform for a haemorrhoid operation.

There would be sad losses, too, for the NZMC in Egypt. On 13 August 1915, well-known Auckland surgeon Major Thomas Savage, a member of No. 2 New Zealand Stationary Hospital, which had left Wellington in June, died of spinal meningitis. 'What a loss to our company and New Zealand!' wrote one of the orderlies who attended his funeral. 'He as surely gave his life for his country as any man killed by a Turkish bullet!'[60] The 41-year-old had cabled his wife on 25 July to announce his safe arrival in Egypt; two days later he was seriously ill. He left behind four children. According to fellow surgeon William Barclay, Savage had come to New Zealand 'because of asthma — London fogs were bad for him'.[61] As his *New Zealand Herald* obituary said, 'he was regarded as a man of strong character, who would always express his opinions frankly and courageously'.[62] On 29 December 43-year-old Christchurch surgeon Captain James Bell, of the Mounted Field Ambulance, died suddenly at Pont de Koubbeh from cerebral haemorrhage. 'We lost one of the best-liked men in the force,' wrote fellow MFA doctor Robert Withers. 'All along he was a particularly fine man; always most obliging and ready to do anything and everything for anybody. Nothing was too much trouble, and his advice and practical hints were always invaluable to those of us who were less experienced.'[63]

The medics were still busy in March 1915, when the Abbassia hospital was 'well filled'. There were a number of deaths from pneumonia, but the major cause of sickness was a problem that would challenge the army and the medical staff throughout the war: venereal disease. On 26 March 206 men with VD were sent, under escort, to Malta. Carbery was inclined to blame the prostitutes of Cairo: 'young men probably of the very best fighting stuff, trained to the pinnacle of physical fitness and warlike spirit, brought to disgrace by the irresistible temptations of a sensuous oriental city.' He did, however, concede that preventing VD was 'a thorny subject' and 'forever insoluble', 'so beset by "Moral Considerations" and prudish disdain, so much a problem of the soldier's life and the tempestuous wilfulness and devil-may-care of men, possibly doomed to die, who have been wrought to a pitch of overmastering fitness and exuberance by skilful training for war'.[64] By February 1915 Lieutenant-Colonel Batchelor of the NZMC had been 'doing very good work in Cairo . . . running an inspection of European prostitutes for the whole garrison . . . He has got a bldg. as a hospital and three nurses already.' When he visited the venereal camp on 2 April, he found that 196 new cases, mostly Australian, had been admitted in the last fortnight. The 12 infected New Zealanders identified the nationalities of the women involved, which Batchelor carefully listed in his report.[65]

The problem, and the tendency to hold women responsible for it,[66] had started at home. On 14 November 1914, Godley had noted that 'Most of the venereal has been on the Athenic . . . I don't know whether this means that the Christchurch ladies are less to be depended on than those in other cities, as most of the troops on the Athenic come from there.' A month later he was telling Allen that VD was the 'only real trouble' he foresaw. He prophesied a loss of about 10 per cent of the men and was 'arranging privately, without putting anything on the subject

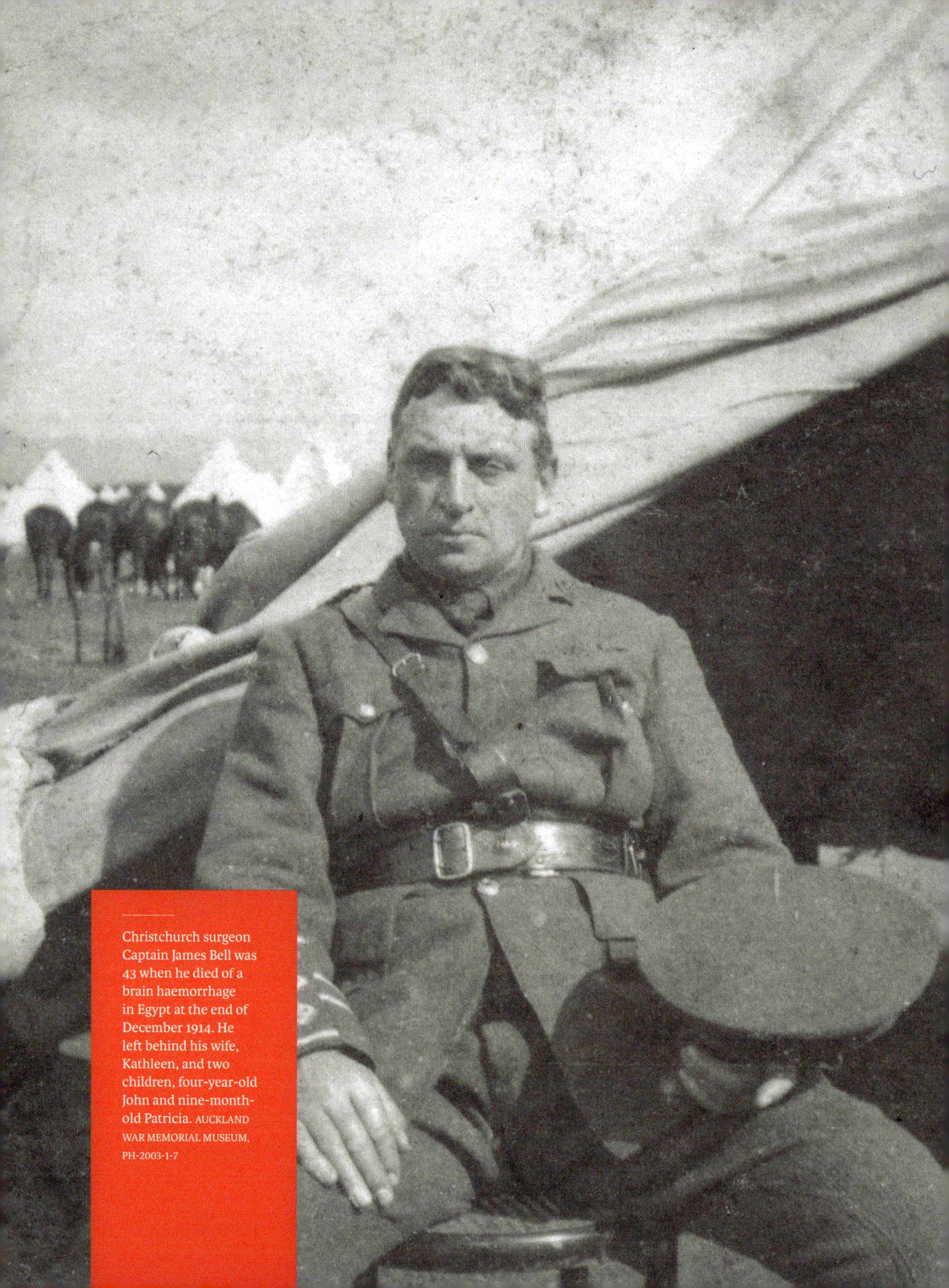

Christchurch surgeon Captain James Bell was 43 when he died of a brain haemorrhage in Egypt at the end of December 1914. He left behind his wife, Kathleen, and two children, four-year-old John and nine-month-old Patricia. AUCKLAND WAR MEMORIAL MUSEUM, PH-2003-1-7

on paper', for each battalion to have ointment and syringes on hand.[67] There had been, and would continue to be, difficulties in the New Zealand training camps. Despite many lectures by the MOs, accompanied by alarmingly graphic magic lantern slides, in mid-1916 a 'lock' hospital for VD sufferers, surrounded by a high barbed-wire fence, was set up at Featherston camp.[68] Drunken soldiers on leave were consorting with prostitutes and frequenting the fairly modest red-light districts, especially in central Wellington. There was talk, too, of prostitutes hanging around the camp gates. Morality aside, the incidence of VD at home and, soon, overseas, reduced the number of men fit to fight, especially as it took some time to be treated.[69]

Venereal disease had been the focus of much discussion before 1914, especially following the 1910 repeal of the 1869 Contagious Diseases Act, which had exposed prostitutes, but not their clients, to compulsory medical inspections. The outbreak of war, however, put VD firmly in the spotlight. There were two chief areas of concern: 'the need to safeguard the fighting manhood of the Dominion from infection and the need to safeguard the Dominion from those members of her armed forces who were infected.'[70] There was cause to worry: although exact figures cannot be settled on, throughout the war New Zealanders, overseas and in the camps, 'had the dubious reputation of the highest rates of venereal disease among the empire's soldiers'.[71]

Also fighting the battle against VD was William Pettit, an 'ardently religious young doctor' who had volunteered as an NZMC officer at Featherston Military Camp after returning from medical missionary work in India in 1915. He convinced the army that he should lecture soldiers on the 'perils of venereal disease'; they also published his booklet on the subject.[72] His effect on his military audience was minimal, apart perhaps from some salutary fright caused by his illustrations of the effects of gonorrhoea and syphilis. As a correspondent signing himself 'N.Z.M.C.' wrote to the *Observer*, possibly as advertorial, 'They're absolutely "bobby dazzlers," those slides . . . They're the most gruesome things I've seen, and, after having seen them, a man would be apt to think twice before succumbing to temptation. Seems to me that it wouldn't be half a bad investment for the Government to secure a few good prints from the doctor and affix a selection in the front of each soldier's pay-book. There's a heap of deterring logic in one of those pictures.'[73] Pettit's urgently moral message had appeal for the general public and he toured the country, lecturing to packed (all-male) houses.

Sensationalist Pettit might have been, but Norman Gray, reading of the lectures in France, thought that '90 per cent of the men who have spent any time in Cairo . . . would corroborate Willie's assertions'. Although the transgressors lining up outside Egyptian brothels might consider themselves cured by the time they returned to New Zealand, 'the germs were still retained in the blood to possibly reappear at some future time, to contaminate a man's wife so that her life was a living death, or cause his children to be born blind, crippled, and insane'.[74] Not sending the infection home was vital. In January Allen had assured Godley that 'if any do come back to us they will be restrained until it is safe to let them loose. We are not going to permit the spread of this horrible disease through the medium of returned soldiers if we can possibly help it.'[75]

Despite further admonitory lectures from doctors on the transports, and warnings from

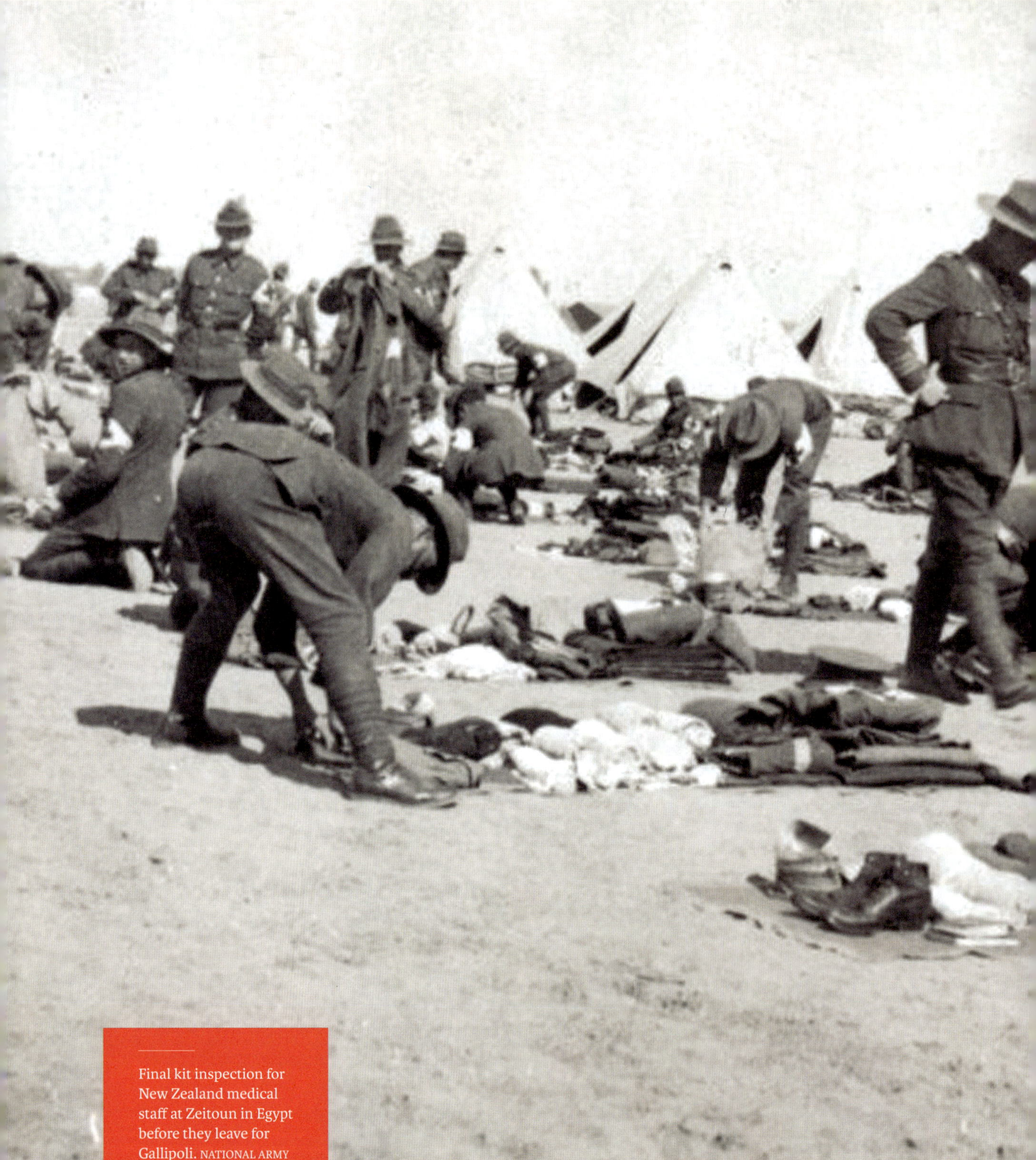

Final kit inspection for New Zealand medical staff at Zeitoun in Egypt before they leave for Gallipoli. NATIONAL ARMY MUSEUM, 1992.772.1

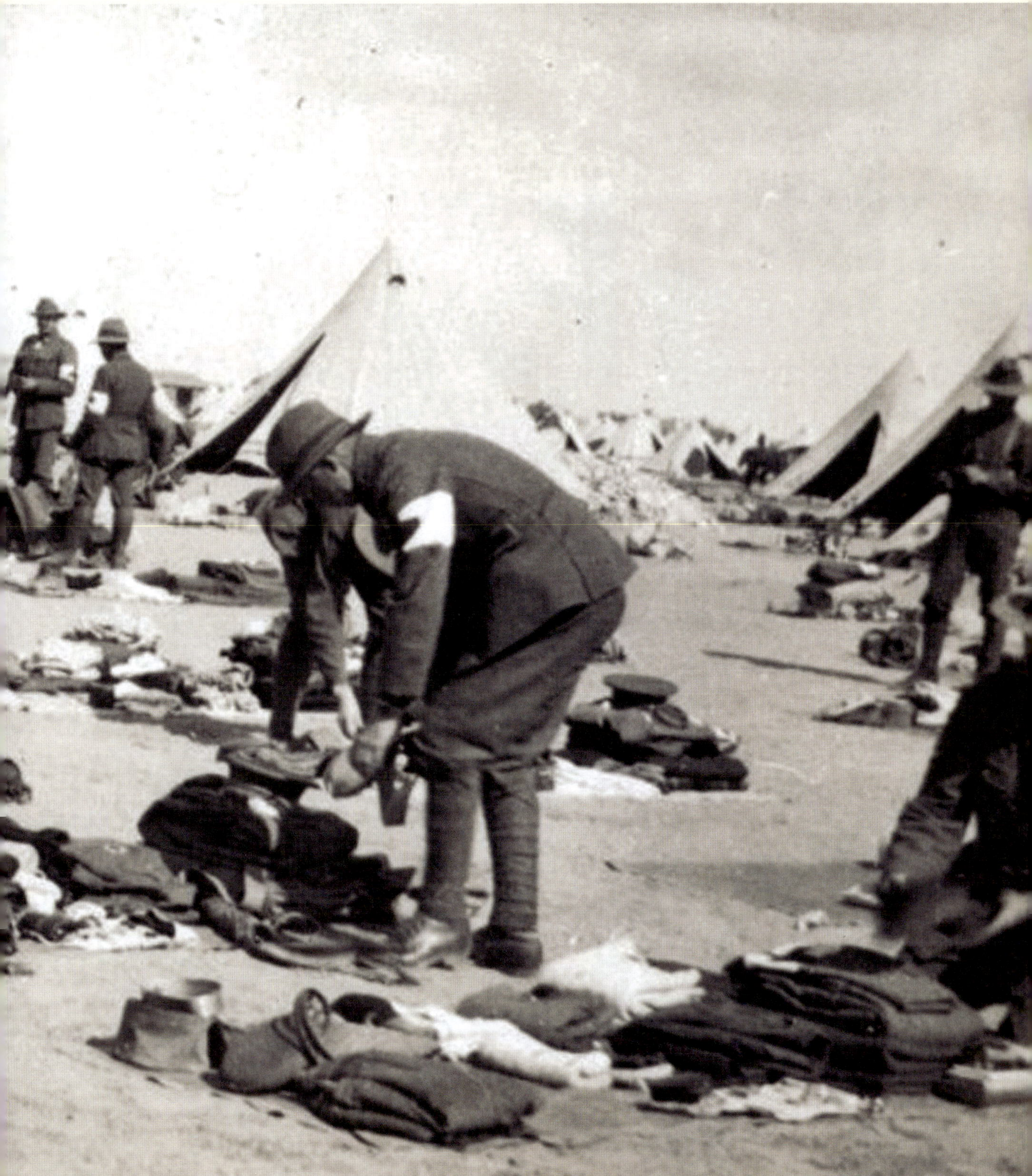

Godley himself, Egypt provided too much temptation for many NZEF men, most of whom were young and single. 'We have been warned to exercise care while on leave,' Thompson reported on 5 December. 'Veiled women must on no account be addressed.' But 'everyone made a dash for Cairo'.[76] In this city of astonishing sights, sounds and smells, what most 'staggered the imagination of the average New Zealander' was the 'plain open fact' of women 'exposed for sale as freely as any other merchandise . . . They sat in rows in the street soliciting custom, beckoned from the windows . . . and accosted passers by.'[77] These women were, of course, a different species from the wives, girlfriends, mothers and sisters left at home, who were not, as John A. Lee put it, 'brought into the conversation. They belonged to a departed world where soldiers had been fathers and husbands and sons and brothers.' John Moloney summarised the problem. 'Many soldiers have paid the price and now languish behind the wire. Who can blame them. Tomorrow they may be sent to the Peninsula and a soldier's grave. Why not make the most of the shining hour. The tragedy of it, is that they should be the victims of such a terrible hotbed of iniquity. Sodom and Gammorrah have their prototype in modern Cairo.'[78]

This exotic, filthy, immoral place offered young men plentiful alcohol (and drugs), and plentiful sex. The number of VD cases exploded, partly, in Malone's view, because of the way the working day was organised to avoid the afternoon heat. Left with nothing to do between 2 p.m. and lights out at 10 p.m., the troops 'naturally go off to Cairo and get into sore temptation'.[79] Fenwick, a few months later, suggested that the men have time off only in the afternoons, when they would see that prostitutes 'unassisted by artificial light are extraordinarily ugly'. Improving visits to interesting places like museums would help, as would talking to the men. The strait-laced Malone was horrified to discover that Godley had 'approved certain measures for preventing certain frightful consequences of vice . . . so as to enable them to indulge in the vice with no fear of disease . . . To do what is proposed is to destroy all moral restraint and lead to worse things.'[80]

Godley was driven principally by the fear of losing fighting men: he knew that many Egyptian women were infected and took the pragmatic view that effective prophylaxis was the most sensible response. But despite preventatives, and Godley's harassing of his officers, medical staff and chaplains, the incidence of VD was 'still very bad' in mid-January 1915. A month later, Godley could report 'a considerable decrease', which he put down to 'the men having had a taste of active service [at the Suez Canal], which has had undoubtedly the effect of making them look after themselves and their morals better. Those that have not been able to fight because they have got venereal are very sorry for themselves.'[81] But the problem did not go away. When Fenwick wrote privately to Allen from Zeitoun in October 1915, he was concerned about preventatives 'not merely from a conscientious, but from a practical point of view. As a surgeon of many years standing, I know that the ointment issued is not a definite preventative . . . [and] not of much value against the excessively virulent infection found in this country.' He was concerned, too, that men would sleep with prostitutes *because* they had been issued with ointment: '"The Doctors gave us this stuff so it must be all right."' The women hated the ointment because it gave them blisters, so the men sold it; Fenwick had heard that the 'natives' found it 'very useful for curing lice in their hair'. 'It is,' he sighed, 'practically impossible to order a mass of thousands of men to clean their teeth. It is an equally impossible task to teach careless young men to take even the slenderest precautions to avoid venereal infection.'[82]

At last the time came to leave Egypt. With their equipment loaded onto wagons, on the morning of 11 April 1915 the medical units boarded a train for Alexandria and the ships that would take them to the Mediterranean island of Lemnos, in preparation for the Dardanelles landings. Generally the 'replenished and overhauled' medical equipment was up to standard, but the ambulance wagons — converted delivery vans from New Zealand — had required alteration in order to take the stretchers on which the wounded would lie after they were evacuated from Gallipoli. Carbery had to admit, though, that in terms of both ambulance and general service wagons, the No. 4 Australian Field Ambulance was 'much better equipped than ours'. He was more optimistic when it came to the readiness of the NZMC. Under Begg, 'a most zealous commander and a strict disciplinarian', the men had had four months of training, 'caught a glimpse of real warfare' at the canal, and gained 'valuable and varied experience' in the camp hospital and at Abbassia. They were also familiar with 'sanitary and preventive measures.'[83] Gallipoli, however, would test the members of the NZMC, and the high command's medical arrangements, to an unimaginable degree.

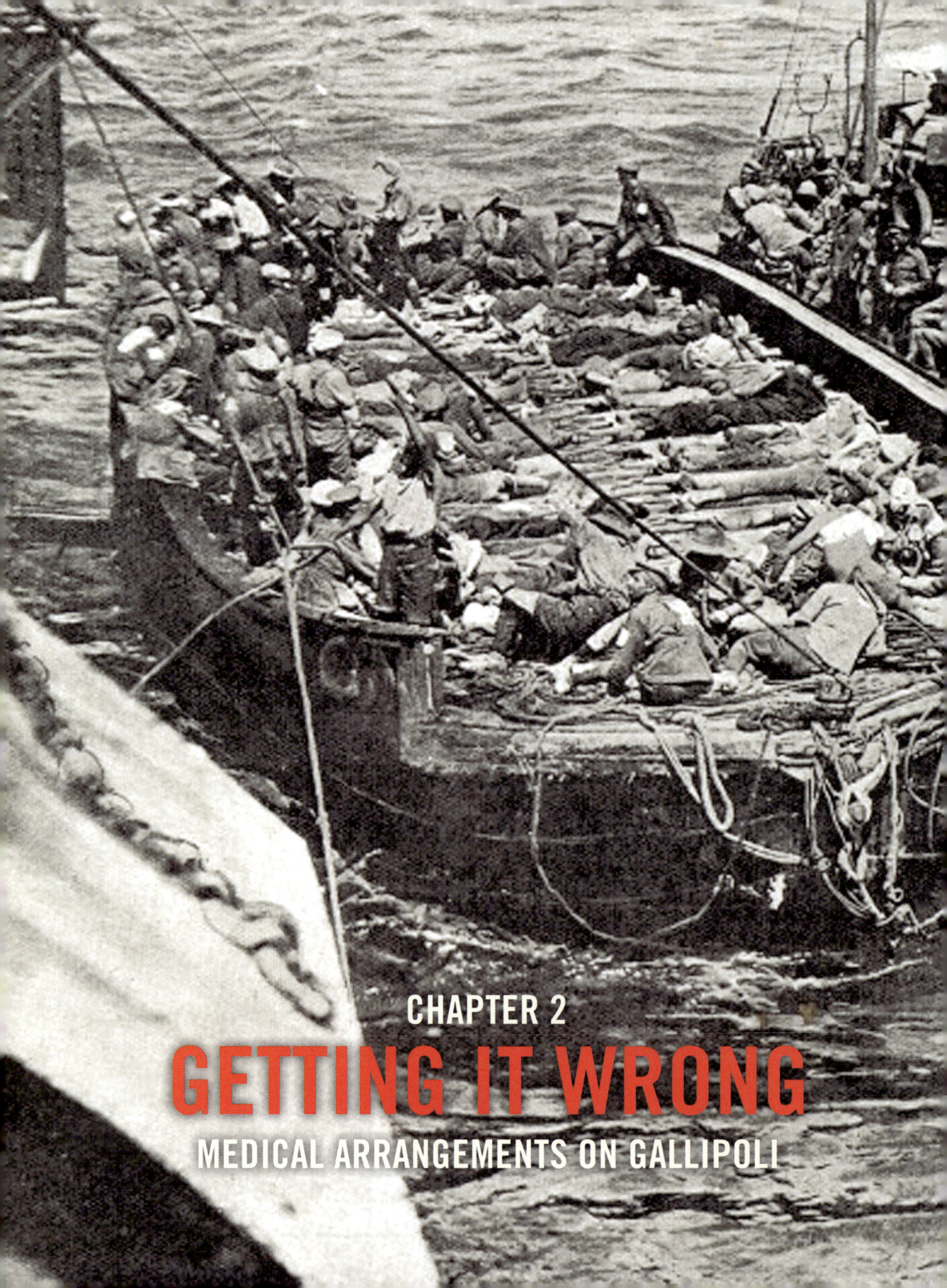

CHAPTER 2

GETTING IT WRONG

MEDICAL ARRANGEMENTS ON GALLIPOLI

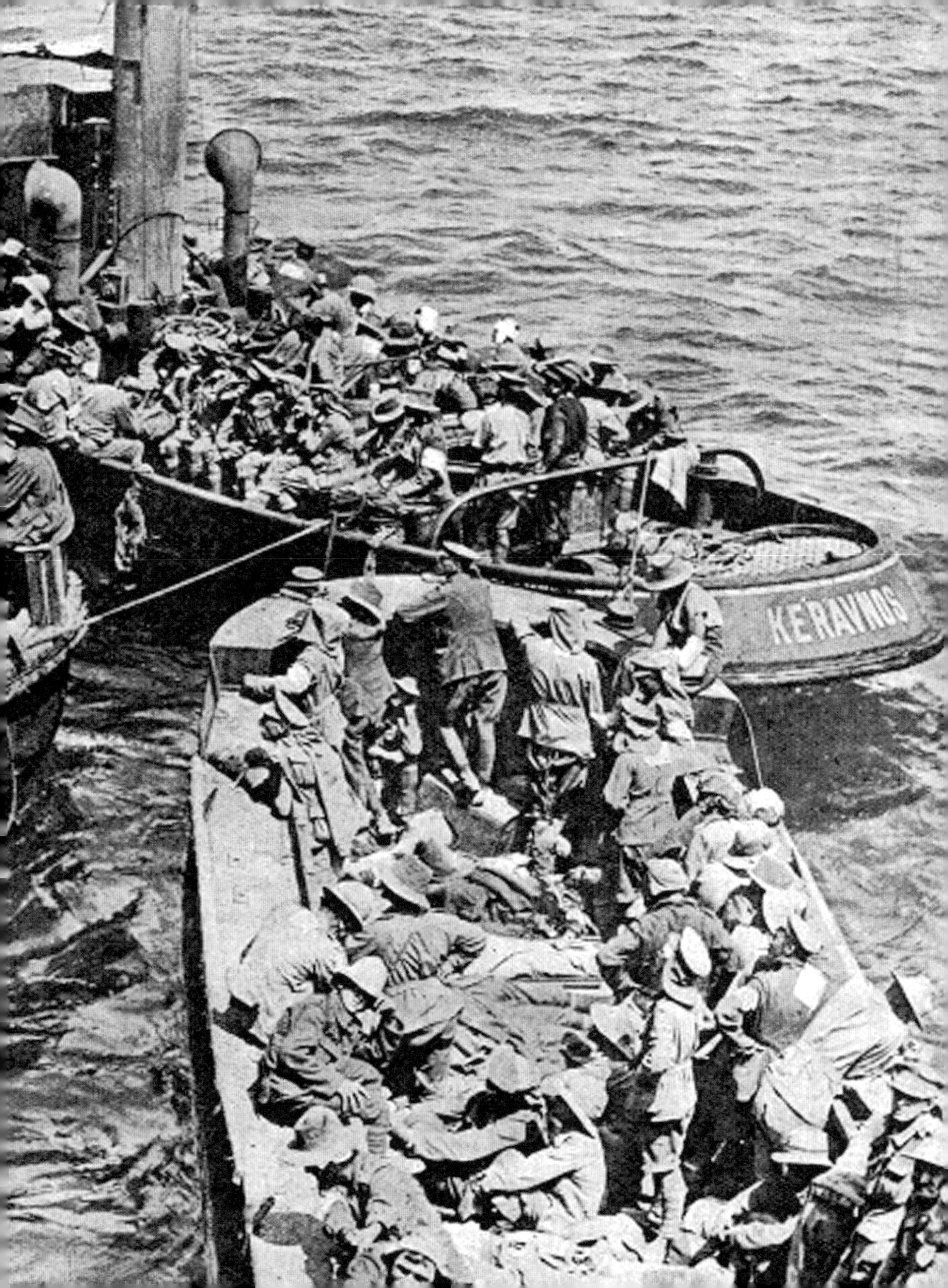
KERAVNOS

previous pages
The barges carrying the Gallipoli wounded out to transports and, later, hospital ships were appallingly overcrowded. To make matters worse, they were unsuited to taking stretchers. NATIONAL ARMY MUSEUM, 1992.760

> Helped out of trench or bivouac, men . . . were sent via the dressing stations to the casualty clearing stations, where they were liable to be hit again by bullets or blown to bits by high explosive . . . In the beginning it was not all plain sailing, and there were not enough hospital ships and not enough doctors and nurses. The toll of human life and limb in modern warfare had been greatly underestimated.
>
> — Malcolm Ross, *Press*, 25 May 1916

'A wounded man's dream of heaven,' according to the official historian Major Fred Waite, 'was to be taken to a hospital boat, get a warm bath, a change of clothes, a bed with clean sheets and a sight of the nursing angels.'[1] But that dream was often a distant prospect for the sick and wounded on Gallipoli, particularly in the terrible days after the 25 April 1915 landing.

The medical arrangements for the Dardanelles campaign were badly botched.[2] The details are complex, and often further obscured by confusing acronyms, but it is all too clear that mistakes, omissions and changes of plan severely compromised the treatment and evacuation of the wounded. Certainly, the landing operation, in the face of a strong Turkish defence, was challenging, as was getting an enormous number of hurt men off the peninsula, but failings of the British high command made matters much worse. Australian war correspondent Charles Bean's diary entries praise the work of the Anzac stretcher-bearers and other medical staff, 'but once the wounded leave our hands there seems to be the same general muddle which is the main thing that impresses you with almost everything this British staff has done'. He was enraged by the 'dull, stupid, cruel bungling that was mismanaging the medical arrangements', which he described as 'a sheer scandal. They have foreseen nothing.'[3] As medical historian Mark Harrison puts it, rather more temperately, 'unusually severe . . . difficulties . . . were magnified by an inflexible command structure and the failure of GHQ to consult senior MOs or respond to their requests'. Especially in the early part of the war, civilian doctors who had enlisted were not always well regarded, or listened to, by senior military commanders.[4]

The problems began at the top. General Sir Ian Hamilton, commander-in-chief of the

75,000-strong Mediterranean Expeditionary Force (MEF), which included the Australian and New Zealand Army Corps (ANZAC), did not sufficiently inform and include those responsible for the medical arrangements. Some key personnel did not even reach Mudros, the harbour on the base island of Lemnos, in time to contribute to the final landing arrangements. Before the end of March, one telling error had already been made: it had been concluded that Lemnos was an unsuitable site for a full stationary hospital — as Godley wanted — and that existing hospitals in Alexandria and Cairo would be used instead.[5] It took only about four hours to reach Lemnos; Alexandria was two or three days' sailing away, a punishing extra distance for sick and wounded men.[6]

The failure to consider the medical aspects of the campaign showed, too, in staffing decisions. A deputy director of medical services (DDMS) was required to coordinate the medical work of the ANZAC, but by mid-April — the landing was originally planned for 21 April — there was no one in this essential role. Godley made Neville Manders assistant director of military services (ADMS) to the New Zealand and Australian Division. (This, plus the 1st Australian Division, constituted the ANZAC.) After Manders reached Lemnos on 15 April, it was decided that, despite his reluctance, he would also act as DDMS to the corps. The next day, as ordered, Australian ADMS Colonel Neville Howse 'submitted a tentative plan' for the evacuation of wounded ANZAC men. This outlined a number of sensible concerns, including 'strong objections' to using transports, since they all carried horses and it would be impossible to clean them properly in the short time between the troops disembarking and the injured being taken on board.[7]

When Surgeon-General William E. Birrell, director of medical services for the MEF, arrived at Mudros on the 18th, however, he changed the evacuation orders. Manders and Howse, still following the original plans, only had 'some verbal notification' of the alterations. An increasingly concerned Manders also pinpointed, in his diary, the 'want of harmony' between Birrell's office and his own, which was entirely due to inadequate communication.[8] Hamilton's headquarters on the *Arcadian* and Manders' on the *Lutzow* were half a mile apart and could communicate only by means of boats, which could not be launched when the sea was rough.

The bad weather postponed the landing and meant that the transports designated to evacuate the lightly wounded could neither be staffed nor stocked with medical supplies. Also out of the question were necessary training exercises such as boat drills and practising the tricky job of manoeuvring stretchers up gangplanks. Confusion continued about which vessels would be available to remove the wounded. Manders, still lacking the full draft of the medical arrangements, was anxious about a 'mix up'[9] and failed to receive important messages in time. Howse, too, was worried and considered the estimate of 5.5 per cent casualties far too low. Manders, to his relief, lost the DDMS role. 'I am thankful to say,' he wrote on 22 April, 'I have no more to do with the Hospital Ships as it is, really, not my job.'[10]

On 23 April, when the new landing date of the 25th was announced, Manders explained the proposed medical arrangements. They were, in Carbery's telling words, 'somewhat as follows'.[11] As military historian Christopher Pugsley has pointed out, the instructions depended on 'a rapid and considerable advance inland and assumed that the wounded would be kept on shore'.[12] A casualty clearing station (CCS), landed early on the beach, would collect and initially care for the wounded; a dressing station would be established nearby. No wounded were to be evacuated until all the arriving troops had been landed. Stretcher-bearers from both the New Zealand and Australian field ambulances would go ashore as soon as possible, then head off to locate and group the wounded and take them to the CCS after nightfall. Evacuation would follow.

The final plan, prepared on 24 April, was not sent to Manders and Howse. Both men stepped onto the peninsula the next day without knowing that just one hospital ship, the British *Gascon*, capable of taking 500 cot cases, would be available for seriously wounded Anzac troops, or that the Australians and New Zealanders had been allotted three 12-man launches, to be towed out to the *Gascon*. There would also be four ambulance transports: the *Lutzow*, the *Ionian*, the *Clan McGillivray* and the *Seeang Choon*. No. 2 Australian Stationary Hospital was supposed to supply all four transports with medical staff but managed only the last, because by the time it arrived at Mudros the other three vessels had already sailed for Gallipoli.[13]

Things went awry from the beginning. The Anzacs did not go ashore, as planned, on a flat section of coastline that could have properly accommodated the proposed CCS, dressing station and wounded, though it would have been exposed to enemy guns at Gaba Tepe. Instead, they struggled, under fire, onto a narrow stony beach. Above, fiercely defended by the enemy, were hills like those at Wellington's Oriental Bay, but, in the words of one NZMC man, 'much steeper & covered with scrub'.[14]

For Percival Fenwick, deputy to Manders, who landed with him at what would become known as Anzac Cove on the morning of the 25th, a 'hellish Sunday' lay ahead.[15] The Australian medics, under Howse, had already set up a CCS at the southern end of the beach, sheltered from direct fire, where rapidly growing numbers of wounded lay under a cliff waiting to be taken off to boats, while troops, mules and ammunition continued to arrive. Fred Glover, with the Canterbury Infantry Battalion, thought the CCS 'an awful sight. Under the cover of a hill, hundreds were lying there groaning, seriously wounded.'[16] The noise from shrapnel and thousands of Turkish bullets was colossal. As one man would recall, 'The hills echo and re-echo the sound and the roar and rattle is frightful.'[17] The unceasing Turkish onslaught sometimes wounded already injured men for a second time.

Fenwick began work immediately, ensuring the wounded were kept against the cliff and dressing wounds, while Howse was 'packing boats and lighters with these poor chaps as fast as possible', though the beach 'kept filling again with appalling quickness'.[18] It was impossible to obey the edict about not evacuating wounded until all the troops were ashore: by early afternoon the barges returning to the ships to collect more fighting men were filled with stretchers and walking wounded. As Henry Winter of the Wellington Infantry Battalion waited to get ashore early on the morning of the 26th, 'the wounded started to come aboard in boat loads . . . The first lot of ours to go off got shelled getting to the shore and some were brought back wounded to the ship within an hour of going off.'[19]

Fenwick and Captain George Craig set up a dressing station further to the north, to take some pressure off Howse. The danger the New Zealand Medical Corps would face throughout the war was already frighteningly apparent. 'It seemed impossible for men to live under the hail of bullets,' Fenwick wrote. 'Capt Craig dressed over 100 cases under fire. One of his assistants had his finger shot off while helping him. Men were hit constantly in our station.' Once darkness fell, Craig and Fenwick were able to get some wounded away. About midnight the latter commandeered 'four big horse boats, which held twelve stretchers on the bottom and I packed in less severe cases along the sides, sitting, kneeling, lying — anyhow, about 120 all told'.[20] Howse estimated that he had evacuated 1500 men that day.

During the landing 'Sergeant X', who later told his story to the *Star* in Christchurch, 'received a piece of lead which put a stop to my progress. I made my way back to a dressing station with the assistance of a New Zealand Medical Corps man. This branch of the service, during those first wild days, showed even greater personal bravery and devotion than our infantry, and they deserve all praise for it. Captain (now Major) Craig especially shone out in that trying test time.' Fenwick, too, admired his colleague. 'Craig has done magnificent work . . . He is the most modestly brave fellow one could meet.'[21]

By the time the bearers of No. 1 New Zealand Field Ambulance, led by Colonel Eugene O'Neill, landed from boats during the afternoon of the 25th, with spent bullets hitting the water around them and shrapnel bursting near the shore — miraculously, no one was hit — there was, in Carbery's laconic phrase, 'much to be seen on the beach'.[22] Not all the bearers landed at once, so, leaving Captain Cyril Tewsley behind to collect the rest, O'Neill and Captain Aubrey Short set off up the steep hill, passing wounded men travelling slowly and painfully down. The bearers worked hard, bringing wounded into the collecting post O'Neill set up. The firing from the Turks did not stop throughout that first cold, sometimes rainy night. The rugged terrain made finding wounded men, and carrying them, extremely difficult. Unable to use their lanterns, the bearers could often neither count nor identify the casualties. Shortage of water was already a problem. The next day O'Neill and his men continued their unremitting cycle of finding and dressing wounded and getting them down to the beach, under heavy fire. RAPs were set up, and on the 28th a dressing station was established in a comparatively sheltered gully about 150 yards from the beach.

When Captain George Home reached the Taranaki Company on Walker's Ridge about 6 p.m. on the 25th, 'they were still under fire and I had to lie flat alongside each wounded man as I dressed him . . . [W]e had to wait for a lull before we could move from one to another.' It was 9.30 before the enemy fire slackened sufficiently to try evacuating the wounded. 'Their position was impossible for stretchers, so they had to be carried, by a half moonlight, down some 300 feet of declivity that frequently compelled one to go on all fours. I and three others of my N.Z.M.C. men carried a 12 stone man with a bullet-fracture femur down this and I never remember a more heartbreaking, backaching job.' They made it to the bottom of the watercourse, where the stretcher-bearers were waiting. It was 2 a.m. before Home, who had been fired at three times by a sniper, saw the wounded safely onto a ship and could lie down on the beach to doze 'coldly, and uncomfortably till daybreak'.[23]

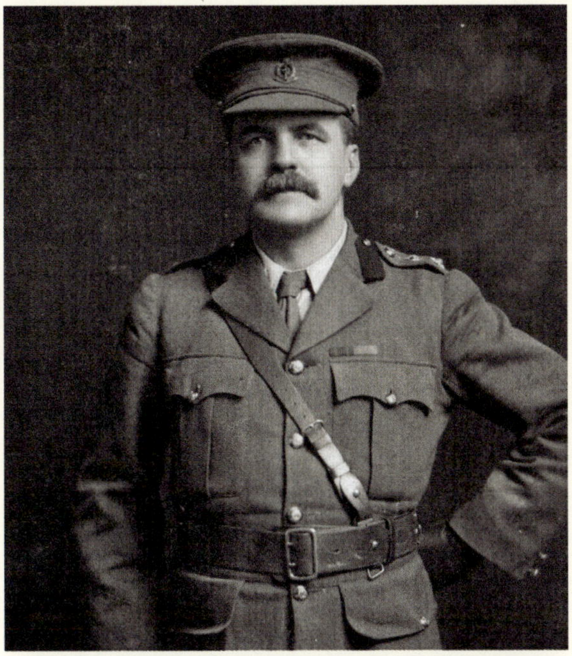

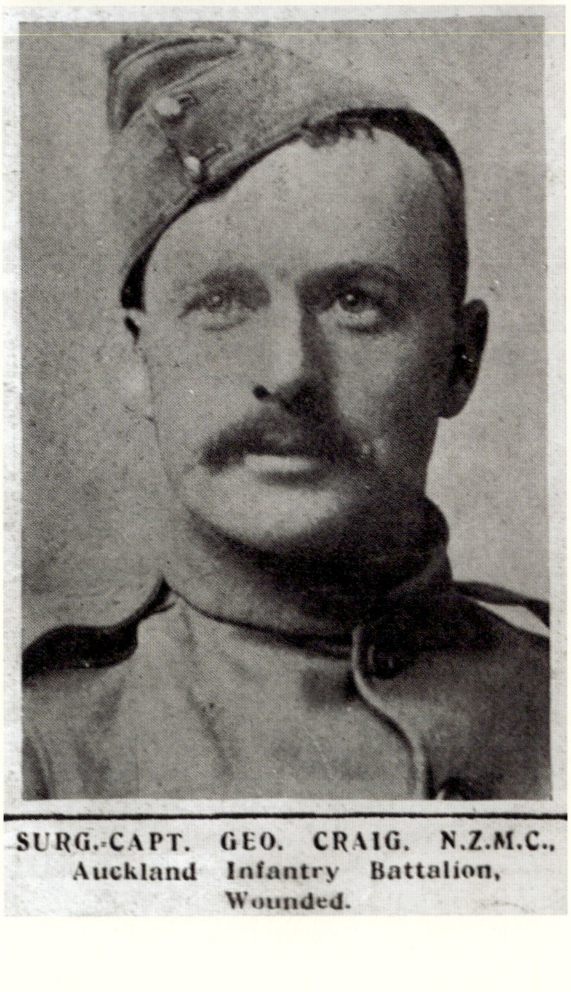
SURG.-CAPT. GEO. CRAIG. N.Z.M.C.,
Auckland Infantry Battalion,
Wounded.

above Lieutenant-Colonel Percival Clennell Fenwick, deputy director of medical services on Gallipoli, was one of the first medical men ashore on 25 April. His diary provides a vivid account of the campaign. COURTESY OF PHILIPPA HORN AND RICHARD FENWICK

below Under the *Auckland Weekly News* headline, 'The Bravest Men I Knew', an unnamed Anzac veteran paid tribute to George Craig in May 1916, recalling how, on 25 April, he 'worked without cessation . . . His conduct, his fearlessness and disregard of danger in the execution of his duty, were splendid.' The writer also singled Christchurch medical officer Neil Guthrie out for praise — 'one of the bravest of the brave'. AUCKLAND WAR MEMORIAL MUSEUM

Glover remembered the 'cries for the stretcher-bearers . . . coming from all around. Ten times the number of ambulance men were required.'[24] After they landed, Sergeant Alexander Lindsay and his men 'were going all night and next day, then we started to feel the strain, and had to take spells in turn. Our boys stuck to their work like bricks, and never growled or neglected their duty as long as they had strength. We had to carry out our work under great danger, and every time one of our squads appeared you would see a shell burst, above or near them.'[25] As Fenwick would point out, their achievements scotched any notion that stretcher-bearing or medical orderly work was less brave or risky than front-line fighting. 'I think the old legend of the uselessness of the Medical Corps has been killed dead . . . our wounded bearers, now numbering at least a dozen, have given their blood to clean that slate.'[26] Those saved by the bearers praised them too. 'Nothing was too hard for them, no spot too dangerous,' wrote Phil Bennett, wounded on 16 May. 'They had no rifles or arms, and they knew that neither their work nor the little Geneva crosses on their arms were any protection in the face of the Turkish fire, but still they worked on. Night or day, it made no difference and I have seen bearers drop from sheer fatigue. But never a word of complaint. A short spell, and they were at it again, getting out some poor beggar.'[27]

Communication problems quickly became significant. Manders, with Divisional Headquarters in a small gully, sent his first message to Birrell on the *Arcadian* at 2 p.m. on the 25th: 'Wounded arriving rapidly, about five hundred. Probably require another hospital ship. Request ships make nominal roll wounded, impossible here.' There was no reply. The *Arcadian* was off the Turkish coast, and Birrell, not allowed to use a radio, could not communicate with the shore or with any other vessel. And there was no one at ANZAC headquarters fulfilling Manders' former DDMS role. He tried again at 6.45 p.m. and twice the following day, but all his entreaties disappeared into the ether. By the end of the 26th he was angry and despairing. He knew that the *Clan McGillivray* and the *Seeang Choon* were 'full and have probably sailed' and that he was 'now dependent on improvised Ship, as no Hospital Ship . . . will be available for one week. This comes of making Alexandria the base and not Lemnos. The medical arrangements made by the DMS [Birrell] are shocking. We have almost 2000 wounded up to date.'[28]

The evacuation of wounded was confused, clumsy and slow. There was no system. At first many launches left the Australian CCS loaded with cot cases, but by the afternoon of the 25th they were perilously overloaded, and crammed barges, unsuited to carrying stretchers, were also leaving from the northern end of the beach. Both severely and slightly wounded were ending up on transports, untallied.

The resulting failure to submit anything like accurate casualty returns would continue to create anxiety and anger back home. 'I hope,' Godley would tell Allen on 6 June, that 'you will explain this to all the people, and make them realise that it is not from any carelessness, or idleness, that the returns are not sent at once.' In September he was still pleading for understanding. It was often impossible even to ascertain if men were killed and missing — 'or

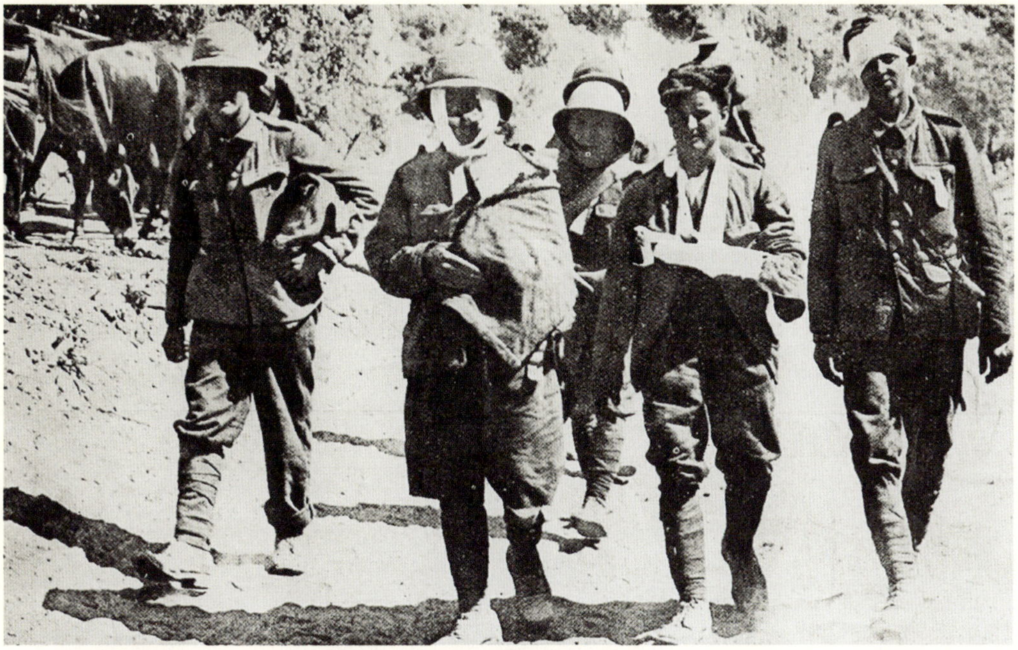

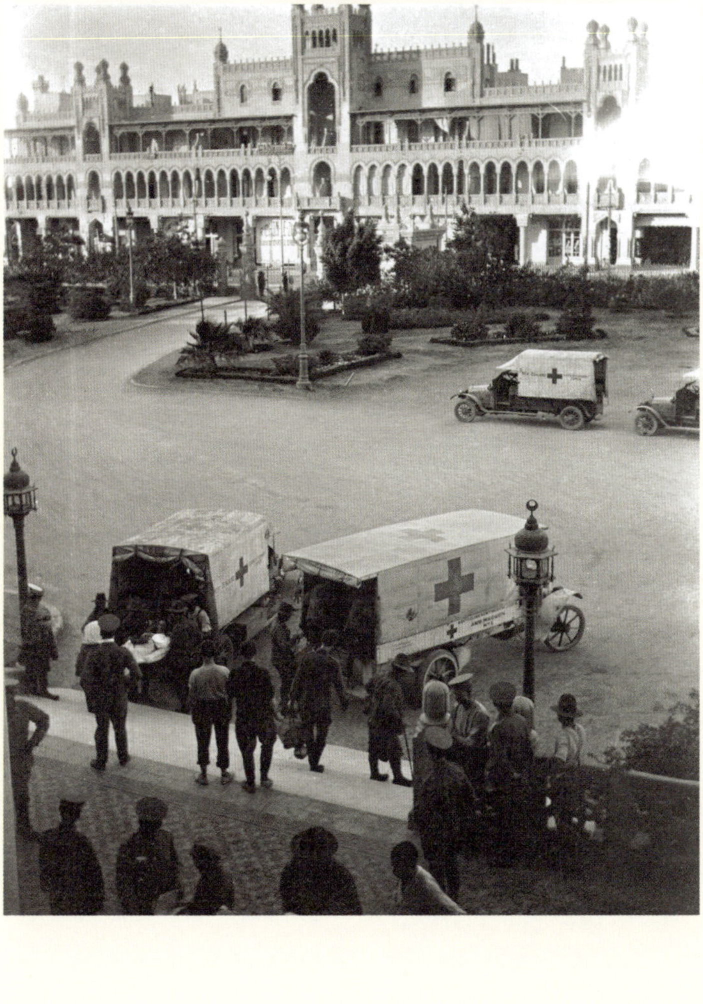

above The caption on this 1915 *Auckland Weekly News* illustration reads, 'Wounded soldiers returning from the first dressing station behind the firing line'. Many were too severely hurt to walk down to the beach. AUCKLAND LIBRARIES, AWNS-19150916-46-1

below New Zealand Expeditionary Force and Australian Army Medical Corps ambulances being unloaded outside No. 1 Australian General Hospital at what had been the grand Heliopolis Palace Hotel. AUSTRALIAN WAR MEMORIAL, P10997.020

slipped away during the first 24 hours, wounded, without any record of it, possibly to Malta or England'.[29]

By dusk on the 25th the *Seeang Choon*, still with all its troops on board, and the *Clan McGillivray* were overflowing, as was the *Lutzow*. From then on, the tows of barges, laden with wounded, visited vessel after troop-filled vessel — sometimes six or seven — but these, not forewarned and usually lacking medical personnel, could take either no wounded or not enough of them. Jacob (Jack) Moller of the Wellington Infantry Battalion, anchored a couple of miles off Anzac Cove, looked out on 'barges and boatloads of wounded as far as the eye could see . . . I personally helped to hoist 65 on to our boat.'[30] Because even the designated transports lacked suitable equipment for lifting the wounded on board, transfers were slow and painful. Men already in agony, and often without blankets, had to endure cold and seasickness as they tossed about in open boats awaiting their turn to be taken onto a vessel. Some perished before this happened.

Because the sole hospital ship, the *Gascon*, was readily identifiable with her white and green paint, red cross and brilliant night-time illumination, she was both a natural magnet for boatloads of wounded and free of enemy attention. The same did not apply to the transports — the 'black ships' — which were unmarked and unlit. They had to sail further from shore to avoid being fired on, and became scattered. After being shelled while loading at Anzac Cove, one ship then 'capsized a boat load of wounded that were alongside. Two were drowned and the others floundered around for a few minutes until picked up.'[31]

Glover, wounded in the head about 6 p.m. on the 25th, made it onto the *Seeang Choon*, 'along with many more'. 'It was very awkward transferring the patients to the transport; all the stretcher patients had to be carted up the gangway.' A bed was made up for Glover on a table in the messroom. 'Every bit of floor space was covered with wounded, some in an awful condition . . . There were only three doctors and a few ambulance men; they were unprepared for this, and had to work very hard all night on the serious cases.'[32] As Colonel Charles Begg would later explain, the *Seeang Choon*, which he reckoned had 700 on board, was 'totally unsuitable for carrying seriously-wounded cases. She was a very old ship, and should have had a thorough overhaul even before she could be made suitable for the accommodation of lightly wounded.' There were only 31 beds in the ship's hospital, no operating room and an 'utterly inadequate' staff of 20 orderlies.[33]

Those on the troopships, like Moller, did their best, but in the overwhelming confusion medically inexperienced crew members mingled critical and non-critical cases, placing them on straw palliasses or mattresses or simply on bare decks. Walking and sitting wounded managed reasonably well, but those with abdominal wounds, bad lacerations or smashed femurs needed urgent surgical attention and the care of trained nurses, neither of which was available. Such patients had been given oral morphine on the beach, but once that wore off they were in severe pain.[34]

The failure of even medical orderlies to take mutilated or dying men off their stretchers so these could be returned to shore increased the pressure on the already beleaguered bearers. To make matters worse, two men sent out from the peninsula to retrieve stretchers from the transports were co-opted for other duties. As Fenwick noted on the 28th, 'The Engineers made us forty [stretchers] of canvas and rough wood, but they don't last long.'[35] In practical Kiwi fashion, the bearers improvised stretchers, using rifles and puttees and even overcoats. (At Sari Bair in August, Te Rangi Hīroa would fashion a stretcher from 'a Turkish overcoat and two rifles'. Because the latter were too short, he lengthened them 'by fixing sheathed bayonets in place and trusting they would not work loose as the patient was being carried'.)[36] Oil sheets were also used. When a Dunedin ambulance man was hit in the hip by a bullet, 'The next difficulty was to get me out of a two foot-wide trench under heavy rifle fire . . . but . . . with the help of an oil sheet I was dragged through from end to end.'[37] In May, to overcome the problem of negotiating narrow trenches, George Craig was 'trying to fix up a long rope and a blanket cot, by which a man can be slung down the trench on the rope'.[38]

The plight of the wounded was little better on the transports intended to take casualties. The *Lutzow* was overloaded and the only men on board with any medical training were veterinary surgeon Major Alexander Young and 22-year-old teacher Ormond Burton of No. 1 Field Ambulance. The *Lutzow* also still contained some 150 horses: Australian surgeon Colonel (later Sir) Charles Ryan would call her the 'dirtiest, nastiest boat I have been on'.[39] Until two NZMC doctors, Robert Walton and Francis Scannell, and a naval surgeon, arrived to help on the evening of the 26th, Young and Burton dealt with an unending stream of badly hurt men.[40] Burton later described the 'very dreadful' voyage to Alexandria, which began at 5 p.m. on 27 April. 'We had stretchers in long rows in all the holds. Any able to walk were crowded into cabins, or anywhere else we were able to get them. The doctors improvised an operating theatre where they were able to do the most urgent things, and at least get clean dressings on broken men.'[41] According to Walton, the *Lutzow* had sufficient medical dressings and drugs, but acquiring such necessities would prove a problem on the peninsula. 'Our supply of surgical equipment is very low,' Fenwick wrote on 21 May, 'and A.D.M.S. is cabling Alexandria and hunting for ships with medical stores on board.' In August MO Alexander Trotter noted, 'Went down to Anzac this afternoon to Medical Supply Depot and managed to obtain some essential drugs.'[42]

Burton found himself in charge of a hold full of seriously wounded men, a number of whom were dying, 'some very horribly, and painfully. There was so much to be done, and so little that one could really do . . . Most of the wounded were very patient and pathetically grateful.' The following morning, in a deck cabin, Burton did what he could for the walking wounded. Over the next two days, 'the line of men shuffling up never ceased'. The 'marvellous relief' of landing at Alexandria did not last long. As soon as the bloodstained blankets had been removed, the stretchers washed down and the drugs and dressings replenished, the *Lutzow* returned to Anzac Cove.[43] She now had 'the skeleton of a trained staff', although the conditions remained unspeakable. Because stretchers 'could not be manoeuvred round the narrow passage ways . . . all seriously wounded men had to go into the great holds which were far from clean, badly lighted, and utterly devoid of all necessary conveniences'. The orderlies slaved for 12-hour stretches. None of the wounded had been washed; many were still in their blood-covered uniforms; some had bandages applied two or three days before and sepsis was setting in. Burton never forgot the cries of pain and the calls for water and morphine.[44]

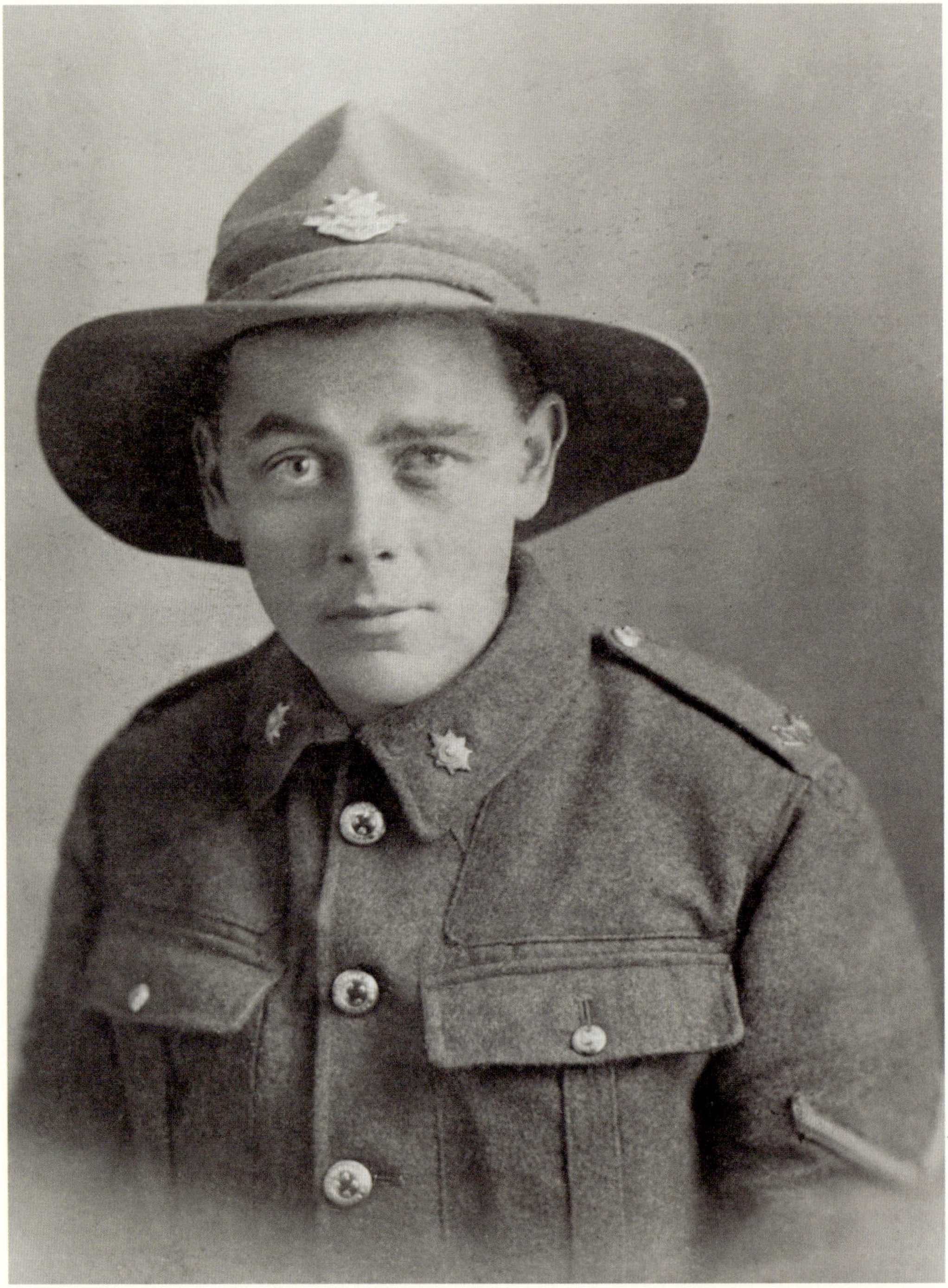

Ormond Burton (1893–1974) had been a teacher in Bay of Plenty before he joined No. 1 Field Ambulance. His experiences as an orderly and a stretcher-bearer, and later as a combatant, would help to shape his conversion to Christian pacifism. ALEXANDER TURNBULL LIBRARY, 1/2-148239-F

On the ship that took Private Robert Capstick, 'shot through the windpipe and through the lungs', back to Egypt 'there was one doctor for 600 wounded, and he could only go round and give morphia to the worst cases'.[45] After being wounded in the leg on 27 April, Herbert Hart, and many others, were taken to a transport 'upon which I was hauled up by an ordinary winch ... All the hospital ships were full and away, and we had only 3 doctors and no nurses so the 800 wounded could get practically no attention until we got to Alexandria on Saturday morning [1 May].' During the voyage 28 men were buried at sea. 'A few who were hit in the head suffered intensely and groaned or screamed in agony the whole way across.'[46] There would be problems again in August, after Chunuk Bair. NZANS nurses Mary Grigor and Catherine Blackie were working on the British transport *Caledonia*, which had beds for 800 but took 1375 back to Alexandria. 'I shall never forget that week,' Grigor wrote; 'we worked night and day . . . I had theatre duty, and when we were not operating we were all dressing as hard as ever we could. Some of the wounds were ghastly.'[47]

Loading the boats taking the wounded to the hospital ships was always an excruciating business. In May Gordon Breen saw a shell just clear the first of two barges laden with wounded. When it exploded, the fragments killed men in the second barge. In June Fenwick described boats lying 'at a little improvised wharf just under Hell Point, and here the enemy have the exact range and pour shrapnel down'. He found it 'mental agony' to watch the 'endless nightmare' of the necessarily slow and careful loading process.[48]

The hospitals in Alexandria and Cairo were often unable to cope with the influx of wounded. Capstick could 'get no attention' for some time. Australian No. 1 General at the Heliopolis Palace Hotel was 'crowded to overflowing and I had to wash myself all over in the open. I shivered like a dog in a sack. Now every doctor and nurse who sees me whistles in amazement that I am alive.'[49] (His miraculous survival was not to be repeated: he was killed on Chunuk Bair on 8 August.) After Benjamin Colbran was wounded in the right hand and leg on the night of 6/7 August, he eventually reached Alexandria, then spent two and a half hours on a hospital train travelling to Cairo, where he 'landed at the Lunar [Luna] Park hospital & got practically no examination or attention as it was crowded with wounded'.[50]

Not all New Zealand's medics served on the peninsula. As soon as the Mounted Field Ambulance men reached Anzac Cove about a fortnight after the landing, they were ordered to re-embark and take charge of wounded bound for Lemnos. Then, as Charles Hand-Newton recorded, they were off to Malta on the SS *Ivernia*, working with Australian medical officers to set up 'two quite adequate operating theatres and [fit] up the steerage accommodation for the wounded. There were about 1400 of these, many of them serious cases but all abdominal ones were sent to a regular hospital ship. The theatres were kept going day and night.' After several other temporary hospital ship duties, the MFA was back in Anzac Cove on 23 July and soon established a dressing station under the steep slopes of Chalk Hill.[51]

Bitter fighting in early May, at Baby 700 and then at Cape Helles, added to the growing toll of dead and wounded, which included NZMC men. During the lanternless, muddy night of 2/3 May, when congestion on the route to the beach meant a carry took three hours with four bearers to a stretcher, 34-year-old field ambulance man Private William Heaver was shot in the head while attempting to rescue a wounded soldier. He was mentioned in despatches for his bravery. His name appeared, posthumously, in the *London Gazette* on 5 August 1915, alongside that of Private William Henry, who had been mentioned in despatches and received the DCM for 'conspicuous bravery and devotion to duty' under heavy fire at Anzac on 25 April.[52]

For ambulance man John Thomson, 3 May was 'the most depressing day we have had not from the difficulties or danger but from the number of missing friends and the widespread death and mutilation. Had the unenviable experience of having a man I had picked up die before he could be got to a dressing station. After yesterdays experience I feel that I could shoot any enemy coldbloodedly & without compunction.' Wednesday 5 May was little better. Thomson's colleague Edward Laseron 'was caught in the open and got a shell nozzle behind the ear. He was able to go to the beach on a donkey but Major O'Neill thinks his skull is fractured.' (Laseron would be hit again in France.) Reginald Napier was also wounded by shrapnel that day. It was 'horrible to think that many still alive [from the 3rd] must be there. We wanted to get them but Heaver was killed in the first attempt & neither the infantry or our own officers will allow another.'[53]

As ambulance man Private Frank Loftus recorded in his diary, on 22 May Arthur Perry was 'killed in his bivvy by shrapnel (riddled with pellets)'.[54] James Bennet's death on 11 June 'was a shock to all his friends. He, [William] Sloan & Snowy Will were just outside the dressing station on the beach, when a shell burst over them. Bennet had the arteries of the neck cut & died in a few minutes.' Sloan 'got a pellet in the spine, which has paralysed his legs'.[55] He would die in an English hospital in October 1916. Will was unharmed. Donald Currie was wounded on 14 June, Abraham Wachner next day. The 24th of June was a bad day: Samuel Tozer was shot in the foot and leg, and Wilfred Singleton, who had already earned the DCM, was shot in the back outside the main dressing station at Anzac Cove; the bullet penetrated his abdomen and he died the next day. The NZMC casualties would continue: Carbery recorded 14 deaths from wounds and disease on Gallipoli, and at least 34 wounded.[56]

Also working as a bearer on the night of 2/3 May was 28-year-old builder Harry Keesing, who had belonged to the St John Ambulance Brigade at home in Onehunga, Auckland. After making the difficult return trip from the dressing station to the beach three times in succession, he 'took a spell by dressing a couple of wounds that were waiting until the doctor had finished with the more serious cases'. He then had to take on his back a wounded man unable to walk. When Keesing and his squad got back from their next trip, about 4.30 a.m., they managed just an hour's sleep before working solidly until 10.30 a.m. One casualty they discovered in a little gully 'was wounded in the back, and had the left femur fractured' — and weighed about 14 stone. They 'got the poor fellow on the stretcher the best way we could, and started off'. Fenwick understood the physical effort this required: 'Considering how young our boys are, it

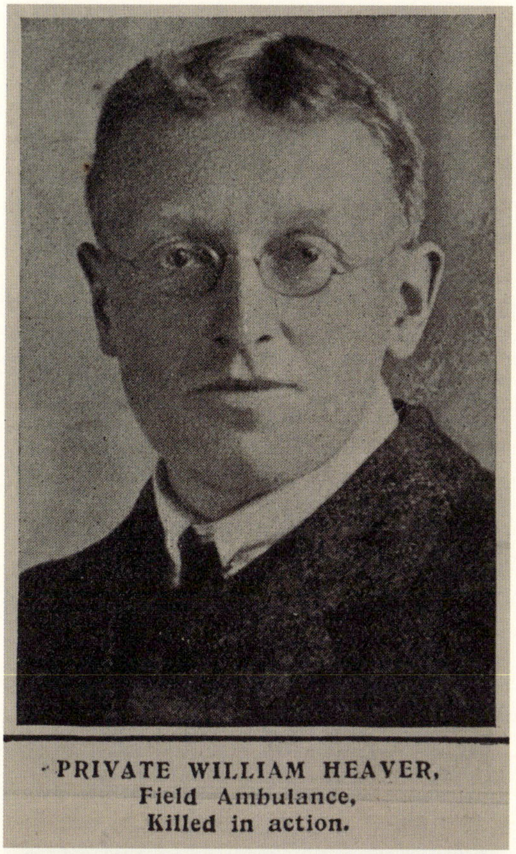

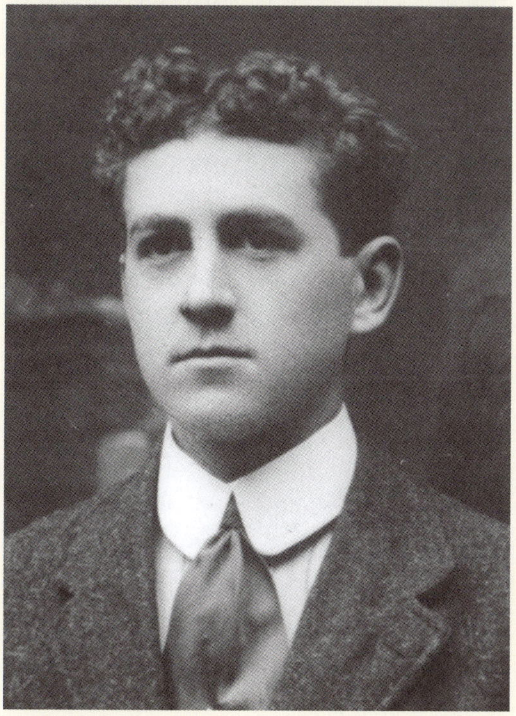

above Before he enlisted, William Heaver, who was killed on 3 May 1915, had been a salesman in Wanganui, where he belonged to the St John Ambulance Brigade. According to a tribute from a fellow member, he could appear 'conspicuously reserved' but his mind was 'highly strung and tense [and] did not readily respond to every fickle breeze'. He had 'indelibly stamped his ardent highheartedness upon the organisation that takes just pride . . . in the unreservedness of his noble sacrifice'.
AUCKLAND WEEKLY NEWS, AUCKLAND WAR MEMORIAL MUSEUM

below Wilfred McMurray photographed in 1914 shortly before he enlisted. Although he was not a stretcher-bearer, he saved badly wounded Frank Shirley from Taranaki, who later wrote: '[I]t is to him I owe my life, for all through that long day while I was lying there and could not get out for the rain of bullets, he kept asking how I was feeling and giving me water. When night came he crawled over to me, and half carried and dragged me over a hill to safety. How it was that he was not hit is a marvel to me.' McMurray was killed in action in the Second Battle of Krithia.
AUCKLAND WAR MEMORIAL MUSEUM CENOTAPH, IMAGE PROVIDED BY NANCY AUBURN

is marvellous. It does prove I was correct when I begged that Amb. Corps should be filled with men of good physique only.'[57]

Keesing found that the only way down was via a gully, in 'pitch dark and drizzling rain'.

> I was at the head, two men at the foot, and the rest wherever they could get. I found my best plan was to sit down and dig the feet of the stretcher into the ground. I had no power to pull back. The poor fellow himself was full of pluck. The chaps at the foot did not have foothold enough to keep the stretcher level, the result being that it was not long before the man was half off. We had no chance of getting him on again, so we got him to hang on to the canvas at the top . . . How he managed it I don't know.

They pressed on, stumbling over boulders, navigating waterfalls, forcing their way through bushes. 'The snipers, who could evidently hear us talking, were sending bullets all round us . . . we would have to be out of it before . . . daylight, or they would be able to pick us off.' They made it, reaching their destination about 5 a.m. Keesing would be mentioned in despatches on 28 January 1916; in 1917 he would receive the Military Medal for acts of gallantry in France.[58]

Non-medical men, too, risked their lives, both in helping their wounded mates when no bearers could reach them and in volunteering to carry stretchers. Frank Shirley owed his life to his friend, 21-year-old Will (Wilfred) McMurray, who stayed with him when he was badly wounded late in April and dragged him to safety after nightfall; he had done the same for another man earlier the same day. McMurray would be killed on 8 May at Helles. Three days after volunteering for stretcher-bearer duty on 4 August, Private Arthur Carbines of the Wellington Infantry Battalion, a professional pianist popular among his fellow soldiers, was fatally shot in the head after attempting to bring some wounded men back to the safety of a trench. He was posthumously mentioned in despatches.[59] When a badly hurt Australian fell on Jack Moller in a trench, he put on a tourniquet, applied a field dressing to 'a wound you could almost put the palm of your hand in', and then 'slung him over my shoulder, fire-brigade fashion, and carried him round to old Doctor Home, our MO'. A member of the Maori Contingent was decorated for carrying nine men under heavy fire in August 1915.[60]

There were some very close shaves. Alexander Lindsay was talking to a field ambulance colleague 'when we heard a shell coming straight for us, we were both thinking the other would stop it when it burst about 30 foot from us and the casing landed right at the man's foot, and missed both of us by about six inches'. The day before, a shell had landed beside the door of the dug-out where Lindsay and his mate were having dinner, and exploded in the ground, 'and a man was just about 10 feet in front. We all escaped, except for a shower of dust over us.'[61]

The MOs were always vulnerable. On 7 May, at Helles, 62-year-old surgeon Walter Pearless, serving with the Canterbury Infantry Battalion, was shot through the left thigh. After several weeks in a military hospital in Alexandria, he would return to Gallipoli. During the slaughter the following morning on the exposed stretch of ground known as the Daisy Patch, George Craig treated wounded men in the open, under fire, helped by his orderly. One of the wounded, crying out for a doctor, drew Turkish fire each time he moved. Craig set off, but the wounded soldier proved too heavy, so he called for assistance; two privates immediately answered. As the trio were almost at the trench, carrying the man, a sniper shot Craig through the thigh. One of the privates was also wounded. They all, somehow, made it to relative safety and treatment.[62]

Others, too, were perilously situated. Cyril Baigent and Wellington doctor James Mitchell set up an RAP in 'a small ruined mud hut without a roof and built on high ground and only about 50 yards behind our front line. We had to remain behind the walls in the day time as the Turks were sniping.' Some 40 wounded men were sheltered here until they could be got away after dark. George Home had an RAP in the Sagli Dere: 'about 170 casualties passed through my hands on Saturday night [8th].' On Sunday and Monday 'I did not lie down, don't think I even sat down for over 48 hours'.[63] As Fenwick wrote later that month, 'The more I see and hear of our regimental medical officers, the more enormously I admire them. Their absolute unconscious heroism is a thing to be astonished at. They have no excitement of firing back at the enemy, no thanks for gallantry or endless work; simply and quietly they do their job.'[64]

On 24 October, as two stretcher-bearers were carrying a patient over a rise, an exploding shell threw all three to the ground. MO William McAra, who was nearby, rushed down the hill, grabbing a first-aid dressing from his surgery as he went. 'With help of two plucky fellows dragged bearer & patient towards some sand bags.' As another shell whistled over, and before the next one arrived, McAra ascertained that the patient was safe, but the leading stretcher-bearer 'very quickly collapsed — that awful grey look crept over face — opened eyes once & groaned — opened again with gentle questioning look all round on the peaceful sea & sunny beach — then the pupils gradually dilated and he was gone'. The other bearer survived. McAra was surprised to be cheered on his way back to the surgery, 'as it didn't seem to me that I had done anything very great'.[65]

NZMC doctors on Gallipoli also had to create RAPs and bivouacs, tasks that required hard work and ingenuity, as one RMO explained on 16 May. 'Yesterday the Corpl. Medical Orderly and myself spent the day in fixing up the R.A.P. I managed . . . to get some timber . . . and got a fairly semi shrapnel proof covering up.' The next day, his RAP was 'well fixed up with shelves and cupboards. A tin let into the clay looks very business like with the sterilizer inside. Instruments are left in Soda Solution ready sterilized. Water is scarce but I have a supply on hand.' He also improved his own shelter: 'I now have a partial sandbagged roof, and can sit up inside.'[66] On 8 September, Alexander Trotter was 'busy all day making a most excellent shelter covering it with a couple of blankets that I picked up on the beach and lining the clay walls with waterproof sheets. I have a large piece of mosquito netting to close the entrance so should be able to sleep undisturbed by the loathsome flies.'[67] MOs also sometimes made use of other buildings and of found materials. During the assault on Chunuk Bair, Baigent set up his RAP just below Table Top in a former Turkish kitchen. 'I found a Turkish Medical companion. It was knapsack shaped, and contained dressings, iodoform [an antiseptic], hypodermic syringe and plenty of Morphia.'[68]

By early June, the main New Zealand dressing station, often referred to as a hospital, run by Charles Begg, was still on the beach in Anzac Cove. There were also advanced dressing stations in Shrapnel Gully and at the foot of Walker's Ridge. The former boasted 'sandbagged walls and, at first, a canvas roof, one bell tent pitched hard by, and a few small dug outs excavated by the personnel'.[69] On the beach, Begg and his men 'soon found that the protection afforded by barricades of equipment was illusory, as shrapnel bullets came freely through the roof, and finally a shell . . . burst inside'. They then 'built up the walls to the height of about seven feet, and by breaking up the shattered boats of the first landing party, we got enough wood to cover in part of the roof; over this we heaped earth to the depth of about nine inches'. After building other shelters in the same way, they 'succeeded in making fairly safe cover [for] 60 stretcher cases'.[70] The doctors' quarters were as primitive as their workplaces.

Fenwick described Begg's 'clearing hospital':

> The back of the marquee is the cliff wall; the front is open to the beach and about 12 feet from the water's edge. Two rough wooden uprights, like a country stile, are placed at the end of the tent; these hold the stretchers. A wooden packing-case makes a desk in the corner, and a rough wooden bench holds basins and instruments. [The bearers] lay the stretcher down and wait till one of the trestles is empty. The stretchers are lifted one by one on to the trestles, the wound examined, and immediate treatment decided.[71]

At first, unless to halt haemorrhaging, there had been no operations here; men requiring surgery were sent out to hospital ships. But when Begg discovered, a fortnight after the landing, how poorly serious abdominal cases were faring in this process, and because bad weather often delayed evacuation, he decided that surgery should be carried out onshore. Until mid-June, Begg and his men operated on almost all those with penetrating abdominal wounds,[72] keeping them for up to four days afterwards. 'The conditions for operating were good,' Begg told the *British Medical Journal*, 'except for shrapnel fire, to which one operating tent was quite exposed. The beach in front was shingly, so there was very little dust.' In about 60 per cent of cases 'the condition was almost hopeless . . . As a rule the gut was perforated or torn in from seven to twenty places.' The survival rate was about 25 per cent. The outcome was better for the many head injuries, even though most 'were inflicted at short range and were very severe. In a large number the whole calvarium [skullcap] and contents were blown right off just as if they had been removed by a saw.'[73]

The Turks' increasingly accurate fire proved too great a threat for the medical staff and their patients on the beach. Gordon Breen was on duty when a shell crashed through the wall and buried itself in the ground, 'scattering dust & small stones over a chap whose hand I was dressing but did not damage the persons'. After an underground operating theatre, rapidly excavated, fitted up and lit with acetylene gas, was destroyed by a high-explosive shell, medics and wounded decamped to the Walker's Ridge ADS. Here, though, 'operations were quite out of the question owing to dust and flies', the latter attracted to the mules quartered in a nearby gully.[74] CCSs, too, were vulnerable. When McAra was a patient himself in November, a shellburst 'came through corner of hospital ward . . . The poor orderlies just lay down and dragged rugs over their heads, although that wouldn't have been slightest protection if shells had come near as they were high explosive.'[75]

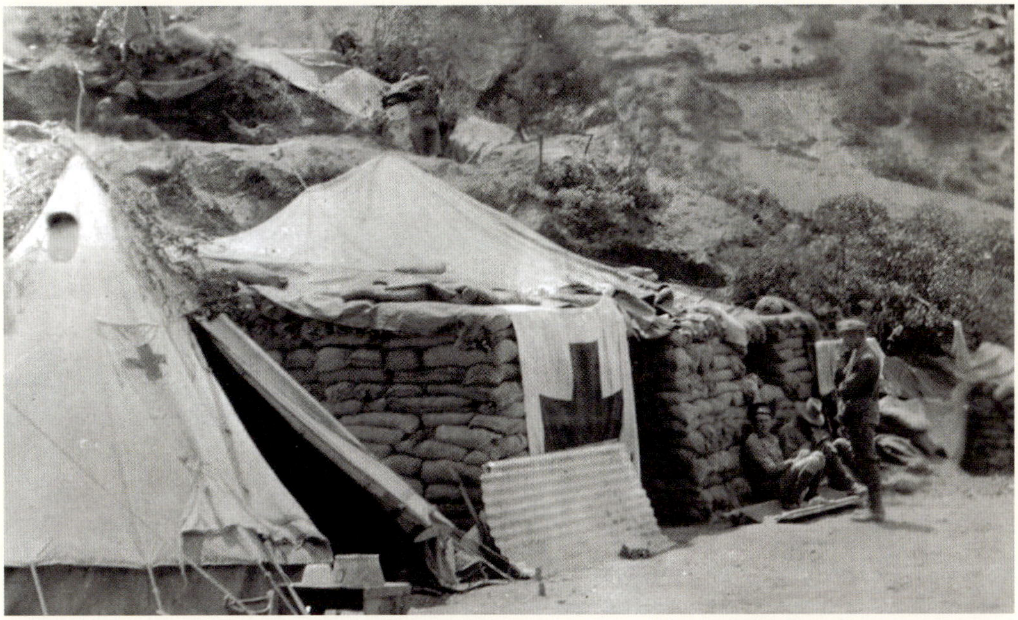

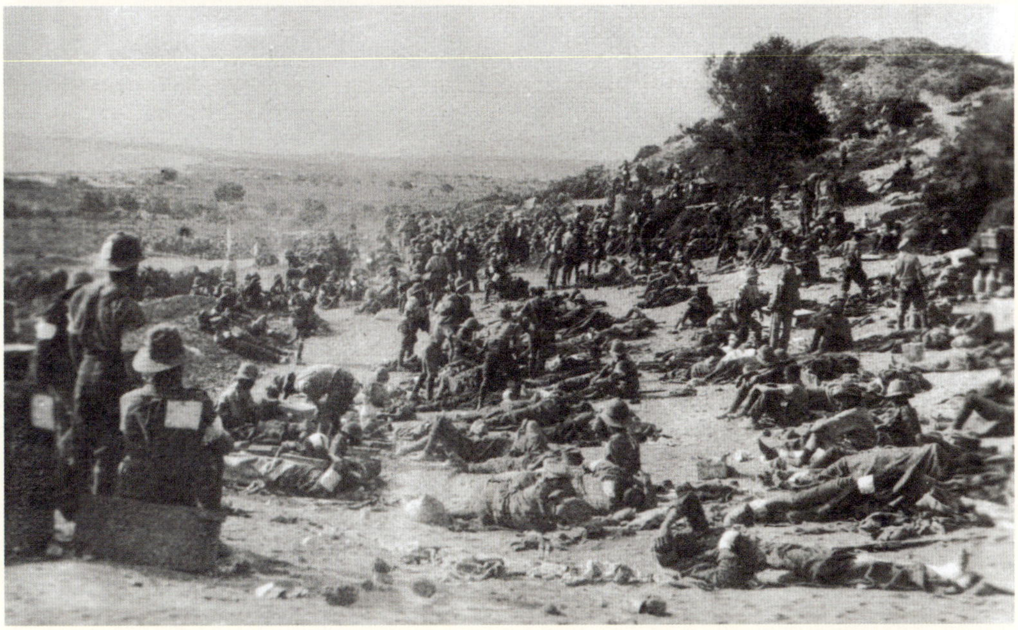

above Sandbags and a large Red Cross offer slim protection at this Gallipoli dressing station. NATIONAL ARMY MUSEUM, 1992.742

below Some of the wounded of Chunuk Bair, photographed on 7 August 1915. For Roy Dalrymple, shot in the thigh, the scene on the beach was 'beyond description'. ALEXANDER TURNBULL LIBRARY, PA1-O-863-03-5

Once the cases Begg and his men had treated left the peninsula, 'it was impossible to get any news as to their progress. They were distributed through the Hospitals of Malta, Egypt, and Britain, and could only be traced by a persevering search of the records.' Such information 'would be of the greatest assistance to the Medical officers, who have the responsibility of early treatment'. And more NZMC men were needed. As Godley told Allen on 23 July, 'No reinforcements seem to have been sent either for the Field Ambulances, which are crying out for them.'[76]

Fenwick, who had initially been proud of his role as Manders' deputy, soon came to loathe it: 'A Staff position is a rotten one if one wants to do good work.' It was his hated task, at 5.30 every morning, to collect the lists of dead and wounded, what he called the 'butcher's bill'.[77] Neither Fenwick nor Manders was, however, content to be purely an administrator. On the afternoon of 16 May a man was hit just above Fenwick's dug-out and another nearby. 'I got the first man down to my cave and dressed him, and then ran down, or rather tobogganed down, to the sunken road. Here I found Col. Manders dressing a bad wound. I finished the job and saw the poor chap off on a stretcher.'[78]

Before the Sari Bair offensive planned for early August, in which the New Zealanders, Australians, Indians and British were supposed to gain control of the steep, inhospitable heights of Chunuk Bair, Hill Q and Hill 971, Manders issued and explained his orders. After the failures of the 25th, everyone wanted a better outcome, and the planning *was* better, but the battle proved a disaster, both militarily and medically. In historian Michael Tyquin's words, 'Some mistakes were repeated, with the same disastrous consequences' — lack of stretchers, for instance, because these ended up on Mudros, and the familiar problem of the least wounded often getting onto boats first. Although less surgery was required and more hospital ships were available, all the ANZAC medical units were understaffed, as were some vessels. There were also the added challenges of sickness and disease.[79] The climate created difficulties too: severely wounded men, wearing little clothing because of the extreme daytime heat, were left lying outside through cold nights. Roy Dalrymple, wounded in the right thigh, was taken to a succession of dressing stations, shivering in his thin shirt and torn pants. 'If ever I have been nearly frozen, it was that night.' When he was finally given two blankets, hot Bovril and morphine, it took him an hour to get warm.[80] Medical supplies were still lacking and two British CCSs sent to help were delayed. The geography proved a significant challenge. Manders had done his best, 'but the narrow ridges destroyed his plans'.[81]

The action began on 6 August, led by the Australians at the Nek at 4.30 p.m.; the New Zealanders started their advance towards Chunuk Bair at 9 that night. Not long afterwards, Te Rangi Hīroa and his stretcher-bearers headed out into the danger-laden darkness to bring in the badly wounded Colonel John Findlay of the Canterbury Mounted Rifles. Once he was safely at a dressing station, the medical men set off again and soon found a group of wounded huddled in a hollow. One was wearing only a shirt and boots, but when Hīroa offered to get him some trousers from a nearby dead body, he replied, 'No thank you, sir. I have dysentery so bad that I got tired of taking my pants down every minute, so I took them off and threw them away.'[82] By the early hours of the 7th there were many wounded. At daylight the troops had to hunker down and the injured were left lying where they had fallen, on Rhododendron Spur.

Overnight the engineers had built two piers, one opposite Chailak Dere (Embarkation Pier) in full view of the Turks, and one opposite Walker's Ridge. A lack of barges caused congestion and delayed and limited evacuation of the wounded, who were exposed to enemy fire. At Hand-Newton's dressing station near the first pier, two wounded men were killed and six were hit again, as were some of his staff.[83] Medical personnel did their utmost at hastily established dressing stations, and too few bearers with too few stretchers worked long hours. When a wounded soldier was discovered on the heights — many never were — he had to endure a 2-mile carry down to the beach. 'The first stage was down a precipitous slope where a man without a load was hard put to keep a footing.' In the second stage, 'through the long and winding Dere', the going was more secure but the route was choked with mules carrying water, food and ammunition to the troops above, as shrapnel and bullets fell continuously.[84] Stretcher-bearers 'had no right of way'.[85]

Although Begg, at the Walker's Ridge dressing station, had 200 wounded men ready to leave, the tide meant that boats could not reach the pier. By nightfall on the 7th, wounded men — lightly clad, without food or water — had been lying out in the open, under a fierce sun, since the previous night; many were in agony, many were dying. As Fred Waite would write, 'In a slight depression behind the line they lay in hundreds. Their tongues and lips swollen for the want of water, with open wounds, tormented by flies . . . With little or no cover, many were again wounded or killed.' The tracks to the beaches were 'lined with wounded, who had collapsed attempting to crawl or drag broken limbs for help; choking on the dust from the hoofs of the pack mules . . . their tongues were stuck to the roofs of their mouths and as the water carriers passed, they beckoned and pointed to their mouths, and there was no water to give them'.[86] The cruel truth, as Ormond Burton knew, was that attempting to move these men 'would have meant certain death. At night [they] might well be missed and so doomed to another day of agony.'[87]

When evacuation at the Walker's Ridge pier resumed at 8 p.m., ships' boats capable of taking sitting but not stretcher cases were the only craft that could get in. Dalrymple knew how fortunate he was to get away to the *Gascon*. 'We were now right by the pier head, and after a long wait a string of boats came in. Luckily most of the sniping had ceased, but there was immediately a rush of walking cases, who were ordered back. Then they picked out the worse cases and about last of all our turn came . . . some poor brutes had been on the shore for days and scores had died, they just buried them in a little patch close by.'[88]

The 8 August attack on Chunuk Bair made matters worse. Former journalist William Hill, who landed on Gallipoli that day, was shocked by what he saw on the beach: 'a big tarpaulin on 4 legs sheltering half a dozen doctors while making examinations of the wounded and in rows outside were the wounded hundreds of them lying in the sun on the bare earth, thickly coated with dirt, sweat and blood to say nothing of the flies which were here in millions'.[89] For Dalrymple, 'the scene . . . was beyond description. No water, very badly wounded (stomach etc.)

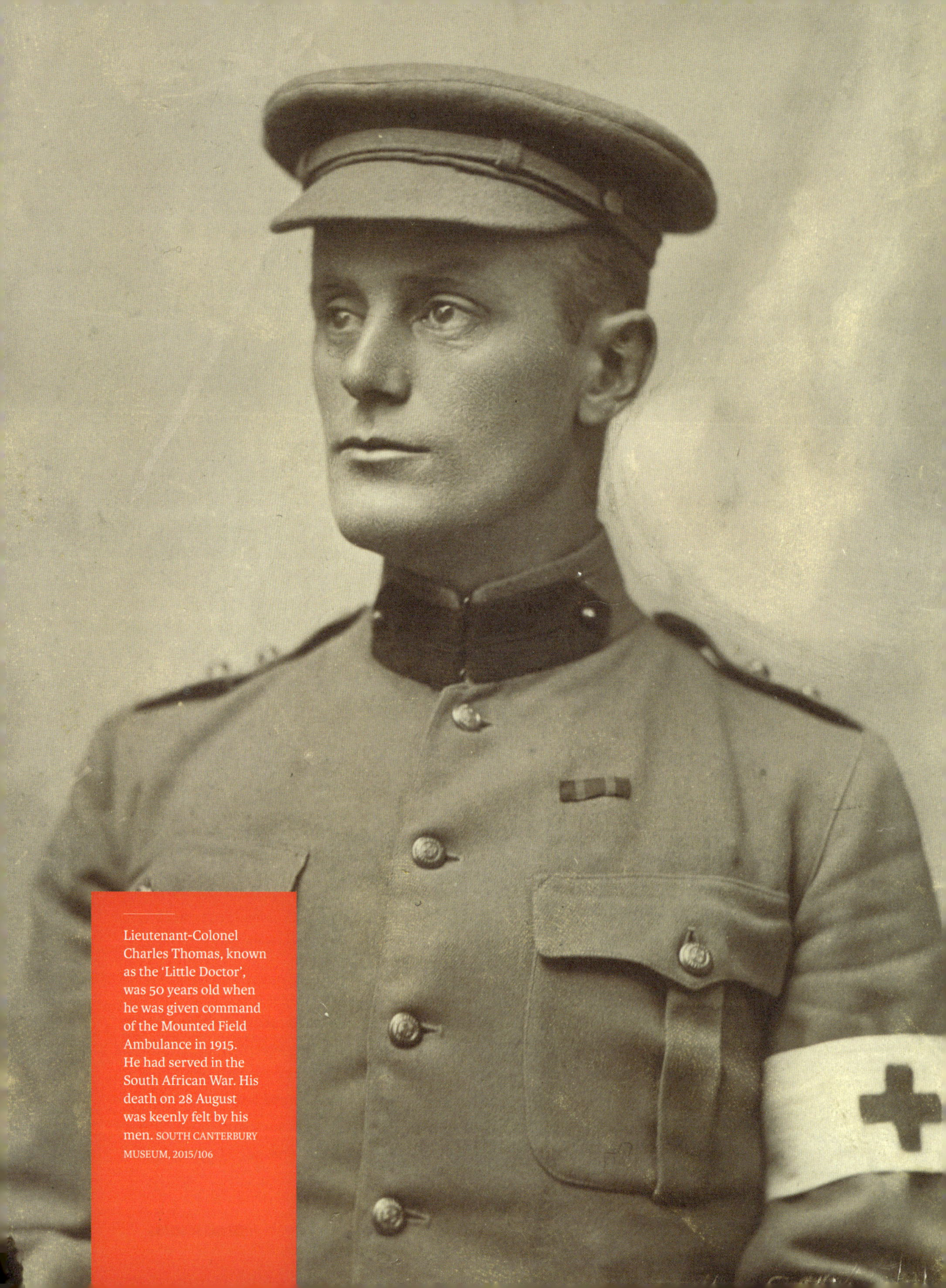

Lieutenant-Colonel Charles Thomas, known as the 'Little Doctor', was 50 years old when he was given command of the Mounted Field Ambulance in 1915. He had served in the South African War. His death on 28 August was keenly felt by his men. SOUTH CANTERBURY MUSEUM, 2015/106

men, Turks sniping the beach and wounding and killing both stretcher bearers and wounded . . . They had to put the wounded down and leave them sometimes, because anyone standing up would be hit.'[90] Not until the night of 12 August was the beach finally almost cleared of wounded, after Begg's desperate request to Godley brought infantrymen to help the hard-pressed medics and more barges arrived.[91]

Once again, the medical men drew admiration. 'Woe betide the man who calls the stretcher bearers Body Snatchers in the presence of any of us in the future,' wrote Hill. 'There is not a man among them who does not deserve the Victoria Cross . . . you cannot honour them enough.'[92] Francis Barber of the field ambulance was awarded the Military Medal for his bravery at Chunuk Bair, bringing in wounded under heavy fire.[93] Medical officers, too, put their lives on the line in this offensive. On 9 August, Hīroa was dressing a wounded Gurkha on a shallow terrace when shells began falling. 'I had to lie flat on the ground beside him to finish the bandaging in the best way I could.'[94] Cyril Baigent was wounded on 10 August: 'About 1 a.m. I was dressing a wounded man, Capt. Craig was close at hand, also busy. He was using a light or an electric torch, and every time he showed a light it drew fire and eventually I was hit.' Neville Manders, who had 'worked so hard to make sure that this battle would not see the tragedy of the wounded at the landing repeated', knew that he had failed. He was killed on 9 August by a spent bullet.[95]

The peninsula remained a dangerous place after Chunuk Bair. Captain Neil Guthrie, the RMO for the Canterbury Mounted Rifles, was wounded for the third time on 21 August. 'I knew I was hit about the back of the neck and retained consciousness, but my legs and arms were not under control . . . I could see my fingers and hands working, and I had a sensation as though I were a glove being vacuumised.' After lying down for a few minutes, he realised 'that the temporary paralysis was due to concussion'. With a field dressing on his wound, Guthrie 'fixed up a fellow with a wounded shoulder' before deciding to create an RAP in the gully where he found himself. He worked until dusk, got the wounded away by 8 p.m. and then went forward with two bearer squads to find, treat and evacuate other men. By this time his neck was stiff 'and I was feeling a little stupid and not fit for much more'. Guthrie finally 'left the completion . . . to others' and made his own way back. It was midnight on the 22nd.[96] He was mentioned in despatches and awarded the MC.

Only a few days later, on 28 August, Lieutenant-Colonel Charles Thomas was killed instantly by a shell while leading two stretcher squads through a sap; four of the men with him were wounded.[97] As William McAra wrote, the men 'stayed right out in open 100 yds behind trenches — shrapnel was bursting all around & everyone seemed to know it was dangerous except Thomas. Finally a shell burst right amongst them . . . Thomas was picked up dead but no bullet or shell had touched him — pure case of shock — must have had his heart affected to go like that.' Mounted Field Ambulance man George Thomson mourned 'Our dear old Colonel — the father of our Company' and next day helped dig his grave 'under a lovely big Olive tree in front of our hospital'. The service was impressive, but 'It nearly broke my heart'.[98]

Reflecting on the 'exasperating problem' of evacuating the wounded from Gallipoli, Andrew Carbery admitted that 'hardship, discomfort, real suffering and loss of life' had been caused by the 'unsatisfactory provisions made for some of the temporary hospital transports'. He felt that adequate deck space, personnel and stores had been allowed for; if the arrangements had been 'carried out in full, much of the hardships and dangers for the wounded would have been eliminated'.[99]

As part of the research for his history, Carbery wrote a résumé of the medical evacuation process. Asked to comment, Graham Butler, the Australian army's 'Medical Collator', pulled no punches. After criticising the rushed and cursory nature of the preparations, he presented a brisk summary of the problems: overcrowding in inadequately prepared, staffed and equipped transports, mixing slightly and severely wounded men so that 'hospital ships were crowded with light cases while serious cases died unattended on transports', too much time before wounds were attended to so that the minimal became fatal, a lack of stretchers and dressings, delays in evacuation, men who might have returned to duty being sent instead to Malta and Egypt, and a lack of coordination that meant boats full of wounded 'took immensely long to find transports to take them'. He was unimpressed by an apparent 'extraordinary absence of adequate administrative control' and astonished at Birrell's lack of involvement.[100]

In reply, Carbery invoked 'military reasons' for such 'inevitable' problems as poor communications. He could not defend the chaos of the first night, but when the situation was desperate 'and failure means further loss of life the position of the wounded can not be too nicely considered. Your Medical situation must be dependent upon the Military.' Finally, he thought it 'impertinent' to apportion responsibility, 'where so many able men failed'. As historians, they should 'show how failures befell and what we think could be done in the future to avoid similar catastrophes'.[101] In his own official history, Butler remained frank. Carbery, also, was often commendably honest in his final published version, but he concluded by firmly toeing the imperial line and criticising those who had drawn attention to the true situation on the peninsula:

> Whatever the extent of the failure of an almost impossible and unprecedented feat of evacuating wounded from a hotly contested and still doubtful landing, the unholy revelations that followed had disadvantageous results on the fortunes of the Expedition. A too ready acceptance by accredited and private investigators of the tales of broken men led to the general publication of crudities and indelicacies better withheld. Only the sordid and nauseous incidents were recalled, not the fact that human energy had been expended to the utmost in an attempt to help the wounded, and that a glowing page of something achieved had been inscribed in the annals of our Empire's amphibious wars.[102]

New Zealand and Australian commentators and participants were not the only ones to criticise the medical evacuation. The medical volume of the magisterial *British Official History of the Great War Based on Official Documents*, after highlighting the failure to properly equip and use transports for the wounded, wrote of the 'utmost confusion' on the beach and the lack of a 'guiding or directing hand'. It mentioned, too, the mishandled classification of casualties: when the *Gascon* sailed for Lemnos about 9 p.m. on the 25th, most of her 584 cases were not serious.[103]

The *Official History* also supported Godley's, Manders' and Fenwick's view that a Lemnos hospital 'would have been feasible . . . and if this had been done in anticipation of the landing on the Peninsula much of the trouble would have been avoided'.[104] Alexander Trotter was of the same opinion. 'What should have been done weeks ago,' he wrote in May, was 'to send all cases on whom severe operations have been done and all cases requiring more than minor surgical interference to Egypt. All convalescent cases and all moderate wounds should now be going to hospitals which should have been made weeks ago on Imbros or Lemnos — with heaps of blankets and mattresses, clean clothes, food, etc.'[105] Not until 26 May did Fenwick record 'four big hospitals' on the island.[106] No. 2 Australian Stationary Hospital moved to Mudros in June. By the end of December, the port boasted two general hospitals, four stationary hospitals and an extensive CCS.

When the Dardanelles Commission set up to investigate the failed campaign delivered its final report in 1919, it considered 'the greater part of the sufferings . . . in the first days after the landing . . . inevitable', though 'some want of organization' had caused delays.[107] As Mark Harrison has suggested, although the commission 'stopped short of condemning Hamilton outright', it clearly held the top man responsible 'for many of the medical and sanitary shortcomings'.[108] New Zealand was aware of what had happened. Lieutenant-Colonel Robert Heaton Rhodes, a South African War veteran and former Cabinet minister, was appointed to visit Gallipoli, Egypt and Malta from October 1915 and report back. Rhodes told Parliament in 1916 that during the April landing and the August offensive 'congestion and consequent delays in getting the sick and wounded away' had been a serious problem.[109]

Although there was less immediate scrutiny on Gallipoli, owing to the absence of civilian volunteers as on the Western Front,[110] facts about the campaign's shortcomings had inconveniently leaked between the jingoistic rhetoric — and the high command knew it. On 5 October 1915, the War Office issued a memorandum to 'Medical Officers and Nurses on Hospital Ships and Ambulance Carriers', who had 'allowed themselves to become too seriously impressed by the stories of young officers and men who have come on board sick or wounded'. Although it was natural that 'these tales should be over-coloured' and that 'contact with so much suffering should incline the listeners to sympathy', such 'enervating influences should be resisted'. More than that, medical staff 'must make it a point of professional honour to maintain a hearty tone of optimism calculated to raise rather than lower the confidence and courage of the fighting men who have been temporarily committed to their charge'. They must, 'under all trials . . . surround their sick and wounded with an atmosphere of enthusiasm and invincible hope.'[111]

CHAPTER 3

SICK AND TIRED

THE LAST MONTHS ON THE PENINSULA

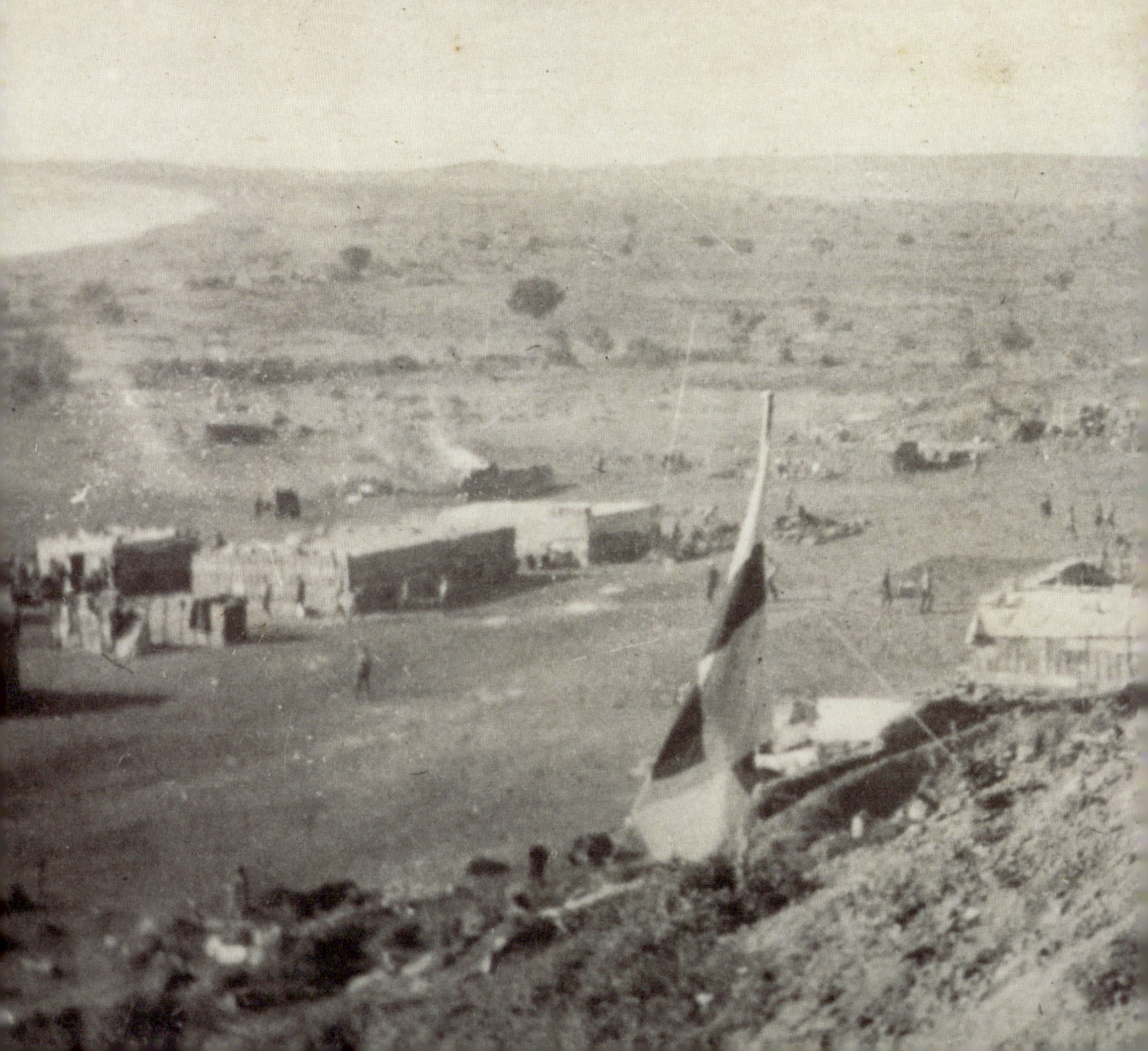

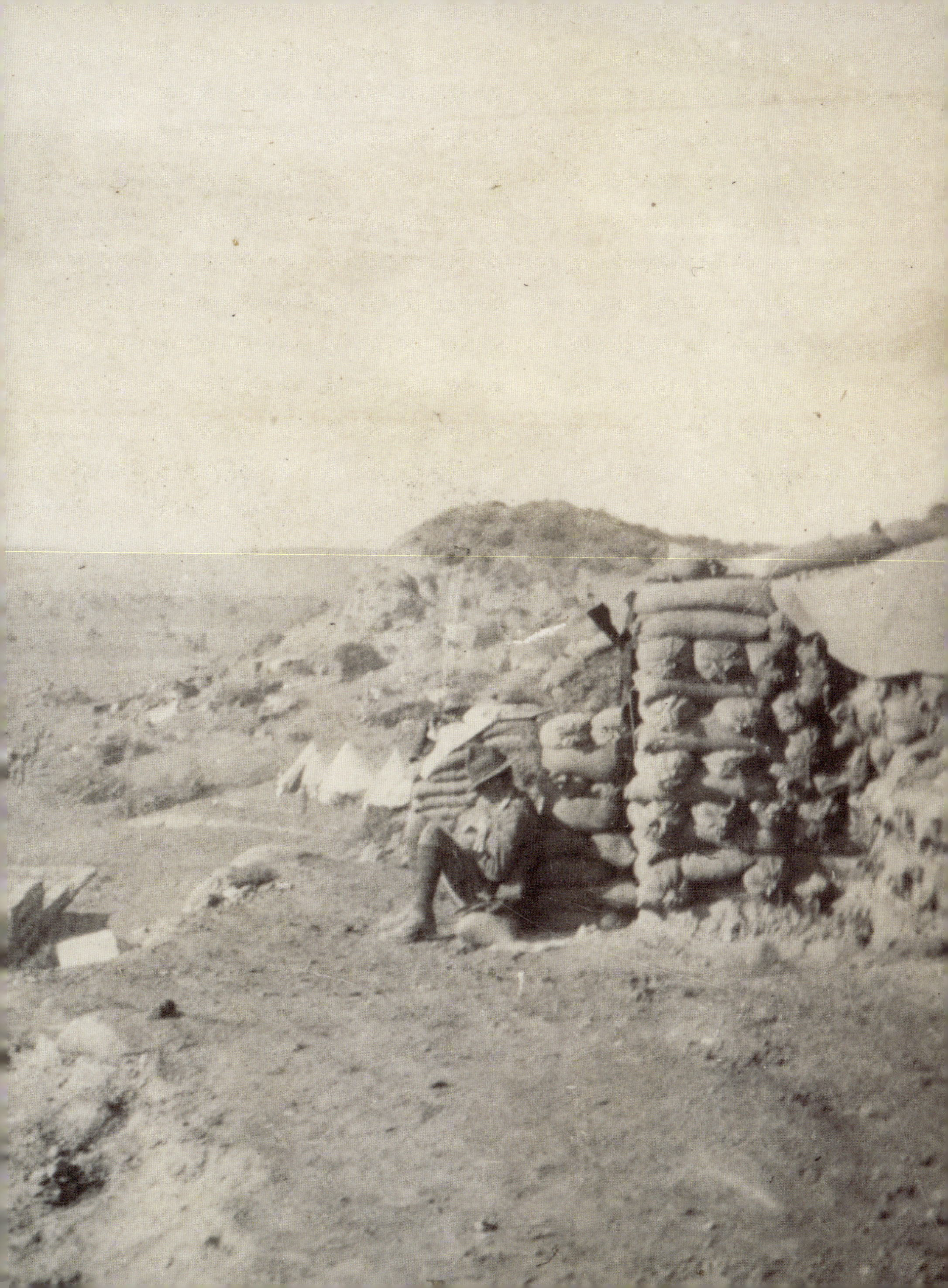

previous pages
The dangerously exposed nature of the Gallipoli environment is all too obvious in this photo of a casualty clearing station (pictured to the right, surrounded by sandbags). Treatment was also increasingly compromised, as drugs and supplies became scarce. TE PAPA, O.040605

And on reaching that war area one came to realize the magnitude and intensity of the epidemic of intestinal infections which prevailed . . . during the summer and autumn of 1915, which was causing men to be poured off on to hospital ships by the hundred, sometimes by the thousand, every week, and which was mainly epidemic dysentery.
— Dr G. S. Buchanan, 'Epidemics of the Eastern Campaign', 7 December 1917

On 3 September 1914, just a month after the declaration of war and six weeks before the Main Body left New Zealand, newspapers reported the advice given soldiers to avoid 'the ravages of disease', which were 'worse than bullets'. 'Never drink any water which has not been boiled,' it stated, and 'Kill flies. Cover food'. Both 'Boils and Carbuncles' and 'Simple abrasions of the skin which fester' resulted from 'Unfitness and want of cleanliness'. It was necessary to clean the teeth daily; 'want of sleep' was apt to cause both frostbite and sunstroke.[1] The impossibility of achieving even one of these well-meant instructions would become horribly obvious on Gallipoli from late May.

As if unforeseen numbers of wounded, and treatment and evacuation challenges, had not been enough, sickness became ubiquitous as the weather grew warmer. Despite some illness, and the trials of adapting to a desert climate, the troops who had left Egypt were generally fit and well, fresh from hard training in the desert.[2] All too soon, however, there was a rapid and serious physical deterioration. By mid-June, three sick men were evacuated for every two wounded; by the end of the month, the 'wastage' from sickness was equivalent to 35 in every 1000 men per week. By this time gastrointestinal disorders, usually in the form of severe diarrhoea, had become 'almost universal'. During the week of 21 to 27 July, 223 sick New Zealanders were taken off the peninsula. Charles Hand-Newton, back on Anzac with the Mounted Field Ambulance on 23 July, put the 'alarming' sickness rate higher than that: he thought about 1000 men a week were leaving.[3] The *Dominion* listed the 54 fatalities since 1 July under the headline, 'Death from Disease, Toll of the Unseen Enemy'.[4] Gallipoli was not a healthy place.

The most widespread problem was dysentery. Caused by flies breeding on unburied corpses and at open latrines, and by contaminated water, this reduced hundreds of previously strong men to skeletons and led to many evacuations and some deaths. As machine-gunner James Rudd recalled, 'I saw men like walking ghosts, all of a sudden excrete and then fall down in their own filth.'[5]

The other prevalent disease on the peninsula was what was generally known as enteric fever or typhoid, which by August was at epidemic level. It was, in fact, usually paratyphoid A or B, which were slightly less serious. Both typhoid and paratyphoid were caused by types of salmonella bacteria found in the blood, faeces and urine of those infected. Transmission occurred through swallowing water or food contaminated by sewage or eating food prepared by someone carrying the bacterium. Lack of water for hand-washing only accelerated the spread of this disease on the peninsula.

The typhoid/paratyphoid confusion, and lack of diagnostic accuracy, were understandable in the absence of testing. As Carbery noted, 'many of the cases were not definitely diagnosed until some time after they had reached remote hospitals in Egypt or Malta'. Apparently a mobile laboratory on Gallipoli had been considered, but not achieved.[6] British bacteriologist Adam Patrick, sent to Malta in September 1915, 'quickly realized the prevalence of dysentery and of fevers of the enteric type' and through further testing discovered a 'really extraordinary' prevalence of paratyphoid A and B. He decided that 'few men who had been on the Gallipoli Peninsula could say with certainty that they had not suffered from paratyphoid'.[7] There was blood testing on Lemnos, too, as Norman Hassell, who had had three different diagnoses of his illness from three different doctors, discovered at a sick parade. 'Take a sample of his blood, orderly!' said the colonel, and next day Hassell was put in an isolation ward: 'This man's bad with enteric!'[8]

There was some controversy regarding the New Zealand typhoid vaccine and its replacement with one that would combat the two paratyphoid strains. A high-powered Medical Advisory Committee, also known as the Sanitary Commission, organised by the War Office, was sent out in May 1915 to advise on the health of the troops in Egypt and on Gallipoli. It decided, using what turned out to be incorrect information, that the New Zealand vaccine came from 'an enfeebled strain or organism' and recommended reinoculation.[9] As Heaton Rhodes explained, however, the vaccine had 'proved efficient in New Zealand during epidemics of typhoid' and more than one make had been used. Also, the term 'enteric' was used in New Zealand Records Office material for both typhoid and paratyphoid.

Once he understood that the vaccine from New Zealand was for typhoid, but not paratyphoid A or B, and that a combined vaccine was required, Rhodes 'lost no time' in obtaining cultures of the two paratyphoid bacilli 'isolated from cases in Egypt' and sending them to New Zealand, where they were used to prepare the correct vaccine.[10] The incidence of 'enterica' decreased after the men were inoculated against paratyphoid from the end of September. In Ormond Burton's view, 'A similar campaign to that of Gallipoli, fought at any other period of history, would have ended in uncontrollable epidemics of typhoid. This was averted for the first time by the new para-typhoid injections . . . [A]lthough thousands were evacuated with abdominal disorders, few died and most of the others recovered fairly rapidly.'[11]

Men sent away sick often hated leaving their friends. When Peter Thompson was ordered to the clearing hospital on the beach on 11 May, he hoped to be back in the trenches very soon. His confidence was misplaced: he ended up on a hospital ship en route to Alexandria. 'No amount of argument,' he wrote on 14 May, 'will persuade the doctor to let me rejoin my unit.' As MO Alexander Trotter noted in August, 'I saw a Sergt. Major the other day with a severe septic throat and a temp. of 104.2 who was annoyed when I sent him off duty to the Fld. Amb. Hosp.!'[12] Some doctors had a different approach. Engineer Charles Wallace described in his diary how a very ill sergeant, the holder of a DCM, had gone to the new MO, only to be told he was malingering. The colonel was forced to command the evacuation of the sick man. 'The doctor has orders to send away as few men as possible, but it puzzles me that a man holding a Captain's rank can so blindly follow the letter of an order, when his experience tells him it is wrong. The order was never intended to keep men like A___ on the Peninsula, dying and useless.'[13]

Diet played a major role in the New Zealanders' poor health. There was enough food but it was monotonous and, as Burton pointed out, 'would not have been well balanced even in a temperate climate'.[14] A 2013 analysis showed the rations to be 'far below modern nutritional requirements for vitamin C intake' and deficient, too, in vitamins A and E. They were too low in selenium, potassium and dietary fibre, but 'excessively high' in saturated fat and sodium.[15] When Frederick Foote and his mates returned to Zeitoun after Gallipoli, they 'had little or no energy . . . I think most of us had vitamin deficiency.'[16]

In the cruel Gallipoli heat the food quickly became inedible. Heading the list of staples, mostly sent from Britain, was bully beef — stringy corned meat, minced and tinned in gelatin; the most common brand was Fray Bentos, imported from Argentina.[17] As John Russell decided, it was passable as an emergency ration, but eaten daily 'it soon became unpalatable & hard to swallow &, in the heat of the day, was in semi-liquid form & quite nauseating'.[18] Also on the roll-call of basic foodstuffs were bacon, jam, cheese ('they didn't know where the cheese came from, but some of them had a pretty fair idea'),[19] tea and a biscuit that was soon legendary for its hardness. On 1 May ambulance man John Thomson noted: 'Our rations are 7 biscuits a day, a very little each of jam, tea, sugar & a very fat chunk of bacon. There's any amount of bully beef but only because it is poor & barely eatable. Have a struggle to get satisfied.' By mid-June, he considered 'monotony and unsuitability of diet', along with the increasing heat and poor water supply, the reasons sickness was 'becoming very prevalent'.'[20]

Almost everyone had something to say about the biscuits. Len Coley thought them 'as hard as the hobs of the place parsons talk about'; Norman Hassell described them as 'great big affairs four inches square and as hard as rock. The only way to eat them was to break pieces off the corners and keep them in the mouth until they were soft enough to chew.'[21] Pulverising them was one favoured approach. With determined optimism, Trooper Len Allen told his sister that the biscuits 'were fairly hard but could be made into a very nice porridge by grinding them down to the consistency of meal'.[22] Sometimes, ground biscuits and bully beef were mixed together to make a kind of rissole that was slightly more agreeable but not good for 'disordered tummies'.[23] Fresh meat, which arrived frozen, was issued, but, as one sanitary officer noted, because it could be cooked only in small mess tins, putrefaction frequently set in before it could be used up.[24] It was often fly-blown, too, by the time it reached the trenches. The hated Deakin's apricot 'jam', which had no nutritional value, was little more than a fly-attracting watery stickiness that could be poured out of a nail hole in the tin. It was popularly known as 'Deakin's Droppings'. Hassell recalled a ration of bread arriving every 10 days from Imbros: a loaf was divided into 10 pieces, each of which was to last one man until the next shipment. When you ran out, it was back to the biscuits. Louis Browne and his Auckland Infantry Battalion mates 'lived on bully beef and biscuits for eight weeks — [we] only had one loaf of bread and three fresh meat stews in that time'.[25] The cheese simply melted into a stinking mess.

Views on the soldiers' diet did vary. On 21 June the Melbourne *Argus* insisted that 'All the troops in Gallipoli speak enthusiastically of the food'; a canned beef and vegetable stew known as Maconochie's was 'very popular with the Australian soldiers'. Just the day before, however, New Zealander George Barclay had noted of Maconochie's that 'a good many complain of being sick after using it'.[26] In July, Colonel Arthur Bauchop considered the rations for his Otago Mounted Rifles to be 'of the most luxurious sort'. He listed, on one day, a ration of '¼ lb figs, 2 oz rice, 2 oz jam . . . ⅛ tin of milk, ¼ lb bacon, ½ lb fresh vegs, 10 oz fresh meat, 6 oz bully (days ration), 1lb bread', and mentioned occasional rum distribution and three issues of lime juice a week.[27] Very shortly after this, however, Trooper Leonard Simpson told his family, 'We very seldom see milk now, but get a tin now and again, just to let us know the taste of it. No fresh meat. Bully bacon . . . from America, bread every other day, biscuits (cabin and army), potatoes, onions, flour now and again, prunes or dates or figs now and then, tea- or lime-juice occasionally.'[28] By September, even Godley was blaming the men's illness and 'general want of spirit' largely on the food. He had the bully beef in his sights, noting, in a 10 September letter to ANZAC headquarters, that it quickly became unpalatable 'and the men prefer to do without meat rather than eat it'.[29]

There was, incontrovertibly, an almost complete absence of fresh fruit and vegetables. The latter appeared only when the men took a rest from the front line, and 'no one had the initiative to send a few light vessels round the Greek islands within easy reach, and buy up the necessary quantities'. In Burton's view, the culprit was 'a War office mentality that could only think in standard terms. If a couple of experienced New Zealand housewives had been made she-generals, and placed in charge, the results could have been very different.' Barclay, too, was mystified: 'Egypt is so close that there should be a supply of green vegetables.'[30] This lack of fresh produce led to malnutrition, gum sores, boils that became septic and 'nasty blood poisoning', which, as Godley noted, 'so many people get here if they get a scratch from the bushes'.[31]

On 12 July, Eric Catchpole 'had a boil on the right arm below the elbow and had to get it lanced, and have had my arm in a sling until yesterday'. Soon after Eric Burnett reached Anzac, he 'tapped' his left leg with the corner of a shovel. 'It only broke the skin but it would not heal up till after I had been in hospital over a month.' A few days later he 'knocked a wee bit

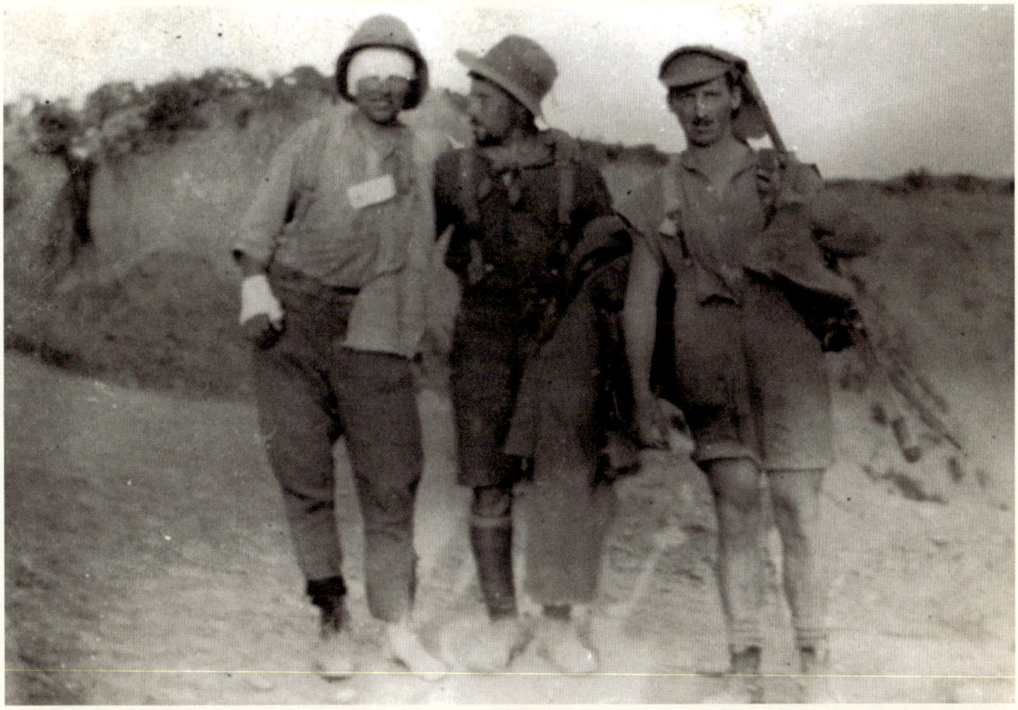

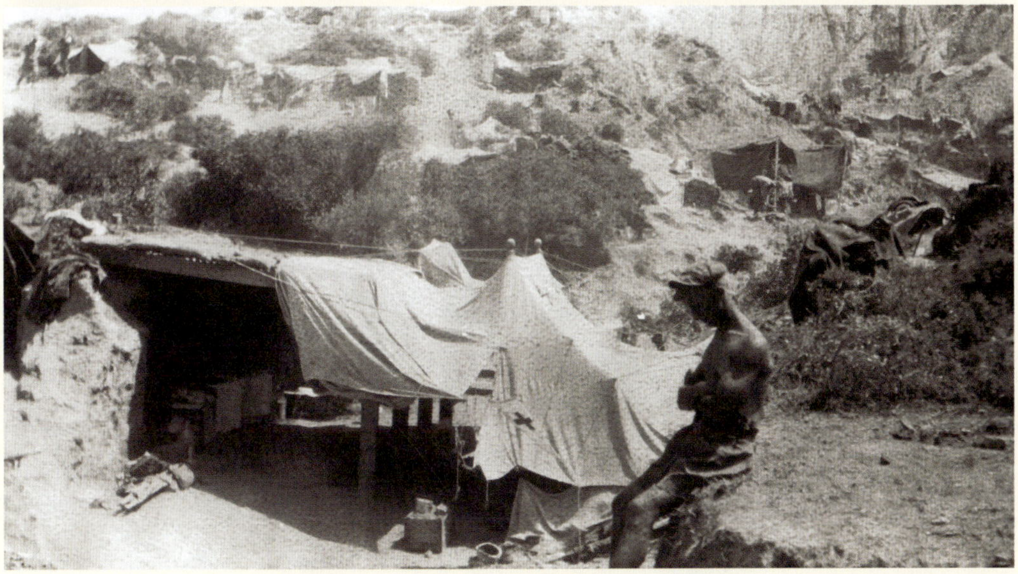

above The wounded man on the left, being led down a Gallipoli hill, has been tagged with a label summarising his condition and any treatment given so far. NATIONAL ARMY MUSEUM, 2001.105

below The soldier waiting outside this Gallipoli ambulance tent wears only a hat and shorts in the fierce heat. ALEXANDER TURNBULL LIBRARY, PA1-O-811-22-3

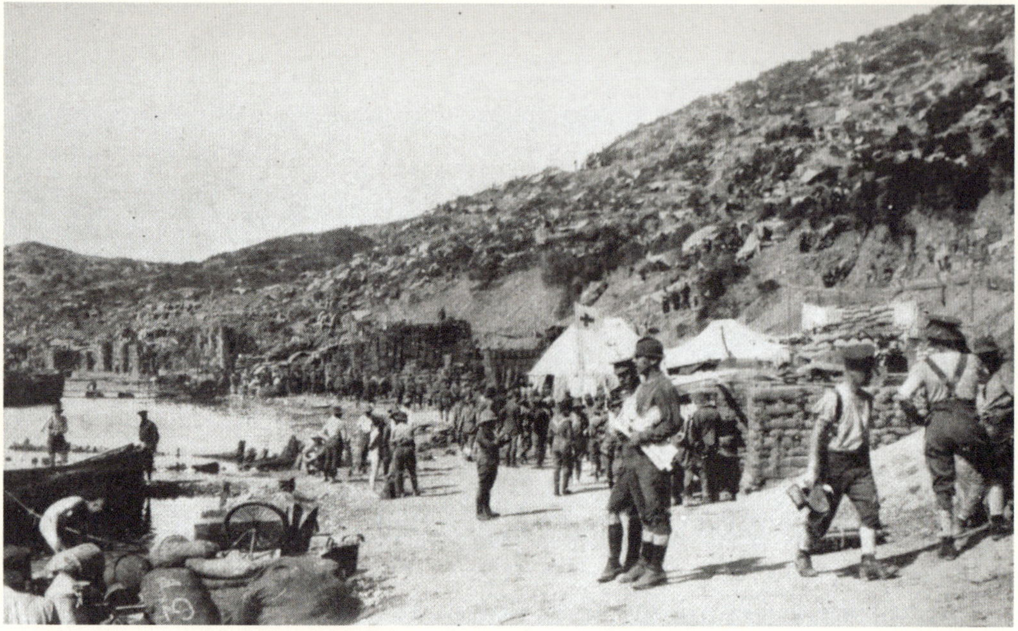

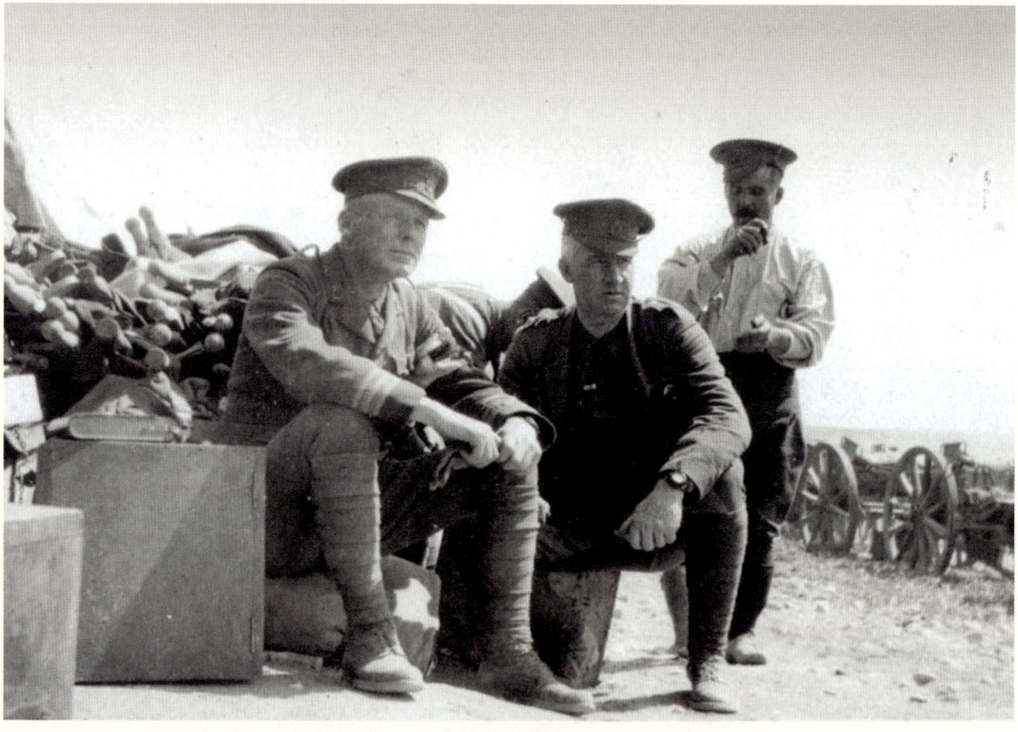

above The Red Cross flag marks the medical tent in this photo, which was originally captioned, 'At the Dardanelles: One of the Beaches'. The cramped conditions on the narrow Gallipoli shoreline are evident. CHRISTCHURCH CITY LIBRARIES, CCL PHOTOCD 3, IMG0047

below Medical staff often had little time to rest. Major Eugene O'Neill (seated left), CO of No. 1 Field Ambulance, and Major Donald Murray (seated right) take a welcome break at the foot of Walker's Ridge on Ocean Beach, Gallipoli, 1915. NATIONAL ARMY MUSEUM, 1992.742

off [his] right shin with a piece of shell'. This wound did not heal until mid-December, and then a 'tiny patch . . . broke out again & got bigger than ever'.[32] Medics were affected, too. On 1 September John Thomson reported 'a great deal of trouble with septic scratches on both hands both knees and right elbow; unable to handle a stretcher so am doing Q.M. [duties] and water fatigue.'[33] As the heat mounted the men refashioned their uniforms, tearing off the lower half of their trousers to convert them to cooler shorts and ripping the sleeves from their shirts. This exposed more of their skin to scratches that could all too quickly become infected.

Men certainly lost both appetite and weight as a result of illness, but poor food could retard their recovery. In mid-October Burnett was on a hospital ship off Lemnos, finally sent away because he had developed jaundice. The MO 'told me I badly need a holiday as I was run down & my blood was thoroughly out of order, and that I didn't stand a hope of getting right if I remained on the peninsula, as I could not get the proper diet'.[34] On 9 November, very ill with dysentery at a CCS, MO William McAra noted, 'Felt very weak, couldn't stand the horrible food they gave me.'[35] Those evacuated from Gallipoli rejoiced in their escape from the rations. When former Taihape clerk Joseph Cody was wounded on 7 August, he was taken to an Alexandria hospital, 'where everything is clean . . . not to mention eggs, butter, roast chicken etc. etc. Quite a change from bully beef, stew, bully beef without the stew, and biscuits hard as the hobs of hell, and microscopic pieces of bacon which represents breakfast, and rice — dinner, while the aforesaid B.B. — tea.'[36]

Over the first weeks the men cooked for themselves, using scarce vegetation from the hillsides to fuel their fires. Instead of resting and conserving energy, they were hunting for water and fuel and the resulting meals were often 'highly indigestible, however appetising'. The makeshift kitchens also attracted flies. 'The large open latrine was a stone's throw away on the crowded hill side, and from kitchen to latrine there was much coming and going all day by the swarming hosts of winged enemies.'[37] The lack of water meant that utensils could not be washed properly, and it was also difficult to store food in hot, dust-filled, fly-ridden dug-outs.[38] Although different food was sometimes bought during leave, and officers had access to better rations, the absence of canteens on the peninsula meant that most of the troops had no opportunity to alter their diet. A primitive canteen was established on Imbros in August, but its supplies were very limited. The Dardanelles commissioners considered that 'had canteens been made available earlier there would have been a reduction in the sickness'.[39]

Both the bully beef and the bacon were salty and thirst-provoking, completely unsuited to a hot environment where usable water was in such short supply that it had to be brought in by lighters. When Fred McKee had a shave and a wash on 29 April, he had 'almost forgotten how to do it . . . But water was scarce, even for drinking . . . by the time you had made two cups of tea and quenched your thirst during the heat of the day, there wasn't enough to clean your teeth with, let alone such luxuries as washing your face and hands.'[40] 'We are on ½ a gallon of water a day again,' wrote William Malone on 5 June.[41] As Douglas Stark (Starkie) remembered, 'The men drank their water issue and let hygiene go where it belongs in wartime. Not that you could call the water drinkable. There were two wells between the trenches and the beach, but both were reputed to be poisoned by the Turks — which left the chlorinated beach water-tanks.

The water was carted up in benzene [petrol] tins, and the men drank shandies of chlorinated lime, benzene, and water.' Desperately thirsty men 'soon learned to suck pebbles in order to promote a flow of saliva'.[42] John Thomson, who found himself 'thinking of the cold streams round Dunedin with maddening persistence', thought it best to 'drink as little as possible during the day and save as much water as possible for a drink after sundown. One is then able to sleep instead of lying awake with a dry tongue.'[43]

After arriving on the peninsula in late May, MO Thomas Ritchie was made sanitary officer for Monash Gully. Although there was 'plenty of water to be obtained by just digging for it', it had to be treated. 'There are hundreds of men buried in the valley, mostly only a foot or so below the surface, & the drainage from them must get into the shallow wells. About half this section is now supplied with water brought from Malta.' Before leaving Egypt, each MO had been given chloride of lime and some hyposulphide of sodium, but Ritchie found that 'only one or two of the medical officers in the valley had any, and all the water was being obtained from shallow wells, with the exception of one deep well'. He also observed that chlorinating water did not prevent diarrhoea.[44]

By July, drugs and other medical necessities were harder to come by, partly because some medical officers were feeding, drugging and treating sick men at battalion headquarters, 'on the off-chance of keeping up effective strength', rather than sending them to the field ambulances — these were overflowing, and Anzac had become 'one big hospital'.[45]

At the end of August a field ambulance quartermaster reminded the ADMS that he had requisitioned arrowroot, cornflour, meat extract and brandy 'every day for the last three weeks'. Because MOs could not 'obtain a supply of simple drugs such as castor oil, salts, bismuth, from the advanced supply depot of medical stores . . . many cases of sickness, especially dysentery' could not be treated on Gallipoli.[46] Stealing of supplies, especially alcohol, did not help. As ASC Captain Frank Parker observed, port wine mysteriously disappeared and cases were deliberately dropped. Percival Fenwick, too, encountered pilfering. 'I regret to say,' he wrote on 9 May, 'that when our two cases of brandy were opened, it was found that the bottles had been emptied and filled with water . . . It hurts to think of the wounded being deprived of this by the greed of a healthy man . . . A dose of brandy may just make all the difference when a man is brought in bloodless and cold all through.'[47]

Sanitation was an enormous challenge. By 27 May, the scrupulous and exacting William Malone was deeply concerned about the possibility of 'some serious epidemics of sickness. The lack of sanitation thro'out this Divn is dreadful. Things are beastly in most places. I can stand a month [of] dead and unburied corpses, but I cannot stand the filthy ways of living beings.' In a diary entry for 5 June he identified the culprits. 'The flies are becoming an awful nuisance. The area is full of them — blow flies — and the small house fly,' but 'general dirtiness' was also to blame.[48] The No. 1 Field Ambulance war diary was of the same opinion: 'it is more rare than the reverse to see men cover their excreta even though a shovel is placed at the latrines for the purpose. Empty meat tins, bits of biscuit, food refuse from meal time, tealeaves, jam tins etc are practically always to be seen thrown about — sometimes in heaps and frequently emitting a most foul smell. Myriads of flies swarm over these plague spots breeding freely.'[49] Bathing in the sea was the only way to get clean but it was a dangerous business, with the Turks firing from above, and men were frequently wounded or killed. John Russell did not take his clothes off for the first six weeks; he had only a couple of swims.[50] During the two months that he and his men were at Quinn's Post, 'Malone became landlord and Quinn's was recognised as Wellington Property'. As well as improving and strengthening the trenches, Malone ensured that his men 'gathered rubbish daily, cooking was centralised, and the strictest standards of sanitation were enforced'.[51]

This situation, however, proved the exception rather than the rule, despite the best efforts of those in charge. As Fenwick wrote on 7 May, 'Given 25,000 men, a very limited area of ground, a poor water supply, and a large number of decaying corpses in close proximity, it is futile to ask for perfect sanitation.'[52] In Burton's words, the flies 'bit like young scorpions and savagely attacked every patch of bare skin . . . Any scrap of food or offal was soon black with them.'[53] As the toll of unburied dead mounted, and the temperature rose, the flies crawled over corpses (which also caused an intolerable stench and attracted vultures), latrines and food, carrying infection with them wherever they went. It was almost impossible for men to swallow their food without ingesting flies. Drinking was testing too. One lunchtime when Herbert Hart 'required the next swig [of his tea] I had first to rescue seventeen flies from the mug, and water is too precious for one to have been able to throw it away'.[54] Moisture was a magnet for the flies: they would cling to the men's eyes, nostrils and ears and the corners of their mouths. Letters, diaries and memoirs abound in accounts of the omnipresent insects. After Chunuk Bair, Leonard Hart found it 'pitiful to see the wounded covered with [flies] from head to foot but too weak even to attempt to chase them off'. One of the most succinct remarks came from Joseph Cody: 'The flies over there are worse than the wildest nightmare about flies you ever heard of.'[55]

By late June, the flies had become appalling. The DMS, William Birrell, made the sensible suggestions that breeding places should be identified and all rubbish quickly removed and burnt, but reduced his credibility by recommending the use of fly-papers. Four thousand of these were 'promptly indented' by a brigade commander, along with 'miles of string so as to festoon the dere'. More practical measures followed. Sanitary officers were appointed (though not always obeyed), 'scrupulous cleanliness was aimed at' in the trenches, refuse that had been disposed of 'promiscuously' was buried or incinerated, wells were controlled and some water holes put out of bounds. Ritchie recalled that the cresol issued to disinfect the water proved 'absolutely useless'.[56] The sanitary officer role was not popular. When Alexander Trotter was briefly appointed, he found it 'a most unpleasant surprise . . . I shall simply have to take it on and get blamed if the flies and dirt and sickness don't disappear.'[57] Thomson thought those responsible for sanitation were doing their best — 'the sanitary conditions are splendid considering the number of troops on such a small area' — but the flies had 'got such a start with so many unburied bodies earlier, that they are quite beyond control'.[58]

Nothing, it seemed, could stop the spread of dysentery, both amoebic and bacillary, and the state of the latrines exacerbated the situation. Early in May, because the hillside above Anzac Cove was 'a rabbit warren of dug-outs' with no space for latrines, Fenwick suggested that 'the only safe way was to use the water's edge, at low tide'. (Ironically, 'most men had constipation for the first few days, as the bowels refused to act under the nerve shock of shelling'. He put the few cases of diarrhoea down to 'impure water near the trenches'.)[59] The small trench latrines that were dug were not popular when the beach was heavily shelled. Latrines became the focus of much attention and discussion, though no type was proof against germs. They were, of course, 'always crowded and many a poor devil could not find a seat. The main latrine at Anzac was a deep trench 6 feet deep and about 20 feet long with trestles at either end which supported the iron pipe we used to perch on. The bottom of the latrine was one seething mass of maggots which rapidly developed into flies by the countless millions.'[60]

Adam Sangster, serving with the Wellington Mounted Rifles, thought 'the hygiene in the trench up on Walker's Ridge was pretty primitive . . . The men with diarrhoea and dysentery had to sit on this rail and you had to be really careful or you'd go over backwards. The flies would come up, crawling over your bare behind!' Many men were 'so weak they fell in and couldn't get out'; others were made so desperate by the pain and indignity of dysentery that they deliberately went to the latrine when Turkish snipers were active. Instead of crouching and running, as most did, 'they'd stand up . . . so the sniper could shoot them'.[61]

There are as many accounts of dysentery as there are of flies and heat and thirst. Auckland schoolteacher Joe Gasparich was among the many 'afflicted with this frightful sickness'. He was initially given 'a "light diet" of preserved milk & cornflour but the trouble grew steadily worse until I felt that my whole alimentary tract was on fire & was periodically being torn from me'.[62] (Flour, cornflour and oatmeal were all common treatments for dysentery, as were milk and arrowroot.) Gasparich was sent to Imbros, where he was 'housed in a great marquee with dozens of others in like state. We slept on the ground.' Despite their condition, the patients were fed ordinary rations, such as stew and tea, 'which we endeavoured to eat hoping to restore our fading strength'. Unsurprisingly, this 'treatment' only made matters worse and compelled sufferers to make agonising hourly visits to open latrines. 'Some men were so weak that they crawled to the latrines & stayed there until they died.'[63]

When Norman Hassell contracted dysentery in September, he tried to cure himself with 'a paste of flour and water, but after a few more days and nights of haunting the latrines I got too bad to even walk about, so I went over to the 1st Australian Field Hospital and asked for treatment'. Put on the floor on an army stretcher with a couple of blankets, he was visited during the night by a doctor, 'who kept sticking a thermometer in my mouth. What I wanted was a cork somewhere else!' After being told he had 'a touch of the "flu"', Hassell left for the clearing station some 500 yards away but lost consciousness and eventually came to on a stretcher on the beach. He ended up in a Canadian hospital at Mudros. 'My stomach, in spite of all the dysentery was swollen to an enormous size and hard as iron. The doctors used to press their thumbs all over it, but couldn't even make a dent in the flesh!'

After 15 days of consuming only a 'pint of hot milk every three or four hours', his stomach returned to normal and he was 'heartily sick of milk'. After another fortnight, and a blood test, he was transferred to a nearby convalescent camp and then to a British hospital before going on to the New Zealand Convalescent Camp at Hornchurch.[64] Henry Clark was also sent to England with severe dysentery: 'the sight of milk almost makes me sick & to think that could I have obtained a little of the beastly stuff on Gallipoli I would willingly have given all my pay & would not have been in my present state'.[65]

Nurse Kate Barnitt from New Plymouth was in charge of the main dysentery ward at No. 15 General Hospital in Alexandria from July 1915. 'The poor fellows from the Peninsular who had the disease twelve and fourteen days and some a longer period still before we received them had a fearful time. They were very emaciated, they had agonizing abdominal pain — distressing tenesmus [cramping rectal pain] — painful and continuous hiccough, frequent vomiting, and the very bad cases hemorrhage; that is more than the ordinary dysentery hemorrhage.' Diet was 'the feature of the treatment', but also used were emetin or anti-dysenteric serum, bowel irrigations, and morphine injections and turpentine poultices for pain.[66] In late September William McAra was trying injections for dysentery and achieved the best results with castor oil and Dover's powder, a drug containing ipecacuanha and opium that was used to relieve pain and induce perspiration. 'Once blood starts to come nothing much good & think they should be given sea-trip at once . . . Been string of stretchers going down to collecting hospital all morning, mostly dysentery.'[67]

The medical personnel were not immune to sickness and exhaustion. On 9 June, Percival Fenwick was 'so thin and so feeble that a few yards walk makes me feel almost collapsed and [I] want to fall down'. By 20 June, he was on his way to Lemnos, 'horribly conscience-stricken' to be leaving but 'as I fall down when I try to run, and get stupid with headache and fever, I suppose I am not much good ashore'.[68] On 27 July field ambulance man John Thomson reported sick with gastric enteritis; by 2 August he seemed 'alright'. 'Diet was arrowroot two meals, rice one with no milk & precious little sugar. It is high time something better was done in this line as the Company is daily dropping in strength from sickness.'[69] On 23 September Kenneth Tapper had suffered from diarrhoea for four days. As his friend and fellow MO McAra recorded, 'Says he can't lie as he has to go his round but feels alright when lying.' When Tapper finally left Gallipoli on 19 October, 'he looked very white & weak — almost on the verge of collapse'. McAra himself contracted dysentery a few weeks later. 'Bad abdominal pain all forenoon, which became so severe that hadn't time to dodge for latrine with disastrous results.' When he reached a CCS, the 'headache seemed worse & they gave me bromides without avail while dysentery went on increasing'.[70]

The stretcher-bearers suffered too. During the assault on Chunuk Bair, Ormond Burton and fellow No. 1 Field Ambulance man Laurie Bell 'dug in under the lee of a projecting shoulder of the Dere. It would be more accurate to say that we 'scratched' in, for neither of us, badly weakened by dysentery, could really swing a pick . . . It was a miserable life. Every few minutes we seemed to have to stagger off to the latrines.' They had to keep working, however, answering the calls for a stretcher party, and making 'a painful journey' down to the CCS.[71] By the end of August, so many NZMC men had been evacuated sick that the two New Zealand field ambulances could muster only seven officers and 74 men.[72]

The sickness on Gallipoli was bad, but it could have been worse. As Egypt had been, and the Western Front would be, the peninsula was home to lice, and their bite could transmit typhus. 'They were,' wrote Burton, 'beasts of prey and of a voracious and ferocious nature . . . They moved slowly, deliberately, surely. They could not jump or fly but they could crawl and they moved with a certain cold, passionless persistence in quest of blood.'[73] Keating's powder, which claimed to 'kill with Ease, Bugs & Beetles, Moths & Fleas', made no impression on them, and nor did attempts to drown them. Only squashing between thumb and index finger killed them, but, as John Russell put it, they 'multiplied at an alarming rate, & those that hatched during the hours of darkness were . . . proud grandparents by the following evening'.[74] Uniforms were not reduced solely because of the heat: less clothing meant fewer seams, favoured gathering places for lice.

Another potential health hazard that did not eventuate was cholera. When Fenwick heard in early May that 2000 Turks were suffering from dysentery, he feared that it might be more serious. 'If this should be cholera it will be a bad thing for us, as we must get water if we advance, and our men are horribly disobedient about drinking water without medical examination.' On 8 June, cholera remained his 'great dread'. He had spoken about it 'again and again . . . and Col. Manders has to my knowledge applied several times for more water disinfectants without result'.[75] By early July, however, Godley was telling Allen that 'we are just beginning voluntary inoculation for cholera. They do not know enough about it to make it compulsory, but we hear that the Turks have all been done, and the results are evidently good.' In August, future DSO and MC recipient Frank Turnbull wrote to his mother from an Egyptian hospital, 'I don't think I told you that . . . we were inoculated . . . two or three weeks ago against cholera, so we are well protected from disease.' Doctors protected themselves: on 3 July Thomas Ritchie gave himself the second inoculation against cholera. John Thomson reported 'a little digestive trouble', for himself and others, after the injections.[76]

As early as 25 July Trotter was frustrated by the desperate situation at Anzac.

> Nearly every man there is sick now worse than at Helles where there is a little room to move about . . . It is to be sincerely hoped that something will be done . . . before sickness still further saps the strength and fighting powers of our men. It is a painful sight every evening to see the sick coming in — drawn and haggard faces, dull eyes and gaunt bodies eloquent of utter fatigue. It has been like this for weeks and weeks and weeks: nothing is being done and the time when rough weather begins is drawing closer . . . What are they waiting for?[77]

By the end of August Hand-Newton, who had headed the MFA since Thomas's death, was 'passing a very large number of sick and wounded through our station, and evacuating them as soon as possible as our accommodation, of course, is very limited and the staff so depleted'. Even those not suffering from dysentery were 'emaciated, haggard and absolutely dispirited'.[78] During the month the New Zealand Field Ambulance had admitted 1693 sick and 1435

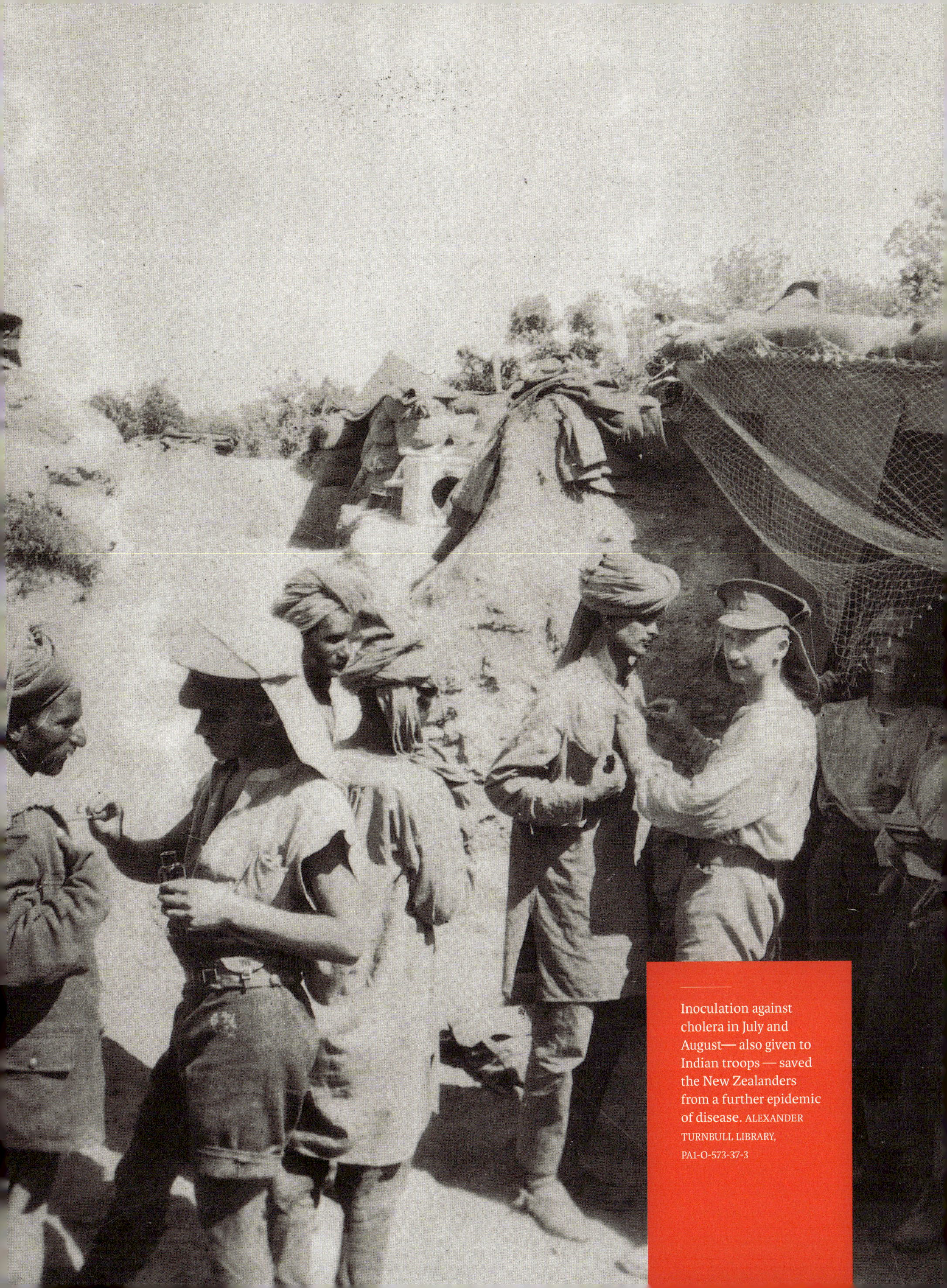

Inoculation against cholera in July and August— also given to Indian troops — saved the New Zealanders from a further epidemic of disease. ALEXANDER TURNBULL LIBRARY, PA1-O-573-37-3

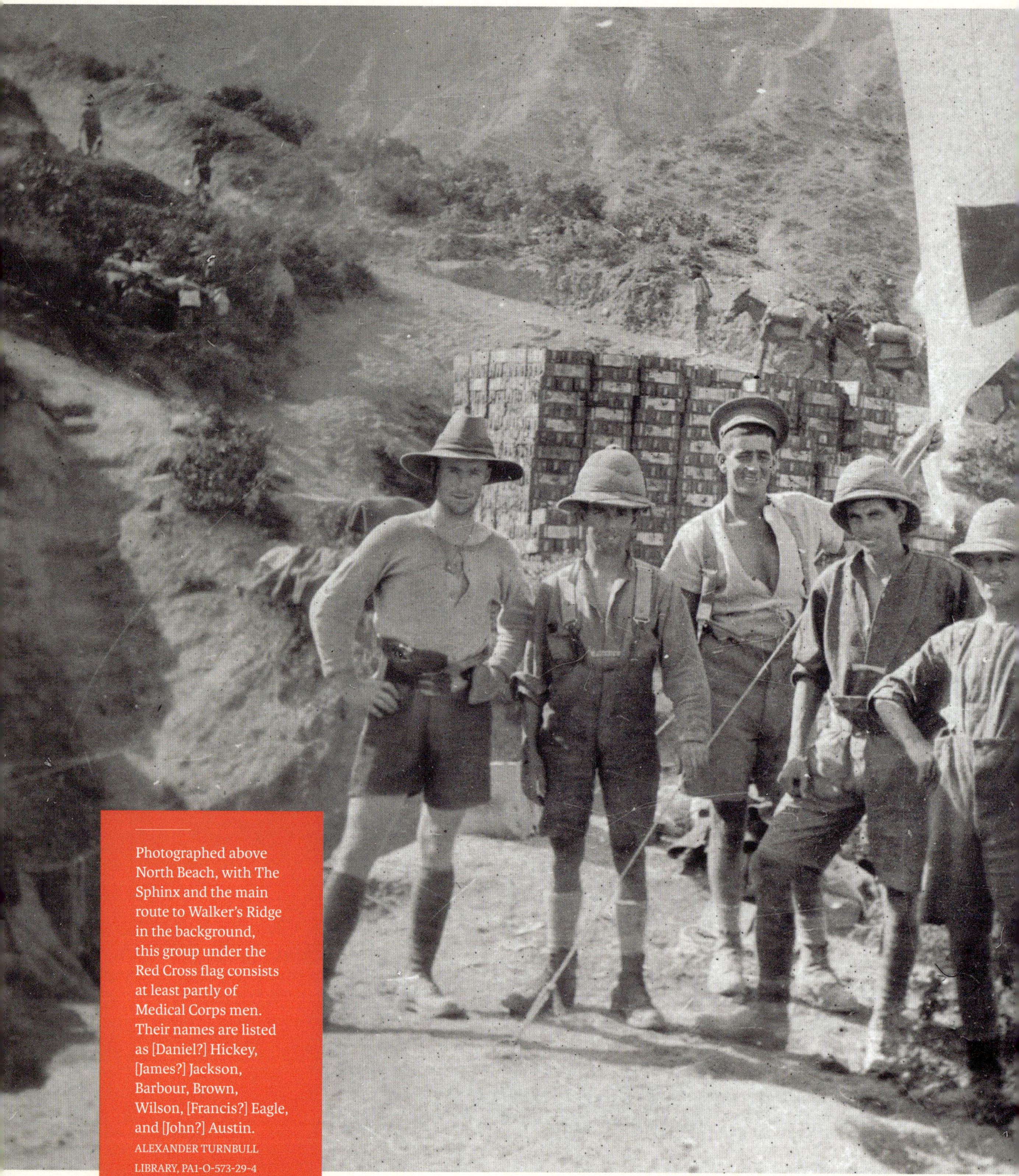

Photographed above North Beach, with The Sphinx and the main route to Walker's Ridge in the background, this group under the Red Cross flag consists at least partly of Medical Corps men. Their names are listed as [Daniel?] Hickey, [James?] Jackson, Barbour, Brown, Wilson, [Francis?] Eagle, and [John?] Austin. ALEXANDER TURNBULL LIBRARY, PA1-O-573-29-4

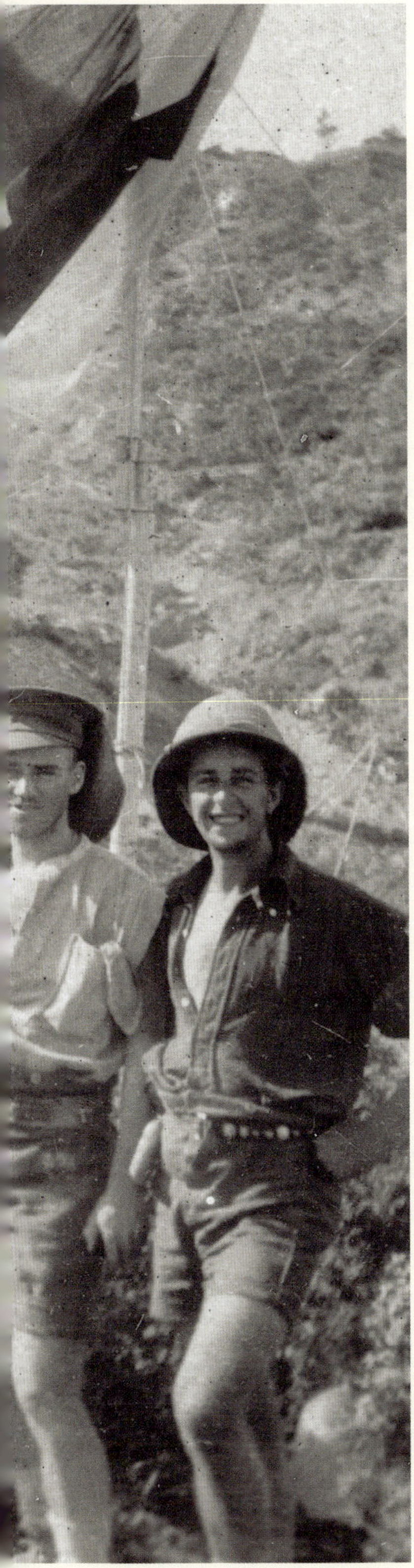

wounded. By the 31st, the Anzac sickness 'wastage' stood at 100 per 1000, or 2578 men, per week. In the first few days of September, 2292 of the 25,175 Anzac troops on Gallipoli were evacuated sick. Disease continued to take its toll in an insanitary environment; exhausted and weakened men were much more prone to infection than fit ones. In an attempt to improve the situation, 'rest stations', sometimes rather grandly referred to as hospitals, were set up in the field ambulances. These amounted to little more than 'a few bell tents' to which the sick brought their own blankets, greatcoats and groundsheets; sometimes a stretcher was available, but most lay on the bare earth.[79] When Herbert Hart returned to Gallipoli on 6 September after a stay in hospital in England, he found his battalion at 'one fourth its correct strength . . . nearly all the men have been wounded, recovered, and returned to duty, like myself. I found everyone very bronzed, thin and most them have a listless, weary, strained look in their eyes. 50% of the men are suffering from diarrhoea and are being sent away in bunches of 7 to 10 everyday, mainly from this cause.'[80]

On 15 September, 900 New Zealand troops were sent from Gallipoli to Sarpi camp on Lemnos for a rest. Charles Hand-Newton and the MFA had arrived a few weeks earlier to run a hospital and inoculate as many men as possible against typhoid. Although the weary soldiers were glad of a respite from the constant noise and sleeplessness, the windswept island was neither welcoming nor well organised. Sarpi 'camp' consisted of a few marquees, and the island's many hospitals and convalescent camps were poorly run and resourced. Clothing and beds, for both the sick and the 'well', were in short supply. Although initially the food was little better than the Gallipoli fodder, once they were paid — for the first time since the landing — the men had access to such treats as grapes and chocolate, and even fresh meat, eggs and condensed milk. But this unaccustomed luxury, and the sudden release from months of tension, combined to make many already severely debilitated men sick. There was, however, a gradual improvement in health, thanks to better food, rest and training. By early November, strengthened by fresh reinforcements from home, the New Zealanders were back on the peninsula.

The strain of the campaign had told on the medical staff as well as on their patients. As early as 27 May, Percival Fenwick had confided to his diary 'a desperate desire to get away for a few days' rest and sleep. The sight of so many men being hit is very saddening and I don't get used to it . . . I believe we are all suffering from nerve strain. It is want of sleep that hits myself hardest.'[81] As Christopher Pugsley has

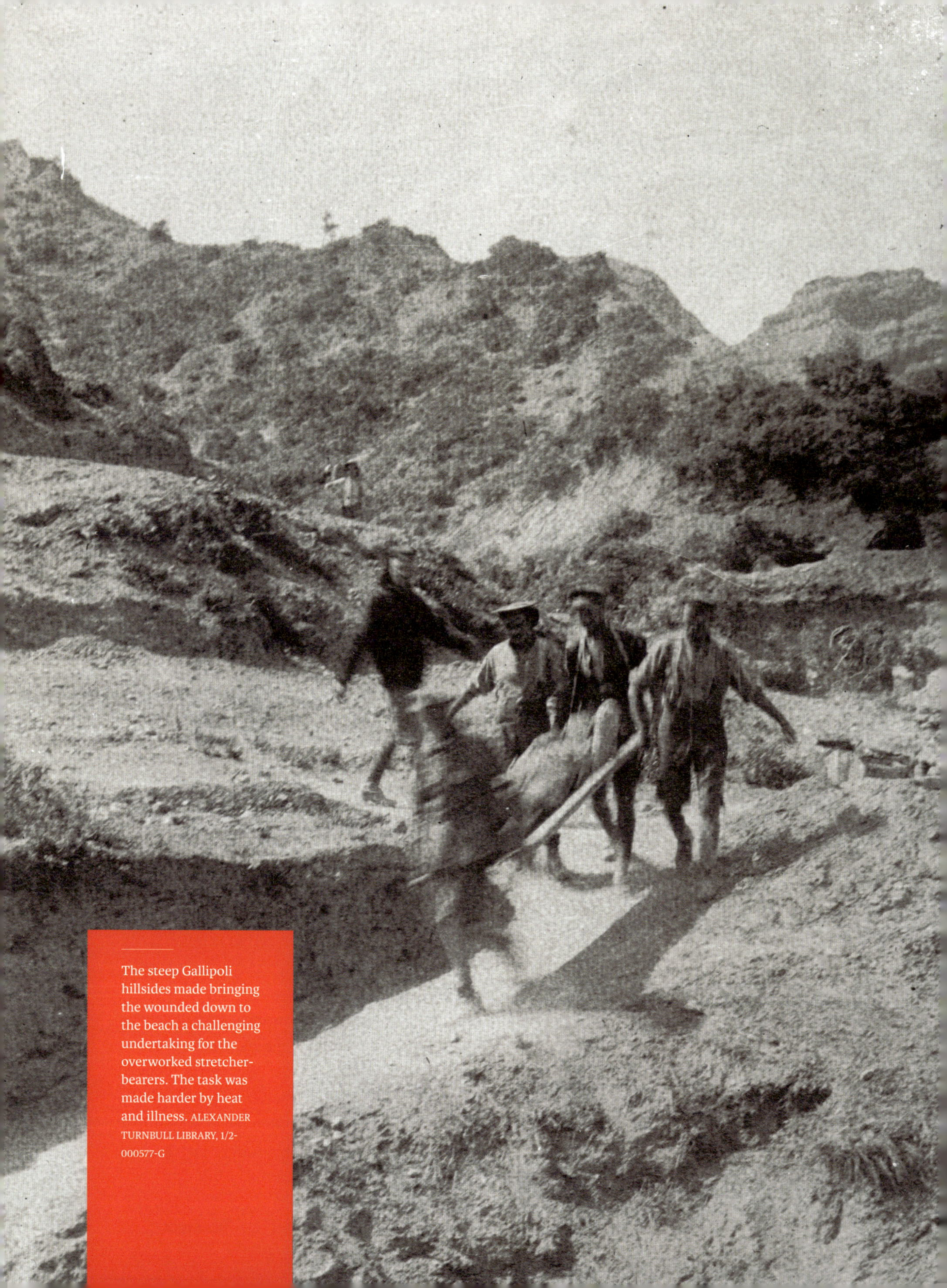

The steep Gallipoli hillsides made bringing the wounded down to the beach a challenging undertaking for the overworked stretcher-bearers. The task was made harder by heat and illness. ALEXANDER TURNBULL LIBRARY, 1/2-000577-G pointed out, 'There was no rest for anyone at Anzac . . . The flies and heat made sleep during the day impossible and the men were always on call to reinforce the line.'[82] Stretcher-bearers were constantly woken for duty. On 12 September, John Thomson at No. 1 Field Ambulance reported: 'Out of the 72 bearers, and some reinforcements of the two sections, all we can raise for duty are 12 . . . Godley is probably largely concerned in keeping us here as he has been blowing up M.O.s for evacuating so many sick men. None of the patients here are fit for further service, nor are any but two or three of our own company.'[83]

Man and mule power, when possible, were the only ways to get supplies and equipment to the front line. Sergeant Charles Warwood of the NZMC, who would die of enteric on 2 October 1915, wrote his last letter home to his mother in Christchurch on 5 August: 'My word, this is some country for alpine climbers. If a fellow is really fond of a stiff climb (under a scorching sun), I can give him all he wants in an afternoon here; it would last him for years. It would add greatly to his enjoyment if he carried a three-gallon can of water in each hand, or a large bundle of stores or ammunition.'[84]

Other factors affected the men's health. One was the amount of gear they were forced to carry. Estimates of weight varied. Writing from Zeitoun on 9 April 1915, Cecil Malthus noted that the 'total weight carried is up to seventy pounds now'. Just before the 25 April landing, Malone reported that the men would be carrying 'close on 75lbs'. Jack Moller thought 'all the equipment, blankets and overcoats [weighed] about 90 pounds'.[85] Some of the medical staff were even more burdened, forced to also carry first-aid kits and stretchers. Unfamiliar and uncomfortable, too, for some was constant shooting with a heavy Lee Enfield. 'My shoulder is aching from firing my rifle at them [the Turks],' Gordon Harper told his mother in July, 'but we are keeping them quiet.' There was little awareness then of the dangers of constant exposure to the sun, although the doctors warned against sunstroke. 'My head gave me fits all day,' wrote engineer Charles Wallace on 18 June, 'and, in the afternoon, I had to stop in my dugout — I could hardly see for the throbbing. Although I had only 6 hours sleep in the last 48 hours, I couldn't even sleep. The Doctor gave me several "Aspirin's" and told me I had caught the sun.'[86]

As the weather finally grew cooler, the flies retreated, but the sickness was not over: an outbreak of jaundice began in October and grew more severe in mid-November. On the 12th, when the *Maheno* was at Anzac for the last time, she was carrying 'nearly all medical cases — 63 jaundice almost all following dysentery'.[87] Then, at the end of that already wintry month, came a fierce blizzard. There had been heavy rain for several days, but the 28th brought snow and viciously low temperatures. Charles Hand-Newton, who had returned to Anzac with his men on 10 November and fitted up a hospital in a 'regular cave' that had been excavated on an 'excellent protected site', wrote that 'the wind was very cold and cut like a knife'.[88] Trenches were soon waterlogged and the slush and snow, which later froze, made any movement treacherous. The roaring gale put paid to vessel–shore communication, and there was no hospital ship in the bay, so sick and wounded, including frostbite victims, could not be evacuated until the 30th.

Determined efforts by the medical officers, 'and a providential issue of gum boots', largely helped to prevent, for the Kiwis and Australians, the severe frostbite and 'several cases of gangrene of the feet' that afflicted the Indian troops on the peninsula. Exposure, and drowning in water-filled trenches, killed many Turks and British.[89] NZMC orderly Walter Carruthers was 'living right down on the beach' when a severe thunderstorm meant 'all my dressings and bandages, etc., got soaking wet'.[90] The storm also hampered the arrival of food and water. Shortage of the latter made useless the only Thresh steriliser at Anzac, which was steam-powered. Without a regular supply of fresh bread, the men were forced to resort to half-rations of the hated biscuits, which were a scourge for the many stricken with gingivitis and other dental problems. Weight loss became common and the number of sick being evacuated rose at the beginning of December.

All this, however, was about to change. The men struggling in the freezing temperatures, and bracing themselves for a hard winter, were not privy to the decision-making under way at the highest levels. The British command was already considering evacuation and after a visit to the peninsula in mid-November, army head Lord Kitchener told ANZAC commander General William Birdwood to prepare, clandestinely, a departure plan. Rumours of evacuation began to circulate, especially as men, guns and equipment left and routines changed. On 11 December the MFA was ordered to evacuate from its hospital all cases except those who would be fit to rejoin their regiment within 24 hours; next day they were 'told secretly to be ready to embark at any moment'. By the 13th, Hand-Newton could note in his diary that the evacuation was 'proceeding steadily',[91] though Godley did not make the final announcement until 15 December.

As well as the sick and wounded, there were some 20 medical units, New Zealand and Australian, to be got off the peninsula, including the New Zealand Dental Hospital. On 12 December, the tent subdivisions of the New Zealand and Australian field ambulances were closed, and the 16th CCS, the Australian Stationary Hospital and three field ambulances embarked. The almost 1000 sick men on the peninsula were taken out to a waiting hospital ship. On that and each following night, some 2000 men left, 'with a proportion of medical units'.[92] By the 18th there were still field ambulance men on the peninsula with the remaining troops, plus two Australian CCSs at Walker's Ridge, to care for the serious casualties expected if the small rearguard there was discovered and attacked by the Turks. As Hand-Newton recorded in his diary that day, 'The whole position now seems absolutely deserted, and hardly a man or mule passes our dressing station.'[93]

The CCSs had accommodation for 2000 cases and sufficient medical supplies, comforts, food and water for 14 days. If these medics had to stay behind to care for wounded, they would be working under the protection of the Geneva Convention. At Anzac itself were 30 field ambulance stretcher-bearers who, with RMOs, would look after any wounded who could not be taken off the peninsula on the final night. The field ambulance tents and the dressing stations, containing blankets, lights, dressings, drugs, food and water, were left standing, their Red Cross flags fluttering as usual.

But the Turks never caught on. With no unusual transport or hospital ship activity in the bay, they had no reason to be suspicious. The rearguard was not in danger, and on the night of the 18th the last New Zealand and Australian ambulance men left safely at 7.20 p.m. As Hand-Newton wrote, 'we silently left our camp, leaving our fires burning'. The wharf from which they departed was 'covered with sacking to dull the footsteps'.[94] Transported by the armoured landing craft or 'beetles' that would remove the last troops the next night, the ambulance men soon safely boarded HMS *Mars*, where 'the officers, especially the surgeon, gave them a hearty welcome, a very good supper, and found them a place to bunk in'.[95] As Herbert Hart recorded in his diary, the abandoned medical facilities served one good last purpose. About 1 a.m. on the morning of the 20th, he and his companions 'drifted over' to one mess 'and made a fine supper . . . incidentally picking up some pyjamas each, a few cigars, cutlery and other useful articles'.[96]

Of the approximately 18,000 New Zealanders who had struggled through this cruel campaign, some 2779 were dead out of a total of about 8000 casualties.[97] The men of the NZMC had worked hard and bravely to help and save as many as they could, but so much was against them — poor medical evacuation arrangements, a hostile environment, shortage of personnel and supplies. At the end, some things seemed sadly the same. NZMC orderly Walter Carruthers left Gallipoli on 14 December and found himself on a German ship, the *Achaia*, at Lemnos. 'I had a bit of trouble getting my medical stuff on board and find that I am the only Medical Orderly . . . and that there is no Doctor, which should not be so as we have about 500 men on board. This ship is the limit . . . We are sleeping everywhere and getting practically nothing to eat.'[98]

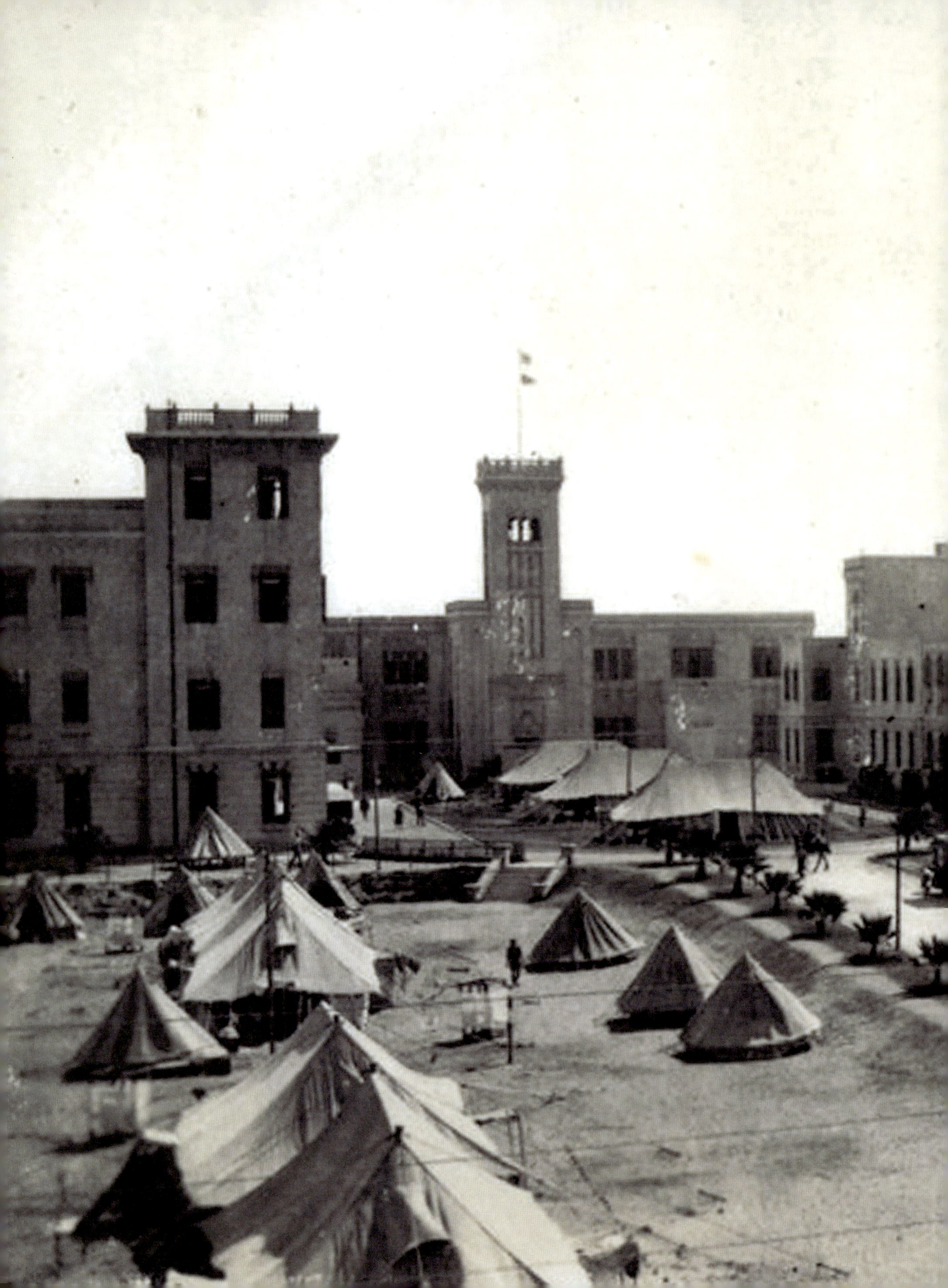

CHAPTER 4

FROM DESERT TO DISASTER

HOSPITALS IN EGYPT AND THE SINKING OF THE *MARQUETTE*

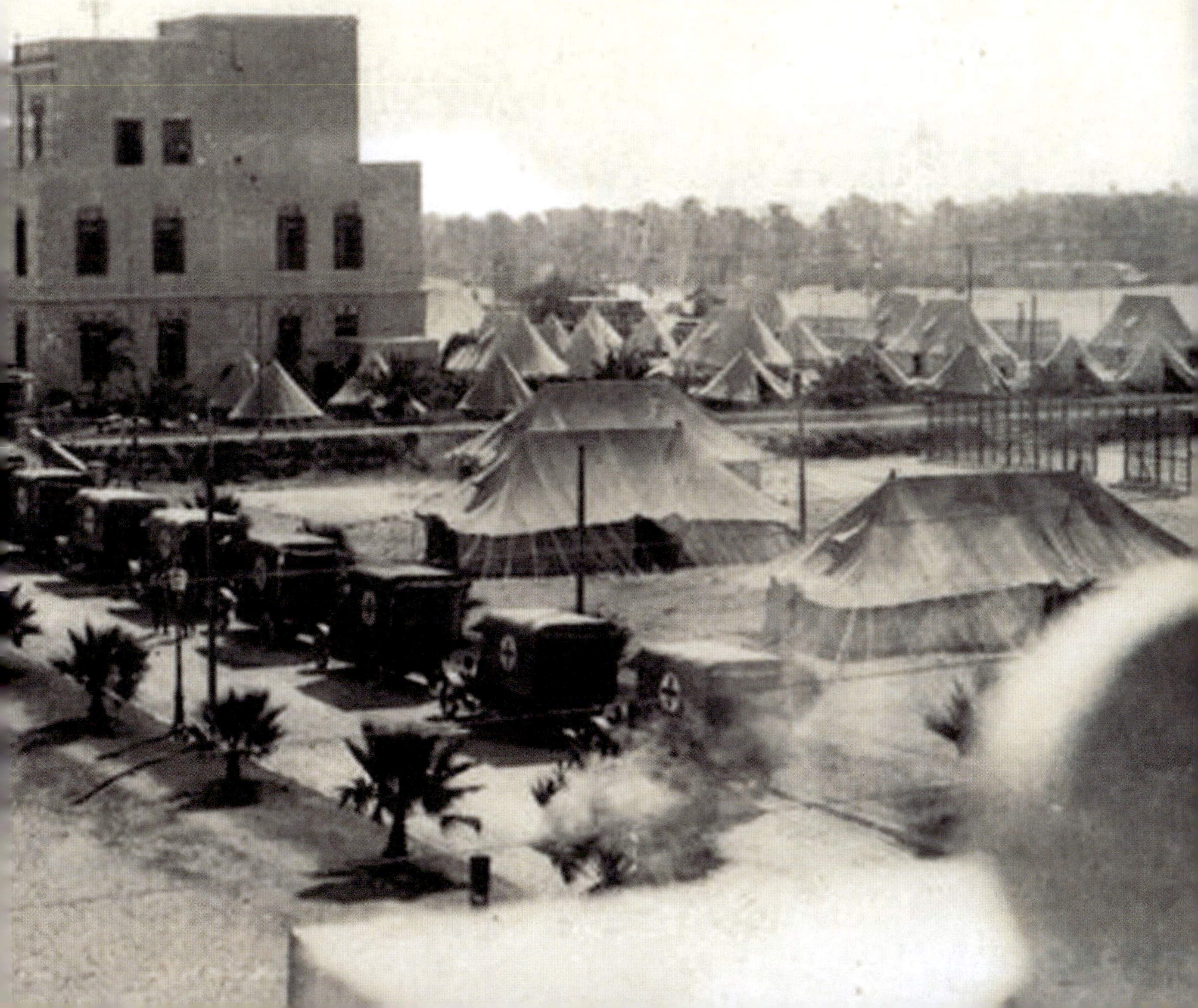

previous pages
Hundreds of sick and wounded Anzac soldiers from Gallipoli were treated at British hospitals in Egypt. This is No. 17 General.
NATIONAL ARMY MUSEUM, 1986.1753

When I first came upon it, it was full of wounded and sick from various parts of the Empire . . . When I saw it again, after months of war, it was just a little bit of New Zealand — sick and sorry, bruised and battered, but still cheerful and optimistic . . .

— Malcolm Ross, describing Pont de Koubbeh, 29 March 1916

No one could have imagined just how bad Gallipoli would be. When New Zealand offered to fight for the Mother Country, it was agreed that the imperial authorities would be entirely responsible for the hospitalisation of sick and wounded troops, but the disastrous Dardanelles campaign, and the large numbers of New Zealand soldiers requiring evacuation from the peninsula, caused unforeseen pressure on hospitals in Alexandria and Cairo — and on Lemnos and Malta, and eventually in Britain.

When the war started there were European hospitals in Egypt, both military facilities used by the British army of occupation and the Egyptian army, and civilian establishments. As we have seen, New Zealand was offered the use of the Egyptian Army Hospital at Pont de Koubbeh, and New Zealanders were also treated in other Egyptian institutions.[1] However, accounts sent back by the troops led to rumblings of dissatisfaction in New Zealand about 'our men being doctored by [British] "Territorials" and nursed by Arabs'. Godley was furious. 'I enclose a report on the Egyptian Army Hospital,' he wrote to Allen from Zeitoun on 9 April, 'and some photographs of it, in order that you may be able to refute the outrageous stories which have been sent home . . . [T]hey have been far better looked after than anybody else in Cairo, thanks to our good fortune in having obtained the use of this Hospital.'[2]

A New Zealand nurse working at Port Said's Egyptian Schools Hospital later in the year witnessed prejudice against non-white medical staff. '[W]e worked under three Egyptian doctors, one English medical officer was over them. It was very strange to me at first, and the other sister, an English girl, hated these Egyptians. However we got on all right though some of their ways were rather weird.' When the daily dressings were done, 'it looked an impressive scene with these dark men in overalls, and the orderlies' funny head-gear'. She initially had 'great difficulty in making them boil up their instruments after each dressing' — they considered a dip in a weak Lysol solution sufficient — but 'taking them all round they were surprisingly good. Sometimes the "Tommies" murmured a bit at being in the hands of these doctors, but not often.'[3]

Allen made sure that Godley's report was widely covered in newspapers throughout New Zealand. 'The hospital is of recent erection, 1906,' said the *Dominion*,

> complete with the most modern arrangements, electric lighting throughout, six large surgical wards, and seven similar medical wards; six special wards for single cases; large dining room and reading room, with library; hot and cold baths, with showers; water carriages, sewage, three operation rooms, electric laundry, steam disinfector, X-Ray room, Pathological Laboratory, and barrack accommodation for 100 orderlies. The building, of greystone, is two storied, with broad, shady verandahs supplied with grass blinds, and is situated in a large enclosure with a pretty, well cared for garden in front.

The article gave the names of all the staff. The New Zealanders among them included X-ray specialist Colonel Ferdinand Batchelor, pathologist Captain Charles Hercus and surgeon Major Arthur Purchas. There was, too, a full nursing staff and several volunteer nurses. '[D]elicacies of soup, wine, jelly, fresh eggs, whey etc. [were] kindly presented daily to this hospital by thirty ladies of Cairo.' While there were indeed some British Territorials on the staff, the care offered was exemplary.[4]

Minister of Defence James Allen was to spend a good deal of time explaining and defending the government's role in, and funding of, New Zealand's medical war effort. On 21 June 1915, for example, he emphasised that there 'need be no anxiety in New Zealand as to the treatment of our sick and wounded soldiers . . . and any stories about lack of hospital accommodation and necessaries should be discredited'. He had 'repeatedly told General Godley that he was at liberty to spend what money was required'; such expenditure was a 'proper charge upon the Defence Department and upon the war loan'. Things 'for a time were not quite satisfactory' — this was a reference to Gallipoli — but all was now well. Allen was also at pains to explain the 'clear distinction between ordinary hospital necessities, conveniences, and provisions for the sick and wounded', which were paid for by the state, and 'special comforts', which could 'be supplied by the generous-minded public of New Zealand'.[5]

By the time the panegyrics about Pont de Koubbeh were appearing in the New Zealand press, the medical situation in Egypt had altered drastically. The sick and wounded pouring in from the Dardanelles quickly filled the existing hospitals, and other buildings were soon pressed into use, chiefly by the British, though there was also an Australian presence. No. 1 Australian General Hospital, created in January 1915 in the impressive Heliopolis Palace Hotel in Cairo, was not far from the New Zealanders' Zeitoun camp, and No. 2 AGH was set up at Mena and Ghezireh. The Australians also used Cairo's Luna Park, with its skating rink and switchback railway, along with the Atelier and the Sporting Club. (One New Zealander who spent a couple of months in Luna Park reported bad conditions 'as to food, ventilation and general comfort'.)[6] Among the British hospitals in Alexandria were No. 15 General, in a large

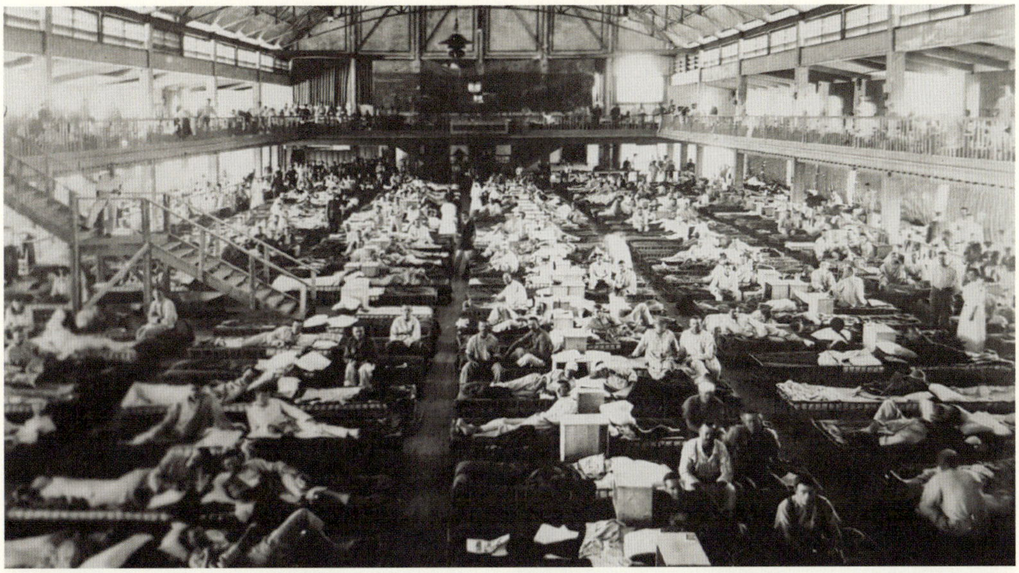

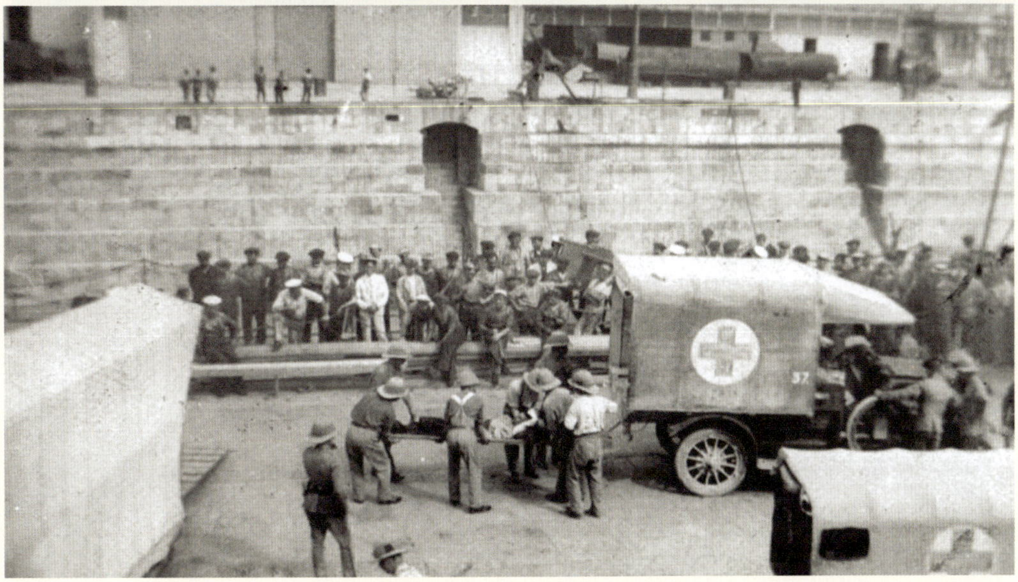

above Built about 1910 as the first amusement park in the Middle East, with a roller coaster and a skating rink, Luna Park in Cairo was pressed into service as an Australian hospital for Gallipoli casualties. New Zealand nurse Ida Willis took this photo. ROYAL NEW ZEALAND ARMY MEDICAL CORPS HISTORY COLLECTION

below Seen from the decks of the hospital ship that has brought them to Egypt, wounded are loaded into ambulances on the wharf below. NATIONAL ARMY MUSEUM, 1992.1149 two-storey building that had been a German school, and No. 19, also known as the Deaconess' Hospital, which had been run by German nuns. As Trooper Horace Haycock, invalided home in mid-1915, explained, 'Practically every suitable building has been convened into a military hospital, and even although a large number of very fine buildings have been so converted, all of the hospitals are overcrowded.'[7] In an October 1915 report on her return from Egypt, Hester Maclean listed, in Alexandria, Port Said and Cairo, 21 'English and Australian Hospitals in which New Zealand Sick & Wounded are Treated'.[8]

As early as 3 March Godley, aware of sickness among his men and anticipating trouble when the Gallipoli campaign began, had cabled Allen to ask for more hospital beds. By the end of that month the Army Council in Britain had accepted New Zealand's offer of assistance — 'the personnel of a stationary hospital would be welcome' — and, to Godley's relief, No. 1 New Zealand Stationary Hospital (NZSH) left Wellington on 20 May 1915.[9] It was established at Port Said about a fortnight after the 50 NZANS nurses, who had left Wellington on the *Rotorua*, arrived in Egypt on 15 June and were posted to local British-run hospitals. A second stationary hospital followed shortly afterwards. By this time, Allen had seen the light regarding New Zealand nurses serving overseas. Although, as was customary, none were included in the stationary hospital, 31 'ladies' of the New Zealand Army Nursing Service sailed with the men in May.[10] Another 69 nurses would leave New Zealand on 11 July in the hospital ship *Maheno*. Early on, however, apart from some doctors and orderlies at Pont de Koubbeh, and the occasional non-NZANS nurse,[11] there was no real New Zealand medical presence in Egypt.

New Zealanders evacuated from Gallipoli were sent to a variety of hospitals. After Private Robert Steele was shot in the right thigh on 25 April, he described a smooth reception in Alexandria. 'Motor-cars met the train and buzzed us to the [Australian] hospital at Heliopolis . . . They entered our names, etc., gave us clothes, hot bath and food and dressed our wounds.' Because Heliopolis was being reserved for serious cases, Steele was transferred to Mena, where he was operated on before having a sociable time with the 19 Australians in his ward. He paid 'a high tribute to the Australian nurses and the hospital orderlies'.[12] Auckland clerk Louis Browne, who had been laid up with diarrhoea for three weeks before he reached Heliopolis in July, thought it 'the best place I have struck since leaving home. You get every attention and comfort. My bed is out on the verandah upstairs and there is a nice cool breeze blowing all the time.' Frank Fougere, however, wounded at Chunuk Bair, reported a much more stressed situation at Heliopolis in August: 'There was very little provision made for the New Zealand wounded. Numbers of them were left just laying out in the desert. Some were in tents and a great many didn't have any covering at all. The doctors were toiling 24 hours a day.'[13]

Ambulances were critical to moving sick and wounded men from ships to the various hospitals. When half the 14 ambulances the New Zealand government had ordered from Britain arrived in Egypt on 10 February, with 15 ASC drivers, Godley considered them 'excellent, and really beautiful cars. Our Ford cars have done extremely well, and are still in good order.'[14] Donated vehicles were also a boon. As thousands of Anzac and British patients arrived from Gallipoli in May and June, without the New Zealand and Australian ambulances 'it is difficult to see how a serious breakdown could have been avoided. The drivers of these vehicles did admirable service.' In the first rush, 'each driver was at the wheel almost continuously . . . for seven days, snatching odd minutes for a hasty meal and having no regular sleep'.[15] Norman Gray got to know many of the cars — 'great Vauxhalls most of them' — and their drivers when he was responsible for admitting men to the Egyptian hospitals late in 1915. There was no specified speed limit; one British ASC man gave Gray the impression that 'all soldiers run the risk of dying anywhere and any time, and might just as well blow out at 40 miles an hour as standing in a trench'. When four trainloads of men from Gallipoli arrived at the beginning of December, most of them suffering from the 'intense cold' on the peninsula, 'every Motor Ambulance in the district was working at top speed'.[16]

'Ambulances on wharf to take us to Hotels,' Palmerston North nurse Mabel Crook recorded in her diary after she and the other *Rotorua* nurses reached Alexandria. 'Everyone gives orders what Hospital to proceed to.' Crook was among 20 sent to the nearby No. 15 British General Hospital, where she was assigned to the officers' ward. MO Cyril Baigent from Gallipoli was one of her patients. By July, when she was night sister, she had '300 patients and only one orderly . . . I was very anxious that I should not miss one sick man, and went with my little Lantern to see with, was perpetually on the go.'[17] Frederick Turnbull was 'quite comfortable' at No. 15 in August 1915. 'The sisters are very nice and capable, as are also the orderlies. Some of the sisters are English, some Australians, and some New Zealanders, though I haven't seen any of the latter yet. This is a huge place.'[18]

The New Zealand nurses sent to the Deaconess' Hospital (No. 19) spoke 'well of the German sisters who have taken over the civil part of the place and attend to the housekeeping'. A Christchurch woman thought it 'really a beautiful hospital, has a lift and many other conveniences which other military hospitals here in Egypt have not got'.[19] The balance of the New Zealanders travelled on to Cairo, where eight joined the Citadel Hospital on the Mokkattam Hills overlooking the city, while Samoa veterans Vida MacLean, Bertha Nurse and Fanny Wilson were among those sent to Pont de Koubbeh. Later New Zealanders were also sent to No. 27 General Hospital in a large converted school building at Abbassia, where Garioch (Garry) Clunie of the Wellington Mounted Rifles went in August 1915 after being wounded for a third time on Gallipoli. 'They are grand . . . these nurses & sisters here, they do anything at all for us. They are mostly New Zealand girls too, so no wonder they are good, like everything else that comes from there.' The care extended to off-duty hours. A New Zealand gunner had been in hospital 'for no more than 15 minutes' when he met a nurse who was 'on the staff of quite another hospital, and was filling in her leisure hours, all too few, in visiting our New Zealand boys . . . All the nurses are doing this, proving themselves angels in reality, and to very good purpose.'[20]

Used to organising their own wards and supervising probationers, and 'not having been accustomed to orderlies and that kind of thing', the New Zealand nurses struggled with the routines and bureaucracy of the British army hospital system. 'I shall be most military,' Edna Pengelly decided, 'when I have mastered the diet sheet.'[21] Fanny Speedy, flat out 'from 7 a.m.

till 11, 12, 1 and perhaps 2 a.m.', had little patience with the red tape: 'There was so much writing to do in connection with each patient that I seemed never to be finished.'[22] Equally unwelcome were bedbugs, which were combated by applying blow lamps to wire-wove bed bases and placing bed legs in saucers of kerosene. At night, the nurses swathed their heads in turbans to keep the insects out of their long hair.

The intense heat was a shock — it was 110°F in the Citadel wards in June 1916, and the previous month Pengelly had recorded a temperature of 123°F in the shade.[23] The climate was always a concern for both staff and patients. As one nurse suggested, 'white women could only stand one summer, and . . . many of the nurses would crack up, because they had been working at the highest pressure'. When 26 nurses returned to England from Egypt in January 1917, Matron-in-Chief of the NZEF Mabel Thurston noticed that 'they were all looking more or less washed out from continued duties in a hot climate'.[24] The medical staff were also vulnerable to the illnesses suffered by the men in their care. On 28 October 1915, 29-year-old nurse Ada Hawken, from Auckland, died of typhoid in No. 19 Hospital.

When the second group of nurses arrived in the Middle East with No. 1 NZSH, they, too, were sent to a number of different hospitals; about 10 remained at the stationary hospital itself. Lily Eddy was posted to Ras-el-Tin, where she worked in a large surgical ward of 66 men. 'We had over 1,500 patients . . . at the beginning of last week,' she wrote on 23 August. 'We don't keep them here any longer than necessary, just get them over the worst, and then pass them on . . . Some poor fellows are frightfully cut about by the awful explosive bullets.'[25] Private Raymond Ward, wounded twice on Gallipoli, enjoyed his time there. 'No noises ever disturb the quietness, except the faint murmur of the waves. Every conceivable attention is given here — the best medical services, the best diet, cool, spacious wards, and a magnificent nursing staff.'[26] One nurse, sent to No. 17 General in Alexandria, found an 'immense' military hospital holding almost 1800 beds, in buildings and in tents. 'I do not know which could be considered worst, the surgical or the medical. Some of the wounds were ghastly, while the typhoid and dysentry cases, which were so numerous, were of the worst type and all very ill patients.' Supplies were a problem: 'Not enough of many things was the frequent cry, especially where soap and sheets, etc., were concerned.' The work was taxing, for doctors, nurses and orderlies, especially when dealing with 'big and dreadful convoys straight off the boats from the Peninsula'.[27]

There were some breaks for both the hard-working medics and men who were convalescing. The nurses were sent, in turn, for two- or three-day stays at the large and roomy Aboukir Rest Home, an hour's train journey east of Alexandria, 'a delightful place . . . lent to the Red Cross Society for the use of Nursing Sisters needing rest and change'.[28] Excursions were popular, too, for convalescent troops, medical men and nurses, especially recent arrivals. When motor ambulances were available in Cairo, their drivers took the women out to the Pyramids and the Sphinx, where they could have their photo taken, perched on a camel. Refreshments were on offer at the famous Groppi's restaurant, or at Cairo's Shepheard's and Continental hotels; many made trips up the Nile. The soldiers' and nurses' letters home were filled with descriptions of their exotic surroundings, but there were less salubrious aspects. 'Most people talk of the "Call

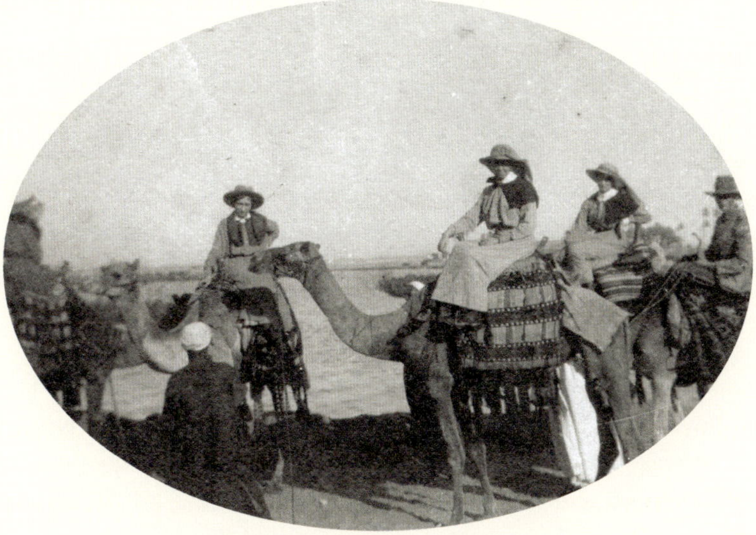

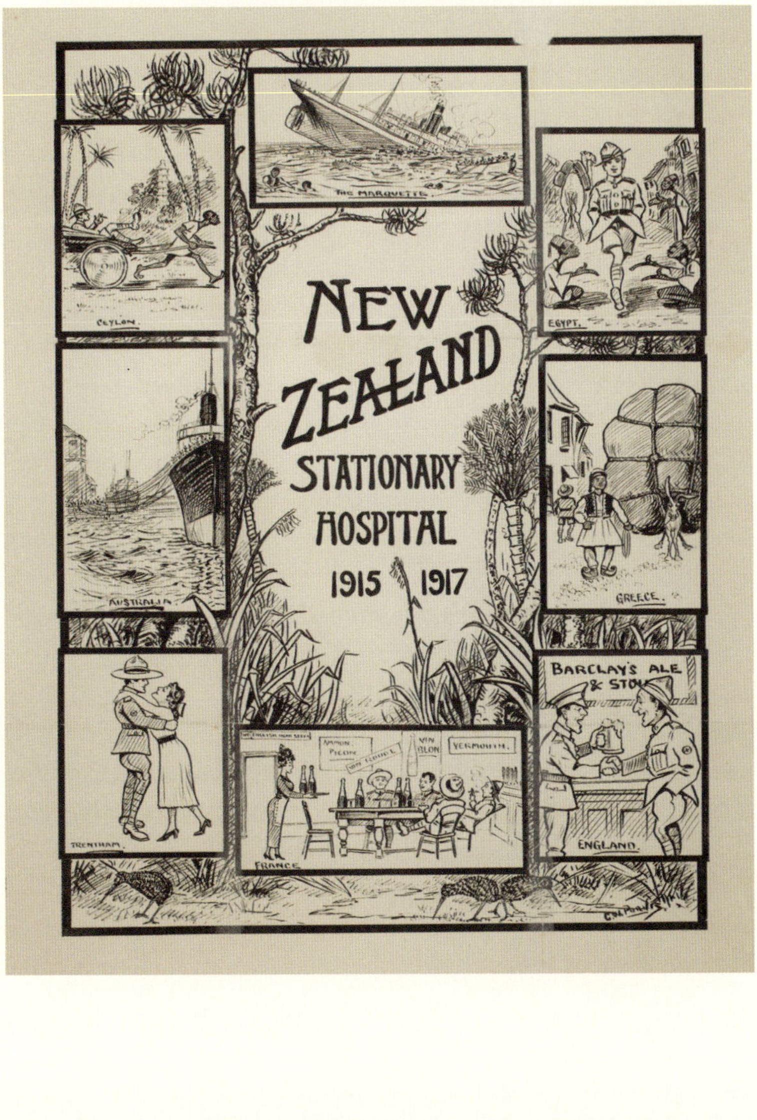

above A visit to the Pyramids and a ride on a camel were de rigueur off-duty activities for busy New Zealand nurses in Egypt. GEORGE CRAWLEY PHOTO, COURTESY DR DAVID RICHARDS

below Created by C. W. Purvis, this poster depicts the adventures of No. 1 New Zealand Stationary Hospital from 1915 to 1917, including scenes of Ceylon, Australia, Trentham, France, England, Greece, Egypt and the *Marquette*. Purvis also drew caricatures of hospital staff members. AUCKLAND WAR MEMORIAL MUSEUM, EPH-PW-1-30 of the East",' wrote Eddy. 'I'd say, 'twas the smell of the East that was most noticeable and most likely to be remembered.'[29]

The NZMC orderlies, too, were kept busy. 'The orderlies work hard,' New Zealand doctor Agnes Bennett wrote from the Infectious Diseases Hospital at Choubra, 'and don't have much of a time.' Owing to a recent order decreeing that 'only 25 per cent of the staff may be on leave at a time . . . they only get out every fourth day at most, and it is hard in these confined quarters. They do good work, and don't get the hero worship the others do . . . they have been absolutely grand.'[30]

No. 1 New Zealand Stationary Hospital, consisting of 200 beds and headed by former Wellington surgeon Lieutenant-Colonel Donald McGavin, included seven NZMC officers: Whangarei's Joseph Frazerhurst; David Wylie from New Plymouth; Duncan Stout of Wellington (son of Chief Justice Sir Robert Stout); Napier's John Leahy; Eric Marchant, an eye and ear specialist from Wellington; noted mountaineer and photographer Ebenezer Teichelmann from Hokitika; and dental surgeon David Isaacs. Among the 86 other ranks on board was Sergeant David Fitzgibbon, who had only praise for the doctors, 'in the highest meaning of the word gentlemen and "white" in every sense of the word. No wife, sweetheart or mother need fear that the boys in our unit are not looked after — in fact, if anything we are "molly-coddled".' Everyone was 'very fond of Dr. Frazer Hurst, who to all hands is kindness personified and who is a paternal personal friend to the young men who are away from home for the first time. He is all energy and keeps things moving.'[31]

When the hospital reached Port Said at the end of June, McGavin 'had at his disposal one house, formerly a school, 25 square E.P. [Egypt pattern] tents, and some huts for messes and recreation room'.[32] What he did not have was equipment: that brought from New Zealand had been offloaded at Bombay. But the hospital opened for 150 convalescent cases from Pont de Koubbeh on 16 July, in Hester Maclean's view 'before it was really ready'; there was no nursing staff. When six nurses did arrive on 21 July, they had 'a very strenuous time' until relieved by Canadians and then other New Zealanders. Maclean later described the building, which consisted of 'a ground floor, basement and two other floors, and there was room with considerable contrivances for the necessary administration offices, store; dressing-room, theatre, sterilising room'. The 36-bed wards on the ground and first floors were 'airy and pleasant with a fine view of the sea'. The remainder of the hospital — when Maclean last visited on 17 August it had 600 beds — was under canvas: 'large tent marquees . . . of three thicknesses of canvas and blue and yellow linings which produced a fairly cool atmosphere with the breeze from the sea blowing through the open sides'. At first the nurses' work was 'extremely arduous' because they had to trudge through sand as the paths between the tents had not yet been hardened.[33] Three motor ambulances were available.

Although, as Methodist chaplain Harry Blamires reported, the men 'are well cared for and go short of nothing within reason' — there was a library, and a games and social hall that offered afternoon picture shows[34] — comforts were always welcome. In September a correspondent

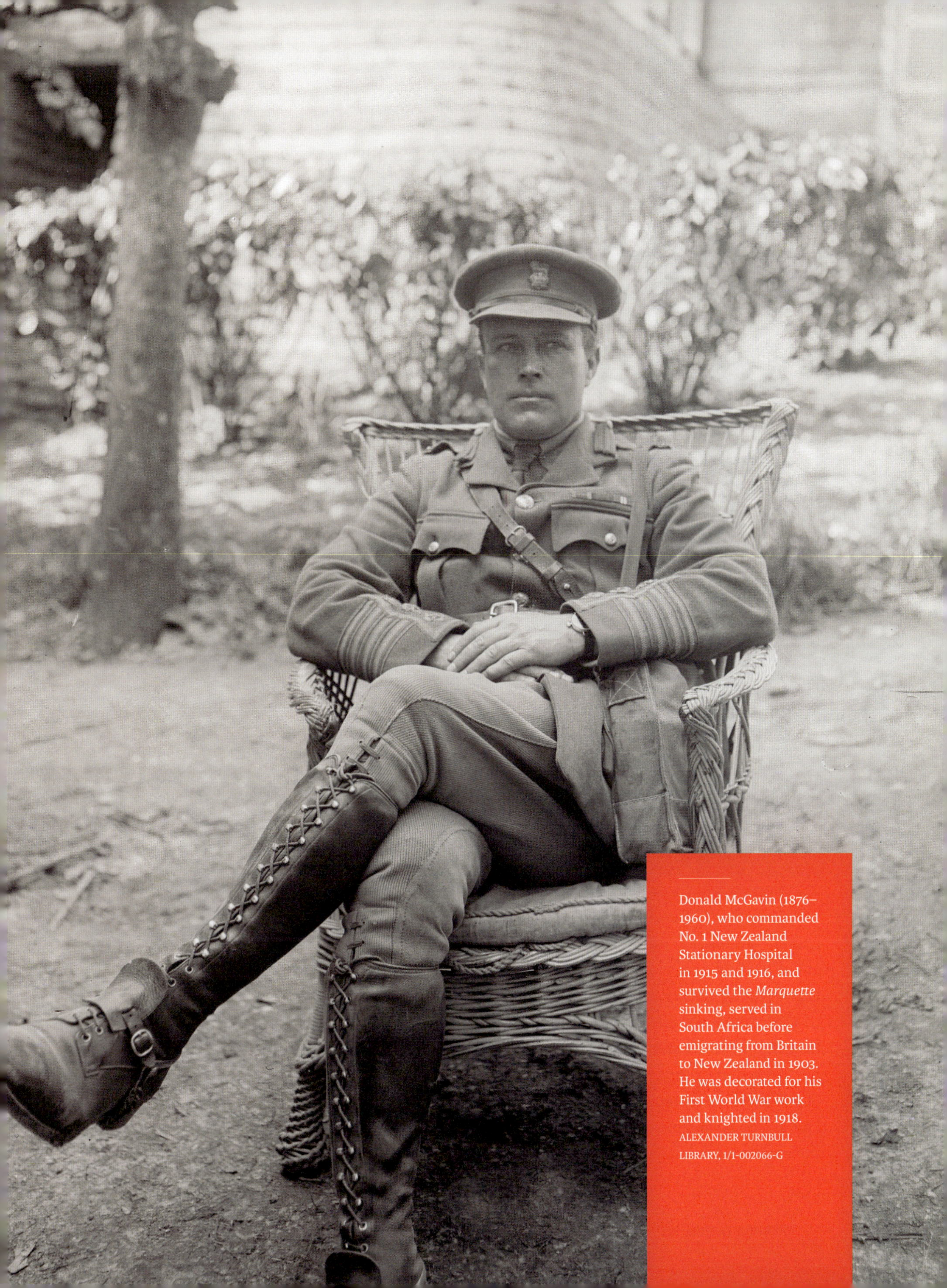

Donald McGavin (1876–1960), who commanded No. 1 New Zealand Stationary Hospital in 1915 and 1916, and survived the *Marquette* sinking, served in South Africa before emigrating from Britain to New Zealand in 1903. He was decorated for his First World War work and knighted in 1918. ALEXANDER TURNBULL LIBRARY, 1/1-002066-G to the *Taranaki Daily News* suggested suitable items for No. 1 NZSH, based on information from 'a special nurse now on duty in Egypt'. Readers should not overlook the medical staff, 'those hard-worked and overtaxed men and women, who are so bravely serving their country'. Among a long list of items were holland bags, 'about 18in. long by 9in. wide, with a draw tape and an inserted flap of calico' inscribed with the soldier's name. Known as 'treasure bags', these contained each man's effects and were hung on the ends of their hospital beds.[35]

No. 2 New Zealand Stationary Hospital left New Zealand on 13 June on the *Maunganui*, under the leadership of Auckland doctor Lieutenant-Colonel William Parkes. It was being organised at Trentham before its predecessor departed, and the *Evening Post* was sure, 'judging by the qualifications of the officers selected', that it too would 'prove a credit to the Dominion'.[36] As former law student Colin Gordon would recall, the orderlies' accommodation on the *Maunganui* was not luxurious — 'built-in bunks, three high' on what had been the first-class smoking room on the boat deck — and he was kept 'pretty busy' caring for 'our sick blokes' and nursing two men who had undergone appendix operations.[37]

When Parkes and his staff reached Egypt on 22 July, he was informed that the Egyptian government had arranged to lend the Pont de Koubbeh hospital to New Zealand, and was asked if he was 'willing to take command of the same, installing my own staff'.[38] Parkes agreed and immediately took over what soon became known as the New Zealand General Hospital, its identity reinforced by its codename, Hohipera — the Māori transliteration of 'hospital'. The New Zealanders were sorely needed. When Joe Gasparich was sent to Pont de Koubbeh, he found his ward

> in the charge of a nursing sister assisted by two male orderlies and two V.A.D.s who came in from Cairo one each on alternate afternoons. The [British] orderlies had been on duty here apparently from the beginning of things and by this time were properly & thoroughly 'browned off'. The attention so many very ill patients needed was utterly beyond their capacity to cope with & they had become adepts at being absent when needed most. To make matters still worse the Nursing Sister was responsible also for another ward across the corridor and reserved for the needs of officers.[39]

This overworked sister was probably Cora Anderson, whom Gordon and his friend Ted Kiely met when they were sent to Medical 1 Ward on their first day. 'We had to do the nursing; she couldn't attend to 70 patients on her own. She showed us what to do and we had to get cracking and do it. God damn it, none of our fellows were skilled attendants! Looking back, I wonder that we did as well as we did and that we didn't have more casualties en route.'[40]

The original 200-bed limit was soon increased. 'The hospital has 400 beds,' Parkes wrote to his wife, 'which are not fully equipped, so will you tell the Auckland ladies that their equipment is to be put to use right away?' They were using 'large, airy tents to accommodate the overflow of patients'. The 20 New Zealand nurses already working at the hospital were 'very fine women, and will be invaluable to us. The work is very strenuous, and most of our operating we do in the early hours of the morning, as it is the only cool time. But we love the work, and hope to do credit to our dear old New Zealand.'[41] In a 5 September letter, Parkes described 'the heavy work entailed and the great strain placed on their resources by extending the accommodation . . . to 600 beds'. Rather than 25 doctors, 'which is the military establishment for 800 beds', they had only seven. He warmly praised the whole staff, 'who were cheerfully working long hours under very unpleasant climatic conditions'. His charges seemed to be appreciative. One wounded soldier told the *Observer*, 'We're not only patients to Dr. Parkes — we are pals.'[42]

Twenty-one-year-old NZMC Sergeant Walter Hopkirk could testify to the toughness of the work and the environment. 'We are very short-handed,' he wrote home on 10 August, 'and when we applied for more men they asked us if we had any orderlies to go to the front at once. All except a few "passengers" [free-loaders] do their fourteen or sixteen hours per day, and you may be sure we are some tired. I could sleep two weeks on end easily just now.' Despite the good tucker — meat, bread and potatoes, plus 8½d a day per man to be spent on such delights as 'butter, bacon, eggs, tomatoes, sago, tinned or dried fruits, plum duff and jam' — everyone was losing weight in the 'very trying' weather: 'we will need plenty of New Zealand dairy feeding to fix us when we get home.' Their quarters were acceptable, but swarmed with bugs and mosquitoes. 'It's quite a simple and uninteresting sport to catch a dozen big black, beetly bugs in the morning. They don't worry me, but the mosquitos have got a down on me, and I lose some of my good points each night.'[43]

It helped enormously that staff and patients alike were New Zealanders, 'so we are all "cobbers"'. It was 'a big job' when the wounded arrived, many of them from Chunuk Bair. 'Then, we all have to move some, for we all must do our best work for those chaps who are straight from the trenches.' On the night Hopkirk wrote, 167 wounded were admitted. 'At 9 p.m. I thought I would rest, so lay down in the corridor. When consciousness dawned again, it was roll call (6 a.m.) — what a lovely sleep it was though I did have my boots on! We are not at the front, but we are at a front, and I think all will agree that we do our little share.' Each day 'we send about 100 patients to the convalescent camps, and then receive 100 more from the front'.[44]

When Dr Charles Maguire was acting as adjutant and company officer for the hospital in November 1915, he was working with 11 other officers, including Major Louis Barnett, who headed the surgical division, and Captain Fred Bowerbank, who ran the medical section. The hospital also had its own bacteriologist, Captain Frederick Armitage from Auckland.[45] Its 35 nurses did 'practically a twelve-hours' day' but had every second afternoon off. Some 120 orderlies, NCOs and ORs, and 'a large number of native sweepers', completed 'quite a large' staff.[46] That month, Dr Robert Hogg from Invercargill reported that they could accommodate between 700 and 800 men, 'with capacity of almost unlimited expansion, by means of tents, if we are pushed . . . [B]y utilising every available corner, the verandahs and balconies, and by means of tent wards and tents for the staff (I am in a tent myself) the accommodation has been doubled.' Hogg was 'thoroughly convinced that our own boys do much better among their own people. They don't fit in either with the Australians or the British Tommy, and the touch of home in our own hospital here, with New Zealand nurses, doctors, and orderlies and last, and not least, the New Zealand flag flying over the roof, goes a long way to give a poor chap who is down and out the filip which starts him on the road to recovery.'[47] William McAra, invalided from Gallipoli, agreed when he arrived on 14 November. 'It is such a treat to be surrounded by all N.Z. doctors & nurses & they couldn't have been kinder to us than they were.'[48]

Staffing could be problematic. Parkes, at No. 2 NZSH, was sent extra personnel in mid-January 1916, but they were not exactly what he had asked for. He had requested 63 orderlies but, to his dismay, also received four officers and a number of NCOs for whom he had no vacancies. This would not be the only example of disconnection between the medical hierarchy in New Zealand and those actually working with the sick and wounded. On 2 February Parkes was awaiting the arrival of Dr Philip Putnam, who, without any consultation, had been promised a surgeon's post. Less than a third of the hospital's cases were surgical and they already had sufficient men to deal with these. 'Our administration would be rendered much easier and cause less personal disappointment if medical officers were sent forward without restrictions.'[49]

When war correspondent Malcolm Ross filed a long article about Pont de Koubbeh in March 1916, he was, predictably, lavish in his praise. The wealth of detail he provided included some impressive statistics. During the preceding year there had been 6506 admissions — 115 officers and 6391 other ranks — including some English and Australians. More than four-fifths of these men — 5325 — were sick, as a 'large number of New Zealand wounded, especially in the earlier stages of the fighting, received treatment in the numerous other hospitals in Alexandria and Cairo, and most of the serious cases returning from the battlefield were not taken past Alexandria'. Thirty-two men had died of sickness and 10 from wounds. 'There had been over 200 operations for gunshot wounds and complications, 35 for hernia, 30 for appendicitis, 42 for varicose veins . . . and 27 for haemorrhoids. There had been 120 minor operations in addition to a large number of abdominal operations.'[50]

It was not always possible, or medically sensible, for recovering men to return to duty immediately. 'More than anything,' Godley told Allen on 13 March 1915,

> what we want here now is money enough to establish a small convalescent home . . . into which we could put convalescent men, with a nurse and a cook to look after them. As it is now, men go straight out of hospital to the sand and dust and flies, and rough and ready cooking of the camp, and it is also difficult to arrange for them to do only light work, and different work from all the others. If we had some place where they could convalesce it would be a great thing.[51]

The GOC's formidable wife, Louisa Godley, who had joined her husband in Egypt, had already organised for some men to recover in private homes, and on 25 March Major-General Edward Chaytor wrote to her, hoping that, 'in view of the great interest you have taken in our sick', she would be willing to oversee the proposed home.[52] In reiterating the need to Allen early in April, Godley also emphasised the pragmatic aspect: 'so many men who come out of hospital with pneumonia or influenza . . . only want a week or a fortnight at a place of the kind before being fit to go back to duty, [but] would, if sent straight back to camp, crack up again and have [to] be sent back to hospital. It is for these men it is required . . . and it will save a great deal [of] delay in getting men quickly in the fighting line again.'[53]

That month a convalescent home was opened in a large unfurnished house with an expansive garden, only 20 minutes' walk from Zeitoun camp. The patients, mainly sick men from the base, were visited each day by a medical officer and followed a gentle routine that began with breakfast at 8 a.m. and ended with lights out at 10 p.m. Lady Godley was also 'very anxious to get a house at the seaside at Alexandria', which her husband considered 'absolutely necessary and desirable, and the cost of it will not be much more than it would be to keep the men in hospital'.[54] By 29 May he could report to Allen on the two 'convalescent homes . . . one in Zeitoun, and one in Alexandria, and my wife is looking after the latter'.[55]

The Alexandria home was, in the view of Colonel James Esson at NZEF Headquarters, 'a splendid little institution'. With room for 30 patients, the 'large and well-appointed building [was] on the seaside, in one of the coolest and best of Alexandria's suburbs'. There were, in fact, two buildings — one for officers and one for other ranks — as the owner of the neighbouring house had offered it to Lady Godley. Such places were 'most necessary' during the Egyptian summer when 'life . . . under canvas or outside a stone building is almost impossible. Yesterday, even in Alexandria, it was 109 deg. in the shade and the sick in the Convalescent camps suffered a good deal.'[56] Thanks to an anonymous offer from New Zealand to fund a 25-bed convalescent home for a year, another home, also managed by Louisa Godley, was opened in Helwan, mainly for cases requiring massage (physiotherapy) treatment.[57] 'It is an extremely comfortable place,' Godley told Allen, 'and the men are very well looked after. My only complaint about it is, that it is rather too comfortable, and I am afraid, therefore, that there may be a temptation for some of them to stay there a little longer than may be necessary. But my wife assures me that she turns them out as quickly as possible, and is much harder hearted than they are at most hospitals and convalescent homes.'[58]

Esson praised Louisa Godley's 'keen and sympathetic interest in our sick', but also hinted at her steelier side. 'I have not met a more businesslike member of the fair sex nor one in whom the faculty of management was so highly developed. Good discipline maintained in the home and of the institution is dictated by the head as well as by the heart.'[59] But the martinet did work hard herself. 'I am glad she is not going to spend another summer at the work,' her husband told Allen in June 1916, 'as the management of the three convalescent homes was really too much, and she wore herself nearly to a shadow.'[60] Louisa Godley would be mentioned in despatches for her work.

Heavy Gallipoli casualties in May 1915 made it clear that more convalescent facilities would be needed. On 31 July, the *Wanganui Chronicle* reported that 'several local ladies' were hoping 'to raise a sum sufficient to enable them to be away very shortly and establish a further convalescent home for New Zealanders in Egypt'.[61] The women acted speedily, gaining permission from the relevant authorities in New Zealand and Egypt, estimating the costs and putting their case to the Wanganui Patriotic Committee. This would provide staff and equipment, and the government the building and catering, so the call went out through the lower North Island for everything from tobacco and cigarettes to stationery, bootlaces, bagatelle boards and gramophone records, beds and linen. All of this, and more, plus generous financial contributions, came flooding in, and on 10 September the staff of the convalescent home, who paid their own way, sailed for Sydney on the first leg of their voyage to Egypt. Three, all from the lower North Island, were trained nurses: Mary Early (the matron), Kate Booth and Nora Hughes. Booth and Early were NZANS members and Hughes was attested in Egypt a few months later; the other women were Ruth Cameron, sisters Betty and Mina McDonald, Mysie McDonnell and Lena McLaren. (Both Mina McDonald and McDonnell would receive MBEs for their work in Egypt.) With them, as quartermaster, went Sergeant George Sleight, from Wanganui's East Town Railway Workshops Ambulance Division.

As Early told Hester Maclean, 'It was, of course, a venture bringing untrained women to Egypt, but I have been fortunate in having on the staff the right kind of women, and as the work here was for convalescents, all trained women were not necessary. In Sisters Booth and Hughes I had two most reliable nurses . . . and the other girls on the staff have been able to help in many ways where trained help would have been wasted.'[62] On 25 November 1915 the 100-bed Aotea Convalescent Home opened at Heliopolis in Cairo — in the former winter residence of an Ottoman prince — close to Zeitoun and the New Zealand hospital. The palace contained some usable furniture, but 'a great many easy chairs' would be needed.[63]

When Eric Burnett arrived a couple of weeks later he found everything 'running beautifully smoothly', apart from some minor plumbing and electrical hiccups. 'This is rightly called a home . . . My word it will be a hard blow going into camp after being here!'[64] Mary Early could soon report that although they were 'going on well', the 'pretty awful' sanitary arrangements made it difficult to take more than 80 patients. There were only two small stoves 'to cook for our large family'; several kerosene stoves had been bought. But the meals were excellent and the patients enjoyed fresh scones every day. 'Owing to the numbers always waiting to come into our home we are only able to keep the boys in for about ten days. It is very difficult, selecting the ones to go out, because we would like to keep them so much longer.' A subsidiary home established at Port Said in 1917 closed at the end of October 'on the advent of the cool season'.[65] Late in 1918 a convalescent camp was opened near Ismailia. On 3 March 1919, Early wrote that 'besides the 5000 on our books who have been passed through the Home', they had, 'in between the busy times', cared for many men from the New Zealand Mounted Brigade, 'who were on leave . . . but required rest and extra feeding'. Although 'we could not put them on our books as patients . . . the rest and extra care they were able to have at Aotea often prevented a breakdown'.[66]

Many hundreds also visited Aotea home, including Trooper Harold Peacocke, as a member of a concert party. (There was entertainment aplenty: Aotea had a piano, and the men were taken on excursions.) 'I cannot speak in too high praise of this excellent Home. For its inmates, it is really home in every sense of the word, except for the absence of their dear ones.' He admired the tennis courts, billiard tables, hot and cold shower baths, 'and everything is as clean as the proverbial new pin. But beyond and better than all this, there are the dear, kind-hearted New Zealand sisters and matron, to tend, cheer and comfort the sick and slowly-mending

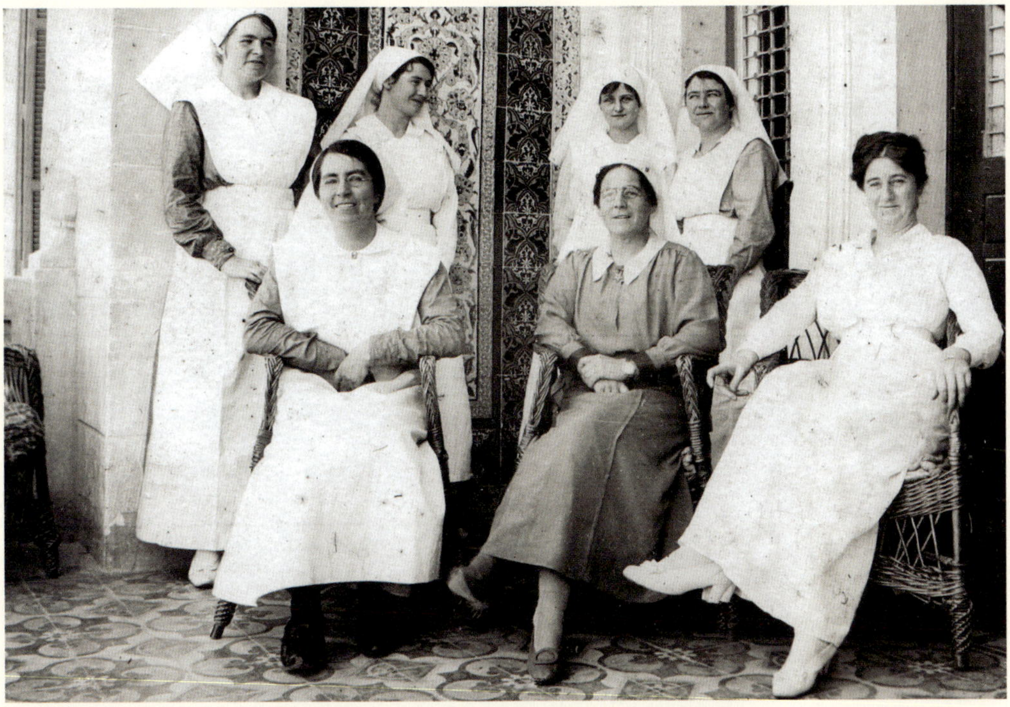

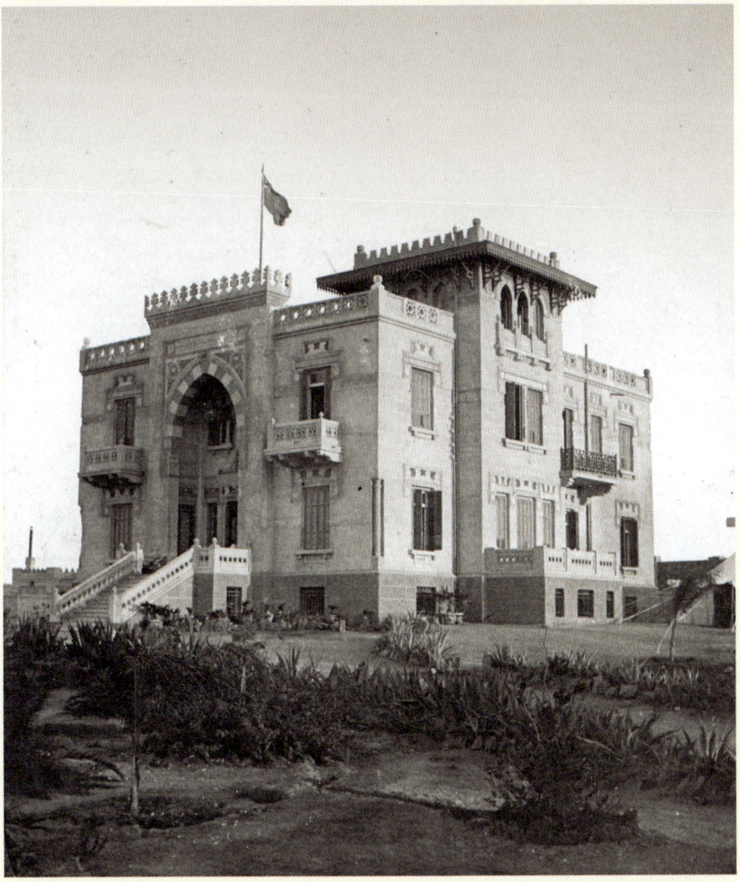

above Matron Mary Early is seated in the centre of George Crawley's photo of the Aotea staff. To her right, wearing glasses, is Kate Booth. GEORGE CRAWLEY PHOTO, COURTESY DR DAVID RICHARDS

below The Aotea Convalescent Home at Heliopolis, with its kind and devoted New Zealand nursing staff, was a dream come true for convalescent Kiwi soldiers. GEORGE CRAWLEY PHOTO, COURTESY DR DAVID RICHARDS wounded men.'[67] The patients themselves loved Aotea. Garry Clunie thought it a 'great place', so good in fact that 'some of the lead swingers [those who made their convalescence last as long as possible] make a home of it'. If a 'chap does not feel well, he had only got to say so & he can stay another week'.[68]

When the New Zealand General Hospital became overcrowded early in 1916, sometimes rather wobbly convalescents such as Eric Burnett, who was ill again with 'Influenza with ________ (big name rash)', were 'shot out of hospital pretty suddenly' and taken to an Emergency Clearing Camp at Zeitoun. Although 'of course . . . not in the least like Aotea', this was 'really not at all a bad place to be in, [and although] the food is very rough, that is practically the only thing against it'. The OC, NZMC Captain William Bruce, was 'a very decent fellow' who did not believe in convalescents being 'too rigidly hemmed in'. There was time for sightseeing and a picnic with some of the New Zealand nurses.[69]

'We are in a hospital constituted of marquees, which are situated on the sands right next to the sea,' wrote orderly Bob Herdman from No. 1 NZSH at Port Said on 5 October 1915. 'At the present time we are accommodating somewhere near 5000 patients, sick and wounded. The majority of cases coming in just now are enteric, dysentery, and diarrhoea. Though the climate is very sultry, etc., wonderful results are attained here.'[70] But as he was penning this letter, decisions were being made to take the hospital to an unknown destination, and on 18 October the staff travelled by 'special train' to Alexandria, where, in the early hours of the 19th, they boarded the British transport *Marquette*. Headed by Donald McGavin, the New Zealand contingent of eight officers, nine non-commissioned officers, 36 nurses and 77 NZMC orderlies were a small minority on the huge vessel. Also sailing were the 500 men and officers of the ammunition column of the British 29th Division, along with 500 mules, some horses and many ammunition-filled wagons. Counting the crew, there were 741 people on board. They were, in fact, bound for Salonika in northern Greece, where the British and French had been fighting alongside the Serbs since September.

There had been talk of submarines, so men kept watch on deck and everyone practised their boat drills, but all seemed well as the *Marquette* crossed the Aegean Sea. Then, soon after 9 a.m. on the cool, grey morning of 23 October, only hours from their destination, a torpedo struck the ship well forward on her starboard side. The nurses, white-faced but calm, went to their designated stations, 18 on each side of the vessel, and the men did their best to follow instructions. But then everything went wrong, as NZMC orderly Lance-Corporal Jack Gillett later told a reporter.

He had been operated on three days before, on the *Marquette*, for an internal tumour, so still had a tube inserted in his side. He got out of bed, took a lifebelt and found his way to the port side of the already badly listing vessel. Some 14 nurses were helped into the first lifeboat, but British soldiers, frightened and inexperienced, failed to lower this properly. Leaving her 'swinging on the davits about three feet from the water, [they] went to the next boat . . . and somehow or other managed to let her come down with a rush' about a foot higher than the first. Then, as the *Marquette* listed further to port, Gillett noticed the forward part of the first boat touch the water and end up at right angles to the sinking ship. Someone let the ropes on the upper lifeboat run out and 'she came crash, fair across the gunwales and about midships' onto the first. Gillett thought 'Nurses [Mary] Gorman and [Mary] Rae were crushed for certain, but of course there may have been more.' Another witness remembered that 'Sister [Catherine] Fox and another New Zealand nurse were injured, and were not seen again'.[71] Although several nurses were helped into the top lifeboat, because her keel was still resting on the first, when the ship lurched 'the boat took a big list and shot all her occupants into the water'. An attempt to launch a boat on the starboard side fared no better. Tipped almost perpendicular, it propelled terrified nurses into the sea. Some of them drowned. Because this boat was badly holed during its descent, it was soon swamped and turned turtle for some time.

Gillett waited with another NZMC man until the water was almost level with the ship's rails on the port side before slipping into the sea. Seeing how close the ship was to capsizing, he 'struck out like fun to avoid being sucked under'. When he was about 20 yards away he trod water and watched as the *Marquette* 'made a very neat dive, bow first, standing perpendicular'.

Hundreds of people were 'clinging on to wreckage, rafts, etc., some of them screaming out for help' in 'a fairly heavy sea' with 5-foot waves. After drifting in the water for around two hours, the pyjama-clad Gillett spotted a lifeboat about a mile away, and set off towards it. Sergeant-Major Geoffrey Baker went with him but was drowned. After hauling himself aboard, Gillett 'at once rowed to where the nurses were in the water, and with assistance . . . managed to get six of them, including the matron [Marie Cameron], into the boat. A few Tommies were pulled on board, also two stewards.' As they were heading towards more struggling women, the boat was holed by wreckage and began to take on water: 'we had to get out three distinct times and get drowning men up to the boat. Finally . . . we had twenty-four all told.'[72] After four hours' rowing, their boat almost swamped, they were picked up by a French vessel.

As Private Bert McGregor recounted, several NZMC men were down in their quarters when the torpedo hit. 'One poor fellow had his legs blown off, while others were bruised and knocked about'; most, somehow, survived. The stairs to the deck were destroyed but as water rushed in through the hole in the ship's side 'they were floated up to the opening on top, and were able to crawl out'.[73] Gillett paid tribute to Privates Harry Pettit and Stan Clark, who 'did heroic work pulling the men up from their quarters. . . Poor [Roland] Pole, [John] Walter, and [Clarence] Perrin were blown down the hold by the explosion, and were never seen again.'[74] Gillett and Pettit, along with Corporal Francis Henderson and Lance-Corporal Melville Mirfin, were 'specially brought to notice' by Godley on 11 December for 'gallant behaviour in assisting to save the lives of others at great personal risk'.[75] Sergeant Alexander Goldsman witnessed 'some marvellous escapes' — one man survived when the raft he was clinging to was cut in two by the *Marquette*'s propeller — but also saw his mates injured and killed. Among the dead was Bob Herdman, who, like Gillett, had been in hospital on the *Marquette*.[76]

Everyone was impressed by the nurses, who, in Gillett's words, 'conducted themselves just as we knew New Zealanders would, without panic or hysterics, and some of them were in real good spirits, even after being in the water over eight hours. Everyone voted them the

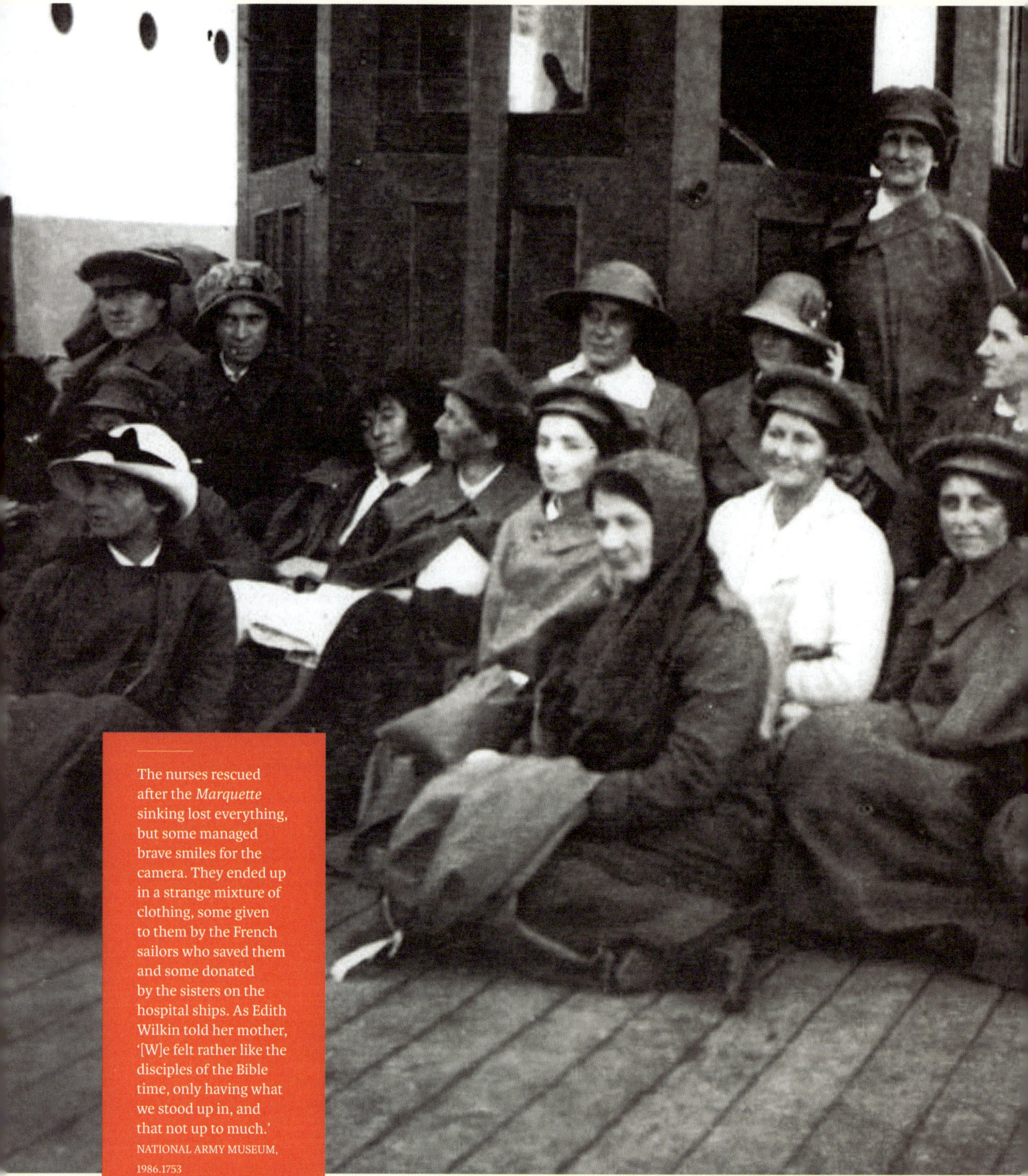

The nurses rescued after the *Marquette* sinking lost everything, but some managed brave smiles for the camera. They ended up in a strange mixture of clothing, some given to them by the French sailors who saved them and some donated by the sisters on the hospital ships. As Edith Wilkin told her mother, '[W]e felt rather like the disciples of the Bible time, only having what we stood up in, and that not up to much.'
NATIONAL ARMY MUSEUM, 1986.1753

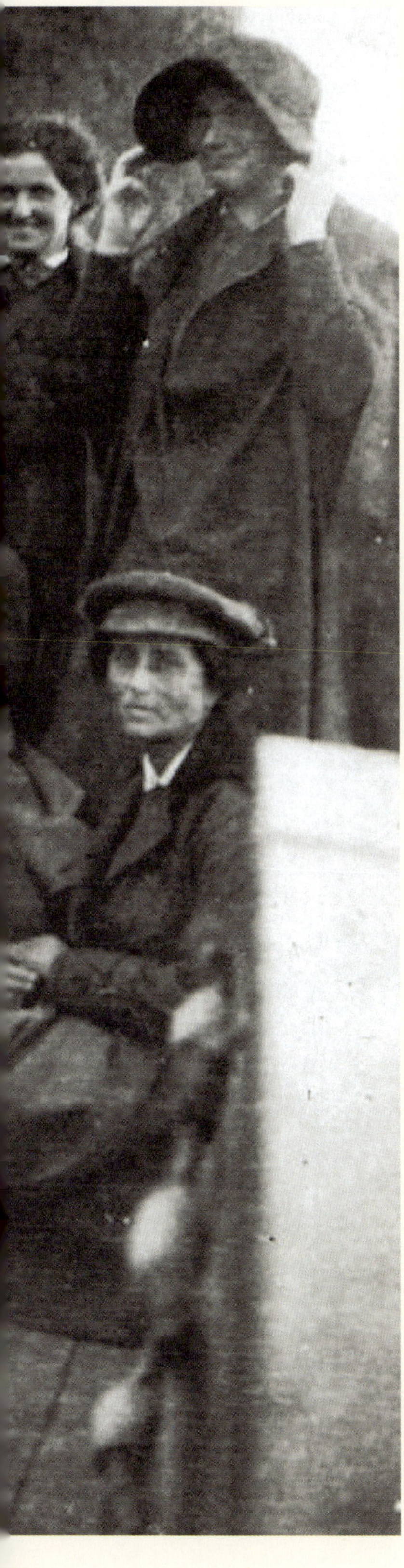

pluckiest girls they had ever met.'[77] Nona Hildyard, badly injured, was 'wonderfully merry and bright, and singing "Tipperary" and "Are We Down Hearted"', before she suffered heart failure and died in the water.[78] Mary Gorman, her legs crushed, knew she would not survive, so removed her lifejacket for someone else to use. Isabel Clark and Marion Brown held hands as they leapt into the water from the deck of the *Marquette*; both drowned.

Help was terribly slow to arrive. A faint SOS signal from the *Marquette* had been received in Salonika, but half an hour later a second message gave a different location, towards which French and British destroyers rushed. This second communication was sent from the submarine that fired the torpedo. Jeanne Sinclair, and an Englishman who had saved her life, were picked up by the French destroyer *Tirailleur*; the crew members, like those on other vessels, were kind and generous, finding coats and slippers for the women to wear. The survivors were taken to the British hospital ship *Grantully Castle* in Salonika, staffed by an English matron and Australian sisters who 'simply robbed their wardrobes on our account and did everything to brighten us up'.[79] By the end of the following day it was known that 10 New Zealand nurses had been killed: Marion Brown, Isabel Clark, Catherine Fox, Mary Gorman, Nona Hildyard, Helena Isdell, Mabel Jamieson, Mary Rae, Lorna Rattray and Margaret Rogers. Twenty-two men had been lost: 19 members of the NZMC and three infantry privates attached to No. 1 NZSH. Of the 741 on board the *Marquette*, 167 were dead and many more injured.[80]

In distant New Zealand, families and friends would only gradually learn what had happened. Understandably, the deaths of the nurses took centre stage — the recent execution by the Germans of British nurse Edith Cavell fed the outrage — but the lost men of the *Marquette*, too, were mourned around the country. The grief was made worse because the tragedy had been entirely avoidable. The staff of No. 1 NZSH should never have been on a transport carrying ammunition, a vessel which, unlike a properly marked hospital ship, was not protected by the Geneva Convention and therefore a legitimate target for U-boats. The rushed inquiry held on 26 October focused only on what happened after the sinking. Despite a great deal of speculation, no one then, or since, has been able to explain why the New Zealanders did not cross the Aegean on a hospital ship.[81]

All the NZMC officers survived, though John Leahy had injuries to an arm and a leg and Hugh Acland 'landed in Salonika in a patient's royal blue serge suit. He was most wonderfully good to the girls.' The

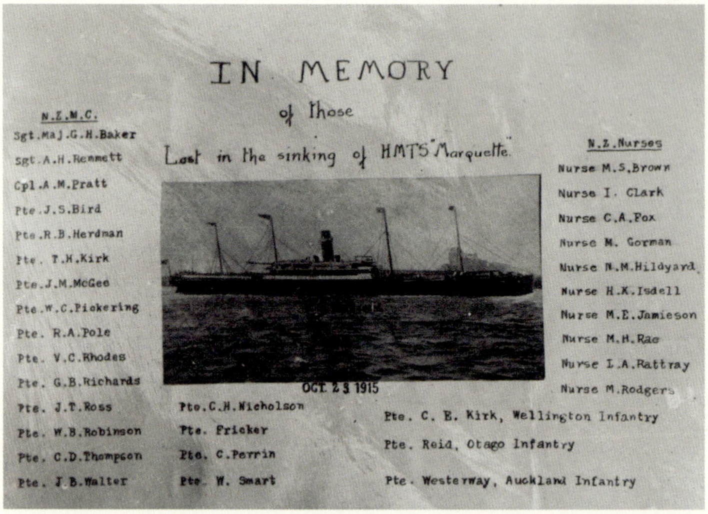

above The names of the New Zealand women and men who were lost surround a photo of the *Marquette* in this commemorative postcard produced in 1915. ALEXANDER TURNBULL LIBRARY, 1/2-000610-G

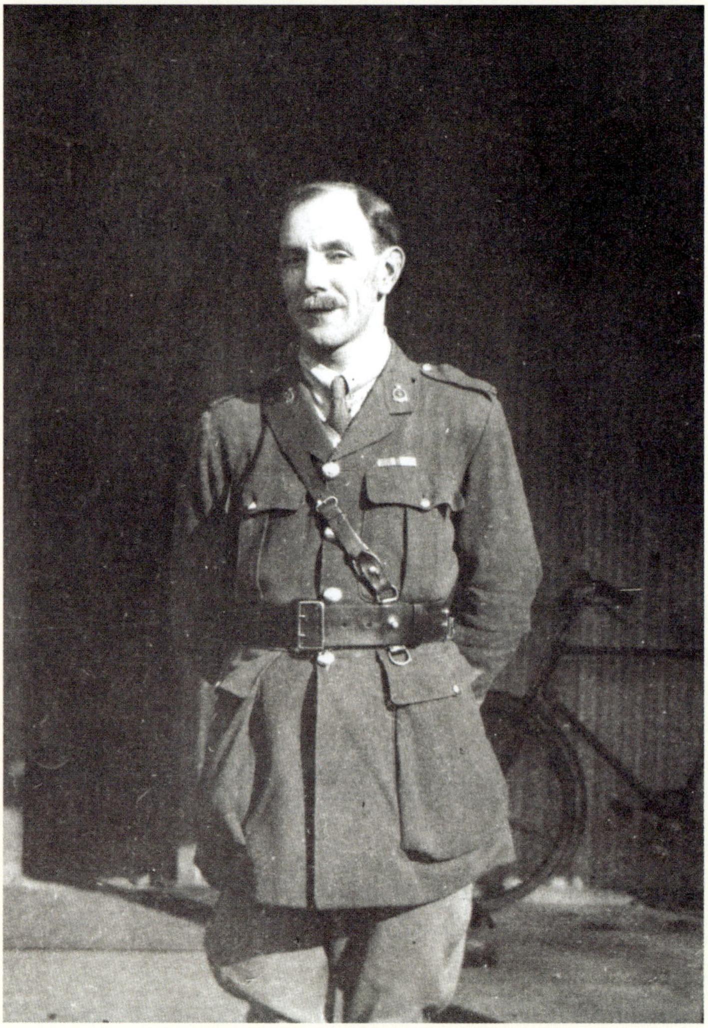

below Surgeon Thomas Duncan McGregor Stout, known as Duncan, survived the *Marquette* disaster. Fifty years later, NZMC man Lance Haggett could not praise him 'too highly . . . he got to work on me, using the then accepted method of resuscitation. I kept coming to and losing consciousness but, in the end, Dr. Stout won the battle.' Stout served with distinction in both world wars and wrote three medical volumes of the Official History of the Second World War. He is seen here at Brockenhurst in March 1919. ALEXANDER TURNBULL LIBRARY, PACOLL-10309-03-034 popular Joseph Frazerhurst, despite 'eight hours partly in the water and partly drifting in a damaged and filled boat, is quite himself again — ever busying himself about the personal comfort of his unit'.[82] The battered and bereaved hospital set about re-establishing itself. On 5 November, Captain Ebenezer Teichelmann reported that the surviving staff were finally in camp at Lembet, a few miles outside Salonika. 'I am still living [in] a few of the garments I had on when wrecked and some Red Cross things, as it is very difficult to get anything here and we have very little money . . . In a few weeks we hope to have our hospital . . . ready to receive patients, but the loss of the original one will, I am afraid, make a great difference to our future plans generally.'[83]

No. 1 NZSH was without its nurses. As Edith Popplewell explained, 'It was hoped enough of us would have been able to volunteer to remain, but only about eight were fit.' On 29 October the nurses were sent to Alexandria, along with David Wylie and Duncan Stout, who were to fetch supplies, 'with a very urgent demand from our officers that we shall be sent back again as soon as possible'. Several of the women, desperate to return, used the £50 they each received to stock up 'on woollens and every possible thing'.[84] *Marquette* survivors and nurses from the New Zealand General Hospital in Cairo were selected to make up a staff for Salonika, but it was decided that they should not go. With two or three exceptions, nevertheless, the survivors served again during the war.

'We have had a great lot of worry,' Leahy noted, 'especially when our new outfit arrived from Egypt (we lost everything), and we were acting as regimental medical officers, field ambulances, clearing stations and stationary hospital, sanitary officers, and two of our company were embarkation medical officers for supervising transfer of sick to hospital ships — 20 were in demand and our help was much appreciated by the military authorities.' The Red Cross had supplied the staff with such sorely needed items as underclothing, socks, towels, handkerchiefs, brushes, and combs, soap and pyjamas. 'I appreciated their gifts very much.'[85] Contributions from New Zealand were vital given that the hospital had lost 23 truckloads of equipment on the *Marquette*. At the New Zealand General Hospital William Parkes 'depleted our stock somewhat, handing over 200 folding iron bedsteads, an X-ray plant, and new surgical and medical panniers. Thanks to the ladies of Auckland we were fortunately able to make a really liberal contribution in bed-linen, bed-clothing, pyjamas, shirts, and the many things of hospital equipment which are so important.'[86] The money and gifts, large and small, that came from all over New Zealand were gratefully received. Louisa Godley told the Christchurch Red Cross, 'You can make us any number more [of pyjamas]. They want warm things and mufflers and balaclavas.'[87]

But No. 1 NZSH's troubles were not over. In early February 1916, to everyone's delight, a 'complete new outfit arrived in the harbour', but before the vessel could berth, it caught fire 'and every stick of the New Zealand equipment was destroyed. The holocaust included about £50 worth of luxuries, for which the men had personally subscribed.' Then 32 cases of goods from the Canterbury–Westland branch of the Red Cross were lost in a fire in another ship's hold in Salonika Harbour.[88] There was also an air raid. 'We had an exciting time,' Private Samuel Swinburne reported, 'when a German Zeppelin flew overhead and dropped five bombs, doing serious damage. The first one was dropped at the back of the doctor's marquee, some distance away . . . The doctor and myself ran outside the marquee, and the next thing I heard was a screeching sound, and another bomb landed on the top of a hill about 200 yards away. A piece of the shell fell at our feet.'[89] After the raid the hospital tents were 'painted mud-colour, and enormous Red Crosses [were] painted on the ground'.[90]

During its time in Salonika No. 1 NZSH made its mark. As one of the doctors reported, 'We started a 200-bed hospital, and now sometimes we have 700 patients, and with staff nearly 1000, which is some family to clothe and feed.'[91] It was, wrote Swinburne, 'a great sight to see forty or fifty motor ambulances drawing up in succession opposite the marquee and discharging their loads of wounded'.[92] The staff treated an impressive 6989 patients, 'including 500 eye cases and 1000 dental',[93] before, early in March, they were given just 48 hours' notice to pack up and leave. The hospital was needed in Egypt: sickness among the troops had reached alarming levels and Pont de Koubbeh was struggling to cope. After a safe journey in a hospital ship, the staff reached Port Said on 9 March, then went on to Moascar, where they took over the auxiliary hospital that had been established in January 1916. A few weeks later, No. 1 New Zealand Stationary Hospital set off again, this time for France.[94]

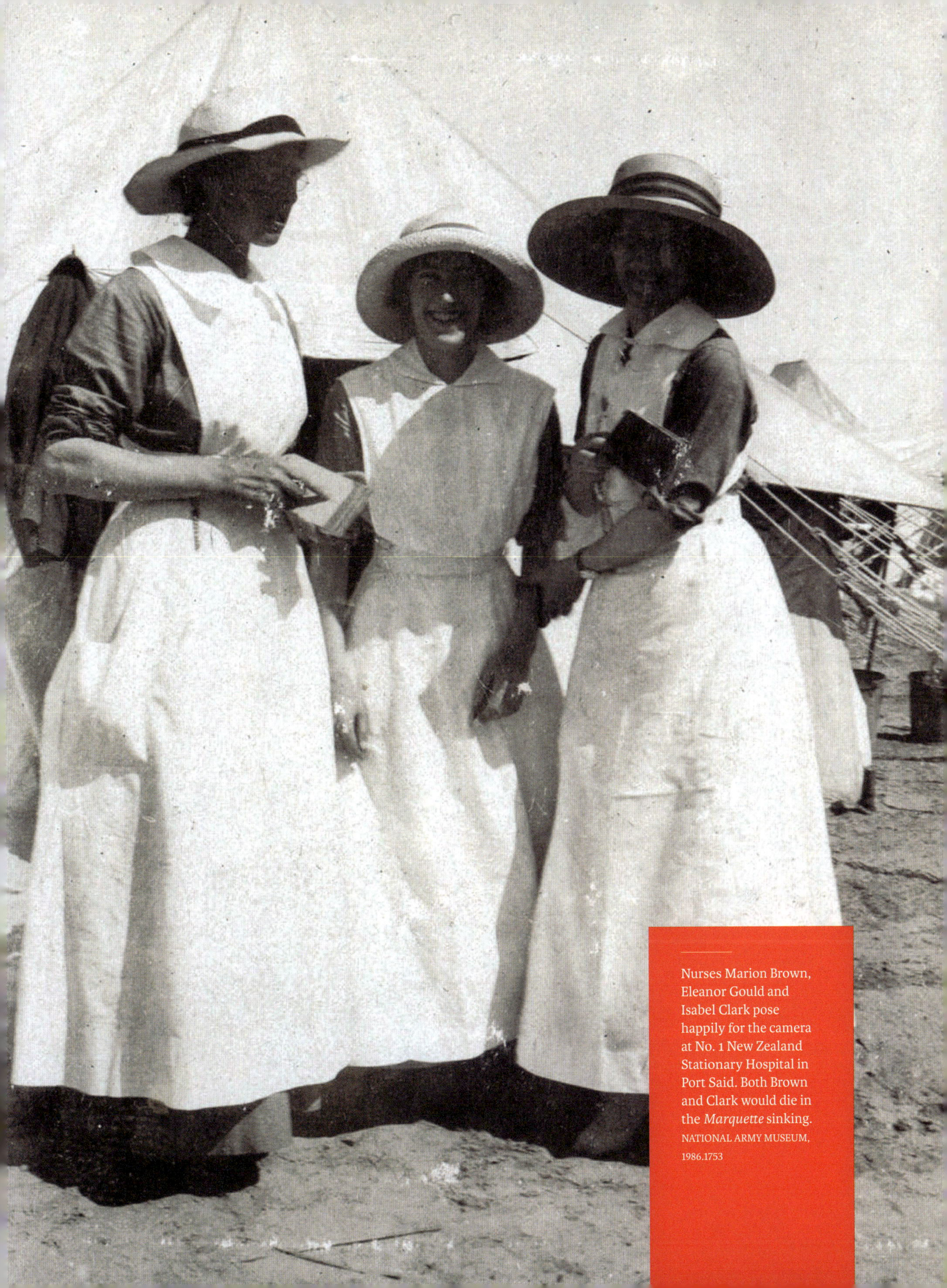

Nurses Marion Brown, Eleanor Gould and Isabel Clark pose happily for the camera at No. 1 New Zealand Stationary Hospital in Port Said. Both Brown and Clark would die in the *Marquette* sinking. NATIONAL ARMY MUSEUM, 1986.1753

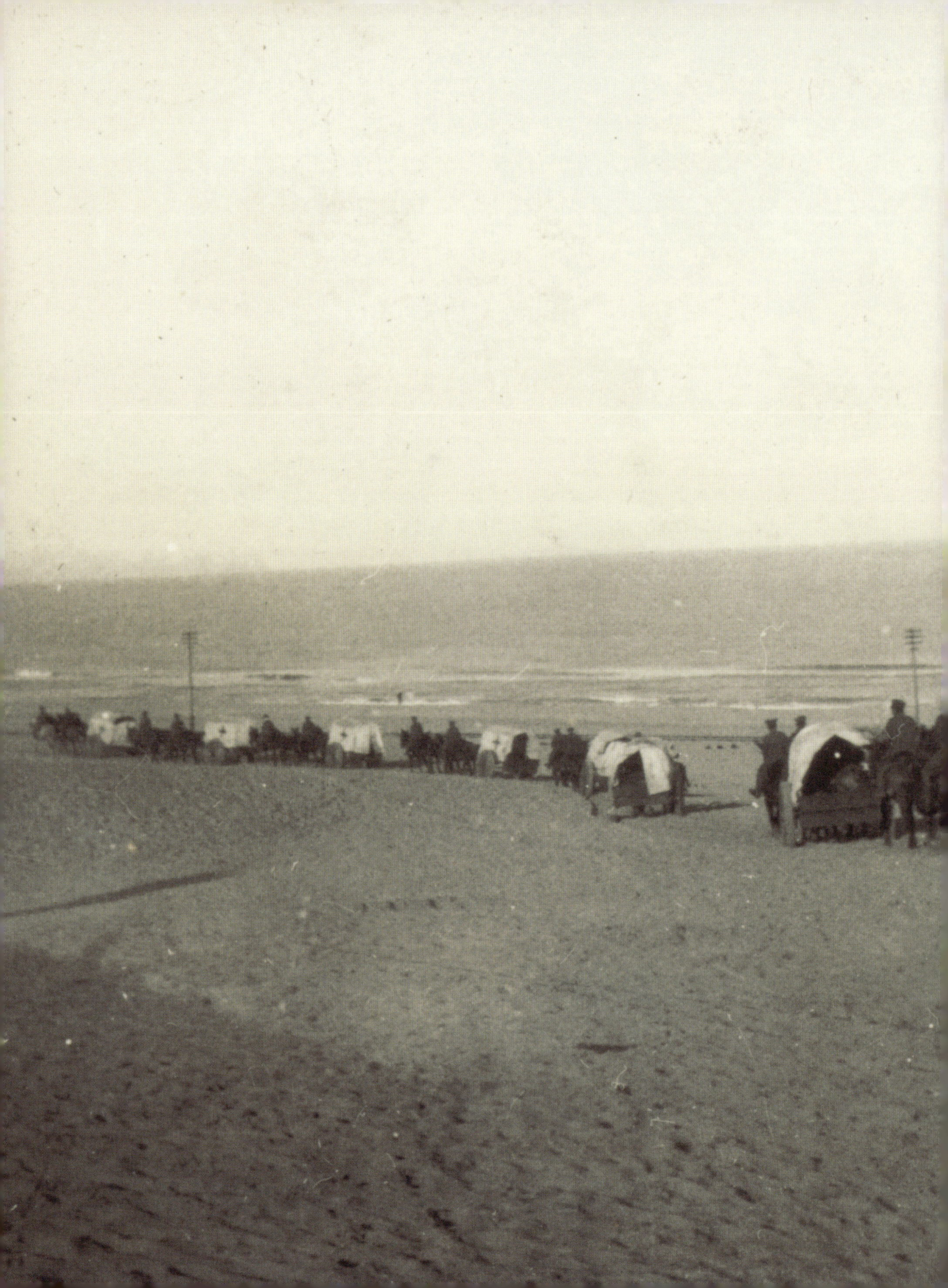

CHAPTER 5

SURVIVING IN THE SAND

SINAI AND PALESTINE

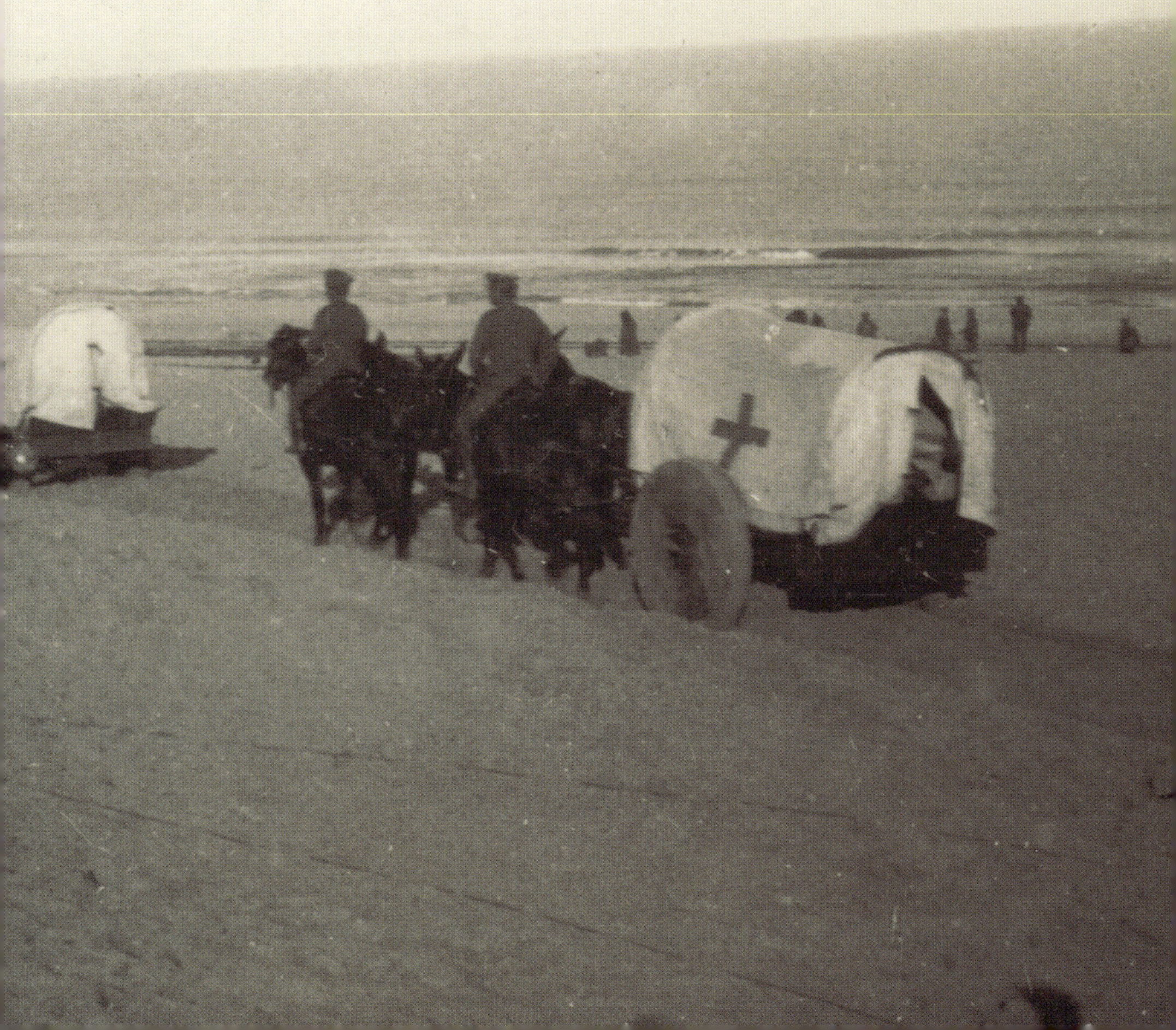

previous pages
The inhospitable environment and vast distances over which the wounded had to travel are evident in this photograph of hospital wagons in 1917.
ALEXANDER TURNBULL LIBRARY, PA1-Q-605-06-1

Can they realise what it is to be wounded under desert conditions; to be brought by rocking camel, by sled, or springly hospital-wagon some twenty or thirty miles to the nearest dressing station. The writer has had the experience and will never forget it. As a result he can the better appreciate the horrors of Dante's 'Inferno'.

— 'One of the Boys', *Evening Post*, 12 February 1918

On 12 February 1918, a letter from a returned mounted rifleman, 'One of the Boys', was published in the *Evening Post*, 'for the purpose of attempting to correct a common misunderstanding of the value of the work done by our boys in Sinai and Palestine, and particularly to point out that hardship is not unknown in that theatre of war'. Since arriving home, he had heard 'odious comparisons between the conditions prevailing in the West [France] and those in the desert'. Although his experience was 'limited to Gallipoli and the Sinai campaign as far as Palestine', he knew men with knowledge of several fronts who 'would rather spend twelve months in France than half that time in the desert'.[1]

Rather like the New Zealand troops fighting in the Pacific during the Second World War, who were often wrongly considered to be relaxing in the tropics, the mounted Anzac troops who fought the Ottoman Turks in the Middle East from April 1916 to September 1918 were sometimes dismissed as enjoying an easy life far from the 'real war' in Europe. In fact, like Gallipoli, this region was completely unsuited, geographically and climatically, both to warfare and to dealing with wounded men. Searing heat, lack of drinkable water, vast distances, the monotony of the desert landscape, problems with transport — all these, and hard fighting, made this campaign gruelling, particularly for the sick and wounded, and those caring for them.

New Zealand's mounted riflemen had fought in the Dardanelles without their horses, and the brigade was sadly diminished, and its survivors exhausted, when they returned to Egypt in December 1915. When the rest of the New Zealand Division, and of the NZMC, departed for the Western Front in April 1916, some 1800 men of the New Zealand Mounted Rifles Brigade stayed behind, as did the New Zealand Mounted Field Ambulance. Alongside the Australians

— together they became the Australian and New Zealand Mounted Division — and with the New Zealand companies of the Imperial Camel Corps, the mounted men were part of the Egyptian Expeditionary Force, which faced, and eventually defeated, the Ottoman Turks, first on the Sinai Peninsula, and then in Palestine. The campaign's main aim was to protect the vital transport route of the Suez Canal from enemy attack; the desert battles were fought in atrocious conditions.[2]

Shortage of water was significant and sometimes dangerous. In May 1916 one Canterbury officer witnessed what happened when desperate men finally reached a desert well. 'The scene here was beyond description. No one who has not suffered thirst can understand it. Men drank with their horses the brackish water out of the canvas buckets. And one bucket did not satisfy some. The look on some men's faces I never wish to see again.'[3] A reconnaissance column riding south from Romani on a day when the temperature reached 126°F by mid-morning had drunk their water, 'and their horses were in extreme distress' when they stopped to rest under some palms at a water supply. When the water proved to be foul, 'the wells had to be picketed by guards with fixed bayonets'. The medical officers at Romani had thought ahead. They loaded camels with fantasses (small copper or tin tanks) of water and headed out to help. 'Some of the men lay comatose for hours. Sand carts were brought out to them and no lives were lost, but over 50 men had to be evacuated to hospital and 500 horses remained sick for some time . . . After that, most men got hold of an extra water bottle and all possible marches were made at night.'[4]

One New Zealand soldier serving in Palestine with the Eighth Reinforcements considered that the water 'is what we would only give to the poor old cows at home, and some of it is not fit for a cow to drink'. Even the newspaper advertisers back home picked up on the conditions: 'PARCHED PALESTINE. Torrid temperatures tempt tired troops to take teaspoonfuls of refreshing "Fluenzol." Palatable and powerful in dispelling disease. Mail your boy a 1s 6d bottle.' Personal hygiene was difficult too, as Charles Malone recorded in his diary at the end of 1916: 'The greatest disadvantage of this life is the inability to wash. One had to clean his teeth, shave & wash up plate out of a mug full of water.'[5]

There were other problems here never encountered in France or Flanders, such as heatstroke and heat exhaustion. A New Zealander interviewed in Sydney on his way home to New Zealand for Christmas 1917 recalled, 'We had to wear spine-pads made of cotton wool, which covered our spine from the neck to the waist. Without this and the big helmets, there would have been hundreds of cases of sunstroke.' In his diary entry for 16 May 1916, Leslie McInnes noted that when the Canterbury Mounted Rifles returned after two days in the desert, 'Forty-five of them were sent to the hospital, forty with sunstroke.'[6]

Eyes suffered too, from the ceaseless sun reflected off the glaring sand. 'On one occasion,' wrote Frederick Foote, 'I went nearly blind for three weeks and my eyes never completely recovered.' In a sandstorm, another trooper reported, 'we cannot see more than a few yards . . . as the flying sand and dust is so thick. Our eyes get a bad time of it and become so sore that one can hardly see out of them. It is so nice drinking our tea with a thick layer of dust and chaff, and all sorts on top of it, for it is impossible to keep it off.' Sometimes, too, the men's elbows blistered 'from constant contact with the scalding sand as they fired their weapons'.[7]

Accidents involving horses were not uncommon. In August 1917 Cervantes Bell recorded two in just a few days: on the 11th, 'George Gibbs thrown today and is in a little pain', then on the 15th, 'Harry Nicholls kicked in the mouth'.[8] Bill Owers suffered a nick to his shin that turned septic and took a long time to heal. Then a frightened horse he was trying to quieten threw him to the ground, whereupon another horse kicked his chin 'and stoved all my teeth in'. The next morning 'the doctor came out and apologised: he had a straight needle instead of a crooked [curved] needle to put the stitches in. It was terrible.'[9] As Hubert Hatrick told his mother, when the wadis (valleys) became 'rushing torrents', a horse could miss its footing '& nearly drown itself & rider before getting out. All men had to remove their feet from the irons in case of accidents.' Foote witnessed a nasty sight in Egypt, when a trooper's horse 'reared up and slipped. It came down and he broke his arm and was away in hospital for a long time.' When the man returned he had 'a great bow in the forearm'.[10]

There was, also, a draining sense of isolation and boredom for those fighting in this remote area, cut off from the rest of the war and unable, like their counterparts on the Western Front, to take regular leave in France or England. After the Battle of Romani in early August 1916, Sergeant Len Armstrong MC told his parents that he was 'having a quiet time away in the middle of the desert . . . with nothing to read and nothing to do . . . We are all pretty much downhearted at being stuck out here.' 'It is true,' wrote a returned mounted man, 'that we did sometimes get to the Egyptian towns, but usually for only three days after a long spell of some months in the desert hell, where men grew so dispirited, so listless, as not to care what happened next.'[11]

Initially, the Mounted Field Ambulance, with Lieutenant-Colonel Charles Hand-Newton in charge, was made up of two sections, each with 35 NCOs and privates, plus six medical officers and 40 ASC drivers. There were ambulance and general service wagons from New Zealand, and seven motor ambulance cars were provided in Egypt, but it soon became clear that a different style of transport would be needed in the desert. The ambulance wagons, which would be useless in soft sand, were replaced by half a dozen sand carts. According to RMO Captain Ronald Orbell, a sand cart had 'two broad wheels, flooring, wire mattresses, and a Cape-cart covering [hood]. It was capable of holding two stretcher cases, and as many as five wounded men could be packed inside.'[12] Camels would also be used to carry the wounded, in a frame called a cacolet, which consisted of 'two rests resembling stretchers, strapped one on either side of a camel, and carrying two patients'.[13] There was also a sitting version, though upright cases were sometimes transported on ready-made chairs lashed to the side of a horse. The cacolets soon became notorious for the agony they caused the wounded.

Camels themselves were a challenge. They were not, in one NZMC man's words, 'quite as nicely scented as they could be. In fact one camel would beat Astley's Tannery [in Auckland] badly, so you can imagine what a few dozen are like.'[14] Asked by Hand-Newton 'to give the men a course of lectures on the camel', the recently arrived Captain George Fenwick 'gazed . . . in amazement and said that before this time, he had only seen them in zoos!' After being handed a book on their habits and care, however, he soon became the ambulance's 'leading expert on these useful but very bad tempered animals'. Hand-Newton also had to lead by example when a shortage of riding horses meant 40 of his men had to ride camels instead.[15]

It did not take the medics long to realise that even their revised transport arrangements would be challenged by the conditions. The sand carts, which needed four or even six horses to pull them through the desert, proved 'too light in construction; the square hood [marked with a Red Cross] was flimsy and soon broke away'. They did, however, prove their worth 'in two years of campaigning on all conditions of surfaces, from deep sand to glutinous mud', and when better ground conditions in Palestine led to suggestions that they be replaced, the ambulance men were reluctant to part with them.[16] But there was an effective alternative from early on: the sand sledge, which was set on wide runners and required only two horses. The prototype, devised by the Australians, consisted of a sheet of corrugated iron bent up at the front, with a wooden frame to hold a stretcher. The New Zealand MFA improved on this and designed what became the standard sledge, with 6-inch-wide runners and a hood for protection from the sun. This was much more successful, especially for seriously wounded and unconscious men — according to one observer, it moved 'with great smoothness and absence of discomfort', at least 'on level, smooth sand'.[17] The desert, however, 'was seldom other than a succession of little sandhills, blown by the strong winds into fantastic shapes and steep and often sheer gradients, and covered as a rule with little bumps of sand blown up about the stunted bushes', and the sledges' 'close contact with the ground surface indelibly impressed upon the occupant . . . the rough nature of the country'.[18]

It was difficult to find anyone who had a positive word to say about the camel cacolets, particularly the lying versions.[19] The original coffin-like cacolet was, thought Australian medical historian Graham Butler, 'perhaps the most uncomfortable form of transport ever devised'.[20] Lying in his oblong box, with his head facing the camel's head, the patient felt, when the animal rose to its feet, hind legs first, as if he were about to fall headlong to the ground. Some men experienced nausea, and even vomited, as the camel moved off, and severe wounds such as fractured hips caused indescribable pain throughout what was often a lengthy journey. Later cacolets were something of an improvement, but they remained a 'distressing mode of conveyance'.[21]

Foote described the 'gruelling time' faced by a wounded man. 'These stretchers would sway, rock and swing as the camel's rolling gait took him across the sand for twenty-four, thirty-six or even forty-eight hours.'[22] One Australian observer suggested that a Blighty, a wound bad enough for evacuation, longed for on the Western Front, where transport was reasonably efficient and hospitals were relatively close, was more feared than desired in the desert. 'In the fierce heat and with flies in thousands, the sufferings of the wounded were of a nature not to be written about. Wounded men, in dread of the cacolet and the sledges, pleaded to be allowed to take their chance on their horses. There are at least two cases of troopers who rode six miles or more in the saddle with a fractured thigh; and one of them did not die!'[23] A. H. Wilkie, in his official history of the Wellington Mounted Rifles, reported 'one instance at

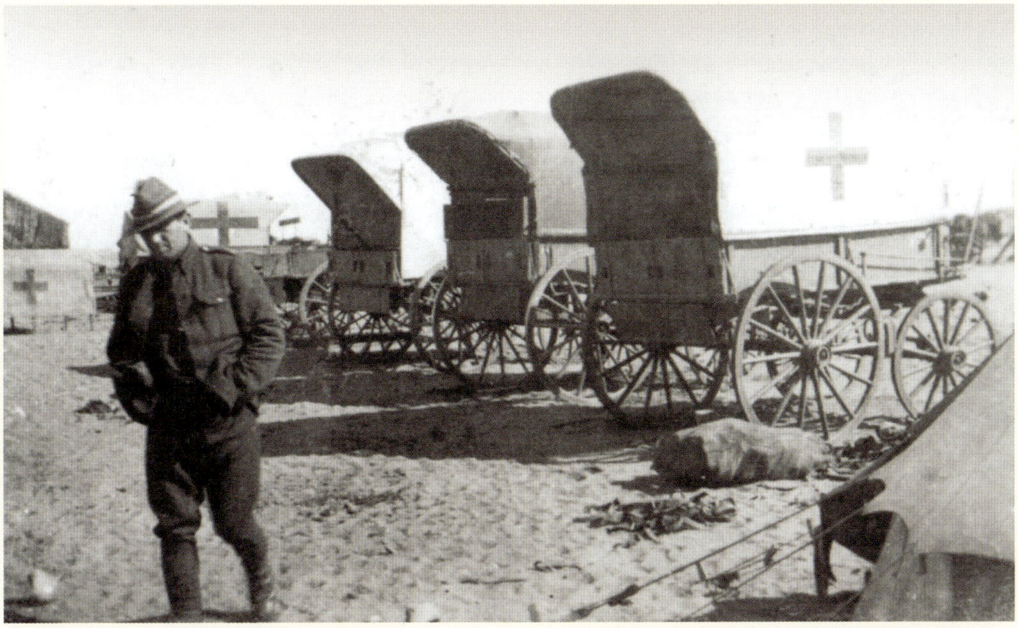

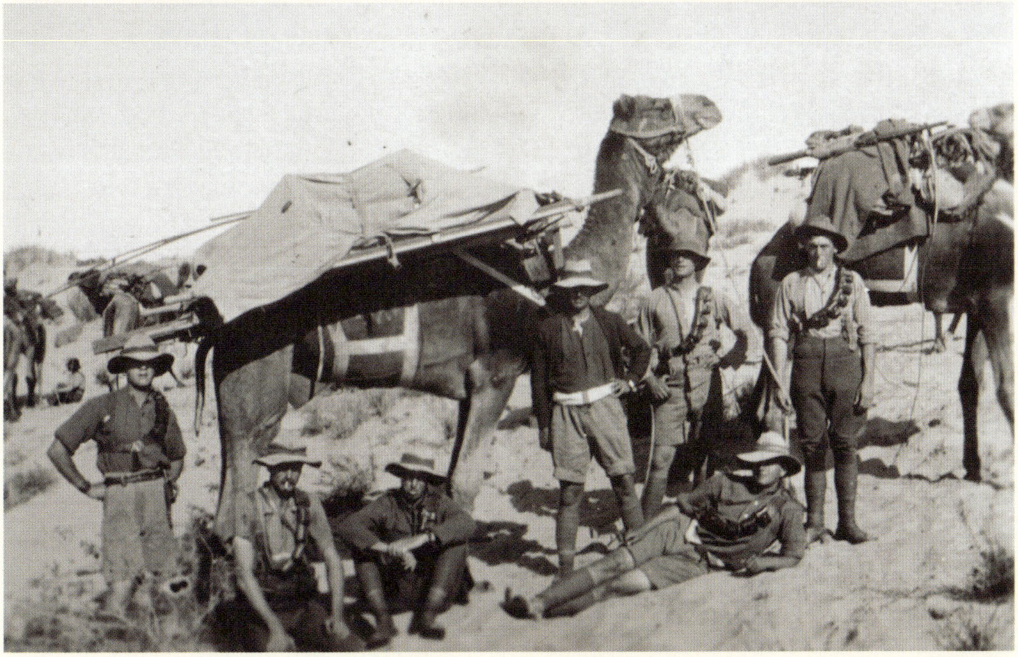

above Wheeled ambulances, like these in the NZMC lines at Zeitoun, were not always a successful means of transport in the desert sand. NATIONAL ARMY MUSEUM, 1992.763

below Being condemned to travel in a cacolet lashed to a camel struck fear into badly wounded men's hearts — they knew the agony that lay ahead. ALEXANDER TURNBULL LIBRARY, PACOLL-6222-12 least . . . of a N.C.O. with a broken thigh having to ride a horse for some miles. Needless to state, he died later.'[24] Following the retirement from Amman in March 1918, seriously wounded men had to be carried 10 miles over rough and slippery tracks on camel cacolets or tied to the backs of horses. This 'agonizing experience . . . was the only available means of saving their lives or preventing them from falling into the hands of the Turks.'[25]

Foote described passing wounded men strapped to camels whose suffering 'was beyond belief'. It was not uncommon for a man 'to appeal to us, if we had any feeling of mercy left in us, to take down our rifle and shoot him so that he could escape the agony of travelling any further. One of our signallers unslung his rifle and was only prevented by his mates from giving way to the appeals of a wounded Australian.' The 'people in charge did all that was possible and gave the wounded every consideration and help', but 'the country we had to travel over, put the wheeled vehicles of those days beyond consideration', and the distances to be covered were considerable: 'We were thirty to one hundred miles or more, out in Turk territory and the wounded had to be given transport . . . We were always many miles ahead of roads and rail, usually around fifty miles but sometimes much more.'[26]

The MFA had planned the familiar style of evacuation. The wounded would be taken to a collecting post, then carried by stretcher-bearers to the RAP for assessment by an RMO. If further treatment was required, this would be provided by field ambulance men at an ADS. From there, for serious cases requiring hospitalisation, motorised or horse-drawn ambulances would take over. Once the wounded reached a railhead, they would be sent to the clearing hospital at the Suez Canal and then on to Port Said, Cairo or Alexandria.[27] But it was frequently impossible, in this hostile environment, to make the usual pattern fit. With almost no built structures available, cover for RAPs and ADSs was at a premium. Initially at least, in the perhaps harsh view of one returned man, 'The medical arrangements were totally inadequate.'[28]

Former bushman Garry Clunie avoided a cacolet but faced a tough journey after he was shot in the left shoulder in August 1916. He had to walk 1½ miles to the horses, then ride some 25 miles to camp, where he arrived at 10 p.m., eight hours after he was hit. After a cup of tea and a sleep, he was taken next morning to the railhead, where his wounds were 'properly dressed'. At 11 that night he was put on a train to Kantara, reaching a CCS there two hours later. He turned in at 2.30 a.m., and the following morning a hospital train finally got him to No. 27 General Hospital in Cairo.[29]

When farmer Fred Dill of the Auckland Mounted Rifles was shot through the lung at the Battle of Rafa in January 1917, he put his survival down to being put 'on a home-made stretcher — a piece of canvas with poles on each side — on the cold sand, and that coagulated the blood and stopped bleeding'. Placed with the men who were obviously going to die, Dill had his dressing changed in the morning but no one was game to move him because of the nature of his wound. It was three days before he was placed in an 'awful rough' camel cart and taken to a Scottish dressing station, where he remained for 10 days. Then he endured a 100-mile train journey to a Kantara dressing station before being taken to a Suez hospital.[30]

On 14 November 1917, soon after the victory over the Turks at Gaza, Frederick Foote was badly wounded by a sniper, who hit his right elbow and then his left upper arm, somehow managing to miss an artery. 'My elbow was completely blown out, the shattered bones were protruding. I was badly shocked and kept falling down with my elbow hanging in the dust and dirt . . . The [regimental] doctor had no equipment for applying dressings to wounds, as it had all been used.' Under shrapnel fire, he staggered towards a dressing station, where he was given a dressing, a sling and a restorative cup of soup. When it was dark, Foote was placed on a stretcher covered with a rug and then, for some 24 hours, 'lay on the floor of a "press the pedal" Tin Liz [Ford] van, with five others sharing the floor with me. We travelled all night . . . I was semi conscious, the jolts, lurching bangs and bumps gave us the torments of the devil; the two beside me died that night and escaped further torture.' When they reached a railhead and a field hospital, he and his companions were taken into a tent theatre — 'a rough table, two Doctors, some orderlies assistants, stretchers all over the floor. Some one asked if they would put me out and one doctor said he would have a look first. He cut some bandage and said, "Whack him out." I woke up back in a marquee ward.'[31]

Foote could remember little of the ensuing train journey to the Suez Canal, which he was taken across by ambulance before being put onto an Egyptian hospital train. Like many wounded men, he was embarrassed by the fresh linen on the train: 'Everything seemed so clean. To us the cleanliness and beauty of that long railway carriage, with its lovely white beds, was overpowering. It seemed a sort of sacrilege to put our unwashed bodies and dirty matted hair in those beautiful sheets and on those lovely pillows.' Foote never forgot the kindness of the sister in charge, 'a middle aged to elderly angel dressed in white'. He was 'in a very low physical state. I was semi delirious, my one arm was in a terrible state, it was so swollen that the wound on the elbow would be twelve inches across.' Foote passed through hospitals in Palestine and Kantara before reaching 27 General on 19 November.[32]

Wounded men welcomed the end of all this travelling. After Charles Sommerville was wounded in the wrist and the shin on 26 March 1917, he experienced a sand cart, a motor ambulance, two hospital trains and a hospital boat along the canal before, on 5 April, reaching No. 31 General Hospital near Port Said, 'where I hope we will be settled down for a while until we mend up a bit'.[33] He remained there until he was discharged on 21 May. Sommerville would die of wounds at Jericho on 2 April 1918.

By early May 1916, midday temperatures reached 110°F in the shade. On the 16th the thermometer hit 117°F, and that was in the MFA's coolest double tent.[34] The combination of pitiless sun and insufficient water soon led to heat exhaustion and heatstroke, especially as the men had to ride, reconnoitre and fight in these conditions. As Ronald Orbell recalled, the situation was 'very trying'.

> The men had to plough their way through soft sand with the heat anywhere from 100 to 120 degrees. The only water supply was carried in bottles and, as a fierce thirst developed rapidly under such conditions, supplies were soon exhausted . . . When it was remembered that a soldier had to carry a rifle, a bandolier, 150 rounds of ammunition, a water bottle, bayonet,

> and haversack, weighing altogether between sixty and seventy pounds, some idea could be formed of the hardships that had to be endured.[35]

The stretcher-bearers, too, initially had to stagger through the sand, until New Zealand decided to follow the Australian example and provide them with horses and mules. Writing from El Arish in February 1917, Aucklander Fred Crum explained, 'I am stretcher bearing now. Got my own horse & have to lead another, a pack horse. The pack on it keeps bumping my moke & then both go mad.'[36] Camels were tried but proved 'too slow and too conspicuous'. Regulation stretchers were too cumbersome to carry on horseback: 'the need of a lighter pattern, or a folding type, was keenly felt by the regimental stretcher bearers.'[37] The light bamboo stretchers introduced later were a great improvement.

By the middle of June 1916, the MFA had reorganised itself. Each cavalry ambulance now formed a mobile section made up of a tent subdivision and a mounted bearer subdivision; this accompanied the troops into action. There were eight sand carts — the only wheeled transport — with 32 draught horses to pull them, plus 10 lying and 15 sitting cacolets. (The numbers would be altered with further reorganisations: Carbery referred to the mounted ambulance transport as 'the never to be settled question'.)[38] The immobile section, in which the remaining personnel served, was responsible for most of the heavy equipment. Mobile could be an elastic term. When a specially organised mobile section of the MFA left Richon-Le-Zion on 13 March 1918, it consisted of five officers, 35 NZMC men, an ASC farrier and four signallers (with a heliograph and lamps), plus six light horsed ambulance wagons, four sand carts, 24 cacolet camels, 37 baggage camels and 10 water-carrying camels. The 'bare essentials' medical equipment comprised 'the most necessary panniers of the Tent Subdivision; extra dressings and splintage, medical comforts, 80 blankets, a Soyer's stove, and a few other stores' — along with one operating and five circular tents.[39]

The Battle of Romani on 3–4 August 1916 brought more lessons for the ambulance men: stretchers proved so hard to carry that they never reached the firing line, and improvised replacements were inadequate; communications had been problematical; bearers were not always in the right place at the right time; because they were slow and constituted 'a very large target', cacolet camels were no good near the front line (though the sledges were); and there was a shortage of the 'indispensable' sand carts.[40]

Although, in such open country, 'bullet predominated over shell injuries',[41] the desert was a perilous place for both the medical men and their patients. During the Battle of Romani, Captain George Wood, who before the war had been a doctor in St Andrews, south of Timaru, and was now RMO to the Wellington Mounted Rifles, was dressing wounds alongside his orderly when both men were fatally wounded. Wood died in Cairo on 11 August; he would be mentioned in despatches posthumously in October. There was danger, too, from the air. On 25 July 1916, not long before Romani, a German plane dropped a 'polite note' to warn the ambulance personnel that their Red Cross flags were 'not sufficiently visible from the air'. In response, the men drew large crosses in the sand near the dressing stations, which Allied aircraft reported could be clearly seen from 7000 feet.[42] Such chivalry was not universal. In

Palestine, early on the morning of 1 November 1918, two enemy planes apparently deliberately bombed a collecting station at which wounded were still arriving, despite 'prominently displayed' Red Cross flags and an absence of fighting troops in the immediate area. 'Bullets and bomb fragments penetrated the tents and bivouacs, tore even the red cross flags, but, by strange providence, the only casualties were one wounded again hit, and one mule killed.'[43]

As they had on Gallipoli, and as their colleagues were on the Western Front, the medical men worked hard and selflessly in the Middle East. On 24 December 1916, after the Battle of Magdhaba, the New Zealand MFA tended to 170 men in 12 hours before, at midday, dispatching the wounded in a convoy of sand carts, sledges and the dreaded cacolet camels, which kept breaking down. The wounded suffered severely during the freezing night that followed, and two died. Not until 4 a.m. on Christmas Day did the exhausted ambulance men complete the handover of their charges at El Arish.[44] As Fred Crum told his mother, 'I was driving in the ambulance waggons, and as we had had no sleep for two nights prior to the scrap, I slept thro' most of it while the chance offered.'[45]

In Orbell's view, 'one of the great difficulties was to get possession of the wounded'.[46] In a hostile landscape, bearers sometimes had to comb a battlefield for wounded in the darkness and removing the casualties to safety could be hazardous. The New Zealand ambulance men also tended to British troops felled by heat exhaustion and cared for Turkish wounded and sick. At the Battle of Rafa in January 1917, the medical corps and stretcher-bearers 'performed splendid work throughout the day, mostly under heavy fire, from which there was no cover'. In the post-Amman evacuation of the wounded in March 1918, stretcher-bearers were frequently hit while trying to cross an area exposed to both shell and machine-gun fire.[47]

The doctors, too, were courageous. After the war Wellington doctor John Gow was given an MC 'for distinguished service in connection with Military Operations in Egypt and Palestine'.[48] At the end of March 1918 he and two other RMOs working in a combined RAP found themselves faced with 20 to 30 wounded men who had been brought down from the firing line. With just two cacolet camels available, the doctors had to lash their patients — many of whom had serious head, chest or abdominal wounds, or broken limbs — 'face down head to tail on their horses'. More camels arrived later, but some men had to endure 'a nine mile journey to the divisional collecting station on a wild night'.[49]

Even in such grim conditions, however, humour was still possible. Charles Powles of the Canterbury Mounted Rifles recounted the story of a wounded man who was being carried by stretcher-bearers when enemy shells landed nearby. Having decided to wait for a few moments in the hope the firing would stop, the bearers put the stretcher down and threw themselves on the ground beside it. 'Evidently this did not agree with the views of their patient. Getting off the stretcher, he proceeded to leg it at a pace the stretcher bearers had no chance of improving on, in the direction of the nearest dressing station. The look of disgust on [their] faces . . . can be better imagined than described.'[50]

As 1916 wore on, sickness became more prevalent: each week between September and November, an average of 12 to 14 men per 1000 fell ill.[51] Dysentery made an appearance and cholera, which had afflicted the Turks, was a concern for the Anzac troops. As Orbell noted, 'The greatest difficulty was experienced in preventing the men from drinking well water, which was particularly dangerous on account of the cholera prevailing among the Turks, who might have used the same water.' Wells were 'pinked' (treated with potassium permanganate), chlorinated or labelled as unsafe. As Charles Powles noted, the Turks marked wells and areas that were a cholera risk: 'These notices were written in both Turkish and English.'[52]

Camping on clean ground and assiduous inoculation prevented more than a modest outbreak of cholera among the New Zealanders. Expert help was at hand to check for disease. Lieutenant-Colonel C. J. Martin, of the Australian Army Medical Corps, who commanded the Military Bacteriological Laboratory in Alexandria, established a temporary bacteriological laboratory which later became the Anzac Field Laboratory. This could test for diseases ranging from cholera and dysentery to diphtheria, malaria, gas gangrene and typhus, and even anthrax in horses. It ensured, too, that wounded men were given anti-tetanus injections.[53] The incidence of VD rose after men went to Alexandria or Port Said on leave.

The Mounted Division's sanitary section did its best to provide facilities for bathing and lice removal, though the latter was difficult to achieve as the train-borne disinfestation plant could not often be brought near enough to the men, who had to rely instead on the old practice of working their fingers down the seams of their clothing or on the 'wholly futile use of N.C.I. or "Oxford" louse powder which served, not at all as a deterrent, but rather as a relish to the parasite in his blood feasting'.[54] Septic sores broke out when men received even a slight skin injury. The nature of the campaign could make it difficult to get proper treatment and the poor water quality did not help; hospitalisation was often necessary. Towards the end of 1917 there was an epidemic of skin disease, caused by their animals, among the troopers of the Imperial Camel Corps. As their historian recorded, 'in one section only one man kept free from the infection. Sometimes the points of irritation turned septic, and men were seen with the whole of both of their arms bandaged on this account.'[55]

There was some respite from the atrocious conditions. Early in May 1917, with assistance from the ubiquitous and indispensable Red Cross, the immobile section of the New Zealand Mounted Field Ambulance, under the command of Major Alexander Trotter, set up a tented Anzac Rest Station on the shores of the Mediterranean near Khan Yunis, in what is now the Gaza Strip. Here, for 10-day periods, weary Anzacs could enjoy swimming in the sea and a much more enticing diet. In Powles' view, the station 'proved a great boon and undoubtedly saved many men from hospital who, though not ill enough to be evacuated, required a spell from the continuous strain and work. Many of the cases of sickness at this time were nothing more nor less than exhaustion, both physical and mental.'[56] The longed-for delight of a Mediterranean swim did not end happily for ambulance man William Vaile from Mangapai when he visited the rest camp. He drowned on 10 July 1917 while bathing at nearby Rafa. A court of inquiry found that no blame could be attached to any individual. Vaile had just turned 21.

Conditions in the Middle East were always challenging, but never more so than during the summer and early autumn of 1918, which the Anzac Mounted Division spent in the Jordan Valley. One Australian journalist described it as 'the threshold of hell . . . With a shade temperature which ranges from 108 at the foothills to from 115 to 120 at the water's edge, the valley is a distressing area in which to exist in peace. Even the Arabs evacuate it during the hot season . . . The heavy dust rides all day in a still and evil atmosphere.'[57] Spiders, centipedes, flies and 6-inch-long scorpions produced painful bites and stings that could easily turn septic, especially in debilitated men whose diet lacked fresh produce — one returned man spoke of the shortage of food and 'famine of vegetables' caused by transport difficulties.[58]

The diet bore a strong resemblance to the inadequate Gallipoli rations: 'tinned beef and stale — very stale — bread or biscuits, and jam, with sometimes a little cheese and a handful of dates'. Len Armstrong described 'living on bully beef and biscuits'.[59] Lack of proper sleep and rest also took a toll. 'We were,' wrote Frederick Foote, 'driven beyond endurance . . . I can remember feeling so weak and tired from lack of sleep that it was an effort to get on and off my horse . . . Riding, riding, day and night battles, and more riding, our eyes were sore, a bath or swim was a thing of the past. We had not seen enough water to wash our faces for four weeks.'[60] Haggard with strain, exhausted men fell asleep as they rode. 'One doses off in the saddle very easily,' wrote Charles Malone, '& several times I woke with a start to find myself falling off.'[61]

Maintaining sanitation was difficult. Although human and horse waste was burnt, and anti-mosquito teams were always on the job, still sickness came: sandfly fever (caused by the insect's bite), five-day fever, stomach disorders of all kinds.[62] New Zealand nurse Eileen Nelson, working at No. 32 British hospital in Basra, suffered 12 days of sandfly fever, with a temperature of 105°F for two days and a raging headache. 'It is like glorified influenza, the fever only lasts three or four days, but it leaves you feeling like nothing on earth.'[63] Arthur Ames 'took sick' at Amman. 'I became so weak that I could not saddle my horse, and fell down in a kind of faint. I reported to the doctor, who told me I had interitis, whatever that may be.'[64]

Most destructive, though, was malaria. The Jordan Valley, with its streams and marshes, was notorious for the mosquitoes that caused malignant malaria. 'The men attacked were suddenly prostrated in high fever . . . and they were often delirious and occasionally maniacal. Unless treated immediately and efficiently with quinine the mortality was high.' Overseen by Major Charles Hercus of the NZMC, a 1000-man working party drained marshes, 'as far as the enemy would permit', cleared streams and cut and burnt out reeds. They also cleared the jungle, filled in waterholes and oiled stagnant pools to kill mosquito larvae as they rose to the surface. This work, and the maintenance work that followed, made an appreciable difference; it was 'hordes of peculiarly aggressive and blood-thirsty mosquitoes' flying in from unprotected areas and enemy lines that did the damage.[65]

An average of 80 men a week fell ill with malaria in June and in August, but from September the disease reached epidemic proportions as exhausted men succumbed. As Carbery put it, 'So ended the war against man and here began the victory of disease.'[66] The MFA dealt with more than 700 malaria cases in the first 12 days of October and the New Zealand brigade lost at least a third of its strength. It was fortunate that fighting in the Middle East ended on 31 October.

'Many a horseman dropped from the saddle during the descent to the Jordan, and many died afterwards in the hospitals in Jerusalem.' As is often the case with malaria, a lot of men suffered relapses and had to be hospitalised again, or invalided home 'with their health badly undermined'.[67] 'The poor boys used to come to us looking utterly broken and old — tremulous and shaky,' wrote Matron Mary Early at the Aotea Convalescent Home in Cairo. 'It was indeed hard to see the woeful change in our sturdy, healthy-looking men.'[68] The ambulance men were not immune. On 17 November 1918, 26-year-old Sergeant John Peat, who had been a chemist in Dargaville before the war, died of malaria at 44 Stationary Hospital in Kantara; he is buried there in the European Cemetery. There were also more than 1000 cases of influenza, mostly likely caught from Turkish prisoners.[69]

Inadequate protection against mosquitoes was probably a contributing factor. Auckland surgeon Captain Alexander Kinder returned to New Zealand from Palestine at the beginning of 1918, but he was already aware that 'the mosquito pest will be greater' in the Jordan Valley 'and there will be more malaria'. The British had effective mosquito tents. 'The New Zealander, on the other hand, merely wraps himself in his netting, or spreads it over his head, and gains very little protection.' Kinder was keen for proper tents to be made and sent as soon as possible, 'so that the troops will receive them before the really severe months of June, July, and August'.[70]

By 1918 the evacuation of sick men to hospitals in Cairo was less harrowing, as it was possible in Palestine to use motor ambulances. After being stretchered to the field ambulance, a sick man would be diagnosed and labelled with a card describing his condition. Next came the Anzac Divisional CCS, 'a little further back in the Valley, handy to the motor road'. Then began the long and dusty motor ambulance journey to Jerusalem, with four stretcher cases per car. If possible, after a day or two of treatment, one of the British CCSs there deemed him fit to travel and he went on by ambulance to Ludd, near the coast, where he could be put on a hospital train. The three- to four-hour trip to Ludd 'over very hilly, dusty roads [was] severe on a man with a high temperature'.

After the train took him to a stationary hospital at Gaza, the patient might move on, also by train, to a hospital at El Arish, then to Kantara and finally to Cairo.[71] Ames, who travelled by hospital train early in 1918, considered it a 'splendid' way to travel: 'You scarcely feel any motion, and they gave us plenty of attention and refreshments on the journey.'[72] Roy McCormack of the Auckland Mounted Rifles was

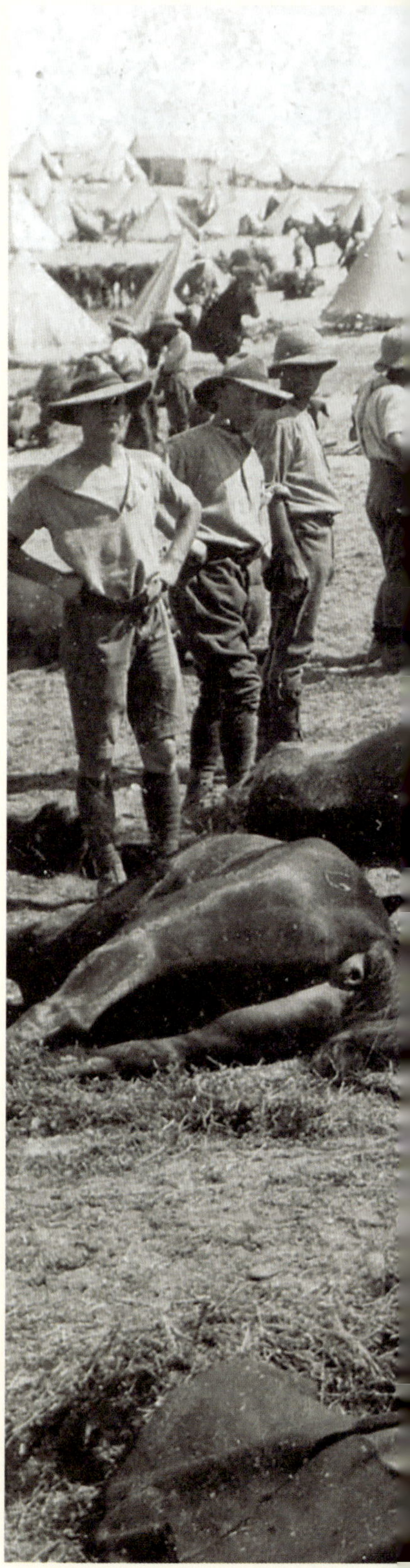

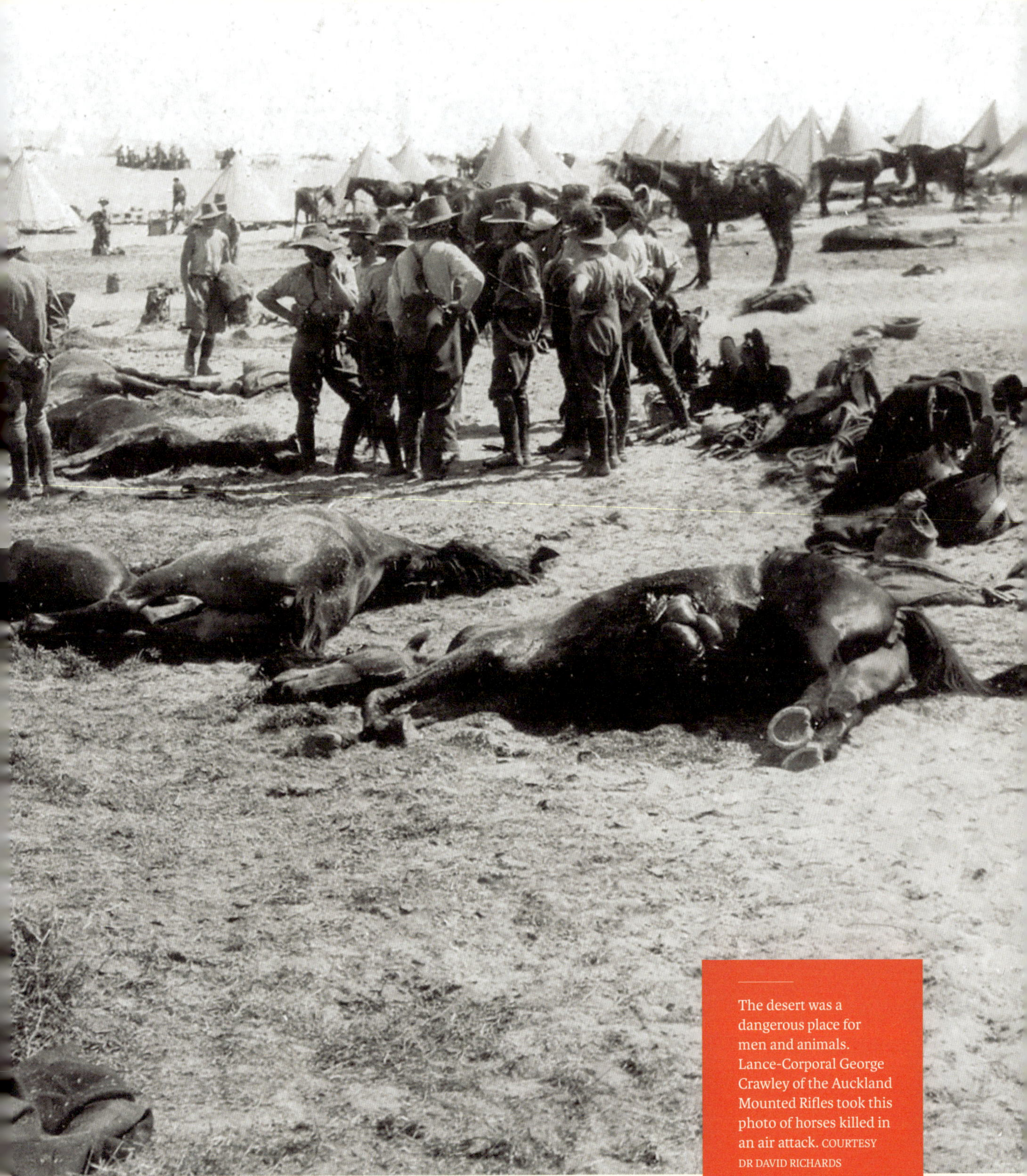

The desert was a dangerous place for men and animals. Lance-Corporal George Crawley of the Auckland Mounted Rifles took this photo of horses killed in an air attack. COURTESY DR DAVID RICHARDS less enchanted when he was evacuated to hospital with heart trouble in May 1918: there were no seats on the train and it was a rough trip.[73]

Without a hospital of their own in Egypt, sick New Zealand troopers went to a British hospital in Cairo, usually the 27th General, where Ames and McCormack were taken. The final step, before the return to the base training camp at Ismailia to regain fitness for the front line, was the Aotea Convalescent Home at Heliopolis. The men did encounter doctors and nurses from home at the British hospitals, and 'remembered gratefully' the care they were given, but 'It was often wished that a New Zealand hospital for the Mounted Riflemen had been possible, where our men could have had the invaluable care of our own New Zealand nursing sisters.'[74]

The physical and mental effects of the punishing desert campaign were clear to others, including those with experience of the Western Front. At Alexandria on 18 August 1918, as the *Maheno* boarded patients, orderly Eric Bardell noticed that 'There are very few patients suffering from wounds, but the following numbers are the results of the Palestine campaign — 410 mental patients, four wards full of venereal diseases and the T.B. ward is full. Give me France every time.'[75]

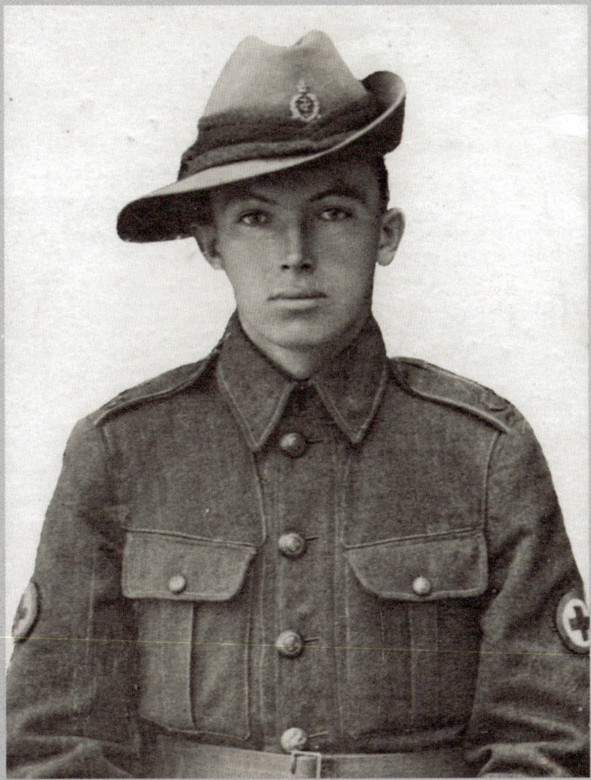

Private Fred Crum.
NATIONAL ARMY MUSEUM, 2008.37

NOT MUCH GLORY

Two NZMC men were killed and nine wounded in air raids at el Belah in May 1917. One of those who died, on the 9th, was 22-year-old Private Fred Crum from Auckland, who was hit while grooming horses. A few days later, his mate, Bugler Thomas Hartigan, wrote to Crum's family and paid a tribute to his 'constant companion'. 'The bomb dropped about 20 yards from him & one piece hit him in the arm. His first exclamation was, "Well, Tommy, I've got a backsheesh one at last." I don't think he knew for some time afterwards that he had another & more serious wound [in the abdomen] and he was unconscious just before he passed away & his last words were of all our folks at home.' As his personnel file shows, Fred Crum was no angel. He had abused an NCO, disobeyed orders several times and missed a roll-call. But he wrote home faithfully to his family, enjoyed a joke and could not speak highly enough of the nurses who cared for him. 'I always found him an upright chap,' said Hartigan, '& although at times he had his little peculiarities, I shall always be proud to know that he called me Friend. Poets & others may rave about the glorious side of War, but when a chap is alongside his pal who has been so severely wounded that there is practically no hope for him, then there does not seem much glory about that. Believe me, these things hit a chap hard.'[76]

PART 2

From Chaos to Care

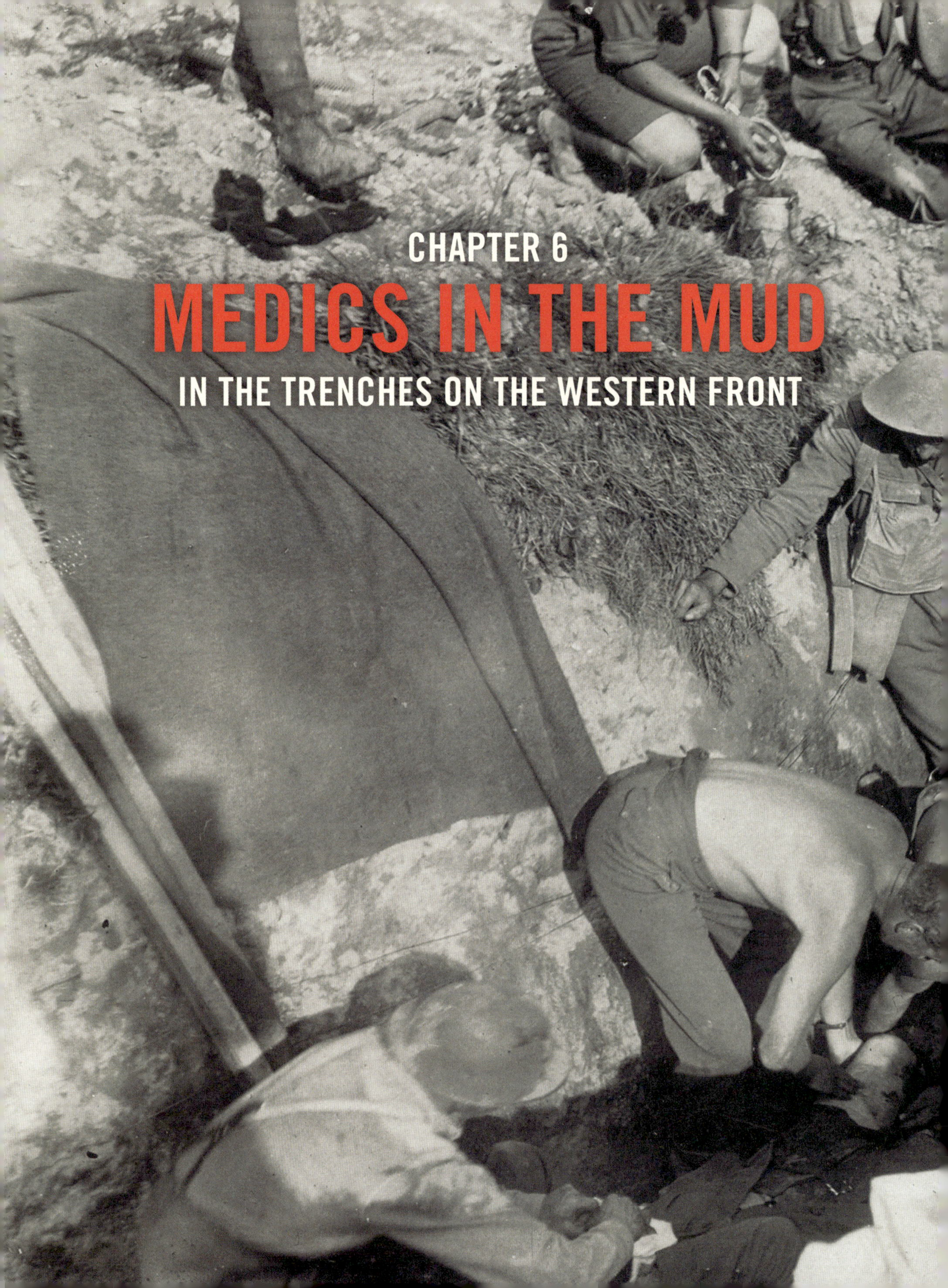

CHAPTER 6

MEDICS IN THE MUD

IN THE TRENCHES ON THE WESTERN FRONT

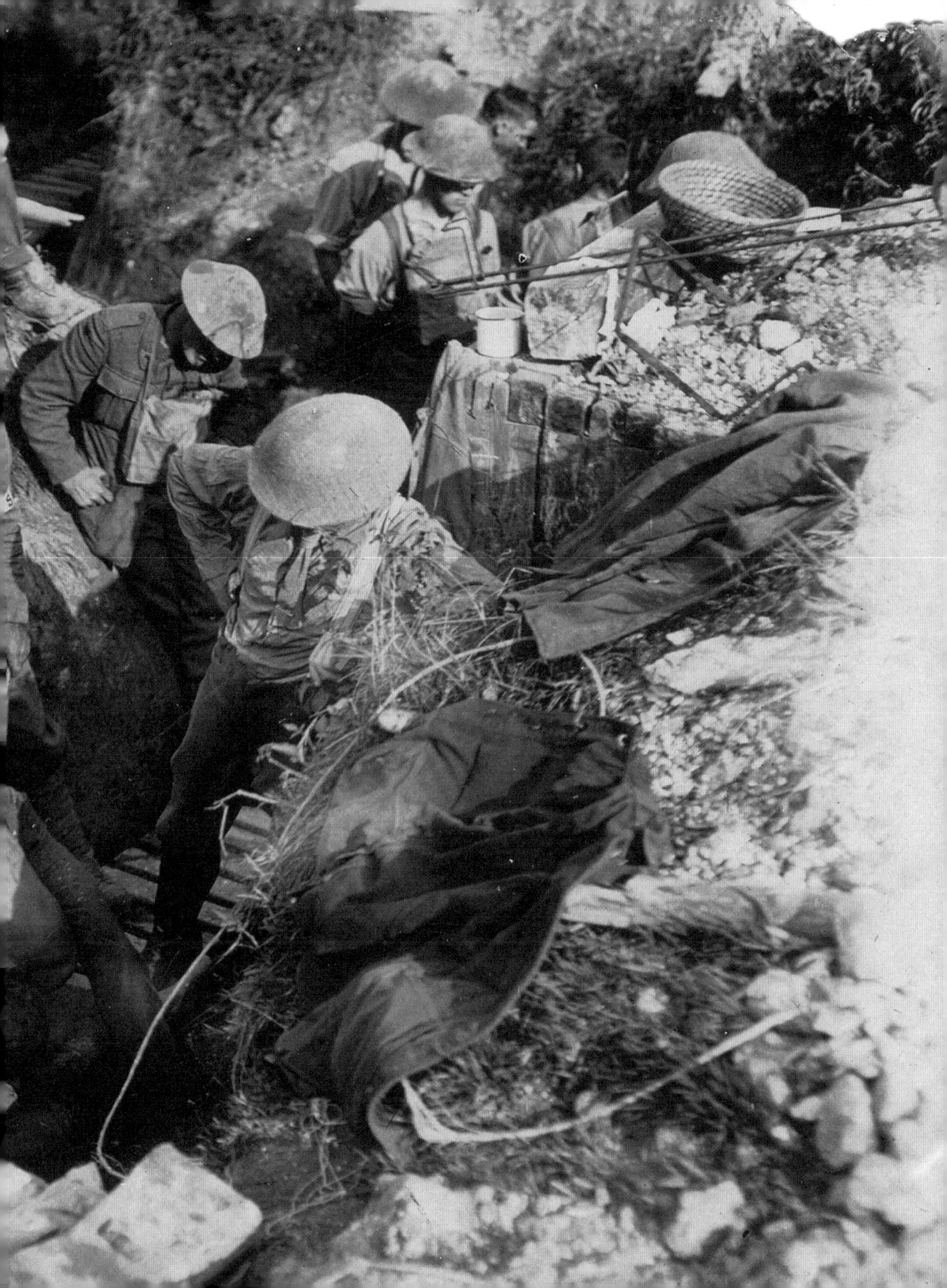

previous pages In a trench RAP, New Zealand medical men, stripped to the waist, tend to a New Zealand Rifle Brigade soldier. The photo was taken at Gommecourt on 16 July 1918. NATIONAL ARMY MUSEUM, 1993-1031, H777

> It is in the C.C.S.s and F.A. stations that the horrors are revealed. There one sees the men brought in with the mud, the filth & the vermin of the trenches still on them, with the worn-out and weary 'God help me' air of utter fed-upishness, brought on by strenuous days & sleepless nights under shell-fire.
>
> — Ned O'Neill, letter from Walton-on-Thames, 22 June 1918

On 22 November 1915, Norman Gray of No. 2 Field Ambulance, newly arrived in Egypt from New Zealand, described a daily training routine that began at 5.30 a.m. and included five 'fairly arduous' hours of drill in the desert: 'It is varied, of course, with waggon loading and lectures and is . . . bearing directly on our work.' On 31 December the medics had a field day: 'We pitched tents for an advanced dressing station and sent our bearers and signallers out to collect wounded.'[1] They were readying themselves for service in France, to which a reorganised New Zealand Division sailed in April 1916. Leaving the Mounted Field Ambulance behind to endure the Sinai–Palestine campaign, Nos 1, 2 and 3 Field Ambulances, one for each infantry brigade, under Lieutenant-Colonels Eugene O'Neill, Donald Murray and James Hardie Neil respectively, left for Europe. With them went the new Divisional Sanitary Section; the lessons of the Dardanelles were to be heeded on the Western Front. No. 3 Field Ambulance had sailed from New Zealand on 4 February and a fourth field ambulance, part of 4 Brigade, would arrive on 1 June 1917, just before the Battle of Messines. Colonel Charles Begg was now ADMS.

After landing in Marseilles, the New Zealanders saw the bright springtime green of the French countryside mostly through the windows of the trains carrying them north to the colder, wetter landscape of Flanders, near the town of Hazebrouck. O'Neill and his No. 1 Field Ambulance established their first tent subdivision at Château de Morbecque, not far from the division's headquarters at Blaringhem. Hardie Neil and No. 3 did the same at the village of Tannay, using a schoolhouse. When the No. 2 men arrived on 20 April, they based themselves at Warne. The first priority was to sort out transport and equipment. The sanitary staff and the engineers got to work, too, checking out the lie of the land, the water facilities, suitable places for building latrines and incinerators, and so on. Such matters were vital in this new environment, where the men were billeted for the first time — in farms, barns, sheds and lofts — and often crowded closely together. 'My "Bunk",' Gray reported, 'is next to the cow shed & is separated therefrom by a wall only.' At Morbecque, an ambulance man who was sleeping in a hayloft over a cow byre fell through the floor onto one of the animals.[2]

When the division moved to the front line at Armentières at the beginning of May, the transport of the field ambulances set off separately,[3] but the personnel went on foot. The French cobbles were hard on boot soles 'worn thin by constant marching over Egyptian sands',[4] and soldiers with foot trouble provided the field ambulances with some of their first Western Front 'casualties'. No. 3 found room for 200 cases at its headquarters in an Estaires convent school. The medics also suffered. William Robson of No. 2 Field Ambulance considered 1 May 'the hardest [day] of my life — and not me alone'. After marching 'thro' the livelong day with a 45lb pack' and only a few stops, by mid-afternoon 'we were all crippled. Fellows were reeling all over the road like drunk gouty old men.'[5] Feet continued to be a problem on the Western Front, and the division soon learnt the value of effective chiropody.

Early on, too, the New Zealanders established divisional rest stations for men who were not seriously ill but needed a few days away from the front line. No. 1 Field Ambulance opened such a place, for 200 soldiers, at Château de Morbecque on 18 April, and from then on a DRS for between 200 and 400 was set up behind the lines. A patient stayed for an average of 10 days and, if still not fit, was evacuated to a casualty clearing station (CCS). In November 1916 Gray was put in charge of the DRS at Nouveau Monde near Sailly, about 4 miles behind the line. 'We have about 30 huts, all with beds, mattresses etc. and about 6–10 men in each hut. Most of the cases are throats, chests, etc.'[6] As usual, there were separate arrangements for officers, in the handsomely appointed château of La Motte au Bois, further from the sounds of battle. Twenty-five officers, and their batmen, could be accommodated here, but there were only 18 in residence when future prime minister Lieutenant Sidney Holland was recovering from pleurisy in April 1917. 'I have a monstrous great brass double bed all to myself . . . We don't do a hand stir of work, simply read the "Daily Mail" . . . and walk about recuperating.'[7]

Effective inoculation, healthier men, better food produced by divisional cooks, clean water and improved sanitation prevented a repetition of the catastrophic Gallipoli enteric, and there was a manageable incidence of such illnesses as tuberculosis, pneumonia, measles and mumps — before the onset of the frightening new strain of influenza in 1918. The rich soils of France that fostered gas gangrene (see Chapter 7) also caused tetanus, although a widely used and effective serum prevented this from becoming a major problem. Scabies, which had first appeared in Samoa, was a considerable nuisance. Caused by a parasitic mite tunnelling under the skin and producing a horribly itchy rash, the condition was easy to detect but hard to treat. When Vincent Jervis, already at a convalescent camp, found he had scabies — 'I very nearly flay myself alive scratching' — it took some time to disappear following steam baths and the application of sulphur ointment. As John Moloney noted, while in isolation in England, 'Scabies is not a nice sounding complaint, so we tell our lady friends we have the "trench itch" . . . Even the best people get it.'[8]

The daily sick parade, run by the regimental medical officer, who was responsible for the health of the men in his unit — and for exposing malingerers — identified minor ailments which could be treated there and then, often with mass-produced pills. The men tended to be cynical about this system. 'Sick parades are just the same old farces,' wrote William Wilson. 'You fall in at medical inspection hut 8.10, wait in the cold until 8.20 for the corp[oral] to come and take your name etc. The Doctor arrives 8.50, has a look at you, an orderly gives you a mouthful of some medicine, and another orderly hands you 6 pills as you go out at 9am. Sick parade is over, about 30 men having been put through the mill. "Oh, oh, oh, it's a lovely war."'[9]

More serious illnesses, such as the respiratory problems and flu common in the freezing European winters, often required hospitalisation. On 11 September 1916, Clifford Collingwood was finding it hard to breathe, and when his temperature topped 103°F he was sent to a British CCS, where the doctor diagnosed pleurisy. As soon as the pain eased, he asked to return to his unit, where he improved with better food and treatment, though he remained weak and short of breath.[10] Things proved much worse for Private Stewart Callaghan, who contracted both pleurisy and pneumonia in December 1917; it later became clear that he had tuberculosis. After time in three British hospitals in France, by 23 April 1918 he was a patient in No. 2 New Zealand General Hospital at Walton-on-Thames. On 10 May, he tried to reassure his sister Tot about 'a third cable saying I was dangerously ill . . . you don't want to take any notice of them'. He had been 'pretty crook', but insisted that he was 'doing all right now'.

A year later he was back in New Zealand, but in the Featherston camp hospital: 'I am getting good treatment here now but it is a slow job getting better.' Not long after this, his father found 'poor Stewart very low . . . much worse than I thought it was possible to be . . . He said last night I will never be able to work again but I will milk the cow and chop the wood for Mum.' The folder of Callaghan's letters in the Alexander Turnbull Library ends with a handwritten note: 'On July 9th 1919 while his father was with him Stewart's last words were "Isn't it Grand."' He had just turned 23.[11]

Rates of venereal disease, particularly syphilis and gonorrhoea, continued to climb on the Western Front. The men were usually infected by British, and especially London, prostitutes while on leave, but also by Frenchwomen. Before departing for France in 1917, Reg Hird decided that 'Cairo with all its immorality [was] a heaven compared to London'.[12] Rather than send VD cases home, as had been done in 1915, docking of leave became the preferred punishment, and a weekly inspection, irreverently known as a 'dangle parade', aimed to identify those attempting to hide their infection.[13]

The alarming medical lectures continued, as did moral coercion from hopeful padres, but it became clear, as Ettie Rout had been pointing out for some time, that issuing condoms was the only sensible and practical way to combat New Zealand's embarrassingly high VD rate. Even though Salvarsan, which was administered by injection, had been discovered in 1906, the old-fashioned treatment with mercury was still used for syphilis; both of these remedies, 'though reasonably successful . . . often had unpleasant and sometimes serious side-effects, such as convulsions and jaundice'; the 'irrigation method' for dealing with gonorrhoea was 'similarly painful and undignified'.[14] Because VD often meant a lengthy stay in hospital, some still regarded it as a welcome escape from the front line. This was one reason why infected men were not sent back to New Zealand after conscription began in 1916, lest they use a dose of VD as a ticket home.[15]

'At the end of a week Guy was lousy and had lost his sense of clean superiority. Like every new chum he was shocked to find that his carcase harboured vermin.'[16] These words from *Civilian into Soldier*, by future Labour politician John A. Lee, could have been echoed by thousands of men on the Western Front. Pediculosis, or infestation by lice — and its potential to spread typhus — was 'almost universal' by the time the division reached France. More arrived with Kiwi reinforcements coming from Egypt to the base camp at Étaples.[17] Later, it was established that lice were responsible for that 'most powerful waster of armies', trench fever, which 'began suddenly with high fever, severe headache, pain on moving the eyeballs, soreness of the muscles of the legs and back' and, often, shins that were agony to touch. Full recovery could take four weeks or more.[18]

The authorities did have a larger plan to combat lice and keep the men clean: the divisional baths, laundry and disinfesting plant established in a disused linen bleach works at Pont de Nieppe beside the Lys River, opposite Armentières. Here huge vats found a new life as bathtubs, the large boilers produced abundant hot water and the remaining equipment was ideal for a laundry. Dirty clothes were washed on the ground floor by 30 local women, then taken in a lift to the next floor to dry in a steam-heated room. On the top floor the clean clothes were sorted, mended and stored. The women wielded hot irons and special steel brushes; underclothes were boiled in disinfectant. 'Roughly . . . 1200 men could bathe, be disinfested, and have their washing done in one day.'[19] William Wilson explained the process. Leaving behind their equipment, rifles and puttees, the men marched to the gates, unlaced their boots, and got 'semi-unclothed'.

> When ready within, you march through the yard in single file, are halted, ordered to undress and take your shirt, singlet, underpants, socks and towel to a window, there get clean clothes and then to the bath. These comprise just huge tubs of warm water containing plenty of Lysol and absolutely thick with soap. Here 30 or 40 men steep themselves for 10 minutes . . . then a cold shower and into your clean clothes and out through another door. Another lot swarm in the moment you get out.[20]

In France, sanitary squads moved with the brigades. Their duties were extensive. In Armentières in August 1916, for example, they

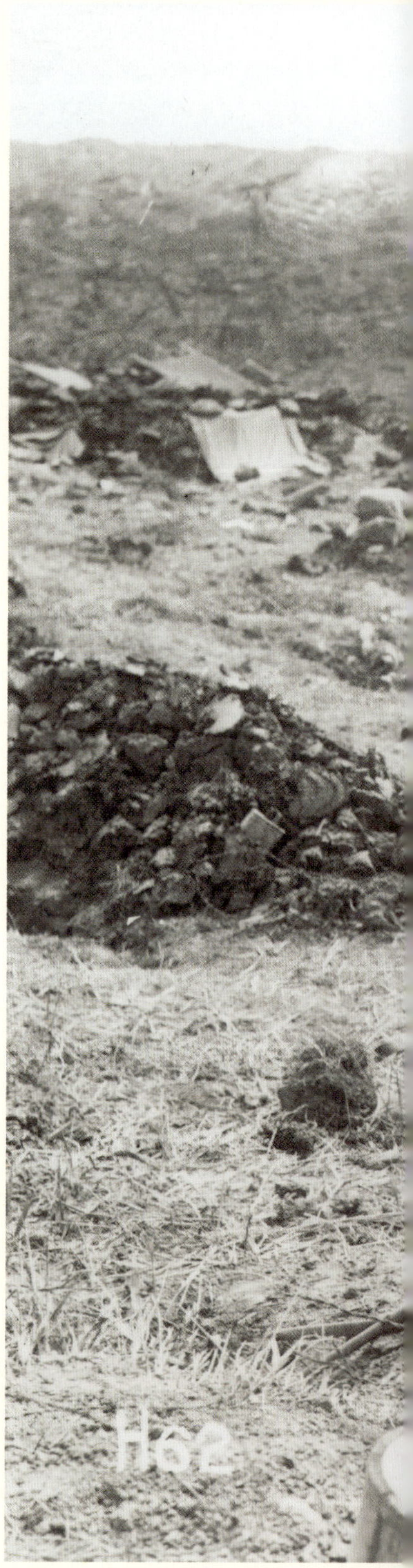

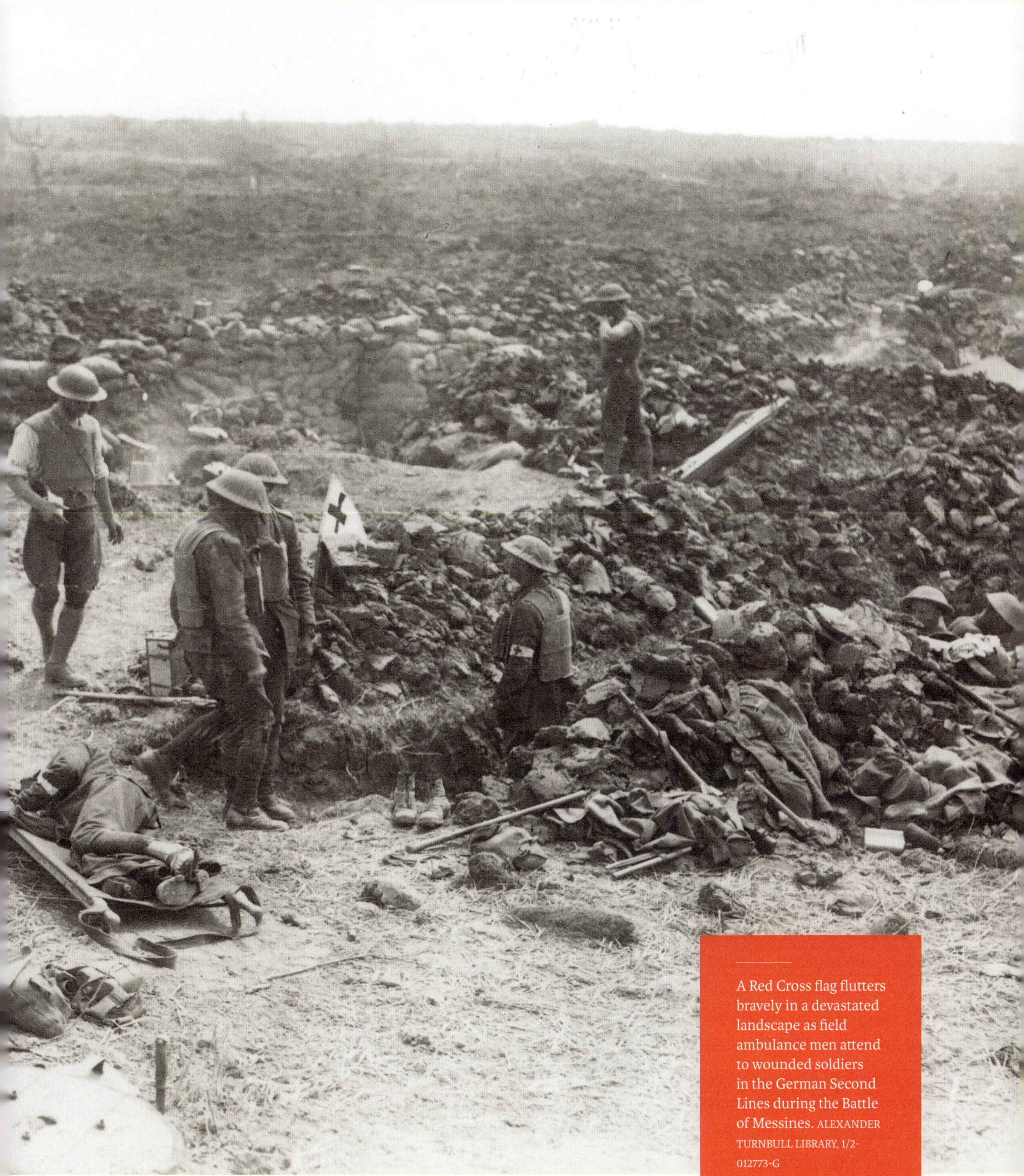

A Red Cross flag flutters bravely in a devastated landscape as field ambulance men attend to wounded soldiers in the German Second Lines during the Battle of Messines. ALEXANDER TURNBULL LIBRARY, 1/2-012773-G buried dead horses, swept streets, removed and incinerated civilian refuse, disinfected billets that had harboured infectious diseases, and inspected food vendors supplying the troops. They also checked out the much-patronised estaminets (small bars).[21] After Edward Dillon was appointed sergeant of the Sanitary Section in Armentières on 12 October, he had 'plenty of work. The place in a very bad state. Streets very dirty.' One of his tasks was fumigating houses: 'Great sport with the old girls. They don't like the Formalin and Cresol being sprayed around.'[22] The section's war diary contained diagrams of incinerators, food stores and latrines; there was even a New Zealand Divisional School of Instruction in Fly Prevention, held in April 1917. Any slackness regarding maintenance of water purity was noted by water patrol officers. Stretcher-bearers were also 'employed on Sanitary work, baths and street cleaning but were always available if required for ambulance work'.[23] Nothing, though, could banish the stench of death that hung over the trenches.

There were other health challenges on the Western Front. The unremitting din made sleeplessness 'the main cause of physical and mental exhaustion. Soldiers became suspicious, restless, unpredictable.' There could be physical damage too. Norman Hassell and a mate both went deaf and had to be hospitalised, 'during which time we had our ears thoroughly probed and sluiced out twice a day'.[24] Rheumatism was common in the damp, cold conditions, as were heart problems, many of which appeared to be more psychological than physical. During the American Civil War, Jacob Mendes Da Costa had identified a syndrome known colloquially as 'soldier's heart', in which men exhibited such symptoms as exhaustion, shortness of breath, dizziness, sweating and even chest pain, but did not prove to have heart disease. The condition, labelled in the First World War disordered action of the heart (DAH), appeared in men with no cardiac history. 'From a military point of view the illness might just as well have been fatal [since it] made a man completely unsuitable for front-line duty, and . . . almost always recurred if a soldier, apparently cured, was sent back up the line.'[25] When Trooper Roy McCormack was diagnosed with DAH in the Middle East in May 1918, 'the Dr scared me a bit telling me my heart was hardly beating & should I get out of bed result possibly dangerous'.[26]

Mercifully, the debacle of the Gallipoli medical arrangements was not duplicated in Europe. Although it could not always be followed in practice, planning for evacuation of the wounded was careful and detailed, and because trench warfare was less mobile and more structured, and British hospitals on both sides of the Channel were more accessible, the chain generally worked reasonably well. The journey from wounding to ward could, however, be long and gruelling. The relative stability of the front also made it possible to create large, semi-permanent CCSs.[27] But the ruined landscape, the treacherous mud and the unrelenting onslaught of artillery and machine-gunners made medical care demanding and difficult.

What New Zealand surgeon Arthur Martin called 'the *via dolorosa* of the wounded' often began, as it had on Gallipoli, with the casualty's mates or with stretcher-bearers, though it could be some time before the latter arrived. 'Sometimes,' wrote William Smallfield, 'the saps are blocked up for long distances by the wounded being given first-aid by their comrades.'[28]

Every soldier carried a field dressing — 'a pad of sterilized gauze with an attached bandage . . . in a compact little parcel'[29] — to apply either to his own wound, if he could manage this, or to another injured man. At Messines, Sydney Stanfield was beside a man hit by shrapnel. 'His face had gone grey and he was trembling. You take the tunic off and have a look, find out where it is and get the field dressing on it as best you can.'[30] If there was no friend to help, or if those who had given aid were forced to move on, it was essential to mark the spot clearly for the overworked bearers. Sometimes it was just too dangerous to rescue wounded men from the battlefield. Stanfield, who worked as a stretcher-bearer at Passchendaele, was haunted by a man he heard crying in no man's land who was never found.[31]

Sometimes, as Len Coley discovered, more than a field dressing was required. When his friend Mac MacIntyre, wounded at Messines, had a leg 'hanging by a sinew or two', Coley 'wrapped a tourniquet above his knee and cut the sinews with my knife'. MacIntyre did not survive, but another mate did. Seeing that his forearm had been almost severed, Sergeant Sandy Weir 'coolly and quickly put the butt of the handle of his clasp knife in his mouth, pulled out the blade with the fingers of his good arm and slashed through the remaining tendons'. He then bent down, retrieved his amputated hand, shook it and said, 'Goodbye, mate, you've served me well.' Weir allowed Coley to tie a tourniquet around his injured arm and bind the stump. 'I admired his bravery, and he admired my handiwork. We both fainted.'[32]

After being wounded at Passchendaele, Claude Weston put an arm around a mate's neck 'and with my stick struggled on'. A few moments later a lance-corporal 'with two fingers shot away . . . very kindly turned himself into a crutch on the other side'.[33] When he was hit in the leg by shrapnel in March 1918, Ormond Burton found a friend who was 'walking well . . . but was deeply concussed. So we teamed up together . . . Between us we made one efficient soldier.' Badly wounded men, buoyed up by 'battle inebriation', could sometimes manage to walk considerable distances, until exhaustion compelled them to become stretcher cases.[34] Those with arm or even shin fractures could manage without a stretcher, but femoral fractures usually left the wounded helpless unless bearers could reach them.[35]

Regimental stretcher-bearers were the first official medical help on the scene. They were part of the field ambulance, a 250-man medical unit attached to each infantry brigade.[36] At the beginning of the war, bearers were often men from regimental bands or those unsuited to heavy labour, but 'experience soon changed this approach and both friend and foe selected strong fit men for this gruelling and responsible work'.[37] Christchurch teacher Harry Baverstock had his femur shattered on the Somme about 2 p.m. on a Saturday. In terrible pain, he waited several hours until two bearers from the Hauraki Company found him. 'Having put me in a shallow funk-hole, they turned me on my back, ripped out the field dressings from inside my tunic, cut open my trouser leg and bound the bandages round the wound, a gaping hole . . . All the while, they were being sniped at.' (Bearers often worked at night to avoid being fired on.) They left for Flers to get a stretcher but Baverstock never saw them again: 'Whether those brave Medical Corps chaps were killed I could not say.' He would not be discovered by two more bearers, with a stretcher, until early on the Monday morning.[38]

However a wounded man reached it, his first stop was the regimental aid post (RAP) just behind the front line. In May 1916 Norman Gray saw five RAPs in Armentières: 'They are only 500–700 yds. from the firing line & consequently need to have cellars and other subterranean refuges when the shells come along.'[39] At an aid post an RMO examined the wound or wounds, replaced field dressings with clean bandages and, if necessary, gave morphine for pain or shock. An orderly attached to the soldier's uniform a tag giving details of his injury and an indication of its seriousness.[40] Work at an RAP could be fast and furious. 'Wounds dressed with all speed!' Burton wrote at the Somme. 'A swift assessment made as to whether a man should stagger on, or be a stretcher case. If the latter, on to a stretcher — we had a pile handy — and moved to one side. Another, and another, and another!'[41]

Haste did not preclude kindness. Dr James Crawshaw had taken only a couple of sips of his hot cocoa when he spotted wounded William Taylor. '"Here," he said. "Drink out of this side. You need it more than me. I'll get another one."' At an RAP in Ploegsteert Wood, a badly hurt Clifford Collingwood encountered MO Philip Benham. The anti-tetanus injection was usually administered to the chest, but Collingwood asked for the arm. 'I was grateful when he agreed. He was very kind and gently turned me over on to my back. I heard him say to his assistant "What an awful mess he is in" . . . He then placed my leg in splints, and I was given two drinks here, and felt much better.' When Collingwood left, Benham 'came out . . . and watched while I was placed on the trolley. As we moved off, I waved my hand in farewell to him, and he answered with a smile.'[42]

RAPs on the Western Front, as on Gallipoli, were often just dug-outs or took advantage of such existing structures as captured German pillboxes (concrete guard posts). At Armentières in 1916, MO Herbert Hutson's RAP, about 500 yards behind the front line, was 'a dug-out made up of several rooms, the largest of which was the dressing room, where all sick and wounded were treated . . . [It] was not proof against any of the heavier shells. There was just sufficient room for a person of average height to stand up in.'[43] Although they were strong, German pillboxes could prove problematical because their narrow entrance prevented stretchers being taken inside, and their solid construction made widening the opening very difficult. The solution was to build, on the lee side, a kind of lean-to, with a corrugated iron roof covered in sandbags and a protective sandbag wall. On the night of 4 October 1917, during the Third Battle of Ypres, Captain Richard (Dicky) Barron, RMO of the 3rd Battalion Canterbury Mounted Rifles, crammed 180 men into a pillbox at Abraham Heights.[44]

Next came the advanced dressing station (ADS), further back from the front line, to which the wounded man was carried on his stretcher, or assisted to walk, by field ambulance bearers who travelled along a communicating trench or sap. Here a doctor, with the assistance of orderlies, focused on halting blood loss, applying splints, preventing shock, rapidly stitching wounds and giving morphine[45] — and made decisions. There were three categories: minor wounds, hopeless cases and 'severe but survivable', who could be helped by surgery.[46] Patients in the first group were given hot soup or coffee and made as comfortable as possible before being taken, usually by ambulance, to the main dressing station (MDS). Although an ADS was not the place for serious operating, the work there could be demanding. In the dug-out ADS at Flatiron Copse near Mametz on 15 September 1916, Norman Gray and his

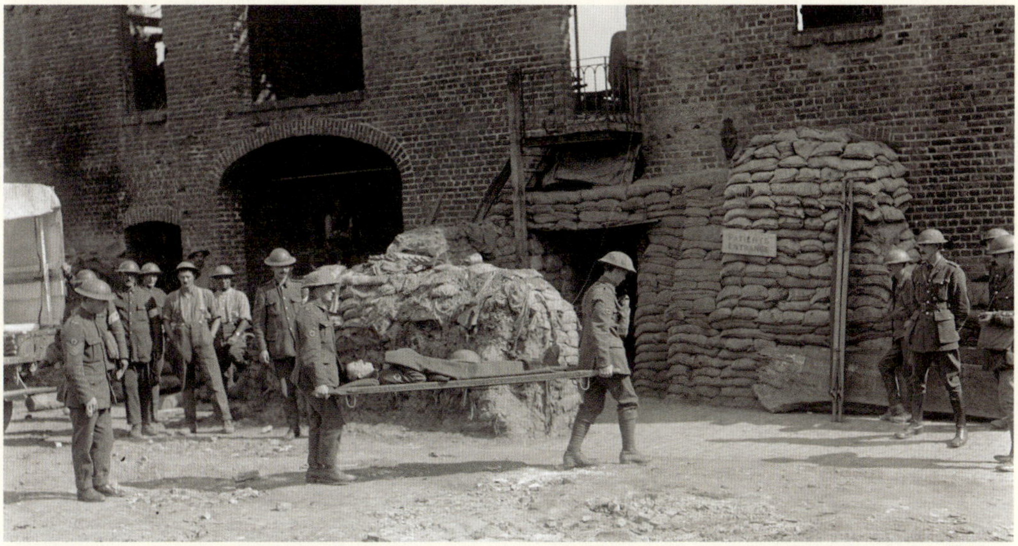

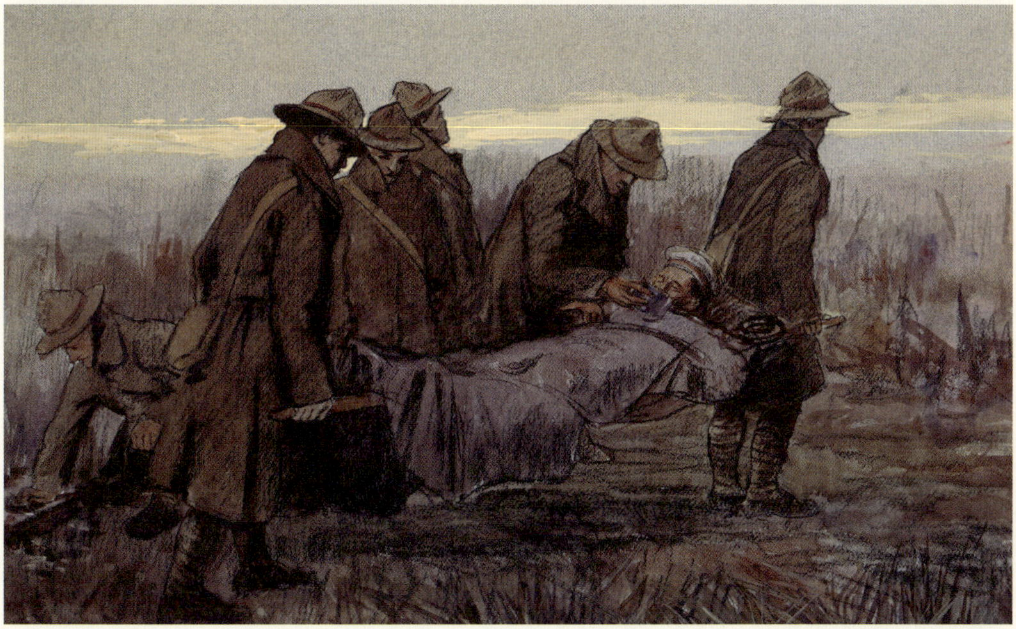

above Sandbags are piled high to protect this RAP at Warneton. Men and officers look on as another wounded soldier is brought in. ALEXANDER TURNBULL LIBRARY, 1/2-012900-G

below As stretcher-bearer Norman Gray was told in July 1915, 'You fellows must have guts of steel to tackle such a job.' George Butler's 1918 painting was titled *The Rescuers* when it appeared in the 1952 Exhibition of Official War Paintings by New Zealand Artists, but it is now known as *Stretcher Party*. NATIONAL COLLECTION OF WAR ART, AAAC 898 NCWA 473

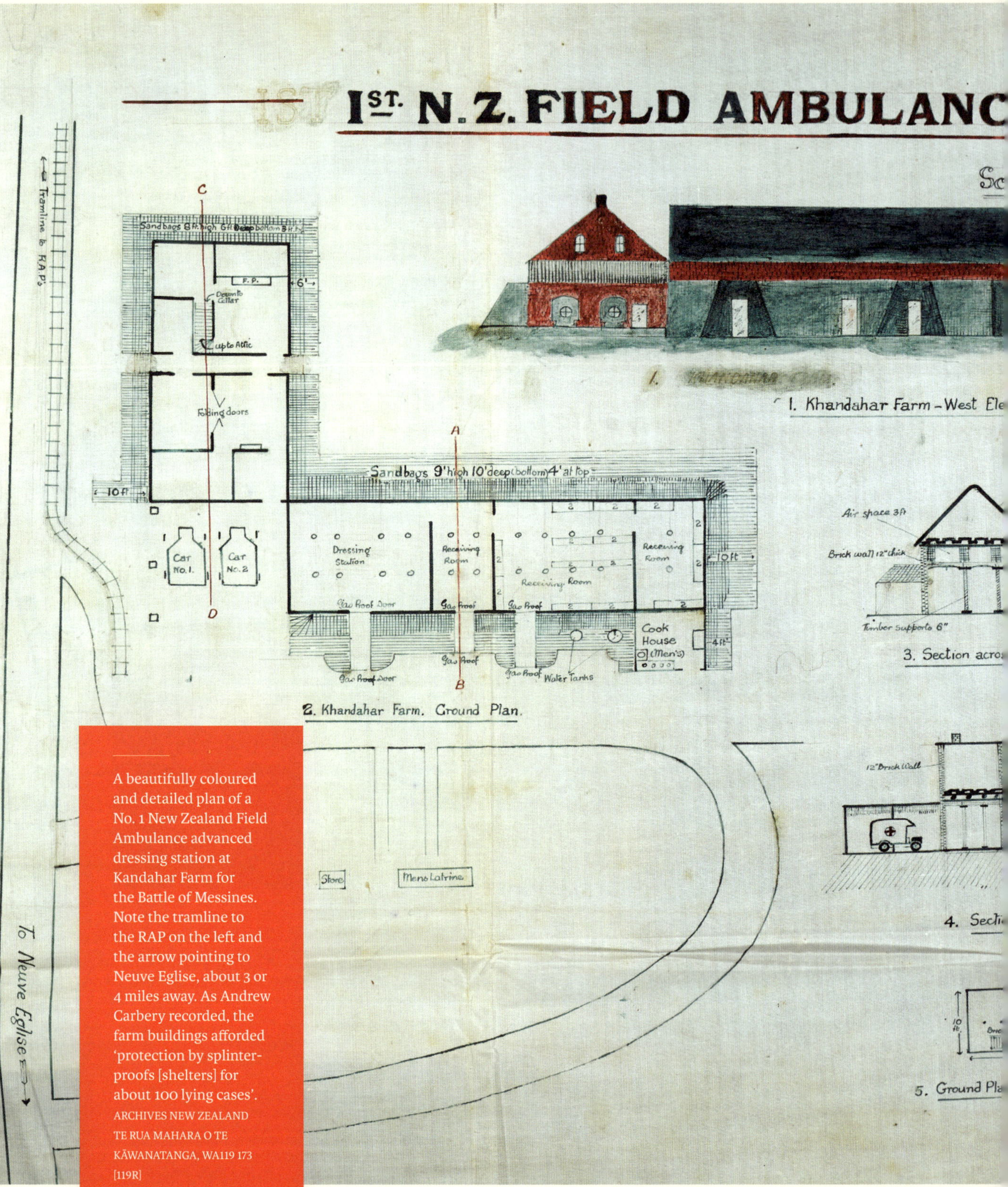

A beautifully coloured and detailed plan of a No. 1 New Zealand Field Ambulance advanced dressing station at Kandahar Farm for the Battle of Messines. Note the tramline to the RAP on the left and the arrow pointing to Neuve Eglise, about 3 or 4 miles away. As Andrew Carbery recorded, the farm buildings afforded 'protection by splinter-proofs [shelters] for about 100 lying cases'.
ARCHIVES NEW ZEALAND TE RUA MAHARA O TE KĀWANATANGA, WA119 173 [119R]

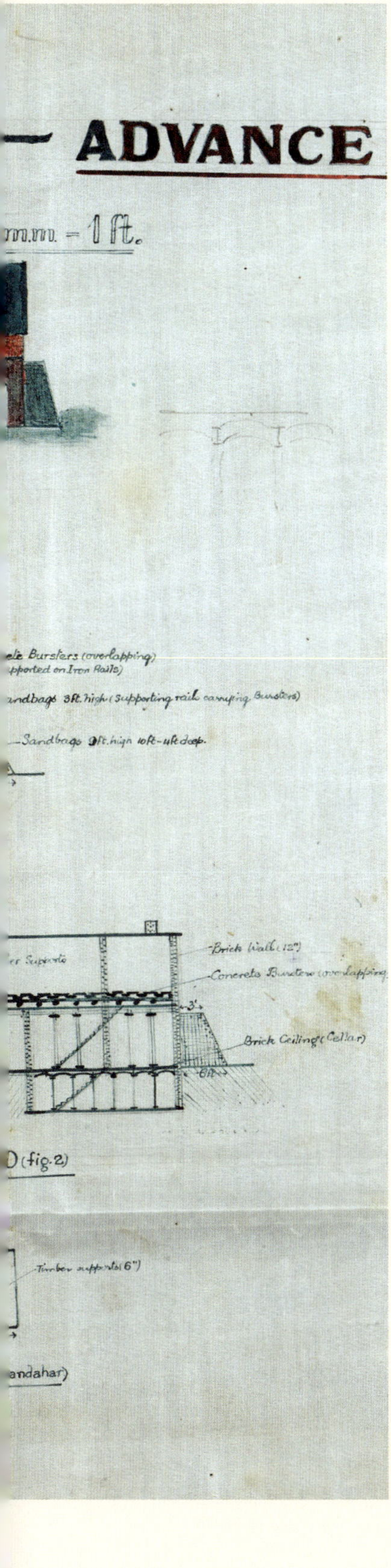

companions worked 'at full pressure', at times with wounded men arriving every three minutes. 'The Capt. in charge gave me a corner . . . and for 24 hours two orderlies and myself dressed without a stop, putting through 69 cases on our "table".'[47]

It was imperative, too, to prevent the potentially deadly effects of shock caused both by the wounds themselves and by cold. Quick, precise treatment helped with the former,[48] and warmth was essential. At ADSs improvised hot air baths were made 'by conducting heated air through a tin pipe from a primus stove into a special folding of blankets', and there were hot bottles and plenty of hot, sweet drinks.[49] When a projectile such as a shell fragment entered the body, particularly the chest or stomach, there was immediate, often copious blood loss and the assault on the patient's entire system could trigger a dramatic plunge in blood pressure and circulatory shock. Without treatment, patients 'turned pale, became cold and sweaty, then died'. The intense pain of broken bones rubbing together, in hip or pelvic wounds, could lead to coma. Even men with minor wounds could suffer from traumatic shock, often born of fear.[50]

According to official orders, operations at an MDS were 'strictly limited to the arrest of Haemorrhage and the removal of shattered limbs'. MOs were also, if possible, to remove tourniquets and ligate, or tie off, blood vessels, though this was 'often an exceedingly difficult thing to do [and] amputation was at times necessary in the case of partly devitalised limbs'. Amputations were performed by the guillotine method — without closing the skin — and patients were kept at the MDS for 24 hours after the operation.[51]

Like RAPs, dressing stations used whatever buildings, or ruins, were available. In Armentières early in May 1916, No. 2 Field Ambulance established its ADS in a big villa in the Houplines area north-east of the town. In an article for his old paper, entitled 'How It Feels to Be a Casualty', former *Dominion* journalist Corporal Arthur Field described being taken there after he was wounded by a shell in June. He wrote of 'a largish house, standing a little back from the road, with a Red Cross flag stuck in its garden railings . . . The dressing station carried on business in . . . a dim and dingy apartment, with a couple of trestle tables and the usual medical appliances.' The orderlies 'soon had my clothing cut away, a comfortable dressing bandaged on, and finally they injected an anti-tetanus serum in my arm' before Field, suitably labelled, went on to the MDS in a heavily sandbagged girls' school near the main road to Bailleul.[52] A young men's club called the Cercle St Joseph was No. 3's MDS. Once 'equipped with beds and head charts and with its white painted theatre and glittering canisters', it 'gave some impression of a modern hospital'.[53] Their ADS was in a brick kiln south of the town. When Arthur Martin was there, he slept inside 'a huge empty boiler, and, to avoid the attacks of the Huns' gas shells, [he] used to hang a towel soaked in some acid over the fire-door of the boiler'.[54] If heavy bombardment was expected, an ADS could be a more complex and extensive undertaking. One established by No. 3 Ambulance at Underhill Farm used 'elephant-iron', concrete slabs and 29,000 sandbags.[55]

For the next stage of the evacuation journey an ambulance, either horse-drawn or motorised, transported the patient to a casualty clearing station staffed by surgeons, anaesthetists and nurses, and chaplains. This was where most of the vital surgery was carried out — amputations, repairing wounds — sometimes, after major battles, at a frenetic pace, with two or more operating tables in use. As well as a theatre 'fitted up with all modern conveniences and instruments', a CCS, usually under canvas, had 'various departments': X-ray, a reception room, a pre-operative ward and a resuscitation ward, where 'patients too ill to be operated upon [were] given salines, morphia, etc.'.[56] CCSs, originally called clearing hospitals and intended as an immediate treatment link between field ambulances and base hospitals, took on a much larger role when it became clear that it was vital to operate, particularly on head and abdominal wounds, much nearer the front line.[57] Sister Ida Willis, working at a CCS in 1917, considered the process of treatment 'wonderful', and the staff's 'brightness and spirit . . . amazing, even after twenty-four hours with only pauses for meals'. With a squad of stretcher-bearers always on hand, 'no time is lost, as one case is lifted off the table another is placed on it'.[58]

From a CCS, a 'much-travelled wounded man' usually went to a hospital behind the lines or near the coast in an ambulance train.[59] Permanently staffed by doctors, nurses and orderlies, and equipped with their own pharmacies and emergency theatres, these trains could carry hundreds of patients in three-tiered cot wards. 'Talk about easy travelling!' said one man. 'That train was perfection.' Vincent Jervis, too, proclaimed it 'tres bon', but Stanley Wood found his trip to Étaples 'very jolty' and Ormond Burton had a 'miserable' journey to the same destination.[60] Because it was 'almost impossible to transfer a badly wounded man from a stretcher to a top cot without causing him acute pain', the upper tier was usually kept for less serious cases.[61] As Clara Cherry discovered while nursing on a British train, it was extremely difficult to dress 'large serious wounds, particularly fractures and amputations', when travelling at 60 miles an hour. 'It means every possible scrap of pluck the boy possesses, and every possible care and atom of patience the nurse is capable of . . . With your two feet planted firmly on the floor, knees jammed tight against the bed board, elbow, if possible, against the outer wall, you commence to work. The lotions swim over the side of the bowl, and the purpose of every other swab is lost.'[62]

To reassure anxious readers at home, in August 1916 the *New Zealand Herald* described the journey from wounding to hospital as 'smooth, expeditious, and as comfortable as this sort of progress can be'.[63] After the first days of the 1917 Ypres fighting, Donald McGavin gave a more realistic summary which revealed the manpower, physical effort and time involved. The front line was then 15 miles from the nearest CCS, and 2½ of those had to be 'covered by hand carriage'. All going well, the stretcher-bearers would take an hour to collect a case. Then came another hour of RAP treatment and perhaps a three-hour carry to the ADS, using three relays of bearers — 18 men. Then there was more delay, perhaps for a splint readjustment, dressings and 'restoratives', before embarking on the 6½ to 7 miles to the MDS, which could take at least 90 minutes, owing to the 'heavy burden of traffic on the roads'. After an hour there, a wounded man faced another 5-mile journey before he reached the CCS. On bad days, the process could be 'prolonged to possibly 24 or 36 hours'.[64] By the time a seriously ill Stewart Callaghan reached Walton-on-Thames at 4 a.m. on 20 April 1918, he had spent '24 hours jolting and jogging about in motor ambulances, boats and trains. I was fair sick of it when I landed here.' Sometimes things went well. Rifleman William Fleming was wounded in the leg at Ploegsteert Wood late in the morning of 24 June 1917 and operated on about 5 p.m. the same day.[65]

The journey to the CCS was often atrocious. Each field ambulance was supposed to have seven motor ambulance cars and three horsed ambulance wagons. The former could take 28 lying wounded, the latter 12 lying or 36 sitting cases. Initially, however, the New Zealanders had only horse-drawn vehicles, though some cars were borrowed.[66] But even though they helped to clear the wounded more quickly from the battlefield, reducing the death rate,[67] these vehicles, with their hard, narrow tyres and vestigial suspension, could be torture for the men lying on shelves. 'The cobbled roads were awful to us now,' wrote Clifford Collingwood, 'for they set up a big vibration through the whole of the ambulance, and where . . . small depressions in the surface were encountered, causing the four of us to clench our teeth and grip the sides of our stretchers in an effort to suppress the screams and moans that were at times forced from us.' After he was wounded at the Somme, William Wilson was 'bumped along over roads that made me howl with pain'.[68] An ambulance driver was in an unenviable position: more speed meant greater agony for his passengers but perhaps a better medical outcome; less speed increased the risk of getting stuck in mud or a hole and having to be pushed out. In Arthur Field's experience, the men 'handled their cars with real feeling for the men inside . . . it must require the patience of a Job'.[69]

Lance-Corporal Leslie Boyd of No. 3 Field Ambulance drove in France during the freezing winter of 1916–17. 'We didn't have any windscreens on the ambulances . . . I've gone out . . . with my heavy woollen undershirt, woollen top shirt, a cardigan, a leather jacket, my tunic and my coat on — and you could still feel the cold.' He also recalled the terrible smell when gangrene cases were aboard.[70]

Correspondent Malcolm Ross described the 'heavy strain on the ambulances' at the Somme in 1916: with 10 New Zealand cars out of action, only 21 motorised and nine horse-drawn vehicles were available. After the British transport broke down on the first afternoon, the New Zealand drivers evacuated both Tommies and Kiwis, carrying several thousand wounded men in 22 days. 'It was nerve-wracking work driving the ambulances, especially in the darkness with lights out. The drivers never quite knew when they might find themselves in a shell-hole or over a bank. The transport between Thistle Alley and the advanced dressing station was often held up by the shelling of the road, and often the ambulance drivers had to bring their wagons down through a hail of shrapnel.' The New Zealand doctors also 'made great use of the ammunition wagons that were returning empty from the field of battle'.[71]

Many cars of well-known makes, such as Ford, Morris and even Rolls-Royce and Daimler, were donated. Their bodies were adapted for use as ambulances, but not all were suitable. 'The [Siddeley-]Deasy motor cars are proving themselves very unsatisfactory,' No. 3 Field Ambulance OC Robert Guthrie reported in March 1917. 'Cars have been into workshops for following defects. Weak springs. Knocking engines. Weak differential. Weak steering arms. Spinning clutches. Loose wheel hubs and locking rings . . . If these cars are to be called upon to do any heavy work similar to the conditions which were experienced at the Somme they will assuredly fail completely.'[72]

Although the cars were usually limited to a few types to make repairs more efficient, exposure to enemy attack, harsh weather and appalling roads meant frequent replacement and incessant repair work — often in situ, as getting to a town or a workshop was impossible.[73] The New Zealand public was keen to help, and both districts and individuals did their bit. While home on leave in 1917, nurse Ethel Lewis organised Māori and European children in the Otaki district, where she had worked before the war, to raise some £700 to buy 'an up-to-date motor ambulance for the use of the Maoris at the front'.[74] As defence minister James Allen noted, as early as February 1915, 'The people seem to have gone rather wild over the presentation of motor ambulances.'[75] There was considerable confusion, however, over how many were required and who was supplying them. Allen, clearly frustrated but always polite, was forced to explain the situation several times to would-be donors and to Lord Liverpool, who headed the Red Cross in New Zealand. A 5 February 1917 reply summed things up:

> I have to state that the Government are prepared to supply all the motor ambulances that are required for the New Zealand troops, or for Hospitals in Egypt.
>
> At the same time the Government has already accepted ambulances from the Hawke's Bay district and other places, and individuals, and in such cases has placed the name of the donor on the ambulance, and has acknowledged with gratitude the patriotism displayed by those who have presented them.
>
> Should your Society, therefore, desire to secure an ambulance, the Government would be pleased to place one at their disposal, and to have the name of the donor inscribed thereon.[76]

Although both the Hague Declaration of 1899 and the Hague Convention of 1907 had forbidden its use in warfare, France, Britain and Germany all had stockpiles of chlorine. The Germans 'were the first to use gas extensively and methodically'.[77] Tear gas, also known as lachrymatory or onion gas, initially deployed in 1914, caused temporary blindness and irritated the nose and throat, but chlorine, which appeared at Ypres on 22 April 1915, and phosgene, first used on Christmas Day that year, were far more severe. And then in 1917 came dichlorodiethyl sulphide, or mustard gas.

Walter Horwell of No. 3 Field Ambulance, seconded to carry a stretcher at the Somme,[78] described what happened when 'Fritz . . . sent tear-gas shells over, mixed with H.E. [high-explosive] shells'. 'We begin to weep and put our gas-helmets on. We begin to suffocate owing to our movement, and take them off. We begin to weep again, but carry on. The tears make little lanes through the dirt on our cheeks — and truly we are a fearsome mob. The gas makes me feel crook inside, sick, spinout, for a few minutes. Sit down for a while, all right, carry on.'[79]

Chlorine reacted with water in the lungs to form hydrochloric acid, which attacked the airways, 'causing swelling and inflammation and making it almost impossible . . . to breathe. A yellowish, thin, frothy liquid was pouring from the noses and mouths of those worse affected . . . Others were suffering acute congestion of the lungs, leading to heart failure.'[80] Men were often blinded, their faces blue and panic-stricken as they felt themselves drowning in the fluid rising ever higher in their lungs. Those who struggled through the initial few hours suffered acute bronchitis and lasting lung and heart damage. Colourless, unlike the disturbing yellow-green of chlorine, and more powerful, phosgene was also an acute lung irritant that caused asphyxiation. Because its effects were often not evident until a day or even two after an attack, phosgene was more deadly, since by then it had infiltrated the respiratory organs and was almost impossible to eradicate. The Germans often used a combination of chlorine and phosgene that was known as White Star.

William Aitken was among the first horrified New Zealand MOs to witness the effects of phosgene in high concentration, at Fleurbaix on 3 February 1917. Fourteen gassed men were admitted to No. 1 Field Ambulance's MDS, and about 20 to No. 3's; all four of the cases Aitken and his colleagues treated died.[81] Young, fit men were gone within a few hours. The medics administered the prescribed treatment — oxygen, camphor and atropine — with little success. Continuous oxygen did help milder cases, but at this stage no suitable apparatus was available.[82] By the Battle of Messines in June 1917 the medical staff had light, portable Novita oxygen resuscitation sets, fitted with a two-way face piece and inhalation bag: 'the regulation of the flow of oxygen was so easily controlled that one orderly could attend to several patients simultaneously'.[83]

Gas masks and helmets were improved during the war, but such protection was of only limited use in the face of mustard gas, which was first delivered at Ypres on 12 July 1917 in an enormous barrage of yellow cross shells. (The Germans had a colour coding system for chemical weapons.) Nor, as NZMC headquarters stated optimistically in mid-July, was 'Complete protection . . . given by properly fitting blanket curtains at the entrance to dugouts.'[84] Whereas chlorine and phosgene affected the eyes and lungs, mustard gas, named for its mild odour, assaulted the entire body, inside and out. Actually an oily liquid with a low boiling point, it penetrated clothing and contaminated any foliage and soil that it touched. 'It rises out in a dense cloud,' wrote Reg Hird at Gommecourt in August 1918, 'and drifts along killing every living thing in its path.' Because it settled in ditches, trenches and puddles, troops, civilians and horses alike could easily be exposed to it. Medical staff were at particular risk: 'At advanced dressing stations cases having gas fluid on their clothes should be stripped before being taken into the station to avoid "gassing" effects on Medical Officers & Orderlies.'[85] As was proved at Passchendaele, stretcher-bearers suffered, too.

The effects of mustard gas, which became fully apparent only after a few hours — or even,

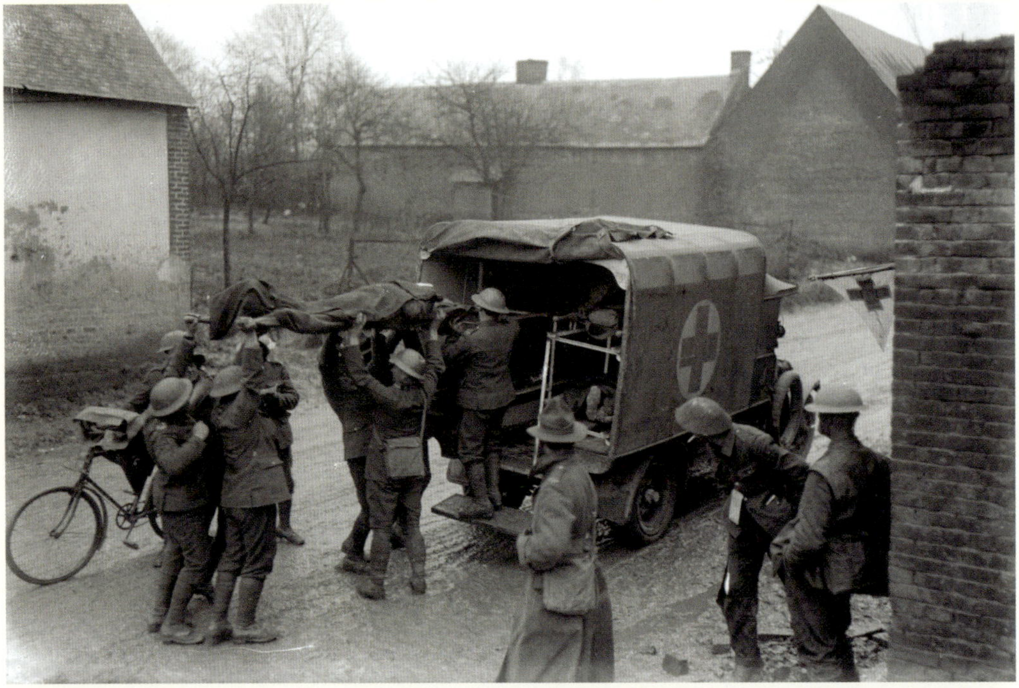

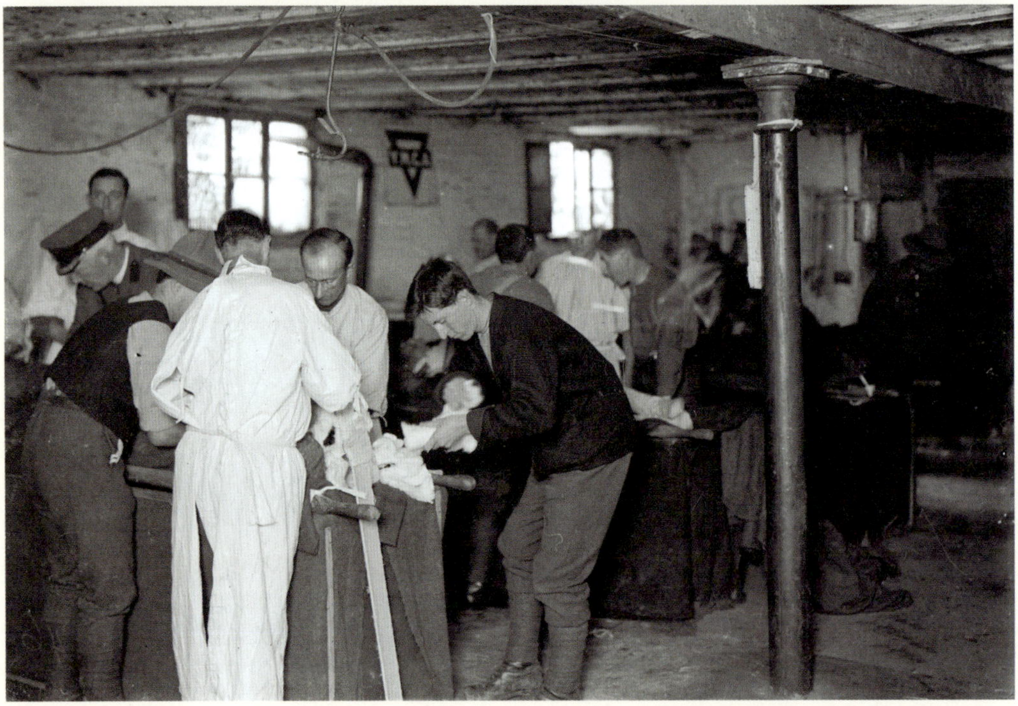

above Care is taken as wounded New Zealanders are placed in an ambulance at the Bertrancourt casualty clearing station on 6 April 1918, but their journey was likely to be bumpy and very painful. ALEXANDER TURNBULL LIBRARY, 1/2-013096-G

below The sense of urgency is palpable in this dressing station in France as a team of No. 2 Field Ambulance men works on wounded soldiers in typically makeshift surroundings. ALEXANDER TURNBULL LIBRARY, 1/1-002082-G sometimes, up to a week, with a lesser dose — were the stuff of horror stories. '[I]t began to rot the body, within and without. The skin blistered, the eyes became extremely painful, and nausea and vomiting began. Worse, the gas attacked the bronchial tubes, stripping off the mucous membrane. The pain was almost beyond endurance.'[86] The excruciating blisters on arms, legs and torsos 'could not be bandaged or dressed, nor could the patients bear any sort of blankets or bedding on top of them'. They could also become infected. If more than half a man's body was affected, 'a slow, agonizing death after four to five days of suffering was almost inevitable'. Civilians were caught too. On 28 July 1917, at Armentières, over 100 locals gassed in their cellars were admitted to the NZSH at Hazebrouck.[87]

The NZMC men at the front had recognised the new gas a week earlier. Some 20 to 30 men admitted to Nos 3 and 4 Field Ambulances were 'complaining of sore eyes and blistering of the skin where the gas fluid had made contact'. In severe cases eyelids and the membrane covering the eye were badly inflamed and swollen.[88] Second Lieutenant John Carswell was 'dosed with mustard gas' in a pillbox on Abraham Heights about midnight on 16 October 1917. Next day, '[I could] only open my eyes sufficiently to see about two feet in front of me, and several of the poor chaps were entirely blind and had to be led by the hand . . . I remained blind for nine days.'[89] Almost certainly in that same pillbox was Edwin Farrell, who was almost completely blind for six weeks until an eye specialist removed 'the fine skin that the gas had caused to envelope both eyeballs'. In January 1918 he was still suffering from 'shortness of breath on slight exertion', his eyes were 'painful in strong light', and he was suffering attacks of nausea.[90]

By October 1917 gas casualties among the Allied troops were so high that the British set up a specialist treatment centre at Brandhoek. The Australians and New Zealanders followed suit on 12 December, establishing a Corps Gas Centre at Dickebusch for all gas cases in the II ANZAC area.[91] Gas of all kinds could have lasting and unforeseen effects: for example, men who had been affected often collapsed while under anaesthetic. Earlier on, at Armentières in 1916, gas cases were given ammonia 'from special glass capsules carried by the stretcher bearers', salt and water to make them vomit. The medical response could be rather more extemporised. When Norman Hassell was gassed, the MO 'worked over me. First he held some ammonia under my nose, then gave me a wallop in the stomach after which I was violently sick . . . [T]his rough and ready treatment ultimately providing a complete cure.'[92] Speedy evacuation from 'the cloud area' was the aim; when patients reached an MDS, they were exposed to fresh air and given oxygen, along with small doses of morphine. At the Somme, Gunner Matthew Roiall hit an unexploded gas shell while digging a shelter. 'When I woke up I found myself in a hospital . . . with a tally round my neck marked "gassed." And I didn't need telling that either for I was frothing at the mouth. I have to thank the inventor of the oxygen pump which brought me to life again.'[93]

Mustard gas victims required more complex treatment. Most important, if possible, was removing the gas from the skin by bathing: otherwise blisters formed after 30 minutes. Men trapped on battlefields far from medical help had little chance of avoiding this. Medical staff were also instructed to bathe the eyes with bicarbonate of soda and shield them from the light; for the skin, the same solution should be used. To ease affected noses, mouths and throats, inhalations of steam and tincture of benzoin were recommended. 'Evacuate early to C.C.S. before acute symptoms develop.'[94]

'By jove,' wrote Rifleman Norman Chadwick, 'all our Red Cross men [bearers were often referred to thus] deserve the V.C. for the way they worked. It is a terrible strenuous job, carrying anyone out, especially over the slippery ground and the shellswept places they had to go.'[95] It was also a dangerous and terrifying job, as Walter Horwell conveyed to his brother in Timaru, using 'a set of little pen pictures'.

> Well, picture 1. Myself and a cobber struggling over three miles of open, shell-scarred country, carrying a heavy man on a stretcher. A heavy barrage on the ridge ahead. We watch how the shells are landing, get through in the weak spot of the barrage, and through to the dressing station properly settled. After a rest we set off again to the aid post, go a little out of the way to dodge barrage, and get mixed up with a wiring party. Fritz sees us and starts sniping with a five-point-nine [howitzer]. Hear a shell coming . . . Hop into old trench and lie flat on a very much dead Fritz . . . Piece of shell goes half-way through my gas helmet — saves me from a wound in the hip. Very much shaken — drop empty stretcher and hook it.[96]

Unlike an infantryman or a gunner, a stretcher-bearer 'was unable to duck every time he heard a shell coming . . . They were rarely deliberately shot at, but in the chaos of battle it was hard to distinguish them from everyone else, and nobody was immune to ricochets and shell splinters.'[97]

When Claude Weston was wounded at Passchendaele, the two bearers helping him were both hit by a shell. 'I . . . saw the bearer at my head falling gently forward with the blood running down his forehead . . . He fell on one knee, and while in that position seemed to recover himself, and with his field dressing bound up his head.'[98] In September 1918, at an ADS at Neuville, No. 3 Field Ambulance treated 38-year-old stretcher-bearer 'Dad' Joseph Vernor. The Oamaru stock agent, who had already been wounded that year, had been hit in the thigh by a shell. 'Before he died he said that he had carried out many who were "for it," but they were, he averred, better men than he. He was typical of the regimental stretcher-bearers . . . whose frightful mortality was the measure of the danger of their work, and who were universally classed with the bravest of the brave.'[99]

After reaching and loading a wounded man came the challenge of manoeuvring heavy, unwieldy stretchers, with splinter-causing wooden handles, through narrow communication trenches that had 'sharp-cornered, right-angle traverses at frequent intervals'. In some of these a man lying on a stretcher could be taken through only by being lifted above the top of the trench. Those who were able to 'sit up at all' were taken out more easily on short trench stretchers, 'but in all cases there was the stream of ordinary traffic up and down the lines to contend with, a slow business where to pass even a single man meant a squeeze'.[100] At the Somme, Malcolm Ross noticed that the first bearers along a trench often carried shovels so

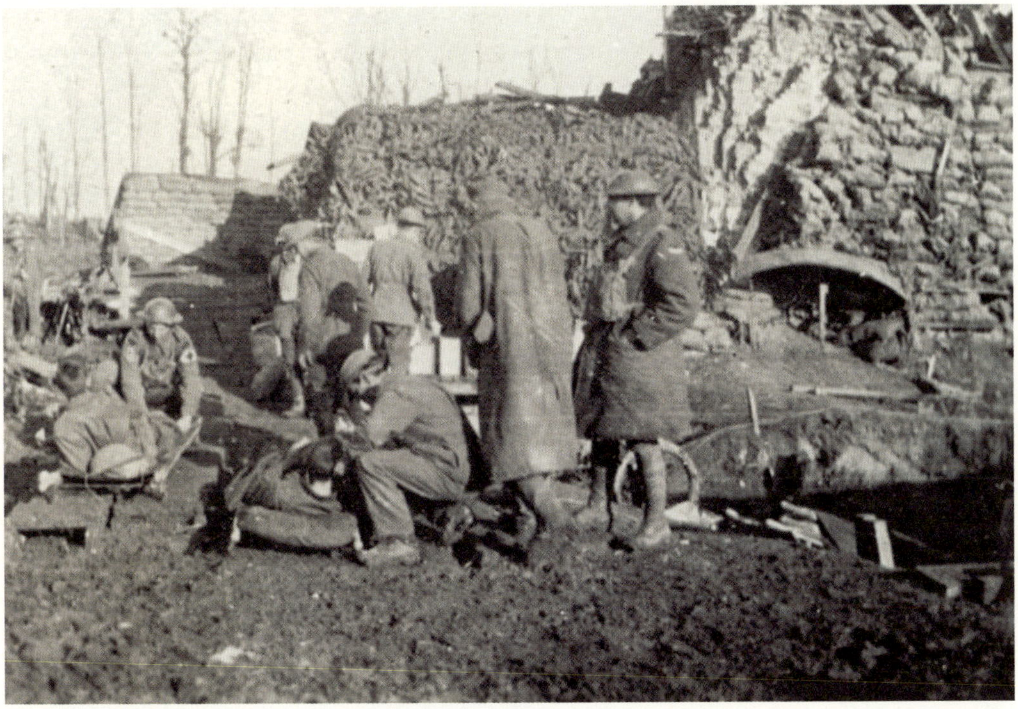

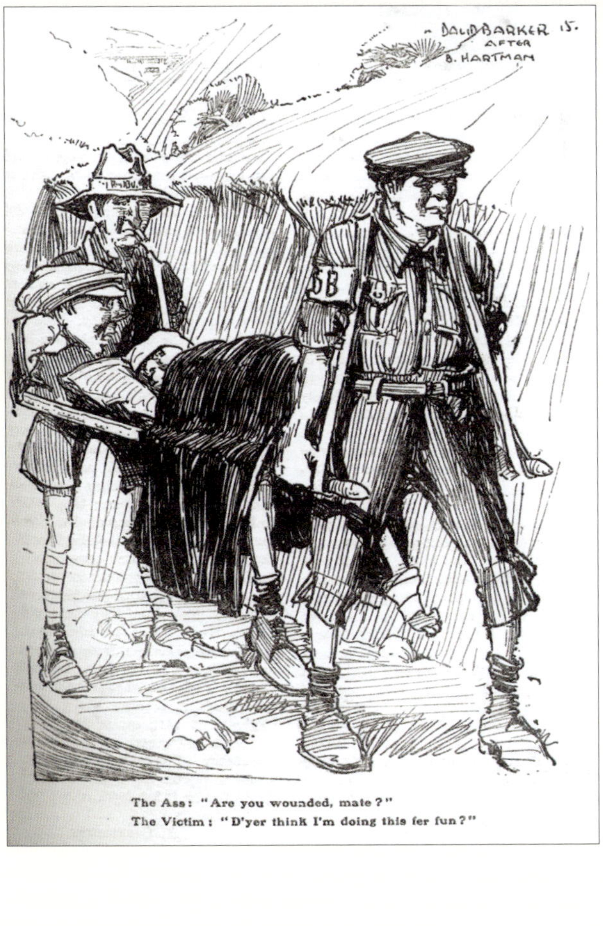
SB
The Ass: "Are you wounded, mate?"
The Victim: "D'yer think I'm doing this fer fun?"

above Mud, chaos and death — a hard-pressed dressing station at Passchendaele. NATIONAL ARMY MUSEUM, 1992.760

below Sometimes black humour was the only way to cope. This cartoon appeared in *The Anzac Book*, published in 1916 by Cassell in London, and the inspiration of Australian war correspondent Charles Bean. COURTESY PAUL WHITE they could round off the corners of the traverses.[101] Stretcher-bearing was brutally hard on mind and body but, during offensives, rest became scarce. In 'Picture 2', Horwell described himself and his mates, 'wet through, miserable, muddy, cold', managing only 10 minutes of sleep before being woken by the sergeant's voice: 'Come on boys, you've to get out.'[102]

Gas added an extra difficulty. Both the PH gas helmets and,[103] later, the small box respirators the bearers had to wear were 'uncomfortable, hot and constrictive', and blurred their vision as they carried stretchers over rough or swampy ground, sometimes through gas-filled depressions and trenches. They also had to make sure that the wounded men's masks were secure. MOs, too, had difficulties with gas protection. While treating wounded in their Fort Osborne RAP at Messines, MOs Frederick Johns and Kenneth Gordon found that 'Owing to the gas shells we had to knock off once or twice as we could not work properly in the box respirators'.[104] Driving an ambulance over rough terrain while wearing a gas mask was not easy, either.

Sometimes bearers received help from an unexpected quarter. A wounded William Wilson was approached by a German prisoner who 'gave me his shell bandages and dressings and offered [to] carry me out'. Wilson 'thought it safer to hobble along as I was', but he observed that 'On account of so many of our Red Cross men being knocked out, German prisoners were utilised to carry stretchers and they did their work with a will, when they saw they were being treated well'.[105] Claude Weston also had enemy assistance: 'The four Germans carried a stretcher easily; they were well-built, dapper little men, and kept step together, as if on a drill ground. And high up on their shoulders I went down the road to the Advanced Dressing Station.'[106]

NZMC orderlies at the front were often in mortal danger, working under constant shellfire in dressing stations. At the Somme in September 1916, two were killed in an ADS on the first afternoon.[107] On 5 June 1917, William Robson 'very nearly stopped a trench Mortar handle which whipped thro. the Dressing Room roof and out thro. the floor about 2 feet from my head'.[108] At a CCS, especially, orderlies were involved in constant bending and lifting, which took its toll on backs and knees, and they also did a good deal of tough physical building work, and cooking, and often marched for many miles to new locations. For untried men, wartime surgery could come as a shock. Leslie Boyd, who had been a clerk in Wanganui, saw his first 'real operation' at Armentières. 'One surgeon started on his leg, the other on his arm. They took off his leg and his arm, and opened his tummy and extracted shrapnel. They said to me, "Boyd, take this arm and leg and put them in the incinerator." I nearly fainted.'[109]

But the worst hell of all, for everyone in the NZMC on the Western Front, was Passchendaele. Here, in a single day, 12 October 1917, 846 New Zealanders were fatally wounded or killed and hundreds were hurt; 138 more would die of wounds over the following week.[110] Wounded lay, sometimes for days, in a vast no man's land of mud and shell-holes, while exhausted bearers struggled to reach them. Controversial military decisions and heavy rain both contributed to the disaster and affected the medical situation. As military historian Ian McGibbon has suggested, the organisation for removing the wounded at Messines had been 'exemplary', but at Passchendaele 'evacuation arrangements collapsed as a result of rushed planning and appalling weather'.[111] When possible, wounded were marked with the sign of a reversed rifle with fixed bayonet, topped by a helmet, so bearers would eventually find them, but many were so weak that they disappeared into the mud, drowned, and were never recovered. Others slipped, became stuck and were sucked down 'agonisingly slowly'. Those soldiers who could 'kept themselves alive with rations from the haversacks of the dead and with filthy water from shell-holes'.[112] Bearers, too, fell victim to the mud. John Moloney saw a stretcher with six bearers sink into mud 'up to their armpits. Ropes were used to pull them out. The stretcher was actually resting on top of the mud.'[113]

As early as 5 October, at Gravenstafel, 'wounded were coming in freely to the ADS — mostly stretcher cases'. From midday on 4 October to midday on the 7th, 1326 were wounded and 398 were evacuated sick.[114] On 12 October, when it was clear as early as 10 a.m. that the attack had failed, more than 1000 walking wounded had passed through Spree Farm by midday, and at 4 p.m. it was estimated that 1200 men would be needed to clear the battlefield of the 230 stretcher cases still unrecovered.[115] And every loaded stretcher had to be carried over a quagmire of shell-holes — often in full view of the enemy. It could take 16 men, in relays, six hours to carry a wounded man back to the ADS. The mud-coated bearers, grim-faced and red-eyed, were soon catatonic with tiredness; men from non-medical units were brought in to rescue severely hurt, often dying men. Moloney and his mates 'had to clear Waterloo Farm which took two days to do. Never have I had such a melancholy experience. It would wring the heart of the hardest man to see the groups of bearers dozens of them struggling along with the poor chaps on the stretcher suffering from the bumps and stops.' Sydney Stanfield helped to carry wounded away from an RAP, where desperate bearers, needing their stretchers, had left the men 'in the wet and cold, just dying there where they were dumped off . . . with an oil sheet tied over them if anyone thought to do that, or if one of their mates could do it . . . We just carried till you couldn't carry more.'[116]

The desperation felt by the beleaguered medics was clear in a plea from Captain John McGhie on the morning of 14 October: 'the cases have been shouting out for stretcher bearers as they have been lying out in the line for some days now . . . Could we please have 540 men to clear these cases in daylight sending 50 every halfhour as after one trip the men are done and the 2nd trip takes four times as long as it ought to . . . Will you please send me as many men as possible urgently.'[117] Charles Begg would record the telling statistic: during the 14 days beginning at 6 a.m. on 4 October, the dressing stations of II ANZAC Corps dealt with more than 11,000 wounded men.[118]

On 12 October several bearers were killed and of the many NZMC casualties, 'a considerable number had been gassed — most of them were exhausted'. In the Gravenstafel and Passchendaele operations, 16 medical men lost their lives and 82 were wounded. Several bearers died later of gas poisoning. The casualties in No. 4 Field Ambulance were 'disproportionately high': eight were killed, two died of wounds and nine of gas poisoning, and 25 were wounded or gassed. There was also a very high sickness rate after the offensive, 'which must be attributed to hardships endured during the Passchendaele operations'.[119]

It was, however, apparently possible to tell a different story. In a letter to Allen on 16 October, Godley wrote of Passchendaele, 'Though not such a big success as Messines or the battle here of the 4th, it was a very good day's work.' Four days later, ADMS Donald McGavin noted, 'On the whole, I consider that the evacuation of the wounded during this action was very effective and rapidly carried out, particularly in view of the difficulties enumerated above.'[120]

One hundred and twelve New Zealand Medical Corps men were killed in action or died of wounds or disease during their service on the Western Front or soon afterwards.[121] Many more were wounded. As Norman Gray noted on 22 September 1916 at Flers: 'Just under 300 of us [NZMC] have been in action, the remainder being in base hospitals etc., and 70 men and 5 officers is the total for eight days.'[122] Of the doctors who lost their lives, the best known, perhaps, because of his popular wartime account, *A Surgeon in Khaki*, was New Zealand-born and Edinburgh-trained Major Arthur Martin. He joined the RAMC when war broke out but enlisted in the NZMC in 1916. He had always held that 'to be really effectual, surgical aid must be given to the soldiers as soon as possible after they received their wounds', which meant that 'surgeons had to be right up in the fire trenches'.[123] Martin was in just such a situation on the Somme at about 3 p.m. on 17 September 1916 when he was seriously wounded in the abdomen, leg, arm and face. Despite speedy attention at the New Zealand Stationary Hospital, where Hugh Acland and Donald McGavin operated, he died that night. Captain Gilbert Bogle, from Hawke's Bay, was killed the same day. He had 'worked ceaselessly in the open, under continual shell fire, for 36 hours, without rest or meals, till killed by a shell five minutes before the battalion moved out. By his extraordinary devotion to duty he saved many lives.'[124] Martin had first been mentioned in despatches in 1915; Bogle received the same recognition after his death.

On 3 July 1916, 29-year-old Christchurch-born Captain Thomas Guthrie, who had gone to Europe with Martin, had been killed by a shell at Armentières. An only son, he had had 'a brilliant University career at Edinburgh, and was regarded in the profession as a fine surgeon'.[125] Dr Alexander Tolhurst was working at an RAP when he lost his life in France on 8 May 1918. He had served as a surgeon on both the *Maheno* and the *Marama* before being appointed to No. 3 New Zealand Field Ambulance. Although 'shells were falling all around and the concussion putting out the lights which lit the place, he went about his work with a quiet heroism that was an inspiring example to us all'.[126] The shell that struck Tolhurst also killed chaplain Alexander Allen. There were severe injuries, too. James Marshall, from Wellington, was struck in the chest by a high-explosive fragment that passed through to a muscle in his back at Petit Bouge in June 1917.[127]

Like Martin and Bogle, many, officers and other ranks alike, received awards for their bravery, sometimes posthumously.[128] Captain Samuel Serpell was killed in action in Belgium on 15 December 1917. He had received the Military Cross in April for attending to the wounded at an RAP while under fire and, after being wounded twice, continuing until ordered to hospital by his commanding officer. 'Always showing great keenness and energy', he had been 'an excellent RMO . . . strict but tactful with the men'.[129] Captain Joseph Venables MC,

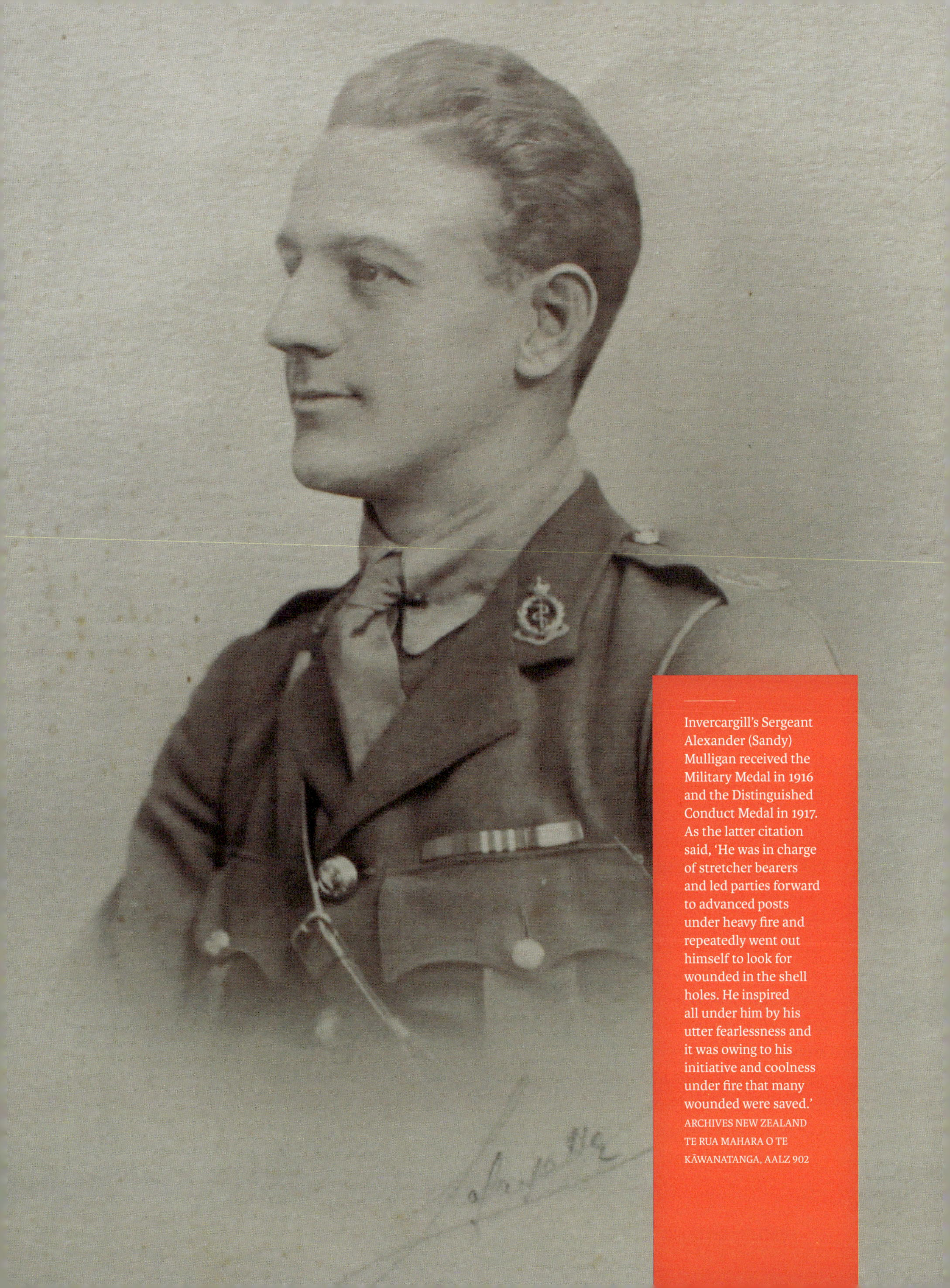

Invercargill's Sergeant Alexander (Sandy) Mulligan received the Military Medal in 1916 and the Distinguished Conduct Medal in 1917. As the latter citation said, 'He was in charge of stretcher bearers and led parties forward to advanced posts under heavy fire and repeatedly went out himself to look for wounded in the shell holes. He inspired all under him by his utter fearlessness and it was owing to his initiative and coolness under fire that many wounded were saved.'

ARCHIVES NEW ZEALAND TE RUA MAHARA O TE KĀWANATANGA, AALZ 902 from Christchurch, died of an abdominal wound on 9 May 1918, and Wanganui doctor Major Frederick Johns MC, 'a fearless bearer commander', was killed in action, with four of his men, near Bapaume in August 1918.[130]

In the view of military dentist Arthur Logan, Masterton doctor Norman Prior, who won an MC at the Somme, was an officer of 'exceptional, and even reckless, courage [who] always behaved with the utmost disregard for his own safety. A man of high moral standards who neither drank nor smoked, he was in no way narrow minded and he had a streak of impish humour . . . He was a great character and a real friend.'[131] Captain John McGhie, who also received the MC and was wounded at Ypres, repeatedly 'took stretcher-parties forward through heavy mud and enemy barrage to the regimental aid posts, and did not stop till he was certain that all men lying out had been collected'. Norman Gray was 'fortunate enough to win a Military Medal for the Somme work . . . This is the 3rd. in our Coy. and I think more should follow . . . The fellows have been good enough to say that it was deserved — and that means almost as much as the honor itself.'[132] At Gravenstafel on 4 October 1917, theological student James McKenzie of No. 2 Field Ambulance earned the MM for his 'untiring energy and capable leadership of his bearer squad under heavy fire . . . bringing in many men who were wounded in shell holes'.[133] Walter Horwell received the same honour.

Some medical men were decorated more than once. Captain Patrick Ardagh, the RMO of 1st Auckland Battalion, already had an MC and had been mentioned in despatches. His extraordinary, sleepless 36 hours of work east of Masnières in the first three days of October 1918, when he continued to dress the wounded, including men from three other battalions, as shells rained down on his exposed ADS, should have earned him a Victoria Cross. Two high-ranking NZEF officers certainly thought so, as did three eyewitnesses, but General Andrew Russell did not agree and Ardagh was given a DSO.[134]

As he told his family, Walter Carruthers of No. 1 Field Ambulance 'got the M.M. at the Somme for going through the barrage for the wounded. I was in charge of a squad. Thanks for the congratulations.' A bar was added to his medal in October 1917.[135] Then there was the remarkable Private Thomas Parsons, a Gisborne labourer turned stretcher-bearer with No. 2 Field Ambulance. He was awarded an MM and bar in 1917, in April and at Passchendaele, then a DCM in 1918. Parsons paid a high price for his bravery. After returning home in 1919, he underwent treatment at Rotorua for trench fever, debility and rheumatism, and then at Hanmer for neurasthenia.[136]

The drivers who risked their lives were not forgotten. Leslie Bryant, a driver with the Army Service Corps Mechanical Transport, and Samuel Downey, a wagon orderly with No. 3 Field Ambulance, both received the MM for their work on the night of 5 May 1917. They safely delivered a carload of stretcher cases to a dressing station after having to turn the vehicle around on a damaged road in the midst of a barrage. Downey 'had a critical haemorrhage case on the car, and showed great judgment in restraining panic-stricken patients'. The episode, like so many in which New Zealand medical men were involved on the Western Front, was 'a fine example of courage, resource and devotion to duty'.[137]

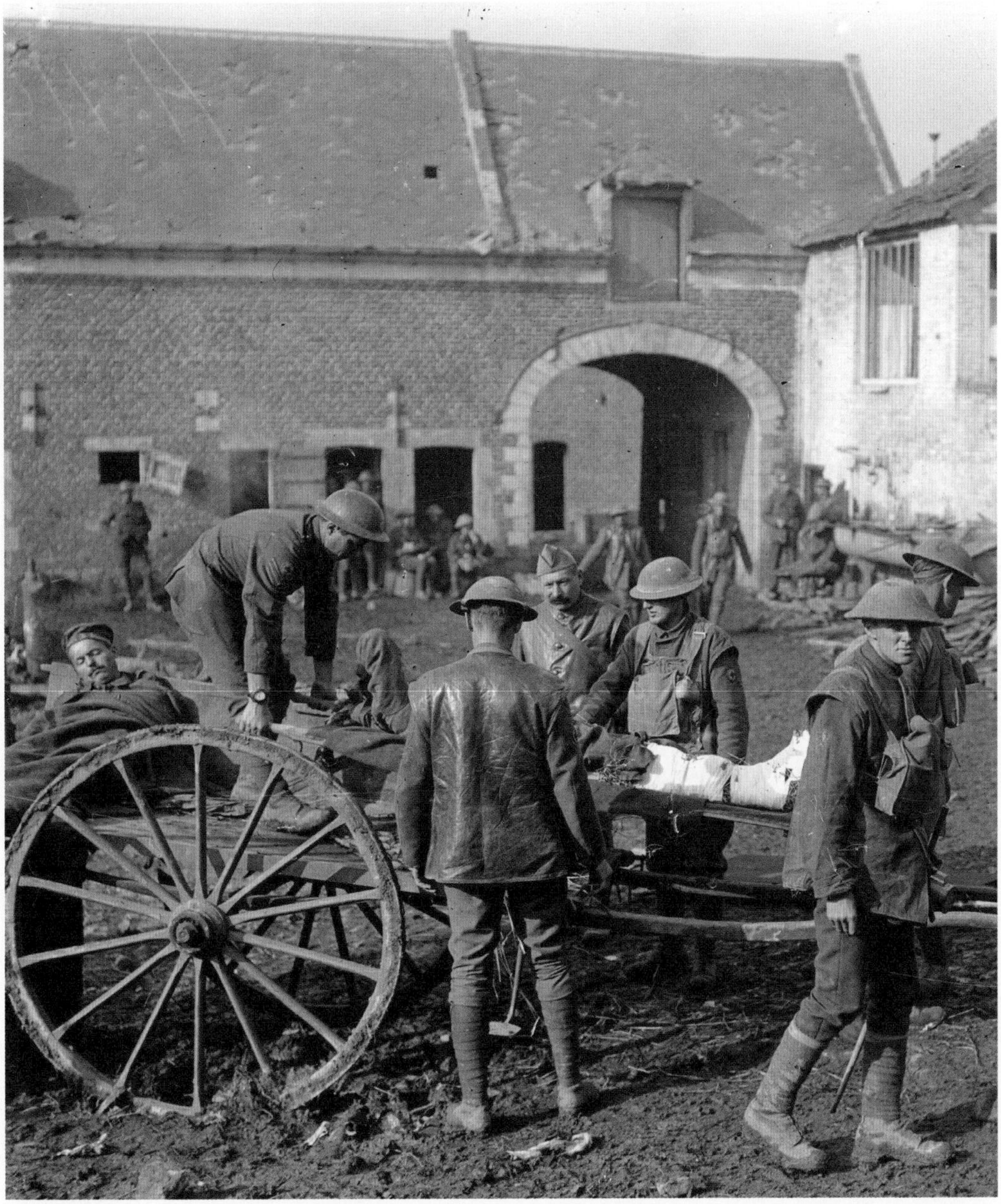

There are no sides when it comes to suffering. At a Pont-a-Pierre farm, not far from Le Quesnoy, badly wounded German soldiers, brought from the front line on a cart, are moved onto stretchers by New Zealand soldiers. The photograph was taken at the beginning of November 1918. ALEXANDER TURNBULL LIBRARY, 1/2-013697-G

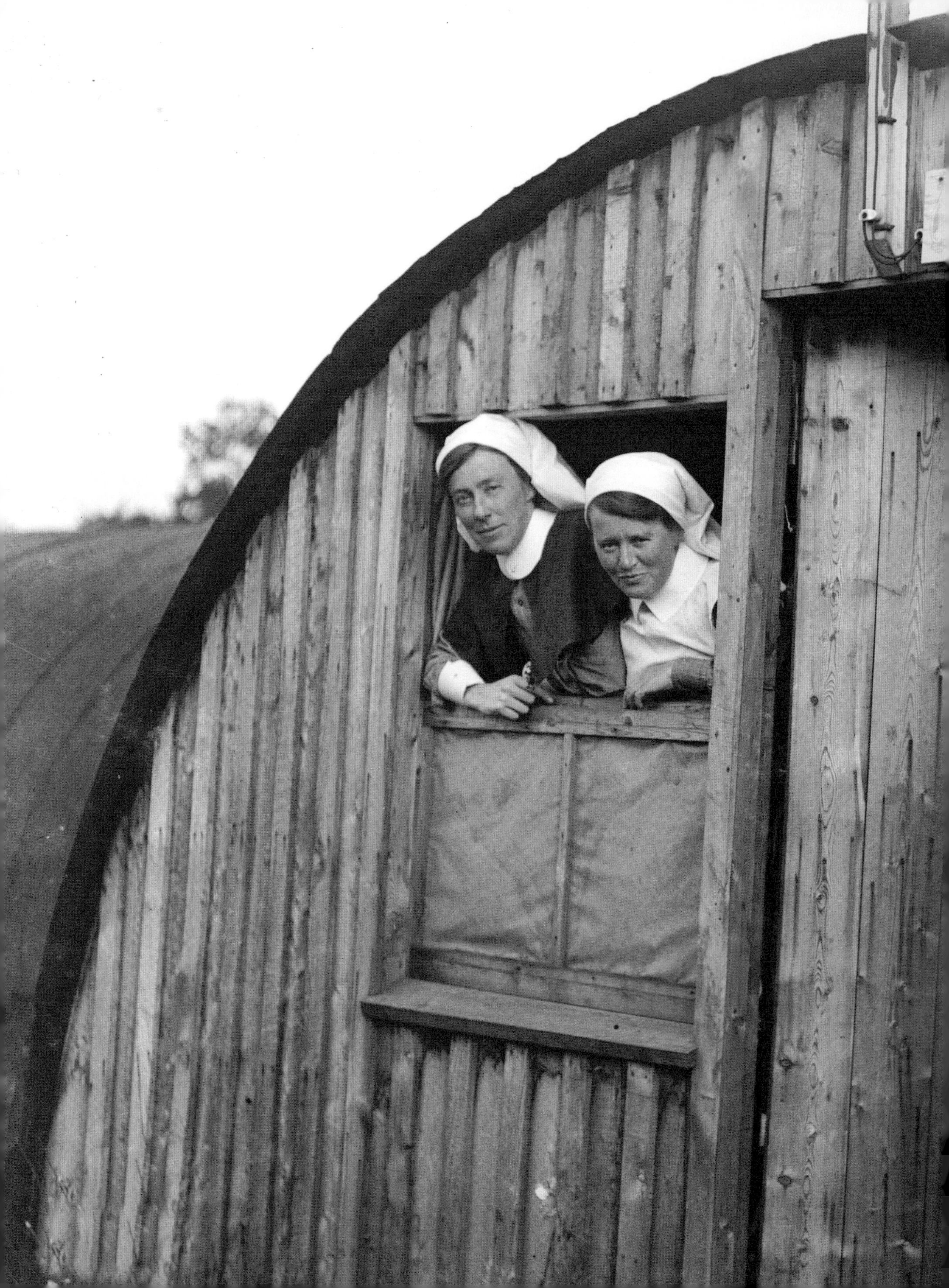

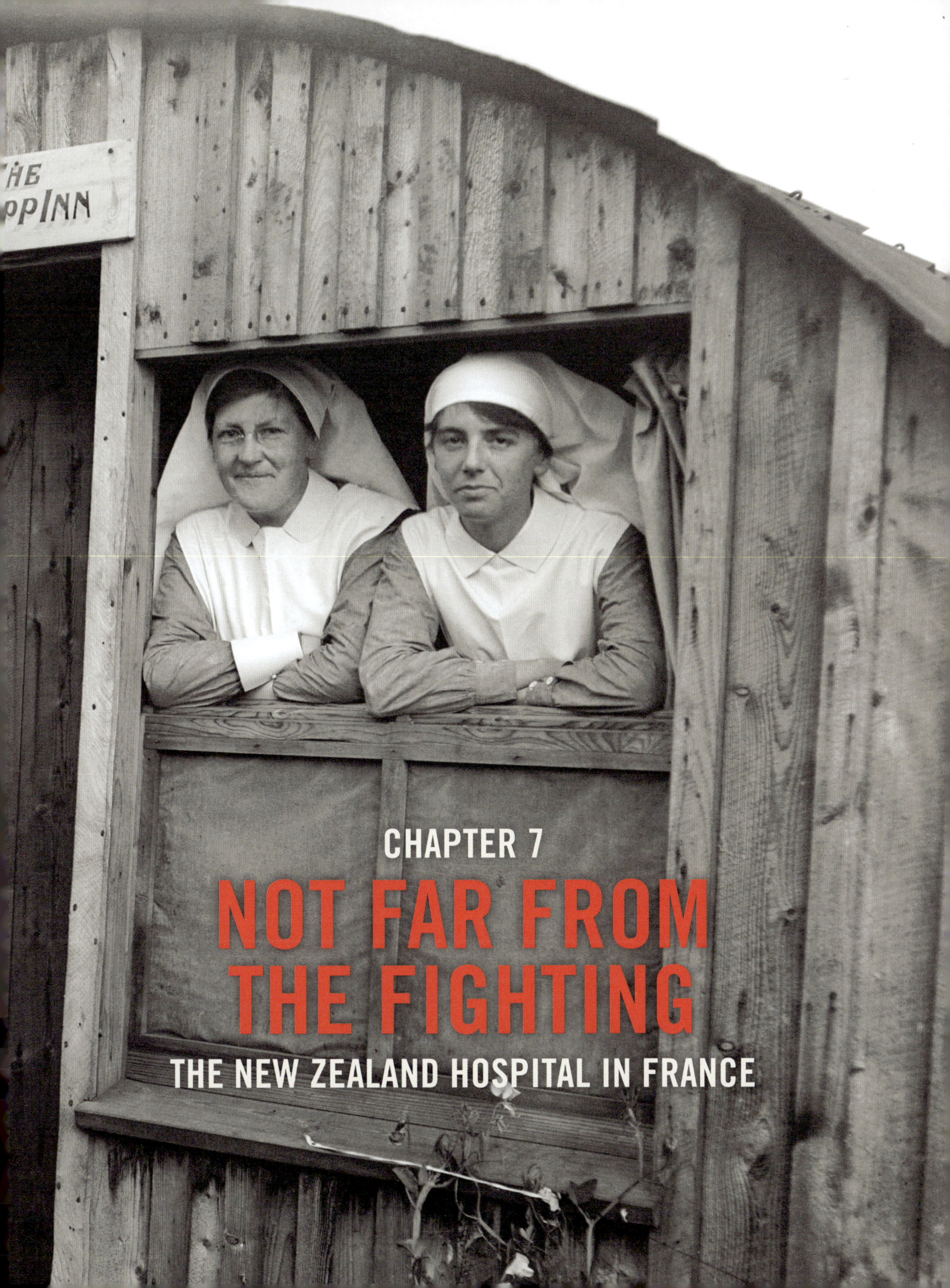

CHAPTER 7

NOT FAR FROM THE FIGHTING

THE NEW ZEALAND HOSPITAL IN FRANCE

previous pages
This famous image shows New Zealand nurses at the windows of their Nissen hut at the New Zealand Stationary Hospital in Wisques, France.
ALEXANDER TURNBULL LIBRARY, 1/2-013482-G

So you are learning a little more now of what a hell war really is. One does not realise it properly even in the hospitals over here. One has to go to France to realise & the nearer to the front line the more one learns . . .

— Ned O'Neill, letter to Staff Nurse Bertha Taylor, 22 June 1918

The end of a seriously wounded man's Western Front journey was the longed-for destination of a hospital bed. Often this was British. Because the NZEF was automatically allowed to use imperial medical facilities, injured soldiers frequently received their first treatment at British casualty clearing stations, and were then sent to one of the many British hospitals in France.[1] 'I know that a few N.Z. boys find their way into your hospital,' Ned O'Neill told his cousin, Bertha Taylor, who was nursing at the New Zealand Stationary Hospital in France in 1918. 'Most of them find their way to Boulogne, Etaples or Le Trapert [Le Tréport] for the Casualty Clearing Stations & thence either to Blighty or the Base Camp at Etaples.'[2] When chaplain Clive Mortimer Jones passed through Étaples on his way to England in November 1917, he counted 17 hospitals, some with 60 wards, and finding New Zealand patients was not easy. 'One may be in one ward of one hospital and two in another ward of another hospital and so on; we also walked 4½ miles each way to another place where there are four more large hospitals. We saw 30 of our men there and it was worth it, for . . . the boys love to see the New Zealand hat and to talk to someone who knows their dear old country.'[3] But New Zealand casualties were also cared for by their own hospital.

Still under the command of Donald McGavin, No. 1 NZSH had sailed from Egypt on the *Dover Castle* two months after the division and landed at Le Havre on 13 June 1916.[4] It comprised a dozen officers and 126 ORs, plus No. 10 Dental Section. After the men had undergone a short period of training and received some instruction in gas defence, Hugh Acland took seven officers and 83 ORs to work as a CCS with No. 2 British General Hospital at Quai d'Escale in Le Havre, helping to ready the large number of Somme casualties for transfer to hospital ships and a Channel crossing. A nurse on the *Marama* encountered the New Zealanders at 'the hospital on the wharf, taking charge of 300 beds, and working very hard'.[5]

The destination for the remaining NZSH members was the lovely old cathedral town of Amiens, where on 13 July they took over from a British CCS part of the convent of Sainte Famille and a nearby girls' school (lycée). As well as the historic buildings, the New Zealanders inherited 100 patients, an X-ray plant, equipment and accommodation for some 700 cases, a mobile laboratory and the Fourth Army Ophthalmic Centre. The hospital set up its headquarters in the convent — 'no rent was charged by the good sisters who cheerfully made room for suitable quarters for the seriously wounded'[6] — and the British nurses who had been working at Amiens were replaced, early in August, by 19 NZANS women from England led by Matron Frances (Fanny) Price.

After a train journey from Boulogne that took 12 hours instead of the usual three, owing to bombing of the tracks, the weary nurses reached Amiens to find that the hospital, on the banks of the River Somme, was conveniently close to the station — 'rather too close', in the view of British chaplain H. K. Bros, an NZSH patient that year, 'because the railway station is the object of frequent air raids'.[7] At the convent building, which contained 350 beds for the more seriously wounded, Sister Jean Ingram, with Sisters Catherine Blackie and Elizabeth Porteous, ran two officers' wards, which could take 49 patients. Initially, almost all the wounded were British: 'We get the very bad cases off the barges [coming down the river], who are too ill to go on.' According to another staff member, the convent was 'suitable for a hospital in most ways, except for the absence of "lifts" and deficiency in water and drainage systems, which applies to the town in general'.[8]

With McGavin in overall command, Acland was in charge of the convent section, working with fellow doctors Ebenezer Teichelmann, William Willis from Feilding and Wellingtonian William Young, while Duncan Stout ran the lycée, a few blocks away, which held another 350 beds. 'It has three stories, and, having no lifts either, transport is certainly a little awkward. The rooms however, are airy and clean, and there is a large gymnasium with 40 beds, making a very cosy ward.' The medical and light surgical cases were treated here, by William Ferguson, Eric Marchant and Angus Marshall. The doctors' mess was in a small outbuilding at the convent, the nurses' in a tent in the grounds. The patients' beds had 'nice blue coverlets' supplied by the Red Cross, and as blue and grey blankets were replaced by red ones, the wards looked 'bright and cheerful'.[9]

The surroundings may have been pleasant, but the work was challenging, with the NZSH functioning as a CCS under the aegis of the Fourth Army. Ida Willis remembered the large 80-bed ward taking 'more than its number of stretcher cases', with medical staff and padres putting in long hours 'in the sorting of them, removing mud and filthy garments from these poor fellows who had come straight from the mud-filled trenches'. In the huge, three-table operating theatre, surgery continued for 24 to 36 hours, with pauses only for meals and coffee. 'Sometimes because of the pressure of work, the theatre staff had no change of garments during 6 to 8 operations, stopping only to plunge and wash their gloved hands under running water and disinfectant.'[10] As Bros observed, during August 'the staff was taxed to the utmost of its powers; frequently 160 wounded would come in daily . . . During the first few weeks of the great advance in the late summer, one of the surgeons was operating continuously for three days and nights, so great was the number of serious cases. To such devotion many will owe it that they are probably not crippled for life.'[11]

The chaplain appreciated his treatment at the hospital — 'a more efficient and capable staff it would be impossible to find' — and had a special word for the sisters. 'Sympathetic, kind, efficient, they seem to fulfil what one has always regarded as the pattern of a perfect nurse. Nothing seems to be able to destroy their capacity for cheerfulness and unfailing attention to every detail which can make their patients more comfortable and contented.' He had written to the newspapers 'because, perhaps, we do not realise what a debt of thanks and gratitude we English owe to the devoted work of the New Zealand medical and nursing profession'.[12] Sister Clare Jordan, working in Rouen for Queen Alexandra's Imperial Military Nursing Service (QAIMNS), was proud of the hospital: 'One of my patients, a medical officer, a week ago not knowing I was a New Zealander, paid a high tribute to the staff there. He said they were a splendid crowd from medical officers down to orderlies. I was delighted, and hastened to tell him that they belonged to me so to speak.'[13]

Besides terrible wounds, the NZSH staff, like all medical personnel on the Western Front, were now facing a new horror: gas gangrene. As British doctor Geoffrey Keynes explained, 'Even with quite a slight wound, when soil and shards of uniform are carried in by the missile, it starts up.' The infection was caused by anaerobic bacteria, *Clostridia*, that flourished in the well-manured, and now extremely contaminated, soil of northern France and developed in the dead tissue left by wounds, particularly compound fractures. Rapid removal of the wounded from the battlefield could help but was not, of course, always possible. If the men had taken several days to reach medical help, 'the wound was simply a mass of putrid muscle rotting with gas gangrene . . . [T]he bacillus that grows in the wound creates gas. The whole thing balloons up. You can tap it under your fingers and it sounds hollow.' There were, too, ominous 'little crackling noises . . . like bubbles'.[14] As Jean Ingram could attest, 'bad gas gangrene cases smell most fearfully'. Less serious cases could sometimes be cured by the removal of all dead tissue and debris, followed by applications of antiseptic Carrel–Dakin solution — Ingram reported that 'so far we have managed to save all the limbs'[15] — but all too frequently the only answer was amputation. Many cases were fatal. The Germans had an effective serum, but the Allies did not develop one until late in the war.[16]

'We have been having a tremendous time; convoys of a hundred at a time two or three times a day all the last week,' wrote one nurse on 18 September 1916.

> Yesterday, we took in three hundred and fifty, and it was immense — three operating tables going night and day. Sisters Willis, [Isla] Stewart, and myself, with three orderlies, have been keeping the theatre going. We just sat in a chair and had a doze for an hour during the night, and the surgeons the same, and now I have just got word sent me of another hundred badly wounded, so it is to be another all-night attack. We are losing a lot of our New Zealand boys, at present we have numbers in here. The convoys the last three days have been most terrible — gas gangrene cases are too awful for words, and the trouble is so advanced before we get them. I never want to see another amputation while I live.[17]

When Matron Fanny Price wrote home in April 1917, the weather was 'still very cold, and snow falling almost every day', after a winter said to have been the worst for 70 years. She described the new 100-bed officers' hospital, which had been opened in January in another school building, three-quarters of a mile away.[18] By this time, more New Zealand nurses had been transferred to Amiens from England, among them Elsie Grey. Along with the severe cold and the dreadful sanitation, she faced the threat of bombing that hung over the New Zealand Stationary Hospital, as No. 1 NZSH had become known at the end of October 1916: 'I cannot realise that we are only 15 miles from the firing line. This is the nearest Hospital.' With a full moon on 1 March, and Zeppelins expected, the staff closed the shutters and readied the cellar. 'We have orders to fly there when two guns go off . . . and the medical officers carry on in the wards. I am sure my legs will not carry me to the cellar.'[19] As Reg Hird, in a Calais hospital, wrote home in November 1917, 'You have no idea what an anxious time it is for all concerned about a hospital when a hostile aeroplane is up dropping bombs.'[20]

During quieter times at the hospital, a surgical team comprising a surgeon, an anaesthetist, a sister and one or two orderlies, sometimes joined a British CCS in another area. In April 1917, for example, Ida Willis was with a CCS near Vimy Ridge when it was taken by the Canadians: 1100 men passed through in the first 12 hours, 'so there was no bed for the theatre staff for . . . thirty-six hours or more'.[21] A few months later, after six frantic weeks in the NZSH theatre following the Battle of Messines, Margaret Davies headed for a CCS in Belgium. Her fellow nurse, Mary McBeth, accompanied an entirely NZSH team, but in Davies' group she and the anaesthetist were New Zealanders, while the surgeon and orderly were English.

At No. 10 CCS, Davies' quarters were a 'queer little' canvas portable Armstrong hut, 'with sheets of some material like gelatine for windows', which 'could be put up and taken down in a few minutes'. Work began before she could finish unpacking.

> It was an awful shock. I did not expect to walk into a strange theatre and start work . . . I seemed to walk over miles of duckboards before I found that theatre, and when I opened the door I found our orderly waiting with a mackintosh gown ready for me, he was holding it up and I just walked into it, scrubbed up, put on gloves, and went over to the operating table. The surgeon had just started an amputation, he greeted me with, 'The saw, please, sister', and that is how I started work at a CCS.

After the operation, the theatre sister showed Davies where everything was kept 'and begged me, almost with tears, to be careful with the towels and swabs and not to change gloves for every operation; but I had been well "broken in" to all this at our own hospital, and had learned the necessary art of economy.'[22] Davies and her colleagues were at No. 10 only a matter of days before they were ordered to proceed at once to another CCS, No. 41, at Godewaersvelde. Their four months there proved fascinating and gruelling. Davies' team was one of four on day duty; the same number did night duty. There were two operating tables for each team, which 'saved a tremendous lot of time, as the anaesthetist was able to have the next man ready . . . as soon as . . . the surgeon . . . was ready to start'. Although the No. 41 theatre was 'just a wooden hut', it was well equipped, with both electric light and acetylene gas if the former failed: 'I have seen surgeons working by the light of a torch only.' The usual hours for the day team were 8 a.m. to 8 p.m., but in busy times they continued until midnight.[23]

Two or three CCSs, made up of different nationalities, were usually grouped together and staggered their work: 'One would take in a certain number of patients, or else for a certain length of time — usually twenty-four hours — and then the next one would start.' The wounded went first to the receiving tent, where their field dressings were taken off and their wounds examined and classified. Some were then taken away for X-rays, while those ready to be operated on moved to the preparation tent, 'where their khaki was removed [sometimes cut off], pyjamas put on, a hyperdermic given, and they waited there for their turn in the theatre'. No. 41 was close enough to the front line 'to have some of the men down, operated on, and ready for the ambulance train within four or five hours of being wounded'. Davies was still at 41 CCS in October when the wounded from Passchendaele arrived 'in a dreadful condition. Solid masses of mud, it was so hard trying to get them out of their khaki, especially when the mud had had long enough to harden.'[24]

Although out of shell range, Davies and her fellow workers were not immune from air raids. Because their CCS group was close to a railway station, where troops were always coming and going, German aircraft came over 'every fine night'. Everyone was issued with a tin hat and a gas mask, and 'as the music of the antiaircraft started', they were supposed to head for a dug-out. If they were too far away or could not leave their patient, 'the alternative was just to lie flat on the ground, for when a bomb bursts the fragments fly upwards, and there is a chance of missing them if one is lying flat'. Twice while Davies was at No. 41, 'we got their bombs right in amongst our tents'.[25] The first time there were no casualties, as the bombs fell on empty tents, but on 20 October the Germans were much more accurate. One bomb landed only yards from the theatre where Davies was working. She and her companions escaped injury, but others were not so fortunate. Working temporarily at 37 CCS was Wellington-born Sister Elise Kemp, who had trained at King's College Hospital in London and was serving with the Territorial Forces Nursing Service. She was killed, along with an orderly and three patients, when a bomb landed close to their marquee; several others were wounded. She is believed to have been the only New Zealand nurse to die on the Western Front.

After rumours of an imminent 'big push' in which the New Zealand Division would be involved, in late May 1917 the No. 59 British General Hospital took over at Amiens and the NZSH moved north to Hazebrouck, near Armentières. The officers and men left first. Among the officers making the eight-hour train journey through the spring countryside on 23 May was chaplain Ronald Watson, who had been with the hospital for seven weeks. 'Since we arrived,' he wrote on the 28th, 'we have been "taking over" from two casualty stations. Our unit has been exceedingly busy getting things fixed up — cleaning buildings, unpacking and erecting marquees. The boys have worked magnificently. I have been proud of them. We are expecting to have 1200 beds so I can see plenty of work ahead for all of us . . . It is grand being as

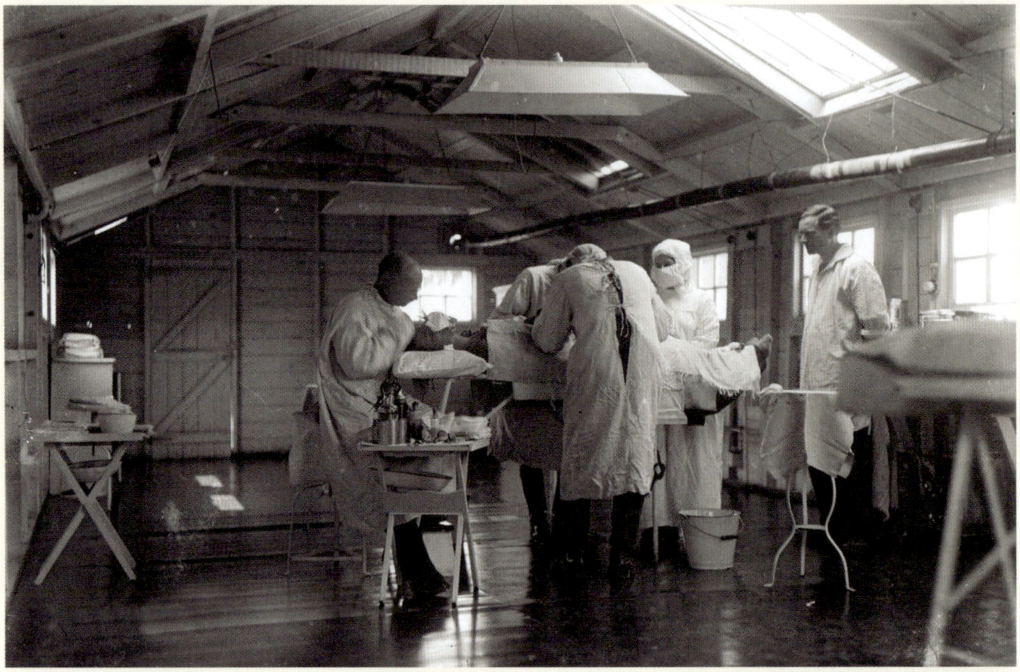

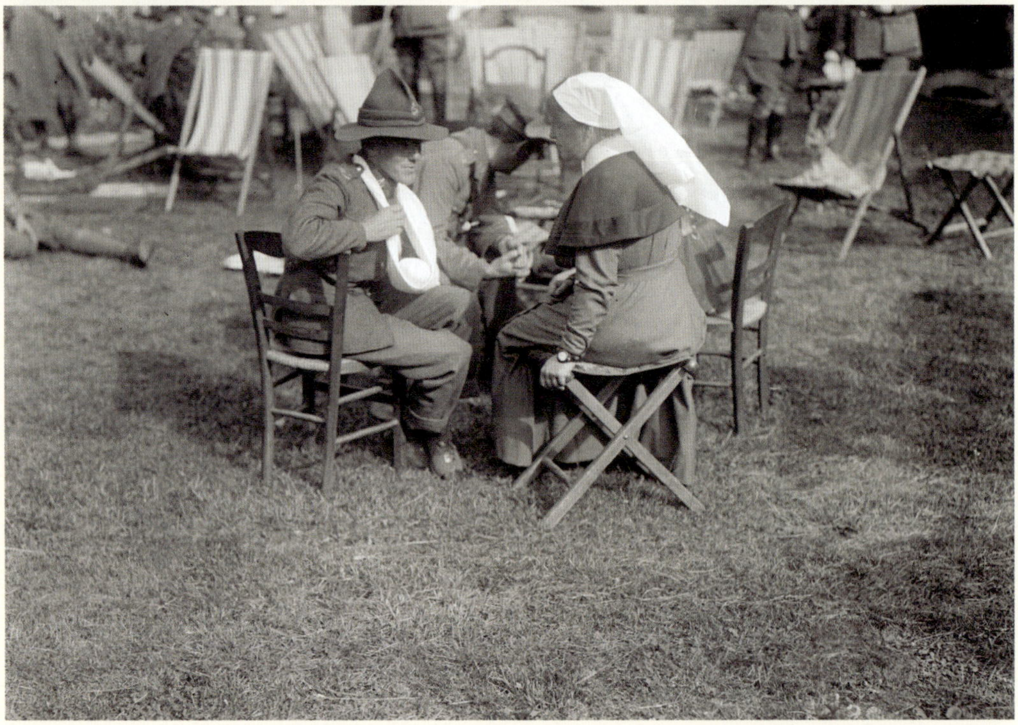

above An operation being carried out at the New Zealand Stationary Hospital. The anaesthetist is seated at the left, a masked nurse assists and an orderly stands by on the right. ALEXANDER TURNBULL LIBRARY, 1/2-013479-G

below A nurse chats to a wounded soldier at a garden party held by the nurses in the lovely walled garden at their Hazebrouck quarters on 24 June 1917. ALEXANDER TURNBULL LIBRARY, 1/2-012800-G near as we are to our Division.'[26] After staying on at Amiens to serve with the British unit until replacement nurses arrived, the NZANS contingent set off for Hazebrouck on 31 May.

During a short visit to France in July, Mabel Thurston decided that Hazebrouck was 'in every way better' than Amiens. 'It is now so much nearer the line that we are able to take in many more of our own wounded.'[27] The old house used as a nurses' home was a 15-minute walk from the hospital. This was set up in two schools and in tents, and the nurses delighted in its 'big private garden, with green lawns, trees, and fruit'. Because most of the women 'had brothers or relations with the division, we were never without visitors when off duty. Picture us with a brother or friend straight out of the line, and the pleasure we had in hunting up new socks and underwear for them. This was easily done owing to our plentiful supply of Red Cross goods, and the boys declared they were new men after a hot bath, change, and meal with us.'[28]

The wards in the 1040-bed hospital were large compared with those at Amiens: four long rows, each of 25 beds. At first there was little for the staff to do, but this changed once the Battle of Messines began on the morning of 7 June. The surgical teams at the CCSs were struggling with the deluge of casualties, so stretcher cases, most of them with gunshot wounds to the head, were sent to Hazebrouck, the first arriving at 4 a.m. on the 8th.[29] As Ian McGibbon has pointed out, there was 'a form of specialisation' at Western Front hospitals, and until December 1917 the NZSH was responsible for the head cases of the Second Army. During Messines, the distinguished American surgeon Major Harvey Cushing, an expert in this area, worked with the New Zealanders.[30] On that first day the NZSH had admitted 10 sick and 187 wounded, and it remained extremely busy, taking in patients every 24 hours in conjunction with a British CCS; three operating tables were in use day and night. Many of the men were paralysed and a number were missing arms, legs or eyes. 'For the first few days they were quite silly,' Elsie Grey wrote, 'lost their reason and some speechless. Oh it was ghastly and desperately busy — we just went on and on doing dressings no hope of finishing. The doctors and padres were awfully good in the wards — taking them drinks and so forth. Crowds died of course [and] 80 were down on the dangerously ill list.'[31]

One of those hard-working padres was Watson, who 'spent time in the Reception Room — where men were admitted, dirty, bloodstained and done, and were prepared for operation — and also in the two wards. I lived in and for the one building alone for several days. I just kept going all day and night, till I was too tired to go on, then in the small hours went off to bed.' He was 'amazed at the perfection of the medical services here, during the Messines stunt. We got some men in the same day as they were wounded. Walton [on-Thames hospital], England, had some in, the night after they were hit. That is *some* travelling.'[32] Adding to the immediate post-Messines pressure were night attacks from a German aircraft. 'Oh it was terrifying,' wrote Grey, 'the shrapnel was falling in all directions.' The whizzing bullets reminded her of howling dogs. Fanny Price had 'put 10 of us out to sleep in two large marquees' but as the firing continued over two more nights, the nurses were taken back inside. 'There didn't seem to be enough between ourselves and glory with just a canvas roof.'[33] Seventy patients were killed and four nurses injured at a CCS just 10 miles away.

At 7 p.m. on the last day of July, a month that had brought the new ghastliness of gas for both

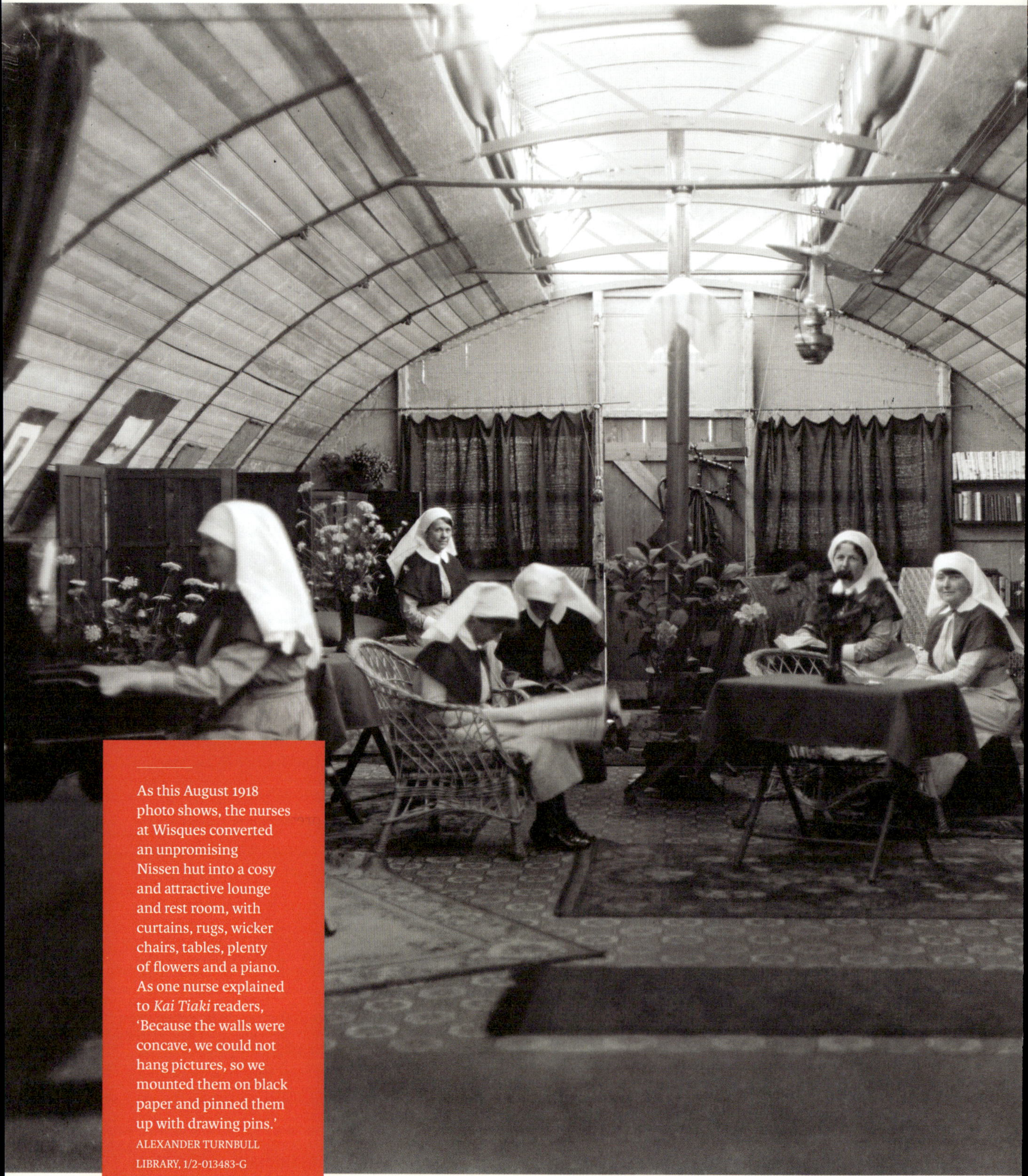

As this August 1918 photo shows, the nurses at Wisques converted an unpromising Nissen hut into a cosy and attractive lounge and rest room, with curtains, rugs, wicker chairs, tables, plenty of flowers and a piano. As one nurse explained to *Kai Tiaki* readers, 'Because the walls were concave, we could not hang pictures, so we mounted them on black paper and pinned them up with drawing pins.' ALEXANDER TURNBULL LIBRARY, 1/2-013483-G

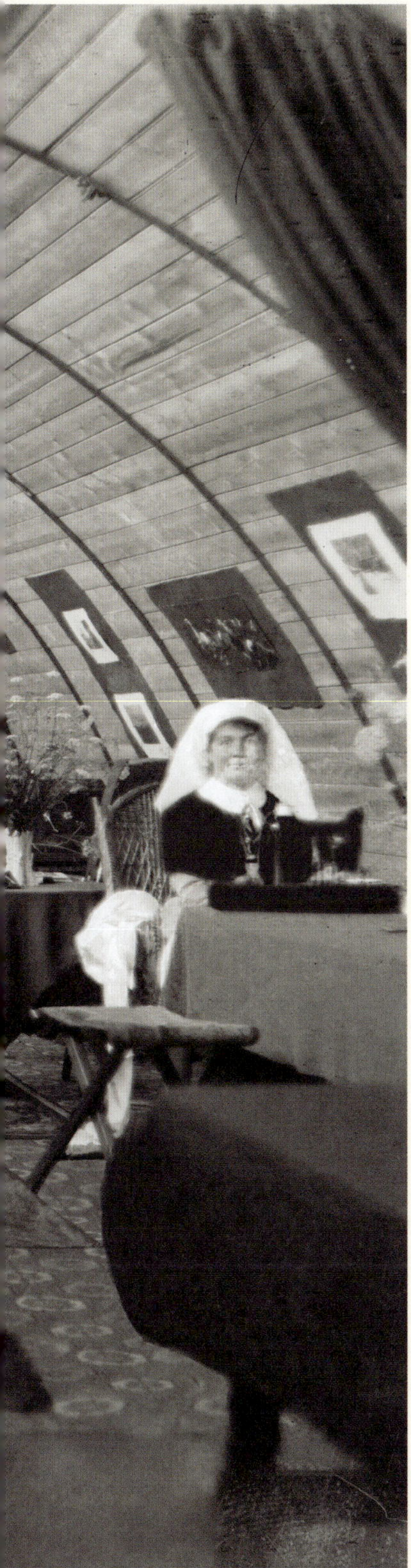

the troops and civilians, the NZSH was shelled. The first enormous explosion was followed by smaller bursts every few minutes for almost an hour and a half. As terrified locals grabbed their valuables and fled, the order came through that, although 20 cases were awaiting operations, surgery was to stop. By midnight between 600 and 700 patients had been discharged, sent away in special trains. Grey thought the 'night sisters all deserve[d] the Military Cross for the way they went on duty' while the attack continued.[34] The nurses departed at 10 next morning, carrying only light luggage, and at 1 p.m. arrived at the 10th British Stationary Hospital at St Omer. They were then distributed across three British hospitals in which they worked for six weeks — some with a break for leave in England — until the NZSH was re-established at Wisques, near St Omer, on 20 September. 'It was a sad staff of sisters that left Hazebrouck, we felt almost as though we were running away.' Apart from a few who remained to care for the locals, the MOs and orderlies arrived safely at St Omer in mid-September.[35]

'We are on the very top of a hill,' wrote Ronald Watson on 5 September 1917, 'and have a glorious view over a wide and fertile valley. It will be an exceedingly healthy place, I reckon.' At that stage Wisques was a temporary camp of marquees and tents on vacant land across the road from the hospital site, which 'will require a great deal of clearing before it is civilized sufficiently . . . There are 60–70 men here now, and we are all busy putting up tents, unloading the lorries as they come up and clearing the ground. I can see weeks of work ahead.' When Watson returned from leave on 2 November he found 'big improvements and enlargements . . . There are now about 650 beds. Electric lighting has begun. We four in our home are still in an E.P.I.P. [European Privates Indian Pattern] marquee — huts to hold 4–6 are being erected for us — but I think I prefer the marquee. There is a great crowd of N.Z. sick in here now — the Division is out [of the line] and near us, at present . . . The long casualty lists for October make sad reading. So many I knew well are gone.'[36]

The nurses, too, were impressed when they saw their new hospital. Initially, they had to live under canvas — fortunately it was summertime — as did their patients, who were accommodated in three long lines of tents, each holding 50 beds. The Nissen huts that replaced these were imported from Canada in sections and took only a few days to erect; each held 48 or 50 beds. The finished hospital had some 18 huts for wards, plus 'one long line of tents; a beautiful theatre, kitchens, pack-stores, and all the usual officers, matrons, P.M.O. [principal medical officer] and post office, orderly room, etc., Y.M.C.A. hall, and a huge receiving room'. All the wards, kitchens, offices, officers' and sisters' quarters were connected by duckboards. One of the wards, 'dubbed "Heaven" by the boys', consisted of two Nissen huts joined together, 'with bare scrubbed floors, usually beautifully white, and a wide piece of linoleum down the centre'.[37]

Rifleman John Moloney was taken to the NZSH at the end of October 1917 when he contracted bronchitis after serving at Passchendaele. 'It was like home at Wisques. The sisters were splendid and couldn't do enough for us. All sorts of people were in my ward, Imperials, Aussies, and even two Americans, who were the star boarders.' He found the Nissen huts 'very comfortable',[38] but as soon as the weather grew cooler, it became apparent that Watson had been too optimistic about the healthiness of the Wisques site. It was in fact damp and swampy; 6-foot trenches were needed around the tents, as were many more yards of duckboards. The Nissen huts were not all completed until the end of 1917 and as the first frosts of a hard winter hit, the tarpaulin floors of the tents proved completely inadequate. As well as catching colds, the nurses and orderlies suffered badly from chilblains and trench foot, which caused the feet to burn and swell. During the first agonising couple of hours each day the nurses, unable to wear their own shoes, resorted to gumboots and men's socks or felt shoes, and rubbed whale oil into their feet.[39]

In early January 1918 Fanny Price was hospitalised for a femoral hernia, a condition often caused by heavy lifting. When she returned to New Zealand on 1 April her place as matron was taken by Eva Brooke, who had been heading the nursing staff at the officers' home in Brighton. From February the NZSH became more of a general hospital, with separate medical and surgical sections, though it reverted to CCS mode when required.[40] As Brooke told the nursing journal *Kai Tiaki* in June, 'We are busy — mostly sick — very few wounded just now: we expect them any day.' On 12 April there had been 600 admissions within a few hours, many with severe wounds. 'They were so tired and hungry that the majority slept for nearly twelve hours: the quiet and comfort was so good after what they had just been through . . . They do appreciate all that is done for them, and it was so satisfactory to see some who were very badly wounded recover enough to be evacuated. Two or three died after they had been with us three weeks. The chest cases and abdominals are kept till the fourteenth day — there were some wonderful recoveries.' Because the NZSH was also then the infectious hospital for the area — its other specialisation — 'we have plenty of infections, including C.S.M. [cerebro-spinal meningitis], and quite a different type to what we had in Trentham. The measles are less acute, although we have had several deaths.'[41]

'At last I really feel I am on active service,' wrote Bertha Taylor when she joined the NZSH early in May, after a 40-hour train trip from Boulogne. By this time the hospital had 1000 beds and there were some 40 nurses, including a few on loan from the British. Taylor was one of six in a 33-bed ward overseen by the popular Captain Roland Aickin, a New Zealand doctor who had joined the RAMC — 'he does excellent work and is so understanding with the boys they all love him'. Dressings were a never-ending task. '[F]our start off with a trolley, nothing boiled, but all well soaked with [disinfectant], instruments and all. We start at the beginning of the ward and do the dressings and that goes on all day, by the time we did a complete round it is time to start again . . . The nurses coming on duty take over as the others leave the ward. Some are done by the Medical Officer himself with a nurse in attendance.'[42]

The hospital staff was in a constant state of flux. 'We are ever changing. The sisters change after a year, the medical officers are always changing, and so are the orderlies, who are mostly P.B. [permanent base] men, and in some cases fit to return for other work after being here six months or so.' As Brooke reminded family and friends back home, their gifts were greatly appreciated, and not just by the patients. On 8 March 1918, NZMC Private Stanley Wallis told the people of New Plymouth that he and his mate had 'had the pleasure of cutting up seven of the fine cakes you sent the staff of this hospital. I wish to thank you, our dear, unknown friends, for the great thought and kindness you have always shown this unit. Last Christmas every member received through you 5 francs, which helped in making pleasure for the boys on that great day of universal festivity.'[43]

New Zealand nurses were also detached to other hospitals. When young NZMC orderly George Tierney, a former Wellington railway clerk, was badly gassed at Passchendaele, the only hospital that could take him was No. 7 British General at St Omer. As he lay in a tent, the nurse who checked his card turned out to be Sister Margaret Drummond, with whom he had worked at Trentham. 'I was in such a state that she couldn't recognise me, but I felt glad I was in her hands as she was famous for her devotion to the patients.' As he realised himself, 20-year-old Tierney was dangerously ill, and he was sure he owed his life to Drummond who, though she doubted her patient would recover, 'was the essence of attention and constantly kept her eye on me'. After a touch and go period, he was moved to a ward in a large monastery. His 'luck was still in', for there he encountered Staff Nurse, later Sister, Mary Reidy, who had been detached to No. 7 from the NZSH.[44] Then in her mid-thirties, this remarkable woman, born in Ireland, had joined the NZANS in 1916 and worked at Colchester Military Hospital, nursing 'men with the mud still on them',[45] before she was sent to Brockenhurst and then to France. She more than earned her nickname, 'Ten Franc Reidy', buying eggs, fruit and other treats for her patients out of her own pocket. 'She didn't care a hang for colonels or anybody, and besides, she knew her work from A to Z.'[46] When Yellow Three Castles cigarettes and Havelock tobacco were not available in France, Reidy acquired boxes of both from New Zealand. On their half-day off, Reidy and Drummond would visit the various hospitals in St Omer, looking for New Zealanders to help.

The last CO of the NZSH was Charles Hand-Newton, who took over in December 1917, arriving at Wisques in a snowstorm after nearly two years in the blistering heat of the Sinai. As the Germans made a final desperate attempt to push the Allies back in the spring of 1918, there were heavy casualties; at one point evacuation of the hospital seemed a possibility.[47] Sickness became the focus of the NZSH as summer turned to autumn. August and September brought dysentery, and early in October, while Bertha Taylor was still nursing the patients in isolation — 'the bug section' — Sister Gertrude Garrard was admitted to an English military hospital suffering from diphtheria. As the weather grew colder and wetter, nurses were back to nursing 'in tents on tarpaulin floors which get mouldy in a few days of rain'. The staff were also noticing a new medical threat: a virulent type of influenza that killed a concerning number in several French convoys that came into the hospital; 'nothing seemed able to save them'. Thirty-four died in one morning. Many of these men had been fighting since 1914, as had four on Taylor's ward who died within a week in late December — 'No resistance,' she wrote sadly.[48]

After two and a half long, hard years, during which they had cared for thousands of sick, wounded and dying men, the time finally came for the men and women of the NZSH to leave the battlefields of Europe. When the hospital closed its doors on Boxing Day 1918, it had just completed its busiest year: monthly admissions had been between 700 and 1200, and the number of beds had risen to 800. Despite the valuable assistance that NZSH teams had given to CCSs, 'it was always a subject for regret' that the hospital, originally raised as a surgical unit, had never really fulfilled this role. Donald McGavin had championed the idea before the division went to France, but the imperial authorities decided that a New Zealand CCS was unnecessary. Still, the New Zealand medical men had acquired valuable clinical experience at 'this much travelled and much storied hospital'.[49]

The departure was hurried but, as one nurse, possibly Eva Brooke, recorded, everyone enjoyed a 'beautifully sunny . . . real snowy Christmas that one sees and hears so much about'. Each of the 20 infectious patients still in the hospital received a small present and the wards were decorated with little Christmas trees. After a morning church service, the orderlies had their festive dinner at noon, waited on by the nurses and doctors, and in the afternoon all the MOs and several visitors had afternoon tea in the sisters' mess. Following a cinema show put on by the Young Men's Christian Association (YMCA), the nurses and MOs enjoyed 'a very jolly little dinner' before the celebrations culminated in a fancy-dress party for the whole staff. 'All the dresses most original and pretty — where the sisters collected the material, I do not know.'

Everyone had to be up by 5.30 next morning to have their luggage ready. 'We only required two lorries and a half — not very dreadful for thirty-eight sisters. Six of the medical officers, padres, and sixty-four of the orderlies left two hours after us; also forty of the orderlies and some of the M.O.'s left for the division.' The OC, adjutant and quartermaster and staff stayed on for another three days. 'We were all very sad at having to break up the hospital, yet one must not be so because the war is over. We were very happy indeed, and it was, after all, a great experience for all who were there.' After a day in Boulogne, the staff endured a very rough Channel crossing and 34 nurses went to Brighton for a few days' rest before beginning their final leave.[50]

Early in 1919 Godley wrote to Charles Hand-Newton, paying warm tribute to the hospital's work in Egypt, Salonika and France. As usual, 'the unstinted praise of the British Medical authorities' was regarded as an important yardstick, but Godley also lauded the MOs', nurses' and orderlies' 'ability and devotion to duty which no amount of overwork could diminish.

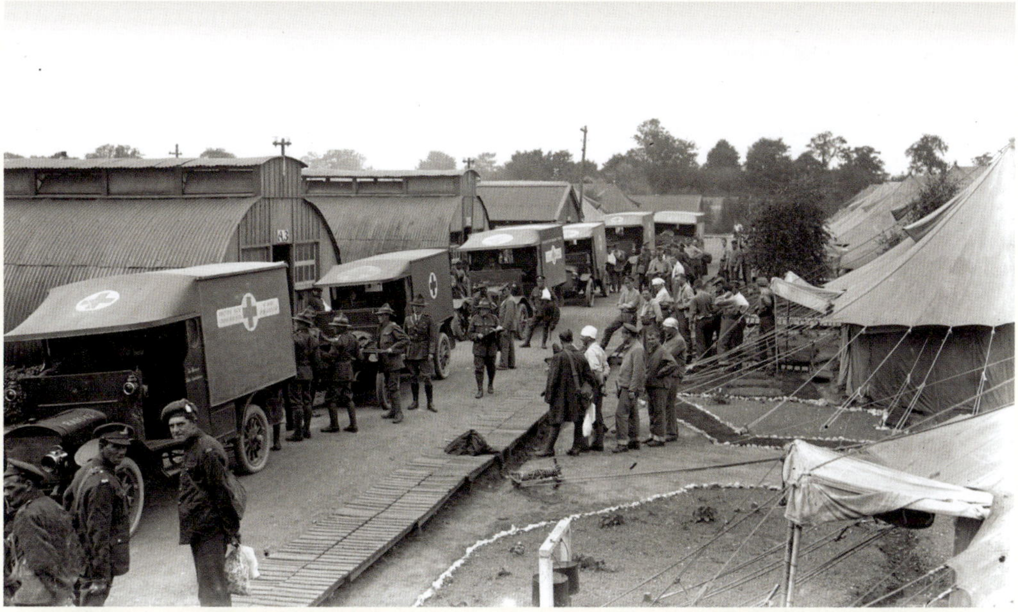

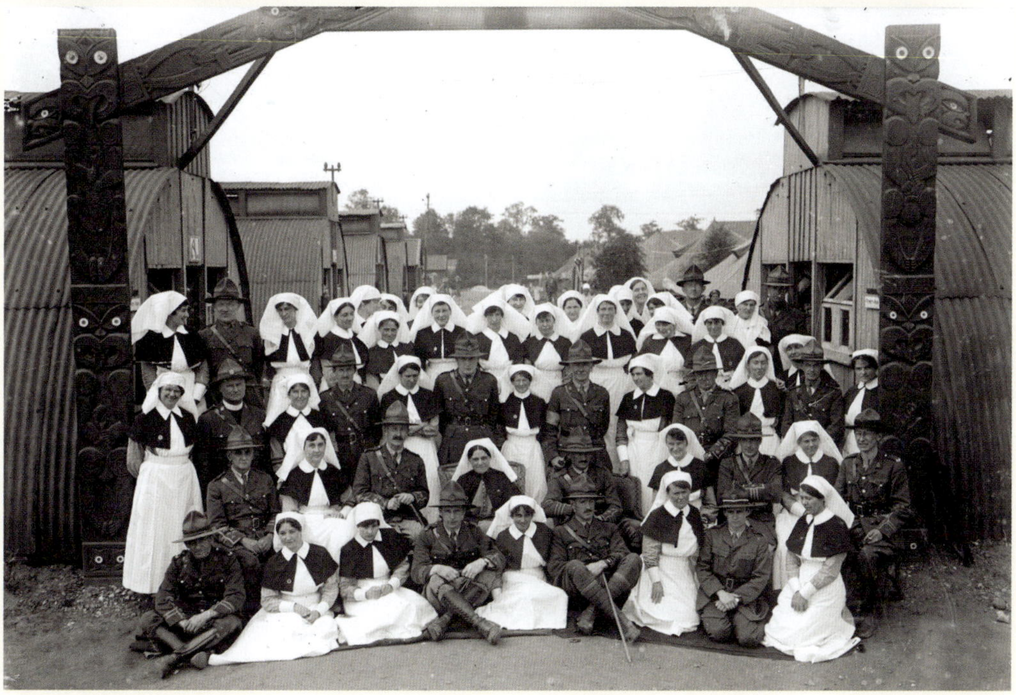

above A convoy of six ambulances prepares to leave the New Zealand Stationary Hospital in Wisques on 16 August 1918, en route for the ambulance train to England. The duckboards so necessary on this damp site can be seen between the tents and the Nissen huts. ALEXANDER TURNBULL LIBRARY, 1/2-013465-G

below The nurses and medical officers of the New Zealand Stationary Hospital photographed at Wisques on 16 August 1918. Matron Evelyn (Eva) Brooke is seated in the middle of the second row. When the hospital closed on Boxing Day 1918, the archway, which had been carved by a Māori patient, was presented to the mayor of Wisques as a memento. ALEXANDER TURNBULL LIBRARY, 1/2-013468-G

The record of the hospital is one of which you, and all those who served under you, may well be proud, and I wish to express to you my congratulations and thanks for all you, and those who served under you, have done.'[51] Terrible and intense though the months on the Western Front had often been, an extraordinary solidarity had developed. Yes, the Brighton home was blessedly comfortable 'after the Nissen huts and the duck-boards, and the cold, and yet we all missed France very much indeed, and would return to-morrow if given the opportunity'.[52]

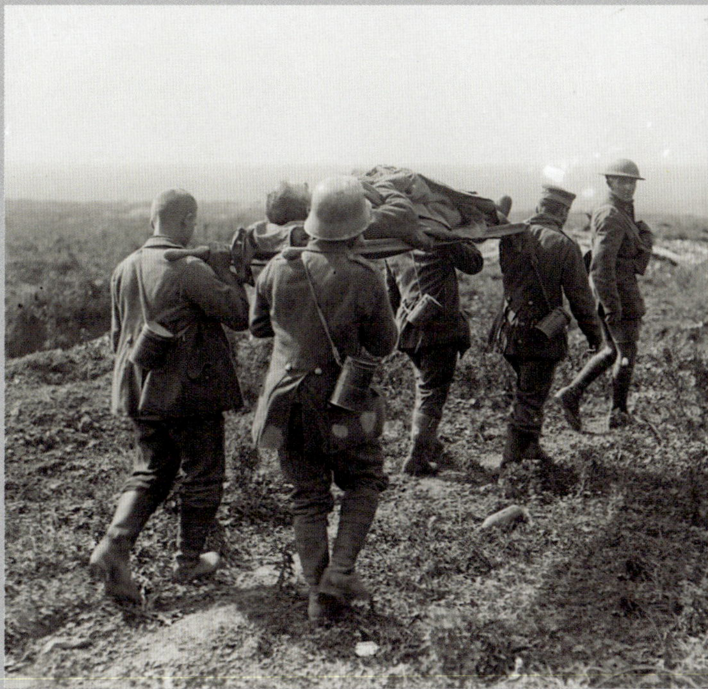

These German prisoners carrying a wounded New Zealand soldier were photographed at Puisieux, on the Somme, on 27 August 1918. ALEXANDER TURNBULL LIBRARY, 1/2-013545-G

HEALING THE 'HUN'

Inevitably, New Zealand medical staff had to treat German prisoners, towards whom their attitudes varied. In July 1916 Millie Tilly, working on the *Marama* at Southampton Docks, described 400 German wounded brought across the Channel as 'a miserable dejected looking lot. Of course their wounds have been attended the same as Tommies. I often wonder if they would mete out the same treatment to our wounded prisoners.' Aucklander Ella Cooke, serving with the French Flag Nursing Corps, found her German patients 'really most respectful to me, and very helpful in every way they can'.

New Zealand soldiers, too, could be sympathetic. 'Some of the poor huns are fearfull sights,' Len Wilton told his future wife, '& seem glad to get taken prisoner.' He helped one wounded German find the nearest dressing station. Louisa Higginson, however, had no charity in her approach when she was working with the QAIMNS at a British prisoner-of-war hospital in June 1917: 'I feel so disgusted & ashamed to think I have to nurse Huns . . . I nurse them because they are Patients, do my duty, no more, no less. I cannot forget the way our poor boys are treated at their hands. I do not bring them flowers or sit on their beds to talk, like some of the sisters.'[53] The previous year, rabid anti-German sentiment at home had led to absurd allegations that West Coast doctor Ebenezer Teichelmann, who had been born in South Australia, had caused the sinking of the *Marquette* by triggering explosives hidden in his luggage.[54]

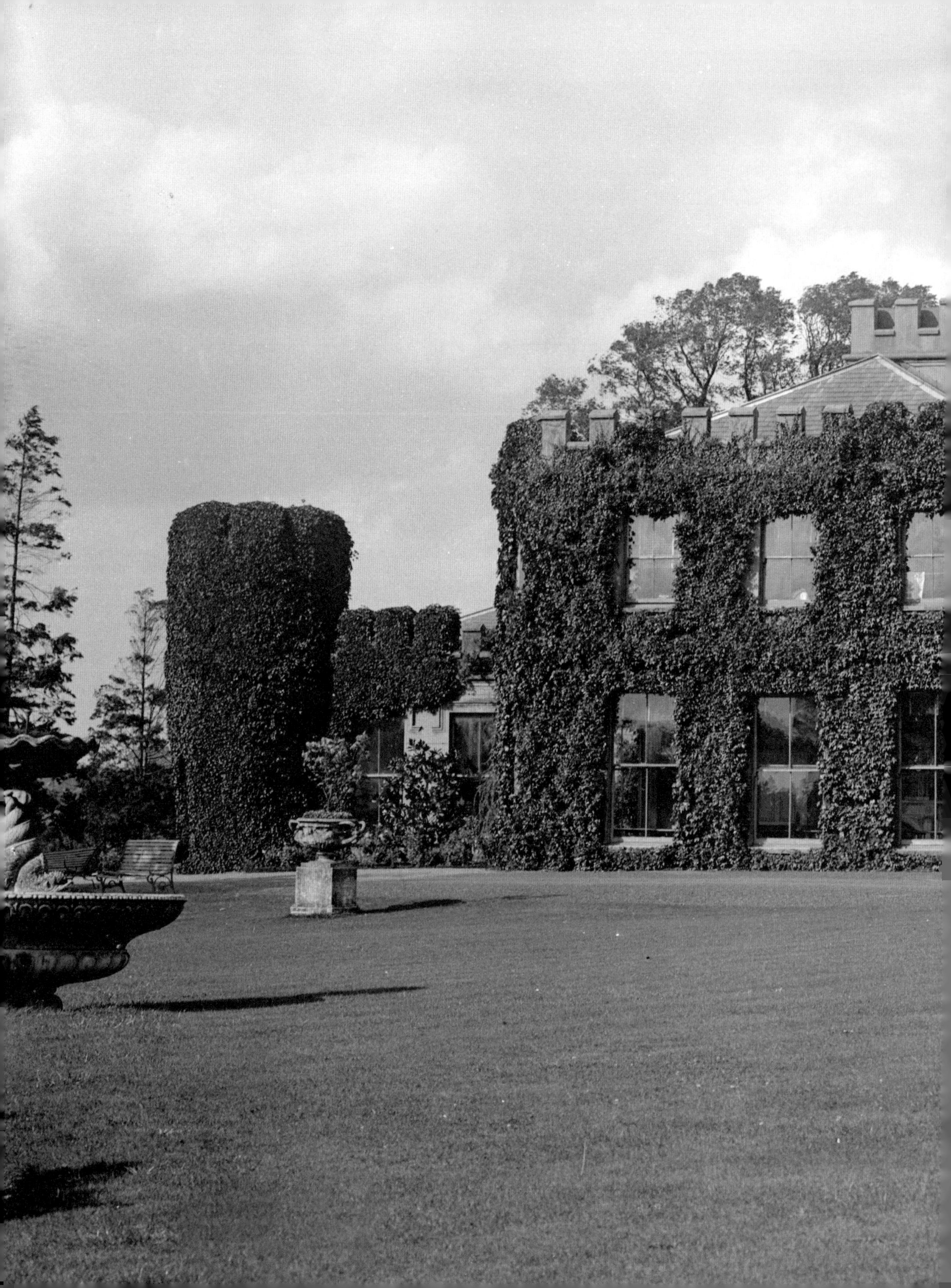

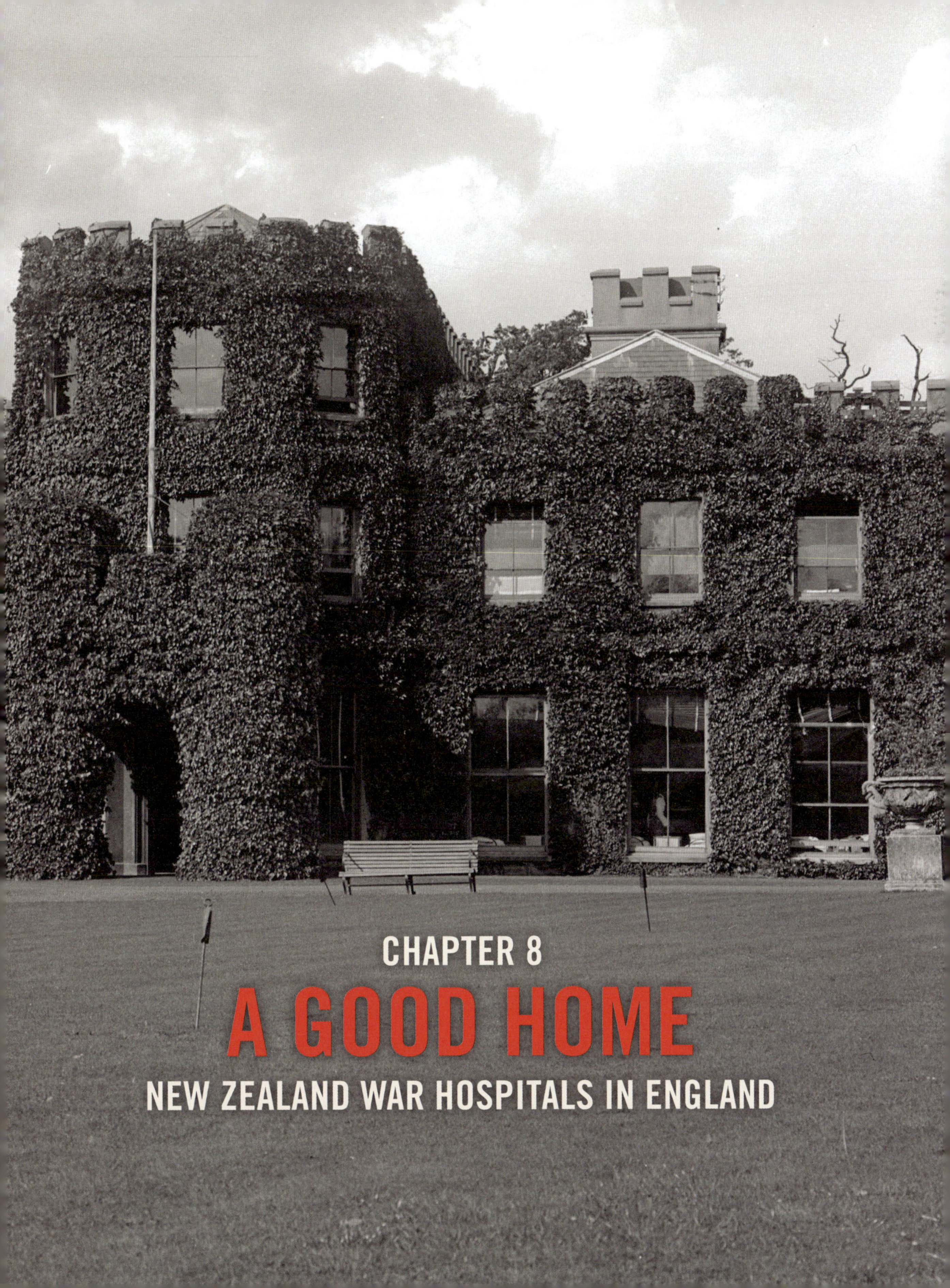

CHAPTER 8

A GOOD HOME

NEW ZEALAND WAR HOSPITALS IN ENGLAND

previous pages
The grand ivy-covered, castellated building at the New Zealand Convalescent Hospital at Grey Towers, Hornchurch, Essex, seen here in 1918, was assigned to officers. The rest of the patients were less impressively accommodated.
ALEXANDER TURNBULL LIBRARY, 1/2-013940-G

My arrival at Walton . . . was a home-coming. I was amongst my own people again, familiar faces, familiar talk and kindness indescribable.
— C. H. Weston, *Three Years with the New Zealanders*

On 17 November 1917, Methodist minister William Lea wrote home from Walton-on-Thames in England, where he was serving as an NZMC orderly at No. 2 New Zealand General Hospital.

> Your readers may know that this hospital is beautifully situated on the bank of the river. The scenery is lovely. Here 1500 New Zealand sick and wounded are accommodated. Considering that convoys of wounded men arrive direct from various battlefields, sometimes to the number of 150 cases during the course of a night, it is difficult to estimate the number of men that pass through this establishment. Very seldom, however, is a patient lost, and New Zealand parents, having a knowledge that their boys are here, may rely upon their receiving the very best of skill, care, and attention. In fact I greet the tired and suffering wounded with the words, 'You have come to a good home now.'[1]

Before Walton-on-Thames opened, initially as a civilian hospital, in August 1915, most of the sick and wounded NZEF men from Gallipoli were dispersed among several British hospitals. When they were convalescent, they reported to the Australian-run ANZAC base depot at Weymouth, on the Dorset coast, where they were either readied for a return to the front or sent home. In the words of Lieutenant Bill Tracy, who had had a finger amputated after being wounded on the peninsula, and did 'light duty' at Weymouth, 'All the crocks come here as soon as they are fit for work of any kind.'[2] When the New Zealand High Commissioner in London, Thomas Mackenzie, visited Weymouth early in August 1915, with his wife, Ida, during a tour of all the hospitals and homes where New Zealanders were being treated, he found some 100 NZEF men, many 'too seriously disabled to return to the Dardanelles'.[3] By the end of September there were more than 2700 sick and wounded New Zealanders in Britain, 'distributed in hospitals from Plymouth to Dundee'.[4]

The congestion at Weymouth, and a shortage of transports to take invalided men home, led to the decision to establish a solely New Zealand camp, and in early January 1916 the New Zealand staff moved to Hornchurch in Essex, just 13 miles from London. The troops were delighted. In place of leaky accommodation in a situation that was 'exposed and bleak in the extreme', they enjoyed 'well-built huts', which slept 30, beside an asphalt drive leading to a gracious country house known as Grey Towers, in which the officers were quartered.[5] And all the occupants, plus the administration and the staff, were New Zealanders.

The New Zealand hospital at Walton-on-Thames began life late in 1914, when the New Zealand War Contingent Association (WCA), a London-based voluntary organisation that oversaw the welfare of New Zealand troops in Britain, considered putting some of its funds towards an NZEF convalescent hospital. The chosen venue was the stately old home of Mount Felix at Walton-on-Thames in Surrey, about 17 miles from the capital. It was ideal, with spacious rooms, extensive grounds, a big kitchen garden and a good rail service nearby. Funded by £3000 each from the WCA and the New Zealand government, and £6000 from the British government,[6] Walton was opened by Mackenzie on Sunday 1 August 1915 as a 110-bed civilian-run hospital. The increasing number of wounded had necessitated the change of emphasis from convalescence.

As well as the wards — named, after the provinces, Auckland, Taranaki, Hawke's Bay, Wellington, Nelson, Marlborough, Canterbury, Westland, Otago, Southland and Dominion — there was the Hinemoa wing, an operating theatre, and quarters for the matron, resident medical officer and staff. The main entrance boasted a 'picture of a Maori carving, and under it the word "Haeremai" in large letters'. Even the ferns and bracken in the gardens 'remind[ed] one very much of New Zealand'.[7]

Major Bernard Myers, then with the RAMC but later a member of the NZMC, who headed the hospital, was supported by a medical officer, an adjutant and two male clerks. The matron was Annie Tombe from Dunedin, who brought with her four New Zealand nurses already working in England. There were also a corporal and four orderlies. The staff increased steadily as the hospital grew: more surgeons, a physician, a radiologist, an oculist, a pathologist, an

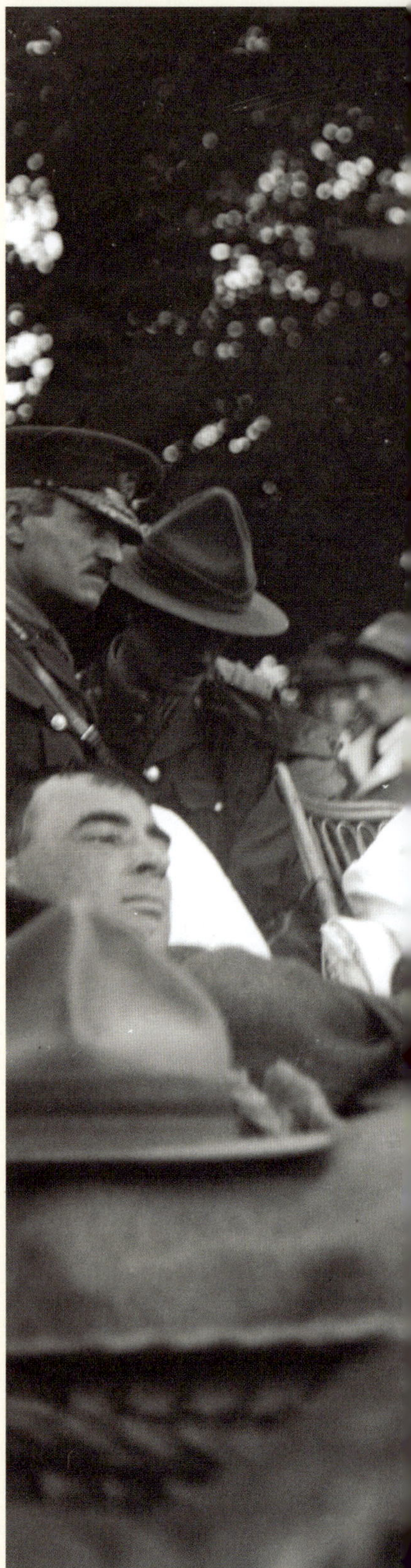

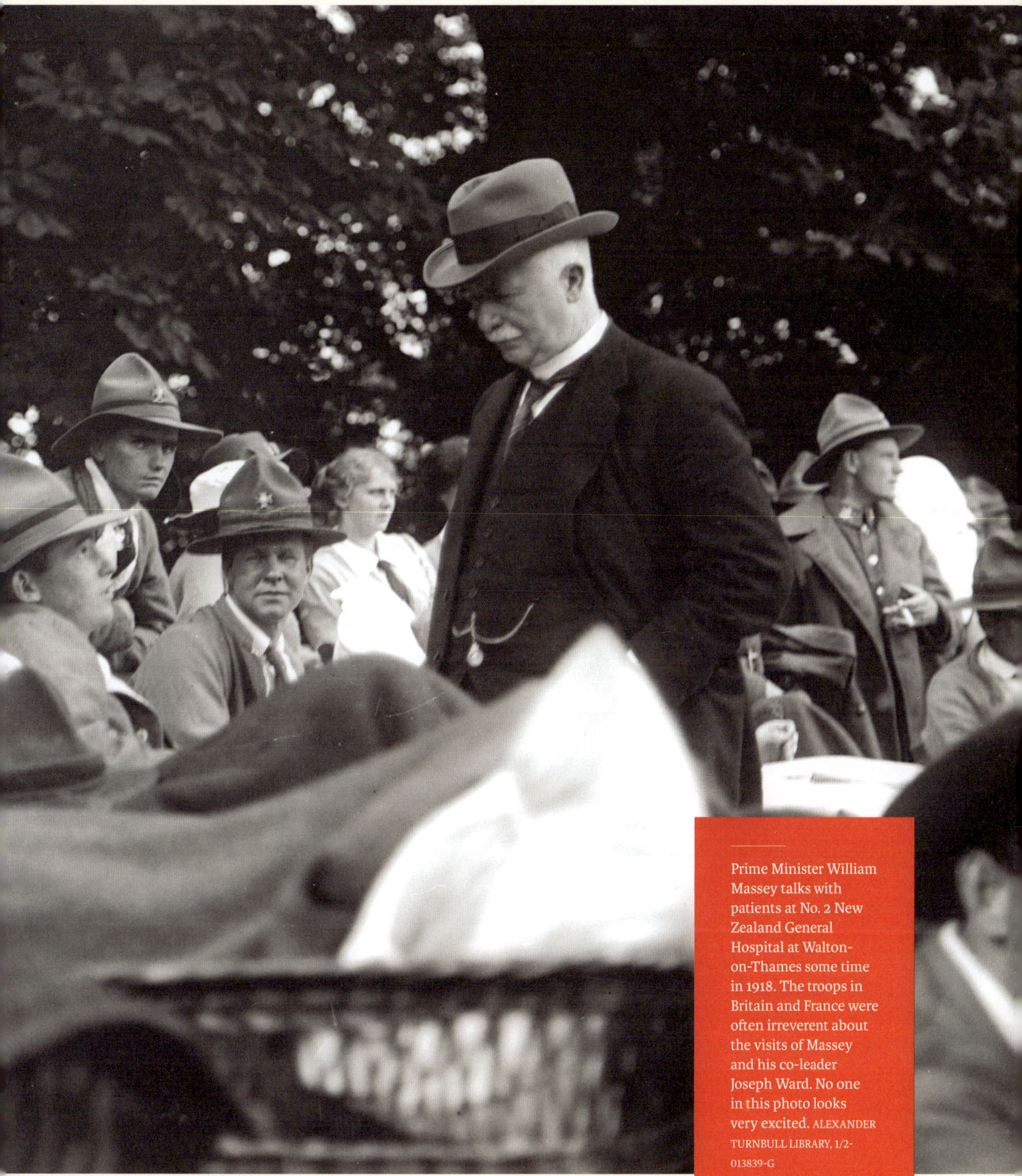

Prime Minister William Massey talks with patients at No. 2 New Zealand General Hospital at Walton-on-Thames some time in 1918. The troops in Britain and France were often irreverent about the visits of Massey and his co-leader Joseph Ward. No one in this photo looks very excited. ALEXANDER TURNBULL LIBRARY, 1/2-013839-G aurist, a dental surgeon and anaesthetists. There was even, by the end of 1915, a trainee female pathologist, 'Miss Durham, a lady of Scientific attainments' who had been 'good enough to offer her honorary services'. She was just one of many volunteers at the hospital throughout the war. By the end of September, X-ray equipment had been installed and 16 patients had been 'skiagraphed'.[8]

One of the first to enjoy the new facilities, and a welcome taste of home, was a Canterbury Infantry Battalion man wounded on Gallipoli who had been hospitalised in Manchester. 'It came as a very pleasant surprise,' he wrote on 7 August. 'Walton-on-Thames is a grand little spot, and just the place for wounded soldiers. The quaint little buildings give it an appearance of quiet and peacefulness that we have not enjoyed for many months . . . no hospital I have been in can compare with our own.' Although he had been 'exceptionally lucky' with his previous nursing, the nurses at Walton were 'New Zealand's best . . . and we are more than satisfied to be under the care of our "own girls" once more'.[9]

As soon as the hospital opened, a 'small New Zealand colony' began to gather at Walton. Lord Plunket, the former governor of New Zealand who now chaired the WCA, had taken a house there, and the Mackenzies had rented a cottage 'for an indefinite period'.[10] Two of their children helped out at the hospital, where another son, Clutha, would become a patient after being blinded by a shell at Chunuk Bair. The high commissioner's personal attention to the care and comfort of New Zealanders in Britain, whether sick or well, won him the gratitude of both the troops and their families. 'My son was in hospital two days before Tom found him out, and when he was well enough, Mrs. Mackenzie had him up at her house,' wrote one mother.[11] Mackenzie's eye for detail extended to checking that the milk being given to the Walton patients came from cows that had been tested for tuberculosis.[12]

The people living near the hospital could not do enough for the New Zealanders. The local cinematograph company offered free showings and sent a car to collect the invalids; the villagers lent their vehicles for outings and gave games, fruit and books. There were concerts at Walton, which had its own piano, and in London. On 24 July 1917, Rifleman George Nuttall from Blackball joined 10,000 other wounded soldiers in the Albert Hall for a show by singer Clara Butt and comedian George Robey: 'Crutches and bandages everywhere.'[13] The men could also enjoy billiards and a London firm sent down a gramophone and records. William Taylor remembered trips up the river that were 'pure delight' and crowds of small craft on Sundays, sometimes with 'a phonograph on a spare seat . . . the music floating across the water was a theme for peace'.[14]

Music could prove a mixed blessing, however. For John A. Lee, recovering in New Zealand's other main hospital, at Brockenhurst, 'Down Texas Way' was 'the hymn of my second nativity' and the gramophone 'the trumpet of an archangel calling to throw away the dust and filth and get up and live' — but the nurse to whom he explained this replied, 'Well, wait till you've heard it as often as I have.' The several Pioneer Battalion patients in Edna Pengelly's Brockenhurst ward 'all love the gramophone, and are always singing, when they are recovered enough, and are full of gags and jokes'.[15] Music could also, however, be distracting. 'I am writing under difficulties,' Alec Hutton told his sister Grace in November 1918, 'for some one is playing the gramophone and that has a detrimental effect on one's concentration.' As Ettie Rout noted, '"Write Home" is a fine motto, but you can't apply it comfortably while the gramophone is advising you to "pack up your troubles in your old kit-bag," and the piano suggesting things would be easier if "you were the only boy in the world".'[16]

The hospital's proximity to a village, and to London, could be problematic. As Myers noted early in December 1915, 'drink can be obtained only too easily from various sources in the Walton district'. The following March, some patients had 'recently been out of bounds in the early part of the evening, and entered some of the empty bungalows opposite, in the company of women'. Myers was confident there would be no further trouble, but emphasised the 'absolute necessity' for a military policeman on the premises. As a patient noted late in 1916, 'Any amount of the boys scale the wall and get out without passes, but the military police are here in scores and you haven't a chance if spotted.'[17]

Walton quickly proved itself 'most valuable as a little corner of New Zealand',[18] but it was soon clear that more beds were needed. By the time Myers wrote his first report on 12 August 1915, 103 patients had been admitted, most of them 'practically healed' surgical cases and convalescents from British hospitals. Two weeks later Mackenzie advised Massey of a proposal to extend the hospital; by the end of the year, Walton was receiving convoys of seriously wounded men directly from the hospital ships. A 200-bed extension was opened on 3 January 1916, and within weeks Myers was suggesting that the committee ask the War Office for 'a daily average of 300 occupied beds throughout the year', with permission to exceed that if necessary. This was agreed to but would, of course, mean more staff.[19] In March Annie Tombe resigned for health reasons. She was replaced by Christchurch Hospital matron Mabel Thurston, who arrived at the end of June. There was a change at the top that month, when Lieutenant-Colonel Thomas Mill replaced Myers, who had been appointed ADMS for the NZEF. When Godley visited Walton in October 1916, he 'had a good talk with Miss Thurston, who . . . seems a capable and excellent woman, and Mill is a great success'.[20]

'On arrival in London,' Thurston remembered, 'I proceeded to Walton that afternoon and immediately took up my duties, as matron of a 300-bed hospital, but it was soon evident that the accommodation for patients was inadequate.' In August she was also put in charge of the nursing service in Britain, doing both jobs until February 1917, when she became full-time matron-in-chief of the NZEF — 'my working day was never less than 14 hours, and frequently 15 and 16' — and Fanny Wilson took over as Walton matron, a post she held until the hospital closed.[21]

With the prospect of many more serious cases once the New Zealand Division reached the front lines in France, a military-run medical base for New Zealanders in Britain was deemed essential and planning began to turn Walton-on-Thames into an official NZEF hospital. The WCA was concerned. At the end of June 1916, Godley met Plunket, Mackenzie and others to discuss the matter. 'They were,' Godley told Allen, 'very unhappy about it, and thought that we were going to ruthlessly tear away all connection with them and not let them have anything to do with it.' But a 'perfectly satisfactory modus vivendi' was achieved, 'which gives us all the necessary control as regards military administration, and still allows the War Contingent

Association to exercise a certain amount of administrative and financial control'. Defence minister James Allen was relieved. Although the WCA had 'done very good work', he feared it was 'overdoing kindness to our troops. I am quite certain that the men who are allowed to remain in England on furlough, ought to be back in the trenches.'[22]

The transformation from civilian to military status initially caused some problems, particularly with pay, but everything was soon resolved: Walton would be a unit of the NZEF and its medical officers and NZANS nurses would be paid at military rates. By the beginning of August 1916, Walton-on-Thames was officially No. 2 New Zealand General Hospital. The No. 1 title went to Brockenhurst, near Southampton, which had opened shortly before. Even with a second hospital, three weeks into August DDMS William Parkes was expecting that all the beds 'will probably be fully occupied soon and my chief difficulty at present is to find sufficient NZMC personnel both officers and men'.[23]

The following month, the New Zealand Division's involvement in the Battle of the Somme led to an enormous number of casualties and convoys poured in daily. To increase Walton's capacity, marquees were erected — eight put up on one day were soon filled with 65 men — as were 70-bed hutted wards. Sister Violet Barker 'had a never-to-be forgotten time . . . during the great rush'. New Zealand nurses en route from Egypt had not yet arrived and until a dozen Canadian sisters came to help, she had to rely on 'three orderlies and two V.A.D.'s from the scullery. The dressing and feeding of over 100 patients was a great business.' There were many bad cases among the wounded: 'compound fractures, abdominal wounds, and big flesh wounds.'[24] Among those who reached Walton, late on 25 September, was William Wilson, whose leg wound had become severely infected, and 'needless to say the treatment I received was wonderful'. By 13 October, he could get up 'but was awfully weak . . . couldn't stand. My mate in the next bed was only too pleased to push my chair. On 14th October I was wheeled up town and saw the sights and the girls and a little bit of old England. It is marvellous how quickly one picks up when out in the air and sun.'[25]

As the casualties mounted, in November 1916 the War Office took over the historic hotel of Oatlands Park, 1½ miles away. By the end of the year, Walton had 1040 beds. 'Ha Ha, a change at last,' wrote Wilson in his diary on 28 November. By now convalescent, he was one of 50 men who helped to ready Oatlands for its new role. Put down as a 'willing worker', he had been recommended for the job by his doctor. 'We are going at top,' he wrote on the 30th, 'trying to get the old mansion into working order. The rooms above are all in first class order but oh, you should see the lower quarters . . . Filthy isn't the word for it.' By 7 December, when patients were arriving daily, Wilson and the others were 'still going strong on the cleaning'.[26] Convalescent patients often helped out at the New Zealand hospitals. 'Am making myself useful in the ward,' wrote Vincent Jervis in September 1918. 'The sister put in a good word for me and said I was very useful they could not do without me.' Alec Hutton, who lost his left foot at Bapaume, visited those he knew in other wards and did 'odd jobs such as cutting up the bread for supper & so forth'.[27]

In the opinion of the *Evening Post*'s correspondent, who visited in January 1917, Oatlands was 'exceptionally well adapted for the purposes of a hospital . . . The old ballroom is now

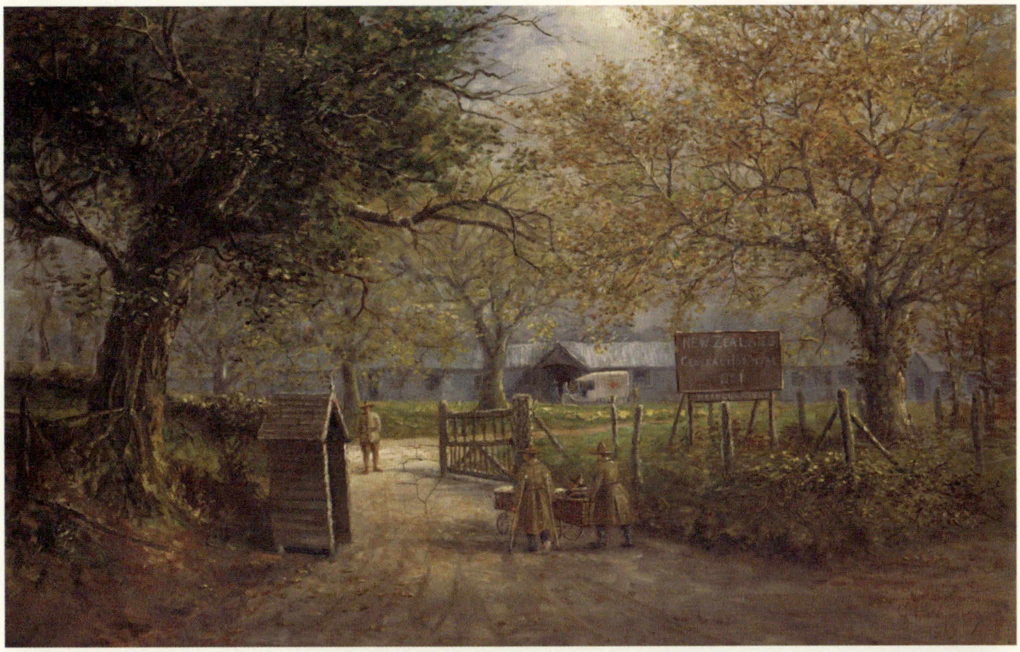

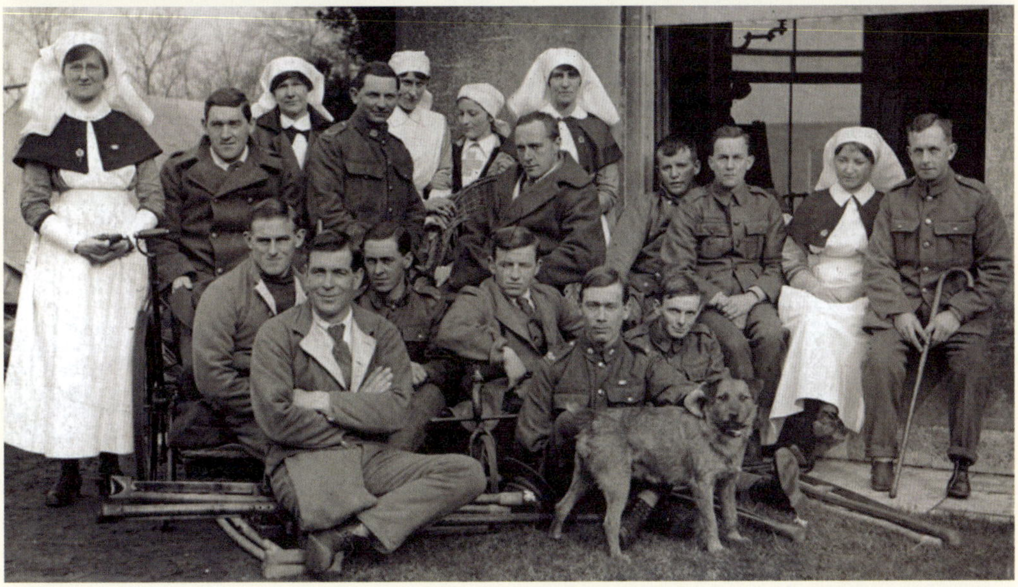

above G. E. Woolley's 1919 oil painting of the entrance to Brockenhurst evokes the attractive and peaceful surroundings that helped to raise the spirits of both staff and patients. The men approaching the gate are wheeling a mate in a basket chair. An ambulance is parked in the background. NATIONAL COLLECTION OF WAR ART, AAAC 898 NCWA 547

below Nurses, amputees and a friendly dog pose for the camera at Oatlands. NATIONAL ARMY MUSEUM, 1986.2657 the dining hall, where 250 men can sit down to a meal at one time, and the bedrooms and coffee-rooms make large and airy wards.' Although there were three storeys, the 'limbies' like Hutton occupied the ground floor, 'so that there is no trouble climbing stairs'. A 'taste of home' was not just metaphorical here: 'all the meat, butter, cheese, and a good deal of the sugar is brought from New Zealand.'[28] A large recreation room, funded by the WCA, was being built in the spacious grounds.

With marquees added at Oatlands, by April 1917 Walton could cater for some 1500 patients. Many of the available beds, *Kai Tiaki* reported, were in 'hutments, which are considered rather wonderful and much admired by professional visitors, for apart from their pretty aspect, they are very serviceably built and have every convenience'. The hospital was, in the matron's words, 'exceedingly busy, tents everywhere. Yesterday we had a convoy of 172 patients straight over from France at 3 a.m., so had to have some of the day staff called. Six of us went to the station and stayed till 4 a.m. giving drinks, etc.'[29] Even when the numbers were huge — in late June Clifford Collingwood arrived in a convoy of 130 vehicles — the medical care and nursing standards never faltered: 'The quilts at night have a pattern of a Chinese boy swinging on a tree, etc all over them, and every quilt must be put so that the patterns all face the same way.'[30]

More tents were needed following the German Spring Offensive in 1918. By 11 April, new cases were arriving constantly, 'and some very sick people amongst them. Our men are having a beastly time. We have over 600 here and are still putting in extra beds.' Two days later they had 700 patients. A bad outbreak of influenza at the end of June was succeeded, from late August, by daily convoys. On 15 September two convoys brought men from the firing line, 'mostly gassed — five days to get here'. On 4 October men were 'still pouring into hospital. All the corridors are full.'[31]

When Sister Edna Pengelly reached Oatlands, she commented on the 'many limbless men . . . most of whom were waiting for the artificial limbs to arrive, and some were learning engineering and other crafts. There were 729 there when I arrived.' The amputees, 'poor lads, are perfect Britons. Many of them do a great deal of sewing, which helps to keep them occupied.' They were 'making great progress at their classes of instruction in shorthand, engineering, carpentry, and woodwork of all kinds. They make all kinds of useful things, and are so game about it.' 'I now go to school in the mornings,' Alec Hutton reported late in 1918, '& am at present learning bookkeeping as I believe it will be one of the subjects to be taught in schools.'[32]

He was just one of several soldiers at Oatlands taking part in a re-education scheme. In mid-October 1917 the *Evening Post* explained that apart from its 'purely economic aspect', the initiative was 'both disciplinary and curative'. In one hut some 40 men, 'almost all wanting a limb, are going through a course of office work — type-writing, shorthand, book-keeping etc . . . Some of them have actually to learn to write again, with the left hand.' Their progress, predictably, was both 'astonishing' and 'exceptional'. In the carpentry area, 'Even the first stool made by a one-armed soldier was a good piece of work; the second was that of a master.'

Some men were placed in suitable businesses to gain experience: a firm of beekeepers in the West Country, for example, or the Vickers factory in Sheffield for 'metallurgy and chemistry in metals' — even the New Zealand Dental Corps.[33]

Concentrating these patients at Oatlands made sense, as Queen Mary's Convalescent Auxiliary Hospital at Roehampton, which specialised in fitting prosthetic limbs, was nearby. By late 1917, when New Zealander Guy Scholefield wrote an article entitled 'New Limbs for Old: Renovating the Cripple', there were representatives from all the dominions on Roehampton's governing committee, and most were sending men to the hospital 'to learn the artificial limb business for the benefit of the thousands who are likely to require subsequent attention long after they have returned to their homes at the ends of the world'.[34]

By the time he got back to New Zealand at the beginning of 1916, Lance-Corporal Frederick Buckley of the Canterbury Infantry Battalion, who had lost most of his right leg on Gallipoli, was walking with only a slight limp. At Roehampton in December 1915, his leg had been 'finally fixed up, and the missing portion replaced by an artificial limb. Within four days he was able to walk about for a whole day without removing the dummy limb.' As he explained to a reporter, 'The wooden leg was affixed four inches below the knee, and the foot was rubber, and so built up of springs that the wearer could walk naturally without the slightest jar.' The prosthesis was built 'so that there was no weight on the stump of the limb itself, but it all fell on the upper leather supports. There were knee-joints and steel parts fastening on to the thigh, the artificial limb finally being supported over the shoulder. The whole contrivance was three pounds lighter than the estimated weight of the missing limb.' This may sound cumbersome, but it represented 'wonderful progress in the science of surgery' for men 'mutilated in a score of ways'.[35]

The process was not speedy, particularly as the number of limbless patients rose. In October 1916, Cecil Malthus explained that a patient 'kept in England to be fitted with an artificial limb . . . is lucky if it takes any less than six months'.[36] By 20 November 1918, Hutton was hoping 'in a short time . . . to be provided with what is known as a peg leg the preliminary to an artificial one. Under existing regulations I shall not be back in N.Z. much before next Christmas i.e. 1919, as we are provided with two legs, one presumably for . . . state occasions.'[37] A man's stump had to be 'absolutely healed and hard' before he was sent to Roehampton to be examined and measured. The Carnes Artificial Limb Company of Kansas City was renowned for making arms.[38] By November 1917, the workshops of the private firms that made the limbs under contract were situated in Roehampton's grounds. On average, it took about 30 days for a man to learn to use his new leg 'freely and with comfort'; arms typically took less time. Even after their artificial legs were successfully fitted, some men continued to have a 'gratuitous limp', a hangover from hobbling about on sticks.[39]

Also headquartered at Oatlands, in the stables, was the Mechanical Transport section, with 'a small but efficient staff of expert drivers and artificers, who are capable of undertaking anything in the motor-repair line'. Although small workshops at Sling, Brockenhurst and Hornchurch could manage minor repairs, all ambulances requiring 'skilled attention' went to Oatlands.[40] When it opened as a military hospital, Walton had only borrowed ambulances, but by early November 1915 it had three of its own, two given by the Red Cross, and one lent by a Captain Macalister. These vehicles conveyed the wounded to and from the railway station. Every ambulance sent from New Zealand received a standard paint job: 'The chassis and under-gear are being painted Dreadnought grey, and the body white enamel. On each side appears the Red Cross with the words in bold lettering, "New Zealand Expeditionary Force."' The ambulance donated by the people of Eltham in Taranaki, 'turned out of the workshops in its new dress' in March 1917, had 'a very effective and smart appearance'.[41]

By the end of 1917, Mount Felix was devoted to wards and boasted, in its grounds, a new operating theatre, an X-ray room and a laboratory. Major Henry D. Pickerill, Professor of Dental Surgery at Otago University, who had joined the Dental Corps in 1916 and then the NZMC in 1917, had set up a department devoted to the treatment of facial and jaw injuries; in 1918 he joined Queen's Hospital at Sidcup in Kent, a purpose-built facility for reconstructive surgery.

When John A. Lee, DCM, who had lost his left arm at Mailly-Maillet in France, was taken to No. 1 New Zealand General Hospital at Brockenhurst, 14 miles from Southampton, in April 1918, he was put into an 'airy ward'.

> Wheeled along a clean corridor I was turned into an airy ward. A white-painted table was covered with spring flowers. From a dozen white pillows heads with cleanshaven faces welcomed . . . I was half lifted, half scrambled on to the white sheet.
>
> My temperature was taken, my pulse tested, my respiration assessed, religion, regiment, name, number and rank were entered in the card above my head . . . Clotted blood, dried mud, sweat, odour, lice, [the sister] sponged away . . . She dressed me in a clean singlet, a pair of pyjamas, propped me in a semi-reclining position . . . The great simple luxuries exhausted me.

In his memory, the sun 'seemed to shine for me all the time . . . There must have been wet days but I lived in my glow of rebirth.'[42]

Formerly a hutted hospital set up in 1915 to nurse Indian soldiers, Brockenhurst, on the edge of the New Forest, took on a new identity when the New Zealand General Hospital arrived from Egypt on the *Marama* on 19 June 1916. 'It is a most beautiful place,' wrote Edna

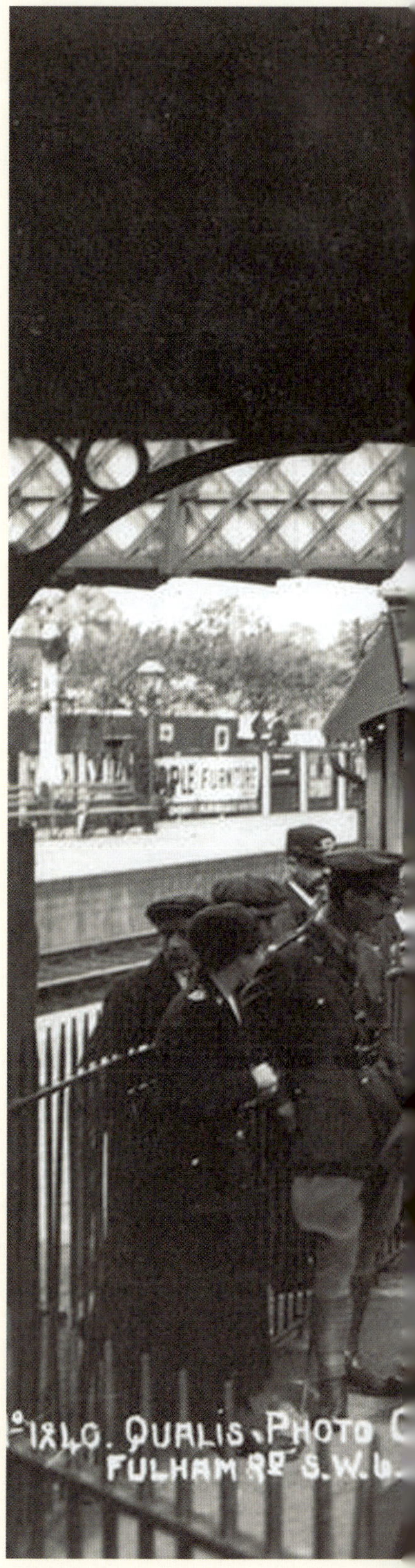

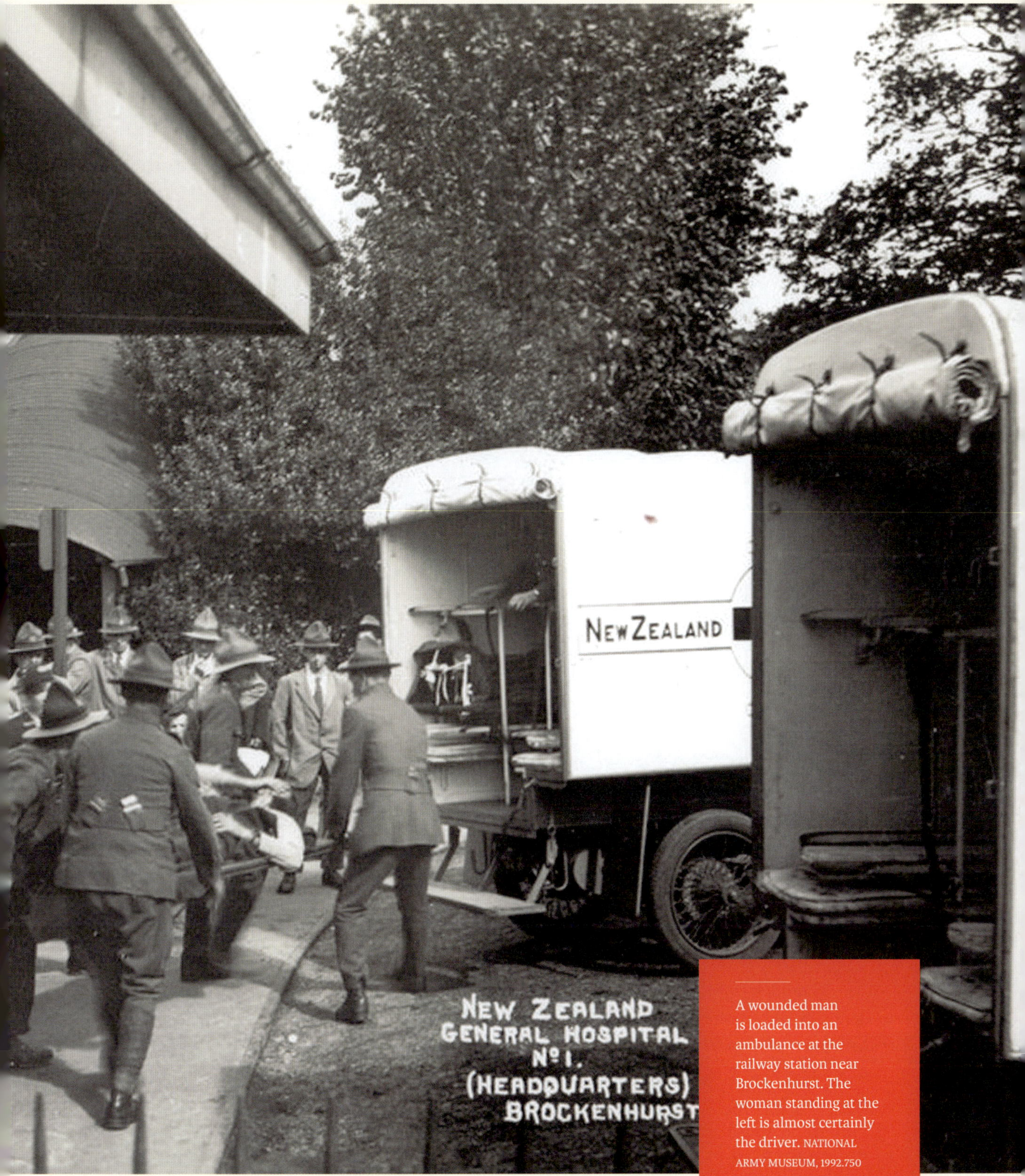

A wounded man is loaded into an ambulance at the railway station near Brockenhurst. The woman standing at the left is almost certainly the driver. NATIONAL ARMY MUSEUM, 1992.750

Pengelly. 'Trees and green grass; live trees and beautiful smell of woodland and hayfields everywhere one goes.'[43] Orderly Colin Gordon helped to ready the vacant hospital for its new role — 'twenty buildings there with nothing in at all, and we had to equip them with the hospital gear and get them ready for patients'.[44] Two hotels in the village — Forest Park, for officers, and Balmer Lawn — were also requisitioned. The main, hutted section of Brockenhurst consisted of two 10-ward wings, each with 36 beds; there was also a central administration block, an operating theatre, an X-ray room, a dental surgery and a dispensary. David Wylie was the OC and Bertha Nurse the matron.

The wounded arriving at Dover were taken to Walton, whereas those sailing into Southampton usually headed to Brockenhurst, though the flow of patients was often irregular, owing to the threat of submarines in the Channel and interruptions to the Le Havre–Southampton ferry service. No. 1 New Zealand General Hospital could, however, be extremely stretched.[45] After returning from some well-earned leave on 20 July 1916, Edna Pengelly and the other nurses soon faced a rapidly increasing workload. By September convoys were arriving every day. On the 20th, 'The whole place is standing on its head — operations galore and scarcely knowing what to do first. If only we could unscrew our legs and put on a fresh pair before going on duty.' Nine days later yet another convoy arrived: 'Poor fellows. They have a rotten time, and some come here only to die.'[46] As another nurse reported late in 1917, 'Beds all full, and Church huts and Y.M.C.A. huts turned into wards. The convoys pour in and often the corridor is a sad sight, lined with weary, grubby-looking bandaged boys.'[47]

As at Walton, the peaceful and attractive surroundings played their part in healing the patients and gave the weary nurses, doctors and orderlies some respite. Former Auckland printer William Smallfield credited the 'splendid situation' with helping his recovery from illness.[48] In both hospitals, the patients added their own dash of colour to the scene. Once up and about, the men wore special blue suits faced with red, white shirts and red ties; they were nicknamed 'blue boys'.

When Arthur Field visited Brockenhurst late in 1916, the patients numbered about 1000. He described the two 'well-built modern hotels' and the headquarters in what was known as 'Tin Town' — 'a big temporary building hospital with about twenty wards, connected up by an apparently endless series of corridors'. The picturesque old Morant Arms accommodated the overflow, who were cared for by VADs.[49] As at Walton, the YMCA was essential to the entertainment on offer, providing games and writing and reading rooms, plus a library with 'a file of newspapers from each of the four New Zealand centres — a very much sought-after corner'.[50] Here, and at all hospitals with New Zealand patients, the WCA organised regular visits — 'I don't know what we should do without them,' wrote Alec Hutton in September 1918 — and supplied comforts from home. Sister Jeanne Sinclair considered Balmer Lawn a happy place, apparently 'considered the "Hospital de Luxe" by the "lead swingers".'[51]

Here, too, YMCA workshops run by New Zealand soldiers permanently unfit for active service were 'a place of serious instruction in future livelihoods, and at the same time a means of curative treatment for others'. Those with leg wounds could learn lathe work to exercise their muscles, and there was 'basket or raffia work for finger-exercise, planing for arms and

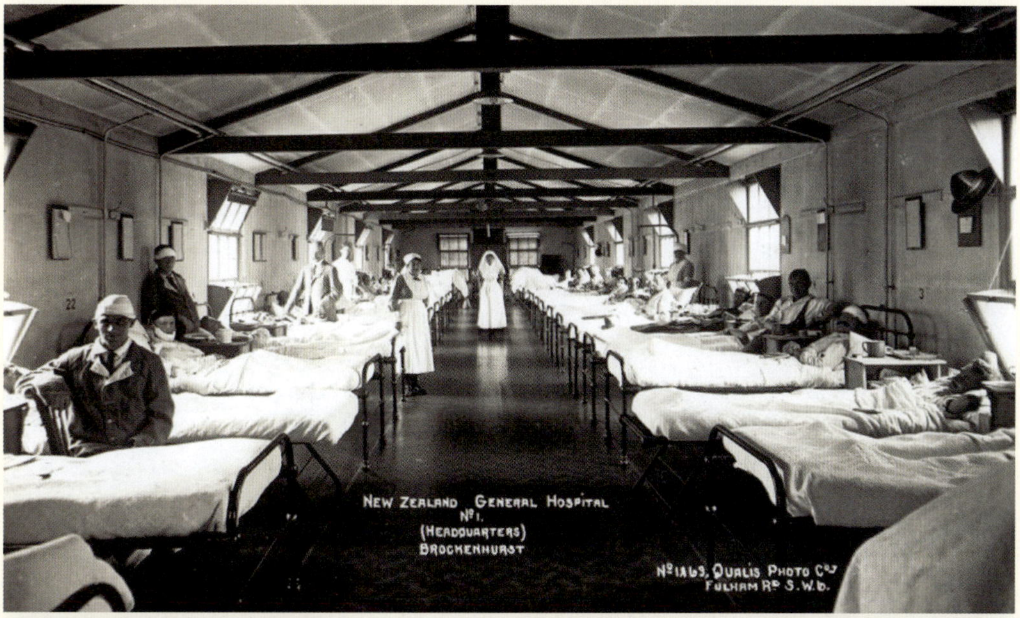

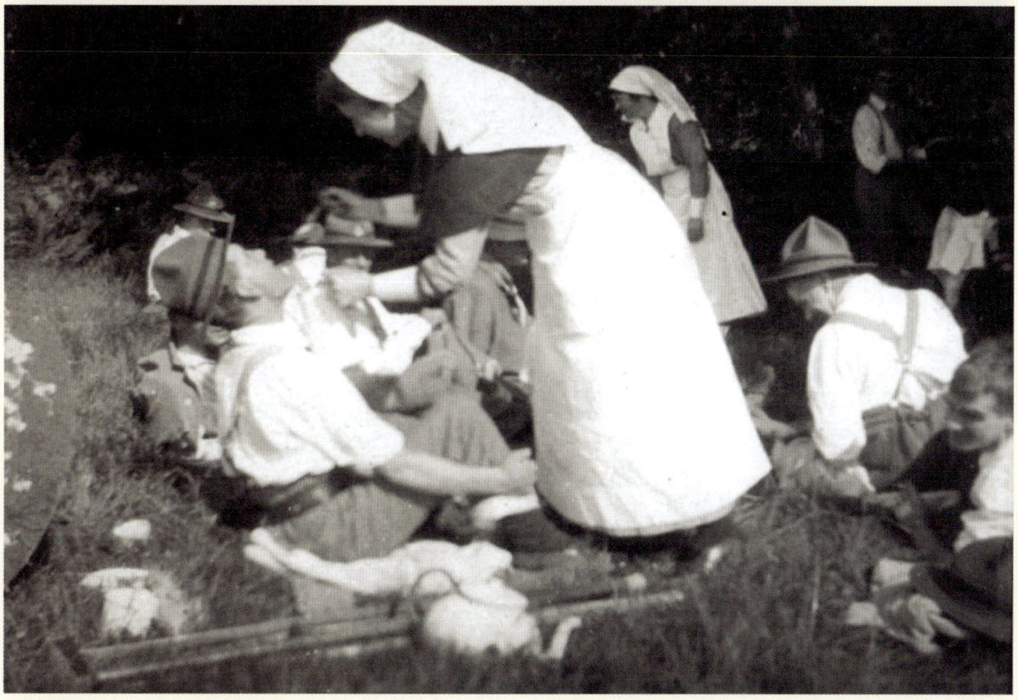

above Neatly made beds and a shiny floor in a Brockenhurst ward. The patients' medical charts hang on the wall above their individually numbered iron-framed beds. The man on the left with the bandaged head is wearing hospital 'blues'. NATIONAL ARMY MUSEUM, 1992.750

below The attractive countryside near the two main New Zealand hospitals in Britain was ideal for enjoyable patient and nurse excursions. This photo, taken in Lyndhurst Wood, not far from Brockenhurst, and titled 'Nothing to be wasted', comes from a series entitled 'Picnic in the Woods — July 1917'. There were also sports days with traditional races and games of tug of war. NATIONAL ARMY MUSEUM, 1992.1156.1

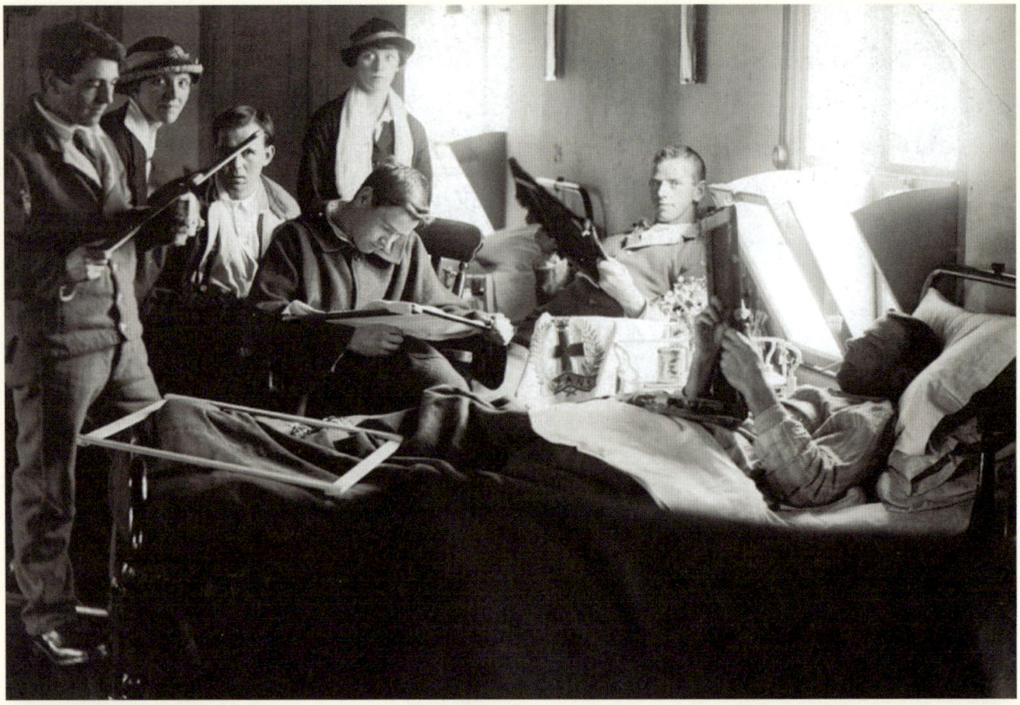

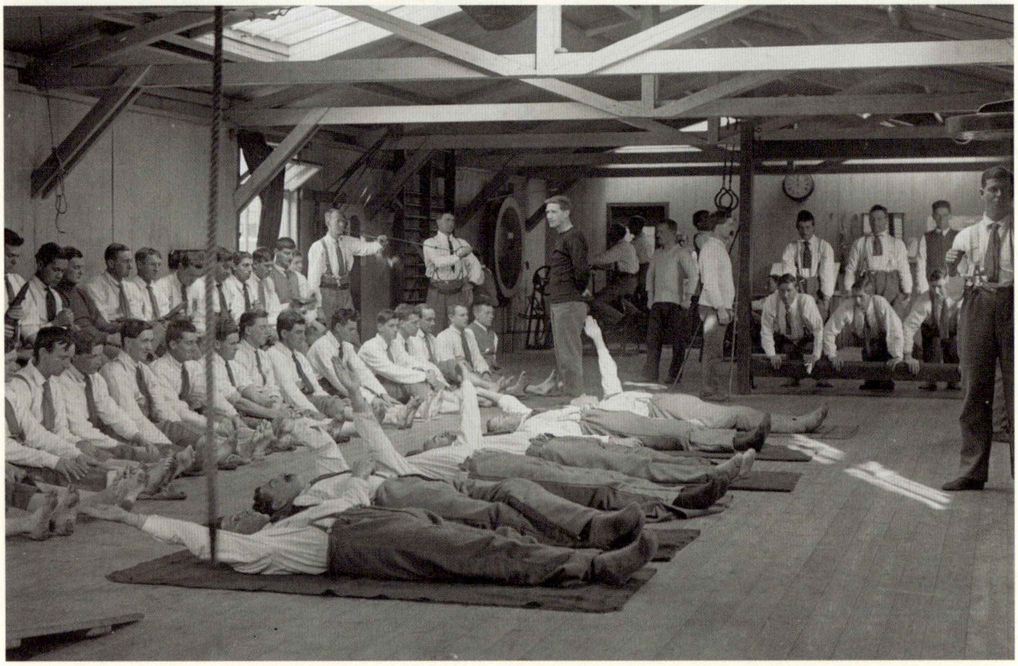

above These convalescent patients are applying themselves assiduously to their embroidery, but not everyone was impressed with this rehabilitative occupation. NATIONAL ARMY MUSEUM, 1994.3345

below Hornchurch offered what Malcolm Ross called 'therapeutic treatment by mechanical exercises of a most interesting kind'. These took place in a 'well-fitted gymnasium' full of 'ingenious appliances and machines to suit the different cases'. ALEXANDER TURNBULL LIBRARY, 1/2-014001-G back, brace-and-bit work for the forearm and shoulders, and so on'. The men turned out an impressive array of metal, leather and wicker work, wood carving, fretwork, signwriting and decorating. They also made crutches and artificial limbs for the hospital, and repaired the patients' chairs and other appliances. Those unable to leave their beds did 'arts and crafts', which included needlework:

> a nurse will ask some temporarily tired-out giant in bed to show you his bit of work, and with a half-ashamed smile, and sometimes with almost a blush, he will pull out from under his pillow or some receptacle beside the bed one of these delicate pieces of work, and you look at its beauty and then at his big rough hands and wonder how it was done! And perhaps you have a fleeting recollection of these same hands, mud-grimed and bloody, tugging a bayonet out of a livid German![52]

Clifford Collingwood, wielding his needle at Walton, was not keen. 'My piece of work was a 6-inch square of net on which I had to work, in wool, some geraniums. On the base of the material there was stamped "Work for Soldiers". "Work" was right, for the article appeared unlovely to me, and it tired me very quickly.' He left it in his locker when he was discharged.[53]

As at Walton, the locals were extremely supportive. 'I do hope you won't worry over me,' Alec Hutton told his mother, 'because we are treated like lords here. People visit us and give us concerts.' Trips to Bournemouth were another treat. As Cecil Malthus explained to his fiancée, Hazel, 'We are only allowed to go in parties in charge of sisters, but ours kindly left us to our own devices in town.'[54] Local stately homes were made available as convalescent auxiliaries for patients 'well on the way to recovery': Hill House at Lyndhurst, Home Mead at Lymington and Avon Tyrrell (owned by Lord and Lady Manners and for officers only) were each supervised by a medical officer and a senior sister.

By 1917 Brockenhurst had both a neurological centre, at Balmer Lawn, and an orthopaedic department. The former, put under the charge of W. Marshall Macdonald in January 1918, had 'grown to be an important unit' by the end of the war.[55] Macdonald, who had supported the nurses' fight to serve overseas, had worked as a neurologist for the French Medical Army Corps, the Service de Santé, for a year from June 1915, before returning to Dunedin. In April 1917 he went to Britain with the NZMC as consulting neurologist to the NZEF: Louis Barnett considered him 'the best man obtainable in the Dominion for work of that kind'.[56] New Zealand surgeons trained in British units brought their skills to Balmer Lawn, and once Brockenhurst perfected 'its physio-therapy and plaster departments, splint shops and curative workshops', No. 1 New Zealand General Hospital became the orthopaedic hub for New Zealand's medical services in Britain.[57]

Like Walton-on-Thames and Brockenhurst, Hornchurch was a delight in spring, but this 'particularly pleasant' place did not last long as a command depot.[58] When General George Richardson took over command of the NZEF troops in Britain early in 1916, his determination to increase the force's 'effective strength' included moving the depot, on 6 July, to the much less alluring location of Codford, on Salisbury Plain in Wiltshire, not far from the hated Reserve Training Camp at Sling. Hornchurch's proximity to London was having a bad effect on the 'invalidity figures', and because the camp could hold only 1000 men, there had been a 'great deal of billeting' of the hundreds more who arrived. Hornchurch would become New Zealand's first proper convalescent hospital; the 'hardening up', as it was known, before returning to the front would take place at Codford.[59]

After his discharge from hospital, a man was medically examined — 'boarded' — and then rated A, B or C. A meant fit to return to service: a short furlough was followed by time at Codford before pre-embarkation training at Sling. B men were likely to be fit for service within six months and went to Codford unless they required special treatment, such as massage or diet, which they received first at Hornchurch. Those with a C classification, permanently unfit and unable to fight again, remained at Hornchurch for 'proper medical treatment as convalescents' until they were strong enough to be sent home or until a ship was ready to take them. Hornchurch became so choked with men waiting to depart that a New Zealand Discharge Depot was established in Devon at the seaside resort town of Torquay.[60]

The boarding and repatriation process could be tedious, as Cecil Malthus discovered. 'The doctor tells me,' he wrote on 16 November 1916, 'he is not at all certain that I shall get back to New Zealand. It seems the latest cry is for "economy of manpower", and the new chief surgeon is very chary of granting discharges.' Although by 14 December it was 'almost an absolute certainty' that he would be going back to New Zealand, his departure would not be immediate: there were 'hundreds ahead of me, and the boats are far between'.[61]

When Rifleman Gladstone (Gladdie) Graham was hit by machine-gun fire on the Somme on 1 October 1916, his right arm was broken in two places and his elbow shattered. He was taken to Walton where, on 21 November, the elbow was 'still full of very fine metal and they expect this to come out with massage treatment I am getting'. By the time he had been moved to Hornchurch, however, no metal had emerged, 'so I shall be here for some time yet'. By 19 August 1917 he had been at Codford for a while: 'My arm is much the same and I have not made my appearance before the Medical Board yet, so am living in hopes.' The next step was the Division Employment Corps for men 'fit enough for [base] duties in France'. By 19 October, Graham was back with his unit.[62] The regime at Codford was 'rather stiff', according to Gallipoli casualty Phil Bennett. When he wrote home on 28 August 1916, he had been there for a fortnight, following several months of treatment. 'To date the hip has stood all tests, and the drill here is rather solid, especially the bayonet fighting. The doctors are watching with interest what they term an "experiment," and their predictions are not too rosy, but I feel that with ordinary care I can get fit enough to get over to France in a couple of months.'[63]

Codford also had a hospital, No. 3 New Zealand General, across the road from the command depot. When Nurse Elsie Grey arrived there in October 1916, she found herself 'in a Valley at the mouth of an Iceberg. My Godfather you don't know what cold is in N.Z.' Her room was 'very up to date' but she was unable to sleep — 'I froze, all the huts are corregated tin stuff and you do feel it. The Hospital is the same.'[64] Mabel Crook reported to Codford on New Year's Day 1917 and recorded in her diary: 'Lakes frozen pipes in home constantly breaking . . . icicles hanging from Sisters' home verandah were two to three feet wide by three or four inches thick. Bucket of water frozen solidly. Hot water bags frozen solid. Water in jug or basin frozen solid — no hot water baths.'[65] There were compensations, though. In summer Sister Clara Cherry was 'able to wander miles over the hills and along the country lanes, and for a while lose sight of the little tin huts. Cowslips, primroses, blue bells, and lilac have in turn decorated our huts.'[66] Temporary escape was possible: Salisbury was 30 minutes away by train, Bath two hours.

As Nurse Isabella Munro found in November 1916, the work at Codford was hard. 'The weather has been so cold and wet, there has been much sickness amongst the boys . . . We have ten wards of 33 beds, and yesterday, some distance from the main building, five new huts were opened for infectious cases, such as measles and mumps, so altogether life is pretty strenuous for everybody, especially for our O.C., Colonel Fenwick, and the medical officers, as they are so few in number.'[67] Some less seriously injured soldiers, unhappy at the prospect of returning to the trenches, swung the lead at Codford but very few, in Bertha Taylor's opinion, got spoiled. 'The boys we get from the late reinforcements are not so strong, many are physically unfit, who have been rejected in the first place and it is not fair to call them shirkers.'[68]

In the view of Gunner Len Wilton, who was at Sling in December 1916, 'The men are treated just like a mob of sheep & as long as they can walk about they are allright. One has to lay down before they will take any notice of him.' One young man 'said he could not go any further if something was not done to him. The Doctor examined him & found his temputure to be 104 & at once sent him to the Hospital & the next day the boy was dead.'[69] Over the bitterly cold Christmas of 1916, Elsie Grey wrote, patients were being sent in from Sling 'absolutely in the last stages of Pneumonia and of course it is too late and we cannot pull them through. It is terrible to see these young boys dying.' By February 1917 Codford was averaging a death a day. As John Moloney, in isolation with scabies at the hospital in March, put it, 'They have left a southern summer, crossed the line and find the bitterness of this English winter too much for them . . . The poor fellows go down with a cold, are sent over to Codford, but when they get here they are too far gone. Day after day they go past. A gun carriage draped with a Union Jack . . . and the band, slowly intoning the solemn dead march.'[70]

When Hornchurch was being set up, 'it was very strongly felt . . . that the presence of a V.D. Section in the midst of a Convalescent Hospital was not in the best interests of the place', so this was moved to Codford.[71] Many of the men in the constantly guarded detention hospital, surrounded by barbed wire, had contracted VD while on leave in London. The flourishing prostitution business in the British capital favoured the New Zealand and Australian soldiers, who were better paid than their Tommy counterparts and could afford to be more generous. In the first half of 1917, 1138 VD cases were admitted to Codford. Of those, only 223 came from France and '50 per cent. of the infection, acquired in England originated in London'. And this was despite the availability of cheap prophylactics at all New Zealand canteens, ablution rooms in each unit and warnings about 'the dangers of infection and the methods of prevention'.[72]

Before going to France in May 1917, a realistic Moloney wrote, 'In a few days we will be in the vortex once more and many will have worshipped at the shrine of Bacchus and Venus for the last time. A blanket and a few feet of Flanders earth will be their portion.'[73] The punitive attitude towards VD was clear even in the official Codford diary entries. On 1 February 1918, 40 invalids and 20 'chronic Venereals' were sent by train to Liverpool to travel home to New Zealand on the *Maunganui*. The men with VD went 'under armed escort'.[74]

By the time former *Evening Post* journalist and NZEF publicity man Lieutenant Henry Drew visited in late 1918, Hornchurch could care for 1600 men and there were often 1000 there. The medical staff comprised 11 doctors and 22 nurses, all New Zealanders, plus 19 masseuses and 118 VADs and other female workers.[75] Patients were divided into three sections: medical, surgical and massage; it was this last area, which included electrical treatment, that became the success story of the hospital. In February 1917 Malcolm Ross described Hornchurch as 'quite a New Zealand colony, where our convalescents are being treated in the most scientific and up-to-date manner'. One man 'will fix himself in a machine that has a sliding seat and enables his muscles to get all the exercise that they would get in a racing boat. Another mounts what to all intents and purposes is a bicycle, and finds his speed registered on a dial. An expert is pattering away at a punching ball with the dexterity of a Jack Johnson. Others are skipping, or working with dumbbells.'[76] By September that year there was so much work that the massage section had to be split into two. One subsection dealt with peripheral nerve lesions, functional nerve lesions, myalgias, neuralgias and trench feet; the other covered joint conditions, fractures and 'Involvements of muscles and vessels except as above'.[77]

Plenty of recreational activities were available, including a swimming pool, but keeping the convalescents busy was vital. 'It is obvious that a man back from the horrifying experiences of the front-line trenches and from the stress and strain of continuous shell-fire, is going to recover much quicker if his mind is filled with continuous impressions of a totally different nature. The less time he has to brood on the past or to worry about the future — when he will return to the trenches — the better.' It is hard not to wonder whether traumatised patients really did 'forget themselves in constructing baskets or knocking together forms or cupboards', or how they felt about making wooden crosses for the graves of those who died in New Zealand hospitals: 'interest for the convalescent and a record for the dead.'[78] From May 1918 there were classes in such subjects as French, English, shorthand, bookkeeping, seed-testing and wool-classing. Because all the hospitals and camps had similar classes, men could continue their studies as they moved from place to place. Both agriculture, particularly potato growing, and poultry farming assisted the aim of making the hospitals as self-supporting as possible. In February 1918, to help with the food supply, a rabbitry was established at Hornchurch with 47 animals. By the end of May there were 300 rabbits and a similar number of chickens.[79]

In Brighton, two houses overlooking the sea and surrounded by attractive gardens constituted a popular convalescent home for New Zealand officers. This had begun in 1915 when a Brighton resident named Knight put his house at 13 Lewes Crescent at the disposal of the WCA for recovering officers. When the NZEF decided to establish an official convalescent home early in 1917, Knight offered both this house and a second in the same street, which was opened at the end of February.[80] 'It was always a great pleasure to visit . . . and see the happiness and contentment written on all faces. The air was good, while the care and attention given by the medical officer and nursing staff, together with the massage treatment, soon made sick-looking officers appear once more robust.'[81] There was swimming, too, in summer. After being wounded in France, chaplain Ronald Watson spent a month at 13 Lewes Crescent in late 1918. 'It is a "bon" home too . . . I am having malt, massage, rest and sea air. So I ought to get my dash back again very soon now.'[82]

The welfare of the nurses was not forgotten, although the home for sick and exhausted sisters in Sandwich had to be moved in 1917 because of frequent air raids. As Mabel Thurston told Hester Maclean, Melrose House, at the Hove end of Brighton, about 3 miles from the officers' accommodation, 'was a large home belonging to wealthy people, and we have taken it over furnished, with beautiful carpets, lounges, pictures china etc. Charming bedrooms are built to catch the morning sun . . . [W]e can accommodate 50 people, that is including the staff.' One, quite separate, portion of the building became the hospital; the remainder was the rest home. 'It is a delightful climate, and the house embodies every comfort. I have long wanted such a place for them.'[83]

The medical officers who headed the New Zealand hospitals in Britain were essential to the spirit and the smooth running of these homes away from home. When Edna Pengelly arrived at Codford in May 1917, for example, Percival Fenwick had been in charge since July the previous year; he was 'very good indeed to the sisters'.[84] These men often had considerable problems to wrestle with: accommodating patients, keeping the administration ticking over and dealing with staff. NZANS Sister Bertha Nurse had provoked Godley's ire when she became matron of the New Zealand hospital in Cairo — he described her as having 'absolutely no ideas of discipline, and only anxious apparently to keep the men in hospital as long as possible'[85] — and his was not a lone voice when Nurse became matron of Brockenhurst. Parkes, Thurston and the hospital CO David Wylie agreed that she was 'incompetent' but, Godley noted, 'neither Parkes nor Wylie will officially recommend her removal, and Miss Thurston told me it was very difficult for her to do so, as they apparently were colleagues together in New Zealand'.[86]

As Mackenzie had noticed, NZEF men nursed in British hospitals sometimes felt lonely and chafed under 'the irksome restrictions imposed'. At the beginning of September 1915, Henry Clark, a patient at 3 London General, 'almost got my head chewed off' after taking an unscheduled afternoon drive: 'they have bundled me straight back to bed again just like a naughty small boy.'[87]

Ned O'Neill, who received a severe compound fracture of his lower jaw in France, was nursed at Walton before being transferred to the Queen's Hospital at Sidcup. 'I cannot say that I or any of the N.Z. boys like Sidcup Hospital . . . There are a fair no. of rules & regulations that we do not like, so our boys let everyone see from the start that some of these . . . would not be observed.'[88] Once he got to Walton, Harry Kitson, wounded on Gallipoli, had plenty to say about his previous hospital in Plymouth. 'The nursing staff looked after me awfully well, but the Doctors & the Major hated all Colonials & made things very rotten for us.' In his opinion, the English hospitals 'have got Colonials well set because we won't stand their petty-fogging ways. Not allowed to have your coat off, must have your collar buttoned up, all sorts of damned rot.'[89]

The atmosphere at the New Zealand hospitals could not have been more different. Kitson proclaimed Walton 'just great . . . & no silly petty rules. You are here to get fit & do as you like, within reason of course.' William Wilson described the high jinks among the Walton convalescents at bedtime. 'Pillow cases are taken off pillows, socks turned into bombs, breakables removed from lockers and all hands prepare for the night raids. As long as nobody is hurt and nothing is broken we are allowed to have our fun.' In September 1918, Alec Hutton, at Brockenhurst, told his sister Fannie, 'We get great treatment here. The nurses are real good sorts and you would be astounded at the fun that goes on. No one is allowed to be gloomy in this place.'[90] The food at the New Zealand hospitals was generally better, too. O'Neill found the Sidcup fare 'very much inferior to what we have been accustomed [to] at Walton, & of course that is one of the main things in Hospital'. At Brockenhurst in August 1917 William Smallfield approved of the midday meal, which was 'a fresh roast joint and plenty of good vegetables, and then usually some stewed fruit'.[91]

Both medical staff and patients relished the company of down-to-earth fellow New Zealanders, with their familiar accent and humour. Often, they even knew one another. When Cecil Malthus arrived at Brockenhurst early in October 1916, his ward sister was 'a Canterbury girl and knew me by name'. When NZMC orderly Private Richard Wilson encountered Dr Robert Hogg at Brockenhurst, he found him 'always so good and attentive to the boys and takes a special interest in all the patients from Invercargill district'. Hutton knew two of the Brockenhurst nurses, all of whom he thought 'simply magnificent . . . they are worked to death but they are always full of fun & some of them seem to possess an inexhaustible supply of jokes & stories'.[92] But the doctors and nurses also had to watch the men they cared for suffer and die. In her diary on 8 December 1916, for example, Fanny Speedy at Brockenhurst wrote, 'Gunner Frederick Fendall, in 17 Sideroom who has been very ill lately died this morning, a very nice boy.' Wounded on Gallipoli, Fendall, who was just 22, had gone on to serve in France, where his diarrhoea had been succeeded by pleurisy.[93]

The numbers treated in the New Zealand hospitals were impressive: according to Bernard Myers, between 1 May 1916 and 1919, there had been 70,000 New Zealand admissions to New Zealand and imperial hospitals in Britain. Walton-on-Thames took in 27,000 patients, and Brockenhurst well over 20,000.[94] The latter was the first to shut its doors. Work ended at No. 1 New Zealand General Hospital on 11 March 1919, when 158 patients left for New Zealand on the *Maheno*, making her last voyage as a hospital ship. Hornchurch accepted its final patients on 14 March and closed in June. Codford followed suit in July, although the last 200 VD patients were not moved to a British hospital until August. The Mount Felix part of Walton-on-Thames closed at the end of June but some 80 beds remained open at the end of August, when Oatlands 'limbies' were still waiting to have artificial arms and legs fitted at Roehampton.

At a special 'break-up' function for patients, staff and other workers on 3 June 1919, Empire

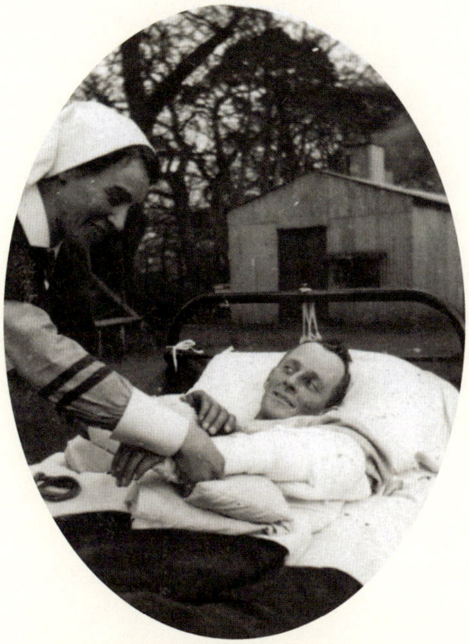

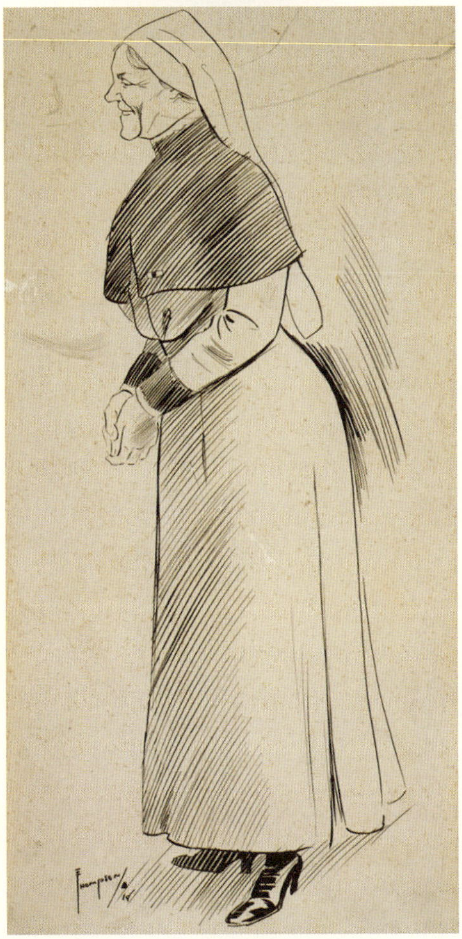

above The easy camaraderie between New Zealand nurses and their patients is captured in this photo from an album thought to belong to Nurse Alice Searrell. NATIONAL ARMY MUSEUM, 1992.1156.1

below 'How are you this morning?' was the title of Ernest Heber Thompson's affectionate 1918 depiction of Fanny Wilson (1874–1958). She served in Samoa in 1914 and sailed to Egypt in April 1915. From January 1917 until the hospital closed, she was matron of Walton-on-Thames. Awarded the Royal Red Cross, first class, in 1919, Wilson was, in the words of her biographer, 'remembered for her tact, her ability to combine human warmth with efficiency, and for being a brilliant and witty conversationalist'. NATIONAL COLLECTION OF WAR ART, AAAC 898, NCWA Q233

Day, not long before No. 2 New Zealand General Hospital closed, Mackenzie announced that only 150 men had died there. Although, as he emphasised, 'that small number spoke volumes for the skill of the surgeons and physicians, and the care of the nurses', the losses, both here and at the other hospitals, cut deep.[95] Myers recalled the fifth funeral held at Walton. The dead man's relatives wished his body to be sent by rail to Scotland. Because heavy snow prevented the gun-carriage and military band from arriving in time, the coffin was placed in an ambulance to be taken the 1¼ miles to the train. 'Behind the snow-covered ambulance marched the men in their blues, their hats snow-laden; the trees and buildings along the route were all white, and from 12 to 15 inches of snow lay on the road. Nought was to be heard except the muffled sound of the wheels. We marched slowly along and at last arrived at the station white in its pall of snow . . . Every man present felt particularly sad.'[96]

Twenty-one New Zealand patients and staff from No. 2 New Zealand General Hospital are remembered at the Walton-on-Thames cemetery adjoining St Mary's churchyard. Among the 19 buried there are 33-year-old Wilmet Annie Bennett, known to her family as Bob, from Masterton, who worked at Walton as a VAD and died at the hospital on 21 November 1918 of appendicitis,[97] and the much-decorated Colonel Charles Begg, who was an influenza victim. Also memorialised on one of the two large stone screens is dentist Captain Charles Ward (see Chapter 10). Ninety-three New Zealanders are buried at Brockenhurst, where a cenotaph was erected in 1927.[98] As at Walton-on-Thames, an annual Anzac service remembers the New Zealanders who lie here.

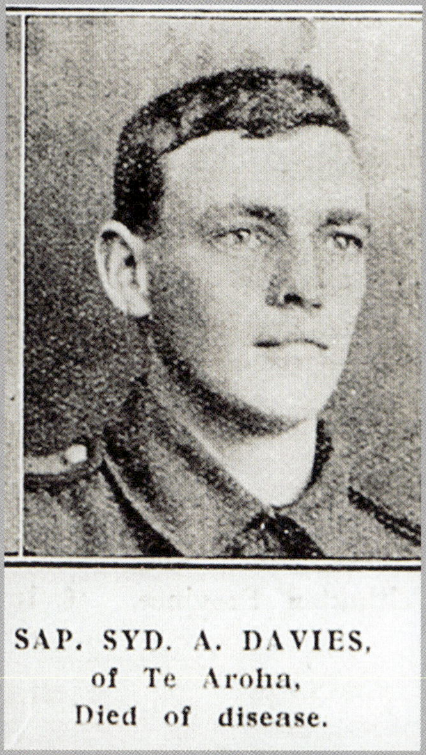

Sapper Sydney Davies. *AUCKLAND WEEKLY NEWS*, SIR GEORGE GREY SPECIAL COLLECTIONS, AUCKLAND LIBRARIES, AWNS-19170816-40-44

POOR BOY

One of the saddest cases nursed at Brockenhurst was surely Sapper Sydney Davies, who died there on 10 July 1917, aged only 24. He had endured a dismal series of medical misfortunes: severe enteritis on Gallipoli, cowpox in France, accidental burns to his face and hands. By Christmas 1916 he had been admitted to Brockenhurst and a medical report on 29 January 1917 told the awful story of what had been diagnosed as severe sinusitis. A harelip had been repaired in childhood but the cleft palate was still open. Davies had worn a diaphragm in it for years, which had caused irritation and produced bad nose bleeds; his right eyeball was proptosed (displaced in its socket). The second of two operations in January had revealed, in the cleft palate, a tumour known as an endothelioma.

Throughout his painful months at No. 1 New Zealand General Hospital the courageous young man was visited regularly and devotedly by the chaplain, John Jacob, and by Laura Pick, both of whom wrote often to Davies' mother. When Pick was unable to continue, Sister Helena Newton took over: 'I call myself the "Pioneer Sister" as I had him when he first came in.' Photos from home revealed the damage caused by his condition. 'What a fine looking man he was,' wrote Newton in a letter that Mrs Davies received after her son's death. 'Poor boy he has altered very much.' Sydney Davies is buried in the Brockenhurst churchyard.[99]

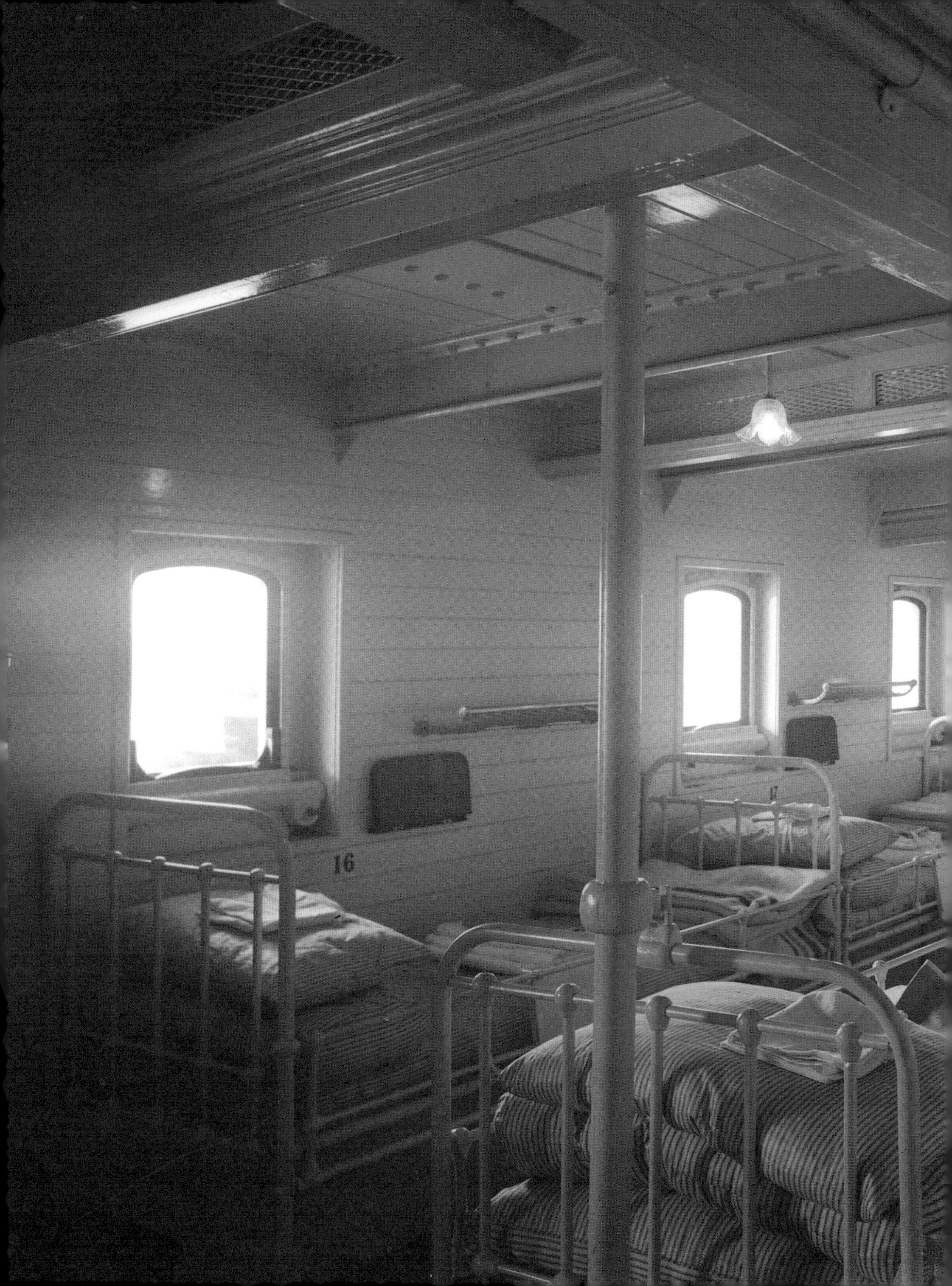

16
17

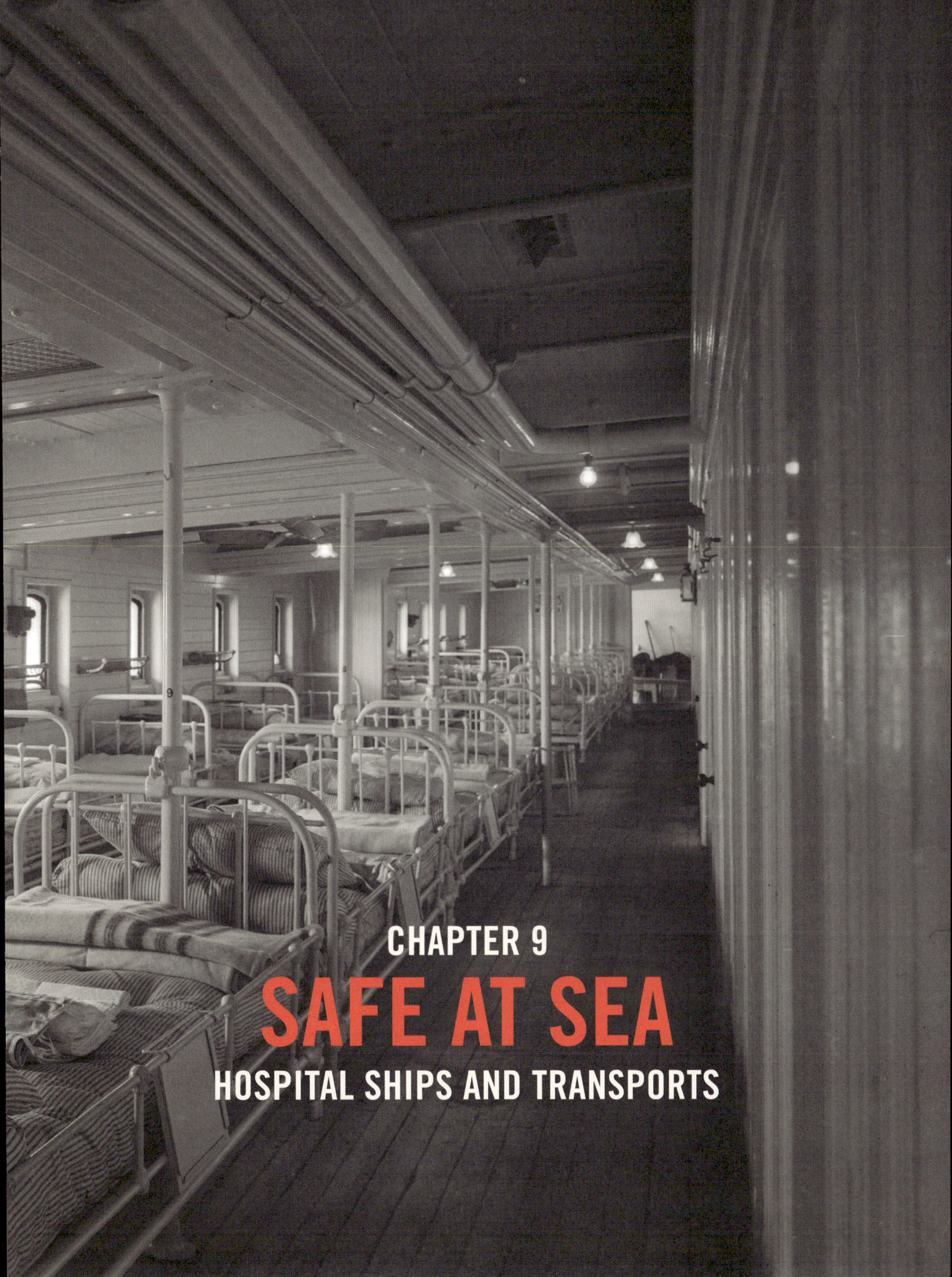

CHAPTER 9

SAFE AT SEA

HOSPITAL SHIPS AND TRANSPORTS

previous pages
Beds in a ward on the *Maheno* await their future patients. As *Kai Tiaki* reported, 'the head pulls out and can be adjusted as a bed-rest, the bed itself can be raised at one end and can even be lifted right out from the frame, mattress and all'. There was also a bracket to hold a basin and a chart-holder that could be turned over to form a small table. After the trenches, these beds were 'heaven on earth. Hair mattresses, feather pillows, clean sheets — what more can the heart of man desire!'
ALEXANDER TURNBULL LIBRARY, 1/1-002216-F

> The Hospital Ship looks lovely at night: a brilliant band of green electric lamps all around her, and a blazing lamp in the centre, just like a Venetian fete.
> — Percival Fenwick, 30 May 1915

Late in August 1915 John Russell and his mates, high on the Apex on Gallipoli, could see, out on the water, a vision of delight:

> [T]he hospital ships . . . were a blaze of light at night, being brilliantly illuminated by broad bands of lights which encircled their entire hulls, while each also had a massive illuminated red cross showing amidships. In the heat of the day when thirst troubled us most, we couldn't help thinking wistfully of the tasty dishes & iced drinks that were being served there, & we agreed that a nice little flesh wound in some convenient part of the anatomy would have its compensations.[1]

Godley had suggested a New Zealand hospital ship, in fact two, before the Gallipoli campaign, but quickly changed his mind, and the idea had also been soundly rejected by the War Office. Seriously wounded men could go to Britain, and the rest could either be sent home on returning troop transports or nursed in Egyptian hospitals before going back to the front.[2] However, the appalling situation on the peninsula, and the alarming casualty lists reaching New Zealand, altered the situation. By 19 May 1915 newspapers throughout the country were reporting a message to the people from the governor, Lord Liverpool, who explained that, at Prime Minister Massey's request, he had asked the secretary of state 'whether there was any particular way in which New Zealand could further assist in the care of the sick and wounded'. It seemed that 'a fully-equipped hospital ship, primarily intended for the conveyance of New Zealanders from the front to the base hospitals, would be a most welcome gift'.[3] The government would hire, fit out and crew the ship, but equipping her would be up to the public. The *Press* was certain that New Zealanders would 'rejoice over the opportunity to do all they can to assist the brave lads who have fallen, and who will continue to fall, out of the fight'. Almost every newspaper in the country took the same patriotic line.[4]

The chosen vessel was the Union Steam Ship Company's 6000-ton turbine steamer, the *Maheno*, which had been carrying passengers back and forth across the Tasman and was, at least in the media's view, 'one of the finest and fastest . . . trading south of the line'.[5] The company not only made the *Maheno* available but also contributed the substantial sum of £1000 to the equipment fund. Money, over £47,000 by early August, and gifts poured in from individuals, clubs and societies, companies and schools.[6] The *Auckland Star*, in an article headed 'Choose Your Task', suggested a daunting list of items that could be bought or made, including pneumonia jackets, cardigans, bed socks (with or without heels), mufflers, quilts, pillow cases (no buttons or tapes), hot water bottles and even jug and cup covers fashioned from butter muslin. The paper was very keen for children to help, but traditional gender roles should not be disturbed: 'The girls might do the work [of making suitable articles], and the boys take up the task of collecting the required money.' Mothers, sisters, wives and fiancées offered their services, all 'impatiently eager for the allotment of their task'.[7]

To rally, or shame, others, subscribers' names and the amounts they gave were printed in the papers. In Wellington a nurse offered to teach women how to tear and roll bandages. Queen carnivals were a popular means of fund-raising: in Hawke's Bay, the 'handsome sum of £6210' was made on 24 May. A group of Wanganui women who gathered the £100 that would equip a bed on the ship 'are desirous that the bed shall be named after their district — the Mangamahu Bed — as they intend . . . to provide for its maintenance during the continuance of the war'.[8] This sense of ownership and identification was repeated throughout the country — the *Maheno* was 'our hospital ship' for 'our wounded'. And the equipping continued throughout the war. On 1 July 1918, the *Wanganui Herald* printed a letter from an NZMC officer thanking those who had responded so generously to a 'recent appeal for music for the hospital ship *Maheno* . . . we start off with a library of over 100 orchestral numbers, in addition to a quantity of violin, pianoforte, and vocal music.'[9]

By 26 May 1915, the governor had presented the public with 'the final list of requisites for the complete equipment of the Hospital Ship', which the major newspapers printed in full. As well as 1200 feather pillows, 1600 pairs of white blankets, 2400 each of sheets and pillow cases, 1000 bath towels and 2800 face and hand towels, the future sick and wounded would need suitable clothing: pyjamas, dressing gowns, bed jackets, felt slippers, flannel waistcoats and flannel drawers ('not too thick'). Sewing items were on the list, too, including '30 gross of various buttons', as were deckchairs, cushions and rugs. Also required was 'an unlimited number of bandages'.[10] On board, the nursing staff would be in charge of all the surgical dressings and hospital linen.

On 4 August 1915, the first anniversary of the outbreak of war, Massey would tell Parliament that the *Maheno* was 'the best-equipped hospital ship in the world' and, even allowing for parochial pride, she was an impressive sight when her five-week refit was complete.[11] Her first medical commander, Lieutenant-Colonel James Elliott, would recall eight wards when there were in fact 14, but he was correct in listing 'two operating theatres, an anaesthetising, a sterilising, and an X-ray room, a laboratory, a laundry and drying-room, steam disinfector, dispensary, telephone exchange, and two electric lifts each of which took two stretchers at a time'.[12] The July 1915 issue of *Kai Tiaki* described the *Maheno* in glowing terms and detailed how the men would be 'conveyed on board through doors in the ship's side' before being examined and sent to different wards, 'according to their injuries'. There they would be washed and put into beds with ingenious 'contrivances for the comfort of the occupant'; some, sensibly, were made to swing with the ship. The nurses' arrangements met with approval, as did their comfortable deck cabins. But the glory of the vessel could not disguise its purpose: 'The sight of so many beds and the realisation that our own wounded men would be the occupants made one's heart ache.'[13] Its future users would also praise the vessel, as did Godley when he saw her at Alexandria at the beginning of September. 'I have been out to visit the Maheno,' he told Allen, 'and think she is beautifully fitted up — I never saw better fittings, and all the staff arrangements seem excellent. The only improvements that one could have suggested were better accommodation for the orderlies, and for Officers who are patients.'[14]

Some disappointment and a sense of anti-climax accompanied the *Maheno*'s departure from Wellington on 11 July 1915. She was to have sailed at noon the preceding day, but concern about possible illness on board meant a move away from the wharf and out into the harbour to anchor off Kaiwharawhara while medical examinations took place. Those keen to farewell their friends and loved ones were deprived of this experience when the vessel left about 1 p.m. She did, though, make a magnificent sight, her 'graceful lines' emphasised by her 'complete coating of white paint . . . with the great red crosses on her sides and the broad riband of green running from stem to stern'. Red and green, too, were the special lanyards worn by the male hospital ship staff.[15]

On this first voyage the *Maheno* was under the military command of Colonel William Collins and carried a staff of 61 NZMC men and 11 NZANS nurses: Matron Eva Brooke, Sisters Louise Brandon and Louie McNie — all Samoa veterans — and Nurses Hilda Burton, Margaret Davies, Clara Hawkins, Lottie Le Gallais, Violet McCosh-Smith, Mary Muir, Jean Muir and Margaret Tucker. Two nurses — Kathleen Cummings and Johanna Edmondstone — were later added to the staff, and Gertrude Garrard replaced McCosh-Smith who, Brooke reported from Colombo, 'has been very sea-sick and has not felt well since being on the boat'.[16] McCosh-Smith joined the 69 passenger nurses who were also on board, bound for the front, under the charge of Sister Ida Willis.

McCosh-Smith was not the only nurse prevented by sickness from working at sea. On the first charter of the *Marama*, New Zealand's second hospital ship, Matron Margaret Brown 'was so sorry to have to exchange, at their own request, three of the staff. They were hopeless sailors, even in calm weather.'[17] The male orderlies, too, suffered. Private Eric Bardell, who sailed on four *Maheno* voyages, 'felt the motion of the ship very much' when he was put in B ward during the fifth charter in 1918. There 'the fresh air does not circulate. I was crook from then on.'[18] The *Maheno* was not the most comfortable of vessels. In the view of MO William Barclay, who sailed on the second charter, she 'had been selected largely for her speed', which was assisted by her yacht-like lines, but these also meant that, 'in a cross sea, she rolled a good deal'.[19] As Willis recalled, when the ship reached open water, 'Almost everybody was sick — some very sick. Three of us went to the pantry and made water arrowroot with a dash of brandy and fed seventy nurses and sixty officers and orderlies.' Willis managed this despite being 'violently sick myself at intervals'. In the memory of one sister, the passenger nurses, 'somewhere in the bowels of the ship', were also 'bruised with hitting the sides of the bunks' in rough weather.[20]

The hospital ship staff were immediately busy. The nurses prepared the wards and gave post-dinner lectures and demonstrations to the orderlies who, as well as scrubbing the ship and doing exercises, had to rehearse the boarding procedure for 'wounded patients', who were impersonated by the doctors. Private Michael O'Malley, struggling with seasickness, reported 'sorting out linen All day' on 21 and 23 July, and on the 26th was 'Working in the Holds All Day Shifting Cargo. At night it was terrible Warm.' After leaving Colombo, there was more seasickness as the ship hit bad weather, but eventually the *Maheno* reached Suez, where, on 17 August, most of the North Island nurses disembarked for Cairo. Two days later, the rest went ashore at Port Said. The *Maheno* left that evening for Alexandria where, on the 19th, O'Malley noted in his diary, 'We have received instructions to prepare our Wards for the wounded who are coming in a day or two.'[21] On 23 August, the hospital ship sailed for the Dardanelles.

After passing such sights as 'three lifeboats, floating, upside down and a number of lifebelts' and seeing 'scores of Battleships and Transports' in Mudros Harbour, the *Maheno* reached the Dardanelles late on the afternoon of 26 August. As 20-year-old orderly Sid Gibb recorded, 'we have anchored about a mile from the shore and

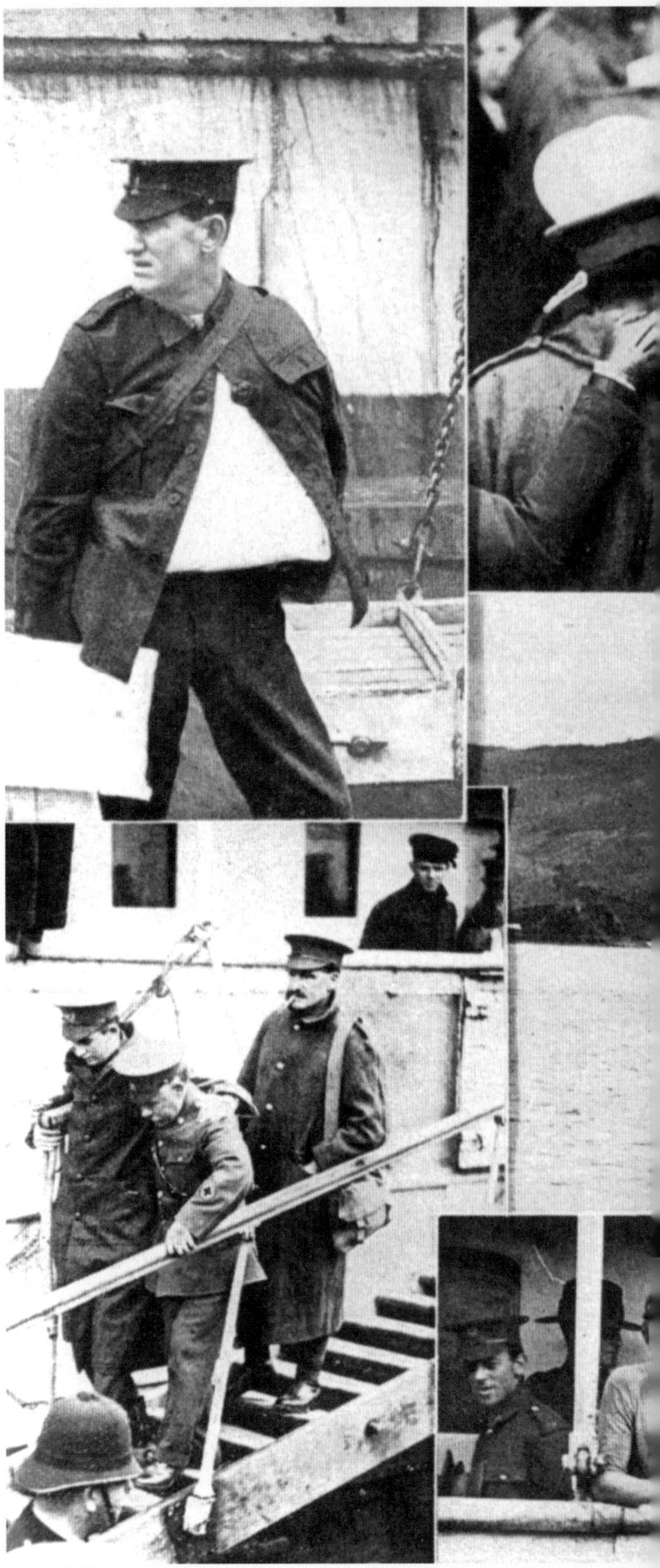

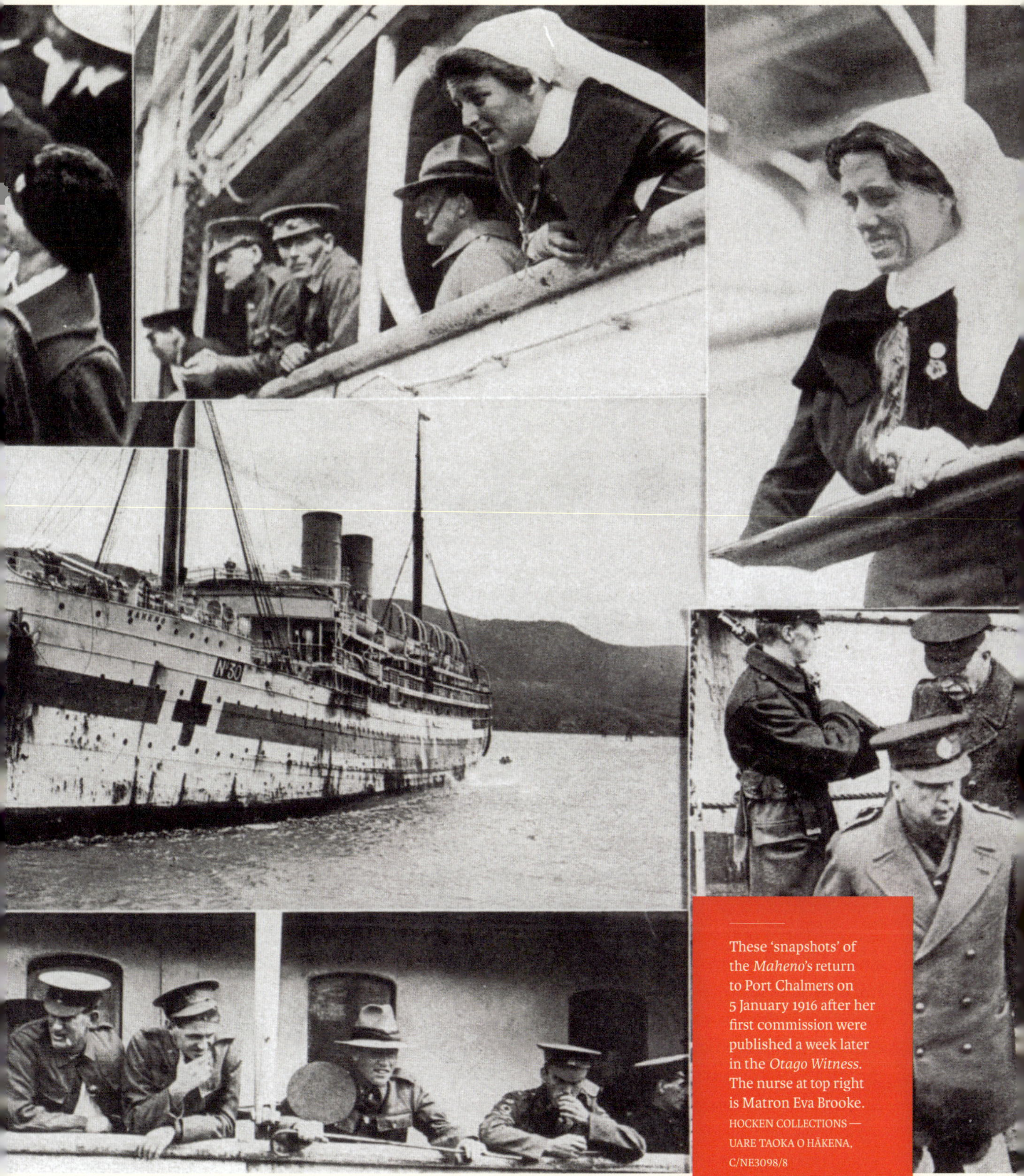

These 'snapshots' of the *Maheno*'s return to Port Chalmers on 5 January 1916 after her first commission were published a week later in the *Otago Witness*. The nurse at top right is Matron Eva Brooke.
HOCKEN COLLECTIONS — UARE TAOKA O HĀKENA, C/NE3098/8

have to wait here till the barges come out with the wounded and sick. On our arrival there was big attack in progress [the battle for Hill 60, which had begun on 21 August] but could not tell how things are going. Just alongside of us there are two Cruisers blazing away good oh, making the old "Maheno" vibrate like anything.' Those, like John Russell, struggling on the peninsula were glad to sight the hospital ship: 'it was very nice to see this direct link with our homeland'.[22]

On 26 July, Third Officer John Duder had recorded in his diary, 'Doctors & nurses spend most of the morning padding splints, rolling bandages & getting everything ready for the wounded. All these things remind one of the awful sights that we shall see.' And now, a month later, he was proved right. The first lighter came alongside with wounded about 7 p.m. 'Poor chaps,' wrote Duder, 'they all look very bad . . . the wounds are really shocking.' The 'horrible part . . . is that they are all run down & as soon as they receive a bad wound mortification [gangrene] sets in'.[23] The experience told on those working desperately, hour after hour, in hot, cramped conditions. Next day brought the second major assault on Hill 60 — 'the heaviest fighting since the landing', according to O'Malley — and the casualties were numerous. 'We received a boat load in one night about 600 patients. We have been working for two days and one night with a spell. When we were anchored in the Bay we were under very heavy fire from the enemy.' Private Colin Reaburn, from Palmerston North, was 'one of the stretcher-bearers lifting the wounded from the lighters to the ship, and it was terrible to hear the groans of the injured men'.[24]

'We arrived here just in time to see a terrific artillery bombardment,' wrote NZMC Staff Sergeant Clarence Schofield.

> Then the wounded began to arrive. I cannot describe the condition they were in, it was awful. Nine poor fellows died within 12 hours; we were absolutely packed and 150 were lying on the deck . . . Despite their experiences the men remain cheerful through it all. What a small sacrifice ours is compared to theirs. They think they are in Heaven when they come aboard our old ship and wonder why we are so kind to them. The need for us here is far greater than I could have imagined.[25]

The following morning, the *Maheno* continued to take on the wounded — and the dying and dead. 'Some of them,' O'Malley wrote, 'are absolutely torn to pieces and only live for a few hours.'[26] Then, with 445 patients and staff 'applying pressure dressings to bleeding wounds, changing the dressings of infected wounds and washing men with the limited amounts of sea water available',[27] the *Maheno* left soon after noon for Lemnos. At 2 p.m. she stopped to bury eight bodies; six more had died by mid-afternoon and another two by the time the ship anchored in Mudros Harbour at 4.30. The wounded — 'except 13 eleven of whom died during the night'[28] — were loaded onto a captured German transport to be taken to Alexandria. Once cleaned and refurbished, the *Maheno* returned to Anzac Cove on the 30th, and then followed a punishing schedule, making many trips back and forth between Anzac, Mudros and Malta, always carrying from 400 to 500 sick and wounded men.

'The bugle calls us to our post of duty,' wrote nurse Margaret Tucker, and 'lighters conveying the wounded are soon alongside'.

> Immediately the stretcher-bearers are seen at the gangway. The medical officers hurriedly examine and classify the patients; on reaching the wards every effort is made to dress any injured limb immediately. Hot drinks are carried round by the orderlies. It is somewhat of a contract to deal with some 60 cases at once. The mention of a bath causes almost a stampede amongst men who have perhaps been in the trenches for weeks and never had their boots off.

The time of departure depended on how quickly the ambulance men on Gallipoli could get the wounded to the dressing station, onto a barge or lighter and out to the ship. This could take three or four hours. 'If bound for Lemnos, another 2 hours and our work of disembarkation begins. As a rule, however, the arrangements at Anzac take longer than this and our patients have been on board as long as 18 to 20 hours.' *Kai Tiaki* may have lauded the nurses' accommodation on the *Maheno*, but Tucker thought it 'undeniably cramped, and accentuated by the length of time in which the [ship] has been our home'. Ward duty began at 6.30 a.m. and work often did not finish until near midnight, but the nurses maintained 'a fine spirit of eagerness to serve and cheerfulness'.[29]

As Jean Muir explained, admitting the patients was 'no easy task': 'There are thirty-four beds in my ward, and the stretchers stream in one after the other until the last bed is full. While I am looking around to see where I will put the various cases that have reached the ward, I can see a line of between twenty and thirty stretchers waiting to close up nearer the ward.' Sometimes the wounded had come straight from the trenches, 'just with their field dressing on. Some of the poor men have never had a wash for weeks, and their clothes are in a dreadful state.' But they were 'so grateful and happy after their bath', and, if well enough, thrilled to be given bread and New Zealand butter and tea. 'They are so good that you wish you had six good pairs of legs and hands.'[30]

The constant heavy work of lifting stretchers and bending to care for patients affected the NZMC men. On 6 September O'Malley wrote, 'We received about 50 Patients for the Day. About 300 Patients come on board for First Dressing and then were discharged . . . My Back went Bad on me today.' Illness was a problem, too. By 15 September O'Malley could record: 'There are at present 12 of our Men in Bed some of them have got Typhoid and Enteric and other Sickness.'[31]

But MO Alexander Trotter was impressed when he visited the *Maheno* early that month:

> She is beautifully fitted up and everything goes very quietly and smoothly — no shouting out and herding of the poor sick and wounded as I have seen. Also when a sweeper came in the afternoon for sick for Mudros they were not permitted aboard by Col. Collins because there were no comforts etc. for the 16 hours they would be aboard. It took my breath away

> rather for I have seen very many worse things than that passed over . . . The *Maheno* has a name already especially among the sailors who man the picket boats and lighters because they are taken on board and given a decent feed. I had a nice long talk with Sister Mac [Louie McNie] who gave me a nip and some cigarettes.[32]

After some welcome leave in England early in October, the *Maheno* staff continued their unrelenting work. One delighted to be on board was MO William McAra, who was invalided off Gallipoli on 10 November. 'Never so thankful in all my life when . . . told that the Maheno was just coming to anchor — what luck . . . It is such a relief to be lying on board here & know that no shells will be coming near me.'[33] Then, at last, this first charter was over and the hospital ship sailed for New Zealand from Suez on 26 November, reaching Auckland in the pre-dawn darkness of New Year's Day 1916 with a 'precious freightage' of more than 300 mostly convalescent patients.[34] There had been challenges for the medical staff en route. At 10.30 a.m. on 8 December, one of O'Malley's Māori patients, suffering from shell shock, 'jumped overboard & was nearly drowned' before a boat picked him up after 30 minutes in the water. That day, too, O'Malley's friend and fellow orderly, Private James Cameron, died of pneumonia after two days in the isolation ward. 'Poor Jimmie was very well liked by all on board and was only 19 years of Age.'[35]

The fervour of the welcome home by thousands of people was dimmed when 189 men recovering from enteric, or suspected of being carriers, had to be isolated in a temporary quarantine hospital. 'Two or three of the heroes,' the *Star* reported, 'were encountered minus limbs, and one had lost an eye. Taken on the whole, however, the health of the men was good.'[36] James Allen, in Auckland for the *Maheno*'s return, was also resolutely positive when writing to Godley: 'by the time she reached us she had only 30 or 40 cot cases. Wonderful what the return journey does for the sick and wounded soldiers. We note this on every Transport that is brought back, and it was the same on the Maheno.'[37]

The jingoism was less determined when the *Maheno* sailed into Auckland in April, during her second commission, with 326 sick and wounded on board. 'Though, happily, most of the men have reached the convalescent stage, and to outward appearances are hail and hearty, moving evidences of the special function of the ship abounded on every hand. Many of the men moved painfully on crutches or hobbled about with the aid of sticks. Others still wore bandages and slings, while one or two wheeled themselves about in invalid chairs.' In the cot ward, for patients confined to bed, a 'prime favourite' was young Trooper William Goldien, from Waipara in Canterbury, who had lost both legs but was apparently 'cheerful and smiling'. Already wounded, he had been taken to a temporary field hospital on Gallipoli, which was then struck by a stray shell: one leg was blown off, the other so mangled that it had to be amputated immediately. Two other men had lost a leg, one an arm; several were missing an eye.

'All the men,' said the *Auckland Star*, 'speak appreciatively of the medical attention they have received on the hospital ship, and express in terms of unrestrained enthusiasm their gratitude to the nursing staff.'[38] They were not always certain about returning without being fully recovered. 'My feelings are very mixed,' Clifford Collingwood wrote on 13 July 1917. 'I want

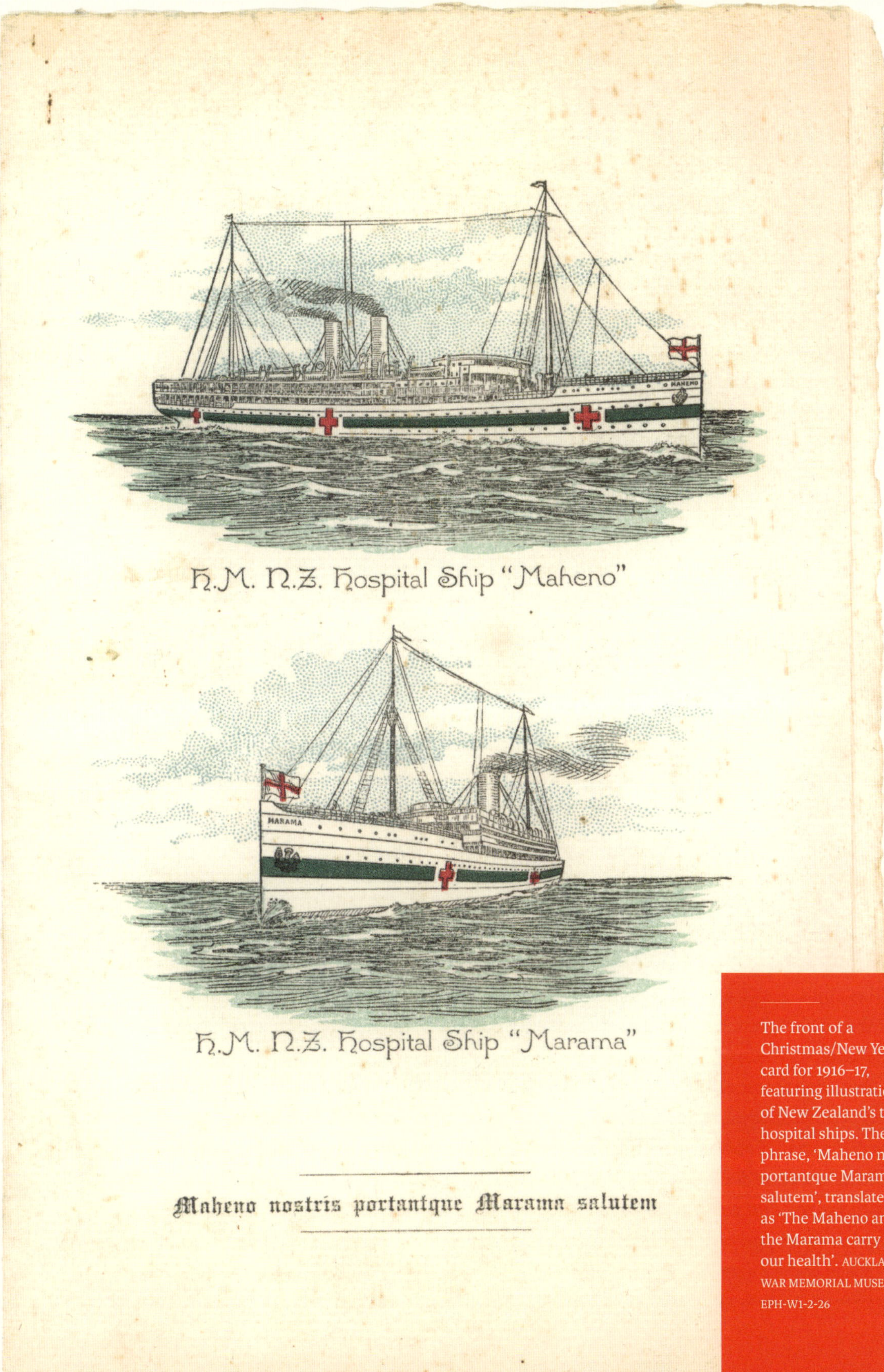

The front of a Christmas/New Year card for 1916–17, featuring illustrations of New Zealand's two hospital ships. The Latin phrase, 'Maheno nostris portantque Marama salutem', translates as 'The Maheno and the Marama carry our health'. AUCKLAND WAR MEMORIAL MUSEUM, EPH-W1-2-26

to go home, and yet I want to stay here rather than go home as a stretcher case.' As his ship reached Auckland in August, he was excited but 'I wanted to go right away until I was healed up and well again, and only then meet my people'.[39]

As part of her second commission, from January to December 1916, the *Maheno* made 20 round trips across the Channel to Le Havre and Boulogne between 4 July and 20 October, to collect the frightening numbers of wounded from the Somme offensive. On 5 July alone she carried 1141 men from Le Havre to Southampton.[40] The walking wounded — in other words, those who managed to remain upright — queued in single file on the quayside before boarding the *Maheno*. 'The mud from the trenches is scarcely dry upon them. The blood from their wounds soaks their clothes. They come forward, still dazed by the crash and roar of rival artillery . . . This man limps painfully, his trouser leg slit to the knee, where the surgeon has adopted the readiest method of getting at this wound. The next man has no sleeve in his coat — it has been similarly sacrificed.'[41] As William Barclay recalled, the tides at Le Havre 'had about a 40 ft rise and fall, and this made the carrying of the wounded quite difficult at times'.[42]

Two tickets were tied to every man's tunic, each with his name, number, rank and unit on the front and a concise statement of his wound or disease on the back. If he had been hospitalised, a brief medical history was added. Most bore the initials GSW (gunshot wound) or SW (shrapnel wound), though many physically whole men 'with drawn faces, deeply lined, the unfortunates whose nerves have gone to pieces under the strain' had tickets saying NYDN (not yet diagnosed, nervous).[43] Common, too, was the acronym PUO, for pyrexia of uncertain origin, probably influenza. One ticket was kept on board and the details entered into the ship's records; the other accompanied the patient to hospital in England. The decks were converted into wards by hanging canvas screens. The staff hardly slept, and they ate when they could.

There would be another three commissions for the *Maheno* before she reached New Zealand for the final time on 22 April 1919. As the *Auckland Star* reported that day, her arrival 'with a contingent of sorely battle-worn fighters closes an heroic chapter'.[44]

'The public will not be surprised,' said the *Press* editorial for 21 September 1915, 'by the announcement that the Government intend to supply another hospital ship for work in the Eastern Mediterranean.' Since the *Maheno* had been sent away, the Gallipoli fighting had been 'harder and heavier', and only a very few of the men on the peninsula had 'not appeared in the long roll of casualties'. The second chartered vessel, the *Marama*, was also from the Union Steam Ship Company, but she was bigger, with beds for 600 patients when her refit was completed, and faster. Although not as much was needed this time, 'the amount of material required . . . is, nevertheless, very large'. When the *Maheno* was fitted out, there had been criticism from some quarters that public assistance was required. The *Press*, therefore, was anxious to reiterate that although such generosity was not 'an essential condition of the despatch of a properly-equipped ship', there was surely 'no better way in which our people . . . can display their gratitude to the soldiers who are facing death and suffering for the honour and safety of New Zealand and the Empire'. The governor, quoted on the same page, had another list of necessities, this time including 'two additional motor launches'. There was, the paper said, 'no time to be lost, and we hope that the public will forthwith begin to send in their gifts in money and kind'.[45] When bringing Godley up to date on progress, Allen added, 'My only hope is that things may have developed so much that she will not be needed when she reaches the Mediterranean.'[46]

Fitted out at Port Chalmers in just over three weeks by hundreds of Union Steam Ship Company employees working night and day, the *Marama*, with her four decks, was a magnificent sight. Along with seven main wards, plus two special ones, one for NCOs and two for isolation, she boasted a superbly equipped operating theatre in what had been the first-class dining room on the upper deck. There was even a 'bacteriological laboratory and a blanket heater'. Other impressive facilities were two electric lifts, a library, a telephone exchange — and a mortuary.[47]

Kai Tiaki approved: she was 'very beautifully fitted up' and the nurses' quarters were 'most commendable'. Godley, who inspected her at Alexandria, thought the *Marama* 'very good, and an enormous improvement' on the *Maheno*.[48] Less partisan observers were also complimentary. 'Our ship,' wrote one nurse on board, 'is much admired by everyone. We are getting more and more fond of her, and the nice things we hear said by patients R.A.M.C. men and officials in ports.' In the opinion of Nurse Kate Stephenson, the *Marama* compared 'more than favourably with the P. and O. and Castle Line hospital ships, in everything except deck space[;] the lovely leather pillows and wide cots are beautiful, and also the food is better'.[49]

As well as her medical staff, which included 27 nurses, the *Marama* carried more than 50 nurses bound for service in Egypt as passengers when she sailed from Wellington on 5 December 1915. Among the staff nurses was 30-year-old Aucklander Barbara Mildred Tilly, known to most as Millie, who was keen to reassure her mother, Maggie, early in the voyage. 'Please Mother do not worry about me because we shall be as right as ninepence. I'll be back in six months to see you again.' When Tilly wrote home at the end of January 1916, from the Bay of Biscay, there were 'close on 600 wounded Tommies aboard + two New Zealanders', who had come aboard at Alexandria. Some of the men, who had come from Gallipoli, Salonika and Serbia, were 'eyeless, some legless & others have mostly ghastly wounds'. Many had severe frostbite. After these patients were disembarked at Southampton at the beginning of February, there was a chance for sightseeing in London before the *Marama* returned to Alexandria.[50]

The *Marama* then continued this first commission, which ended at Port Chalmers in early November 1916, with trips to Marseilles, Salonika and Stavros, where she was used as a base hospital for British troops until she left for Malta, loaded with patients. Then it was on to Southampton again and back to Alexandria. Like the *Maheno*, throughout July and August she became part of the Great White Fleet carrying thousands of wounded men from France across the Channel. The two New Zealand ships often encountered each other at sea or in port. When they were 'lying side by side in harbour at Havre', the sisters, though busy, 'were delighted to meet and exchange news'.[51]

As one unnamed sister wrote to Hester Maclean, in the first 10-day rush the *Marama* carried 1635 wounded soldiers from Le Havre.

> We got in at 1 a.m. and loaded at once. We had a great many bad cases, and got away at 5 a.m. I will never forget the sight of the seemingly endless stream of men along the wharf from the sheds. For a start the Adjutant gave our unit as 900, but one couldn't go with one corner empty and all those poor tired out sick boys standing on the wharf . . . One could hardly move anywhere for tired out men sleeping anywhere we could make them lying space down, under beds, on benches, tables, and stairs. Feeding was a great business, and began at once. They were so hungry. It makes one's heart bleed to see them coming on — all mud, clothes torn to pieces very often, and dried blood everywhere — all black, tired and hungry. They fall asleep the minute they get on the bed.[52]

This description did not mention the stench that clung to the men. Despite having left the trenches as little as 12 to 18 hours earlier, most had wounds that stank and had turned septic, which meant each dressing took a long time. The soldiers also brought sickness with them, which affected the medical staff, and unwelcome visitors: the nurses had to check their own clothes for 'fleas, etc. (the etc. are much worse than the fleas)'.[53] By 12 August, Tilly could report from Le Havre that the *Marama* had transported 10,000 wounded '& that is nothing compared with other ships'.[54] By the time she departed for home at the end of that month, New Zealand's second hospital ship had covered more than 50,000 sea miles and carried over 12,500 patients and almost 600 hospital patients.

When the *Marama* left New Zealand on her second charter, in November 1916, one of the nurses on board was 38-year-old Bertha Taylor from Auckland. In December, with mostly convalescent patients boarded at Malta, the staff still had 'a strenuous time . . . feeding 150 in one ward was a bit of a contract, and we were on duty from 7 a.m. to 10 p.m'. At one point on the *Marama*'s journey, Taylor had written, 'We have boat drill sometimes, our nearest approach to sport, we feel quite safe, nothing diasterous is likely to happen.'[55] But her confidence would prove misplaced. In May 1917, the *Marama* sailed for a time without her nursing sisters, who were ordered to disembark at Suez because of the threat of U-boat attacks in the Mediterranean. A number of hospital ships were mined or torpedoed during the war, and only the previous month the *Salta* had been sunk, with the loss of 130 lives, including nine nurses and five medical officers.

As Sid Gibb, now serving on the *Marama*, explained, 'It is just a new order that has come out that Hospital ships are to have no sisters . . . We believe that the cause of them going off is that the Subs are pretty bad just now and we may strike a tin-fish [torpedo] any time.' The orderlies felt 'very sorry' at the departure of the 'good women' with whom they had served for two years.[56] Although *Kai Tiaki* admitted that the decree was 'possibly justified . . . the sisters feel that where the sick and wounded are, there is their rightful place, and they do not shirk any danger which those they are detailed to care for have to face'.[57]

When Clifford Collingwood was carried onto the *Marama* at Avonmouth on 14 July 1917, with no nursing staff on board, he and his companions were 'warned of the "Submarine Alarm" which would be given by the Ship's siren . . . all orderlies and men must get to their allotted posts, the portholes are to be closed, and the Orderlies to "stand by" in readiness to carry cot

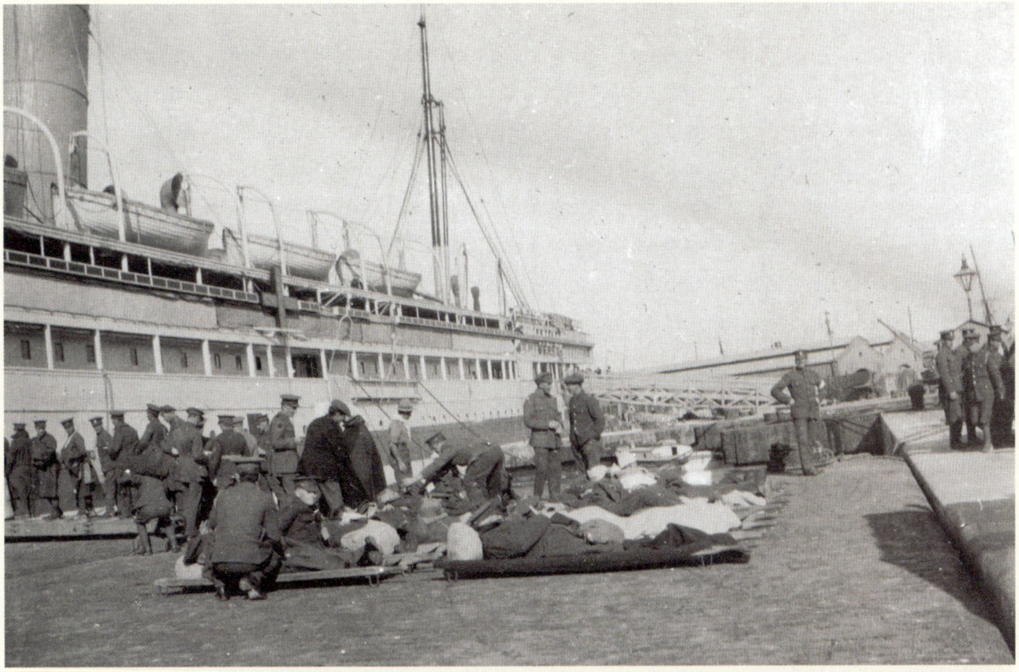

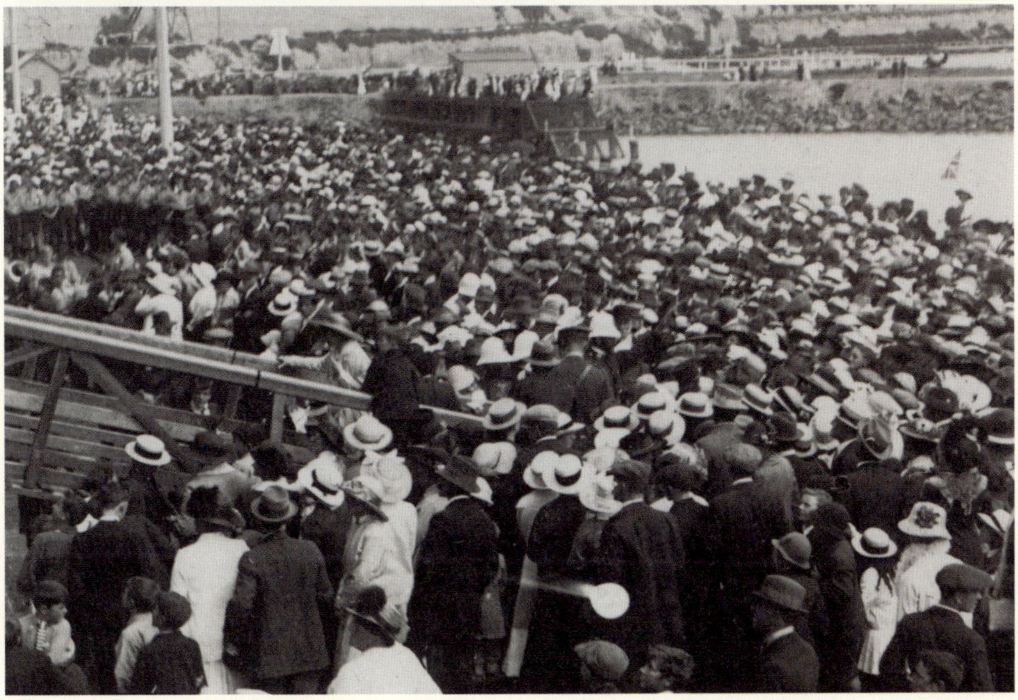

above Bill Yates, an NZMC orderly on the *Marama*, captioned this album image, 'Embarkation of wounded men at Alexandria, Egypt'. WILLIAM YATES ALBUM, COURTESY WILLIAM YATES FAMILY, FEILDING LIBRARY

below Huge crowds, like this one greeting the *Marama* in Timaru in March 1917, turned out to welcome hospital ships and transports bringing sick and wounded men home to New Zealand. WILLIAM YATES ALBUM, COURTESY WILLIAM YATES FAMILY, FEILDING LIBRARY cases up to the deck in the event of the ship being torpedoed. The orderlies tell us they could not shift so many cot cases [some 150] if the ship was sinking — a cheery prospect for us — however, we are in the hands of GOD.' A practice alarm the following day proved 'a very painful experience for most of us with our fractured limbs' — Collingwood was in Ward C, where the swinging cots held the worst cases. 'How helpless one feels.'[58]

The *Marama*'s nurses were sent to work in hospitals in England and did not return to New Zealand with their vessel: 'it was alleged that they could not be got together again and the ship sailed without them'.[59] Nurses in Port Chalmers, about to board the *Maheno*, were recalled at the last minute and left behind. Without the nurses, the orderlies 'were put to a considerable test in nursing severe cot cases, but they rose to the occasion and succeeded reasonably well'.[60] 'Did I tell you,' *Maheno* orderly Eric Bardell asked his brother, 'we have no sisters on board this time? It may mean harder work, but we will willingly put up with that.'[61]

Kai Tiaki allowed that the men acquitted themselves adequately, but pointed out that they 'had had the advantage of some training under the sisters' and maintained that a few patients 'suffered considerably from lack of the special attention the trained nurse alone can give'. Others, like the *Evening Star*, were more generous about the orderlies' work. They had 'won high praise for their care and attention to the sick and wounded in their charge. Their work is arduous, and, contrary to the opinion sometimes expressed, they must be vigorous men in perfect health, else they could not stand the strain.'[62]

With or without nurses on board, the orderlies had it tough, as a correspondent to the *Dominion* pointed out in April 1918. 'Working all hours, from 5.30 a.m., on diseases and ailments, contagious or otherwise, and of all descriptions, extreme climatic conditions, from 120deg. in the shade to points below freezing, high seas and heavy swells for perhaps a month continually, and sleeping in bunks even worse than some troopships . . . These men are now skilled in this particular branch, and in that peculiar to hospital ships — tried and proved.'[63]

There were nurses on the *Marama*, though, when she left New Zealand in September 1917 on her third charter, which ended in May 1918. This was followed by a fourth, before the *Marama* returned to New Zealand for the final time as a wartime hospital ship at the end of January 1919, carrying 557 patients. The 300 cot cases on board when the voyage began had, thanks to the 'untiring attention' of the nurses and orderlies, been reduced to just 70.[64] By the end of the war, New Zealand's two hospital ships had transported more than 47,000 patients from many countries, including Germany.[65]

Important events were not forgotten on the hospital ships. 'J.C.' spent Christmas 1918 'in mid-Atlantic' on the *Marama*, 'in company with about 600 wounded and disabled soldiers'. On the afternoon of Christmas Eve, 'the padres and the matron and Sisters got busy in the several wards. They fixed up flags, and ran colored streamers and paper festoons all over the place. They even had a bunch of good old English holly and a bit of mistletoe to place here and there in odd corners.' That night, a padre brought around 'a carol party, composed of an orchestra and about half a dozen singers . . . The ever-present throb, throb of the screw and the familiar swish of the waters seemed to fade away, for these Christmas carols filled the whole ward; so the Diggers who were talking or playing cards quietly suspended operations, and the men who were sick and weary closed their eyes and lay still.' Next morning each man found a little bag at the foot of his cot, containing 'sweets and raisins and cigarettes, some little present, and a card of greeting . . . "What did Santa Claus give you, Digger?" was the common morning greeting thrown from cot to cot.' Also part of the day was special food such as eggs and bacon, and tinned pears and jelly, plus a concert by the orchestra, 'a fine combination of about 14 N.Z.M.C. orderlies', who offered 'a rare assortment of all sorts of operatic pieces, ragtime selections, marches, etc.'.[66]

Music was part of everyday shipboard life too. On 12 August 1917, Collingwood reported 'several gramophones' on the *Marama* and 'we often have a change of records'. He practised his rusty Pitman's shorthand by writing down the song lyrics. Among 'the tunes we play' were 'Under the Bridges of Paris', 'Little Grey Home in the West', 'Keep the Home Fires Burning', 'Land of Hope and Glory' and 'Because'.[67]

The *Maheno* and the *Marama* were not the only ships that brought sick and wounded New Zealanders home from the war. Thirteen invalided men returned to New Zealand on the *Athenic* on 22 January 1915, along with defaulters and men who had refused to be inoculated against typhoid.[68]

The first significant group of wounded from Gallipoli arrived on the troop transport *Willochra* on 15 July. This Australian vessel had been sailing the Pacific on charter to the Union Steam Ship Company before she was requisitioned by the New Zealand government and converted into a troopship; she had taken part of the Main Body to Egypt in 1914. She made eight further trips over the next three years, four to Egypt and four to Britain, carrying reinforcements from New Zealand and bringing sick and wounded men home.[69]

The *New Zealand Herald* correspondent reported when she arrived with her first cargo of invalids that the two medical men on board, Captains James Mitchell and Robert Withers, had had 'a very busy time' on the voyage, carrying out operations daily. Although she was not a fully equipped hospital ship, the *Willochra* did boast a 'fine X-ray plant', which had been 'freely used. Bullets have been extracted and fractures satisfactorily set, and it is a great tribute to the skill of the medical staff that although many of the men are in a serious condition, and passed through a very trying time in the Red Sea, not one life was lost.'[70]

Reporters did their best to represent the *Willochra*'s arrival in a positive and heroic light, but the evidence of suffering was undeniable. 'Of course, there are among the cheery company of wounded warriors evidences of battle to move one to tears, but nothing terrible to justify the wicked rumors that have preceded their return. It is true that about six men are walking on crutches, and as many more are wearing celluloid patches over an eye, but none are distressingly maimed. Not one is totally blind, and one man only . . . has lost an arm. There are 15 cot cases, rather serious.' The men, 'in high spirits', were 'the very type who win kingdoms'; they 'invest the war with merriment'.[71] Allen was not entirely pleased. As he reported to Godley, 'about 30 of the men were about well enough to go to the front again. I cannot understand why they have been sent back'.[72]

The large crowds and civic celebrations that welcomed the *Willochra* would be repeated for arrival of the *Maheno*, the *Marama* and other vessels. Among the latter was the *Tahiti*, which sailed into Wellington on 11 September 1915, bringing from Suez some 490 sick and wounded men, who had been cared for on the voyage by two medical officers, four nurses and 19 medical orderlies. Nurses did not initially serve on transports, but the absence of their skilled assistance on the vessels taking the wounded off Gallipoli caused a change of heart. When the Sixth Reinforcements departed in mid-August, James Allen could announce that 'Three nurses were going on each vessel, and the staff of doctors was unusually large, as a draft of medical men was being sent to the Egyptian hospitals'.

The transports themselves were better prepared too, to avoid sickness during the voyage: 'Clothing, bedding, and kits had been disinfected, and each member of the force had been medically examined with the object of ensuring that no man with a sign of ill-health about him should get aboard.' The nurses would care for sick and wounded men on the return voyage, or possibly 'relieve other nurses, who perhaps, feeling the strain of the Egyptian climate, will prefer to return to New Zealand in charge of the wounded'.[73]

'Welcome home,' said the *Evening Post* editorial on the *Tahiti*'s arrival, 'to another large company of war-worn heroes from Gallipoli.'[74] Vessels like the *Willochra* and the *Tahiti* also carried men who had become sick during their service on Gallipoli, or after being wounded on the peninsula. Others never reached the Dardanelles, 'deemed "medically unfit" because of conditions identified after they left New Zealand or illnesses contracted en route or once overseas. This pattern continued throughout the war.'[75] When the *Aparima* returned on 16 September 1915 she brought several venereal cases. 'These are all being interned at the Quarantine Island at Port Chalmers, until they are well enough to be let loose.'[76] Newspaper reports mentioned the quarantine, but not the reason for it.

No longer on the *Tahiti* when she arrived, but buried in a Colombo cemetery, was Crowther Garside, who had cut his throat on 12 July. 'Fearful gash,' MO William McAra noted, 'severed trachea just above larynx — could see both carotid arteries pulsing — All oesophagus cut except posterior wall. I put iodine on and stitched skin up — Military Officer took charge after. I got him to shore. He is going to die.' The finding of the inquiry into Garside's death on the 18th read: 'While suffering from a very irritating skin disease & having very broken sleep attempted to commit suicide in a moment

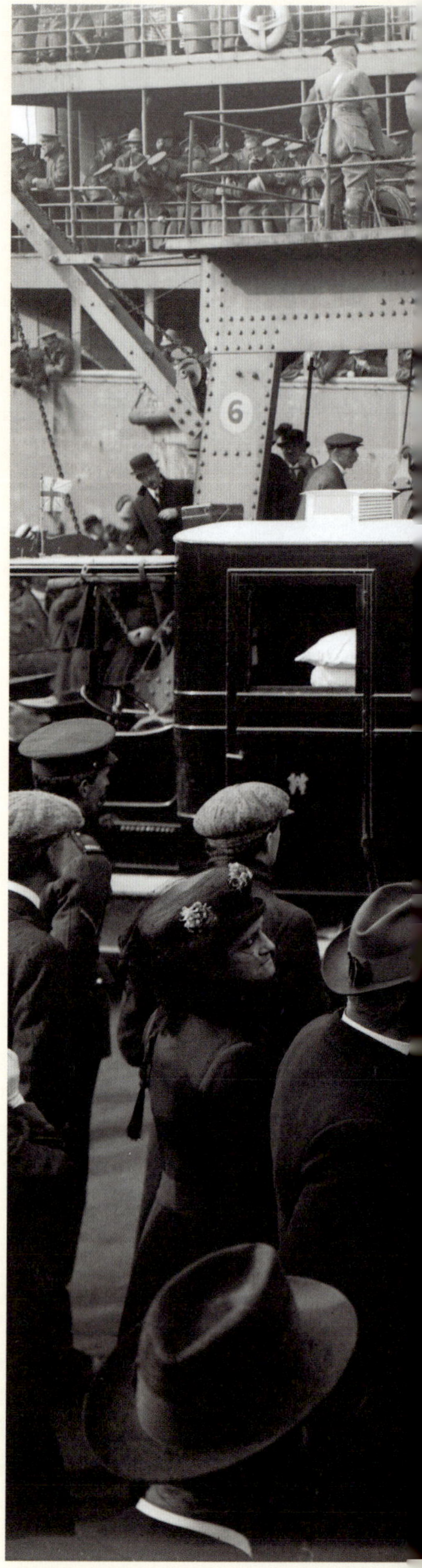

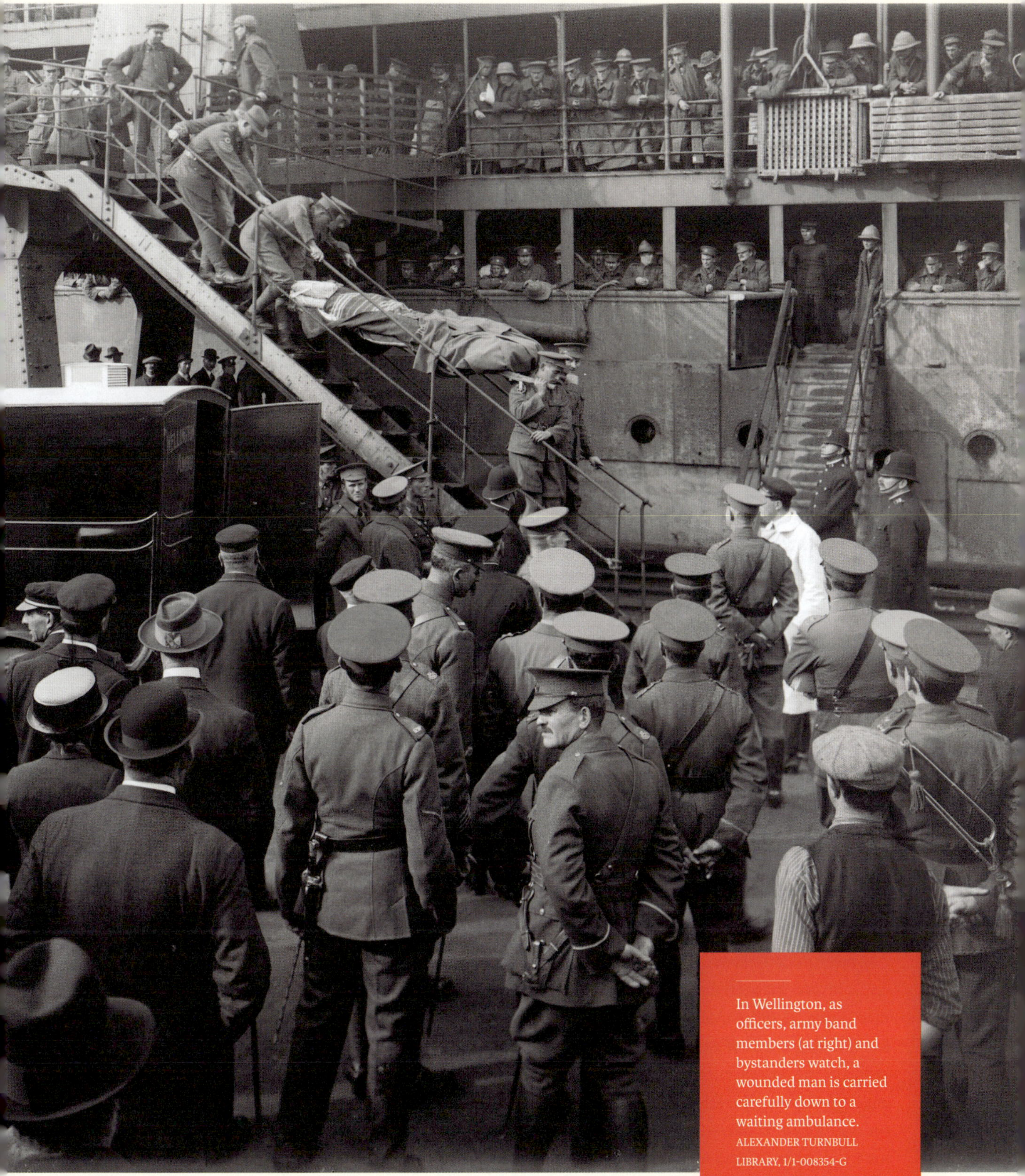

In Wellington, as officers, army band members (at right) and bystanders watch, a wounded man is carried carefully down to a waiting ambulance.
ALEXANDER TURNBULL LIBRARY, 1/1-008354-G

of temporary insanity.' His wife Eliza had petitioned for and been granted a divorce in 1913.[77]

On Christmas Eve 1917 Sister Mabel Kittelty, who had been working at No. 17 General British Hospital in Alexandria for two and a half years, was suddenly told that she and two other sisters were to leave for Suez on 27 December. 'It was a big surprise as we had been looking forward to going to England in the spring . . . yet there was nothing to do but accept the inevitable.' At Suez, an ambulance took the women to the transport *Tofua* which, with a staff of four nurses — Lucy Bowie, Florence Greensill, Kittelty and Hugha Sutherland — was returning to New Zealand with mostly Australian wounded and some 100 New Zealanders on board. 'Some of the men were very ill, and could not be left during the night. Fractured femurs on extension, and one with a Stimins [Steinman] pin through the knee, necessitated very careful handling, but they had to be put in the top bunks for convenience, and worst of all was the hospital being in the extreme bow of the ship. The sea was rough from Colombo, so you can imagine the awkwardness of dressing wounds and the effects on sisters and patients.'[78]

One of the New Zealand patients was Trooper Frederick Foote, whose arm had been severely wounded in the Sinai. He later described how he was taken aboard. 'There was a platform or huge tray on the wharf, my stretcher was put on that and the corner ropes from the tray hooked on to the great cargo hook hanging in the air above. A signal given and the rattle of the steam winch as I was hoisted away up to the mast head, swung over the ship and lowered down on to the deck without the slightest jar or vibration.' He found it 'a bit uncanny, but very gently done'.[79]

Kittelty was in charge of the dressing room, where she and two orderlies 'put through between sixty and seventy dressings every morning. Septic cases were done twice a day.'[80] She had only praise for her charges: the Australians were 'a pleasure to look after' and the New Zealanders 'the very best'. Many who were stretcher cases when the *Tofua* departed 'were able to go off the ship on crutches' when they reached New Zealand in early February 1918.[81] Such improvements wrought by medical staff were often reported by journalists. When the *Willochra* returned at the end of January 1916, bringing chiefly enteric convalescents, the *Free Lance* considered it 'quite amazing that most of them looked wonderfully well. The voyage and the medical treatment . . . have worked wonders, and many of the next of kin, who went down expecting to see a sort of frail invalid, found instead a browned, healthy-looking young creature who seemed glad to get home certainly, but who considered that he was now quite fit to return to active service. They quite forget that as soon as they exert themselves they feel their weakness.'[82]

After a 'weatherbeaten' *Ulimaroa* docked in Lyttelton on 23 April 1916, 'Maimed men were conspicuous by their absence, and the only signs of war and wounds were a shade over one man's eyes, a bandaged hand on another man, and a few limping warriors.' The ship had left Suez with 49 cot cases on board, but 'the sea air and careful attention [had] very greatly reduced this number, and now there are only ten, two or three of these being rather serious cases'.[83] The sea air could also be a liability, however. When Norman Hassell was coming home on the *Hororata*, the ship struck howling gales in the Tasman. 'We had a hospital structure built up on the deck in which four or five patients used to live, but as the waves got higher and higher they were moved below for safety. Two hours after they had been removed, the hospital structure was washed overboard.'[84]

A number of NZANS nurses also worked on British hospital ships and transports. At the end of 1915, Fanny Speedy began transport duty on the *Assaye*, working with several nurses from Australia, Ireland and Scotland and some 50 Australian and New Zealand Ambulance Corps men. The following February she was transferred to the hospital ship *Gascon*, on which all the nurses were New Zealanders, including five *Marquette* survivors. That same month, May Chalmer was the only New Zealander on board HMHS *Glengorm Castle*, which was carrying wounded from Alexandria to Southampton: 'They call me "Anzac," or Sister Ann for short.'[85] While Mabel Crook was briefly on the Royal Naval hospital ship *Somali*, a surgeon told her that 'they could not get two Maori's to eat' and asked if she could speak Māori. 'I said yes sufficiently I think & he took me to his ward & I found them right down & after a few words in Maori they looked up astonished, I told them they were worried at them not eating & they must eat all that was given them . . . they were amongst friends. The last I saw of them was when they were taken off the ship at Malta.'[86]

There were medical staff on the transports that brought New Zealand troops home at the end of the war. Each vessel carrying 1000 men had two medical officers, five NZANS nurses, four female Red Cross workers and 10 NZMC men. Extra women sailed when soldiers' families were travelling with them, 'and supplies of artificial milk devised by [Plunket founder] Dr. [Frederic] Truby King were carried for the use of the babies'.[87]

When they arrived in New Zealand, the wounded could not simply walk, or be carried, down the gangplank into the arms of waiting family and friends. As Allen informed Parliament on 14 July 1915, the day before the *Willochra* arrived in Wellington, the ship would have to 'be kept in the stream for several hours, because the Defence Department had to medically examine every man, check the examinations and records, and issue railway passes, leave warrants and pay books'. Each man must appear before a medical board for an assessment of his medical and physical condition. The process of being boarded was not without imperfections. As Clifford Collingwood noted, when the *Marama* docked in Auckland on 22 August 1917, the medical notes for the cot cases were left on each bed until the board doctors reached them. 'Naturally we all read our Medical papers with great interest.'[88]

The defence minister 'knew that relatives and members of the Press were anxious to get on board at the earliest possible moment, but the details . . . must be completed while the ship was quiet and nobody was about'. The wounded ended up in a variety of places. North Island men requiring hospital treatment were put aboard a hospital train that travelled to Auckland, and 'placed in hospitals nearest their own homes' along the way. Some convalescents were treated either at hospitals or in convalescent homes, while others could be looked after by their families. The men who had recovered during the voyage and were fit for discharge received money and a railway ticket home.[89]

When the *Arawa* reached Wellington on 17 March 1916, 'in the golden glow of a beautiful autumn morning', she had on board both ordinary passengers and 129 mostly Gallipoli men who had been hospitalised in England. The board doctors often went out to the anchored transports, but on this occasion they sat behind 'long makeshift tables' in a shed on King's Wharf. The returned men 'formed a rather sad spectacle, most of them having been "broken in the war"', and already designated permanently unfit in Britain. This re-examination, however, could select those who might be fit for home service.[90]

Finding hospital beds for returned men could be challenging. When the *Maheno* reached Auckland early on New Year's morning 1916, the Military Annexe at the public hospital 'was a busy place indeed, there being two hundred returned soldiers to be accommodated there. The other soldier patients were moved up to the general wards to make room.' Most of the men were able to walk off the ship and were detained only until the medical board and the health authorities 'ascertained that they were no longer typhoid carriers'. The majority were released the next day after 'bacteriological tests'.[91]

Whatever a man's condition, finally being home was often a very emotional experience. When Clifford Collingwood was carried down the gangplank of the *Marama* in Wellington about 9 a.m. on 25 August 1917, wearing his overcoat and hat and covered in a blanket, he could see 'the large crowd of people down on the wharf . . . As I was being placed in the Ambulance . . . I noticed Dad and [his sister] Eva nearby. I could not say much to them, for I felt too overcome for words.'[92]

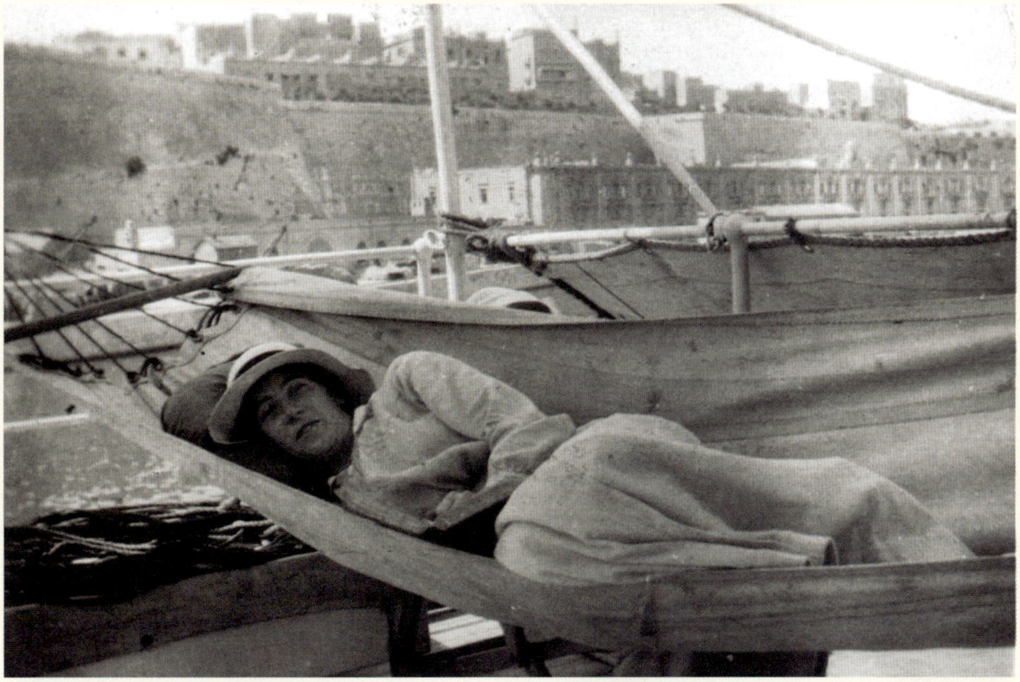

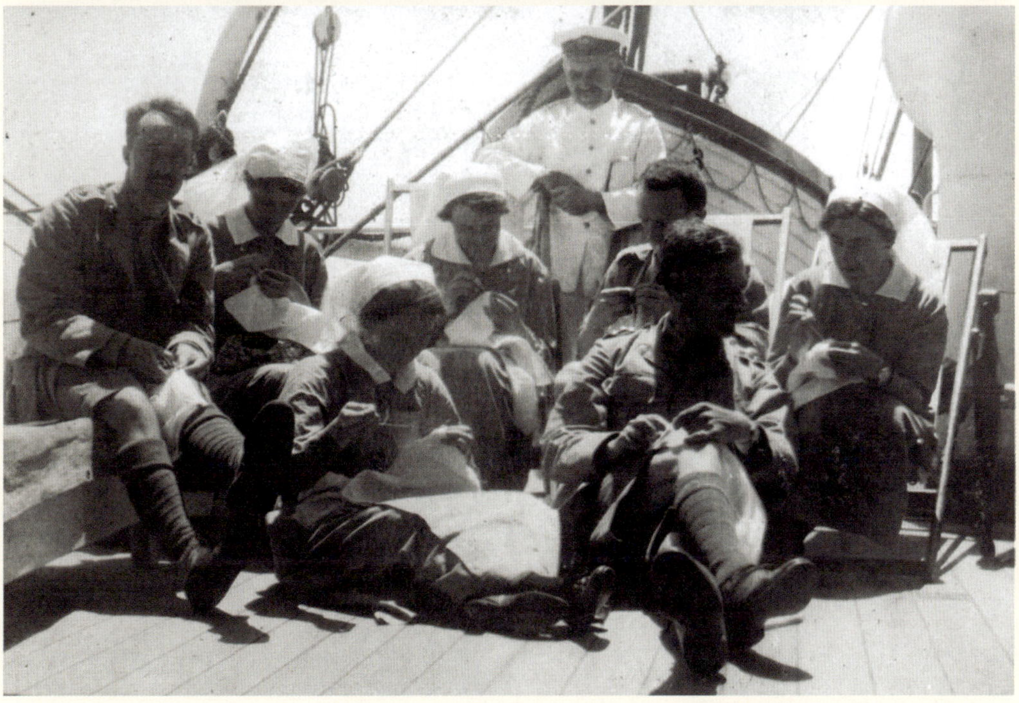

above There was sometimes an opportunity for relaxation on board a busy hospital ship. On a Sunday in Malta Harbour, New Zealand nurse Eleanor Gould rests in a hammock on the British vessel *Gascon*.
NATIONAL ARMY MUSEUM, 1986.1753

below In her photo album, Eleanor Gould called this photo 'The Sewing Class' — British officers and New Zealand nurses enjoy a break on the *Gascon*.
NATIONAL ARMY MUSEUM, 1986.1753

PART 3

Unexpected and Unsung

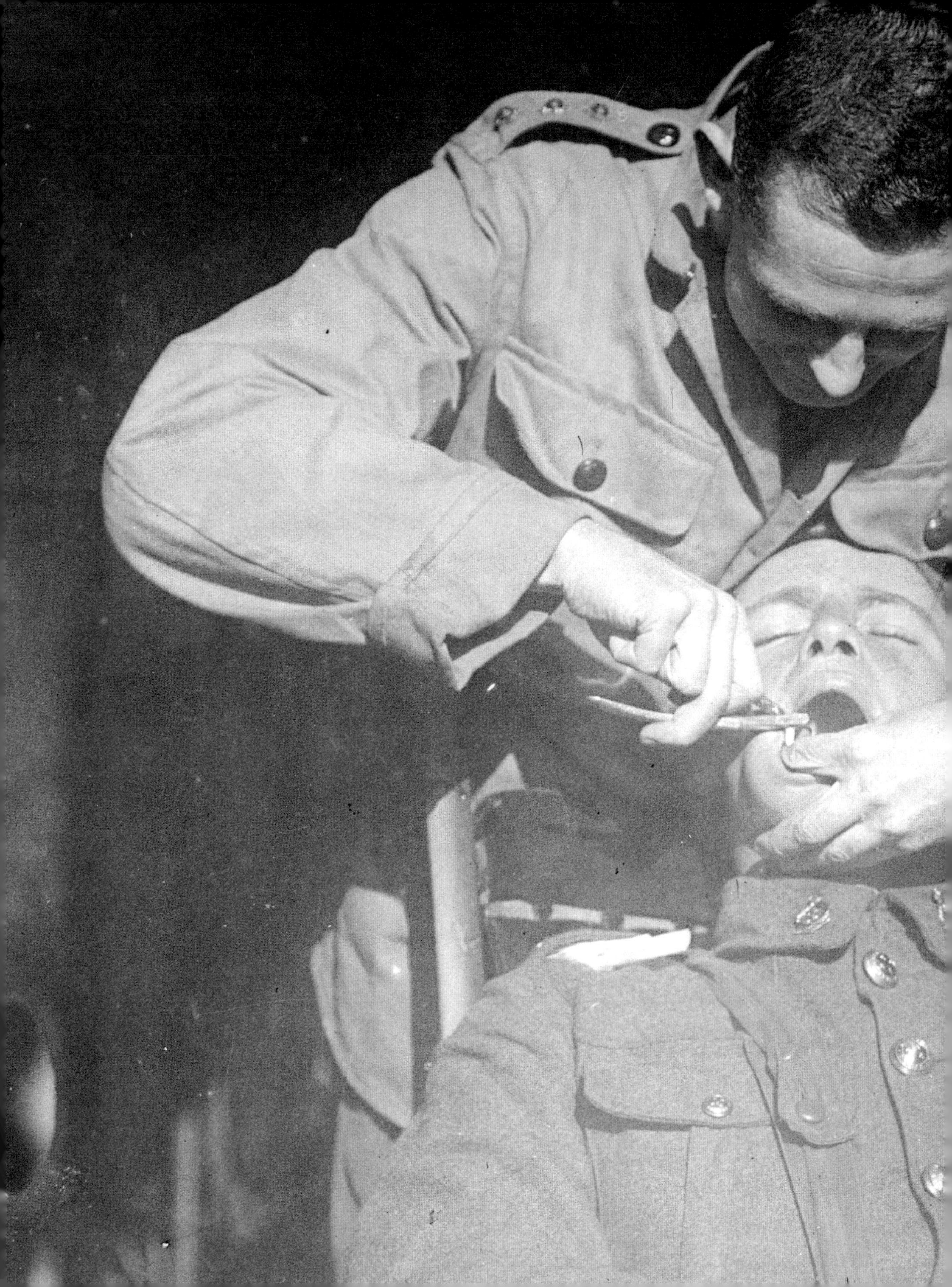

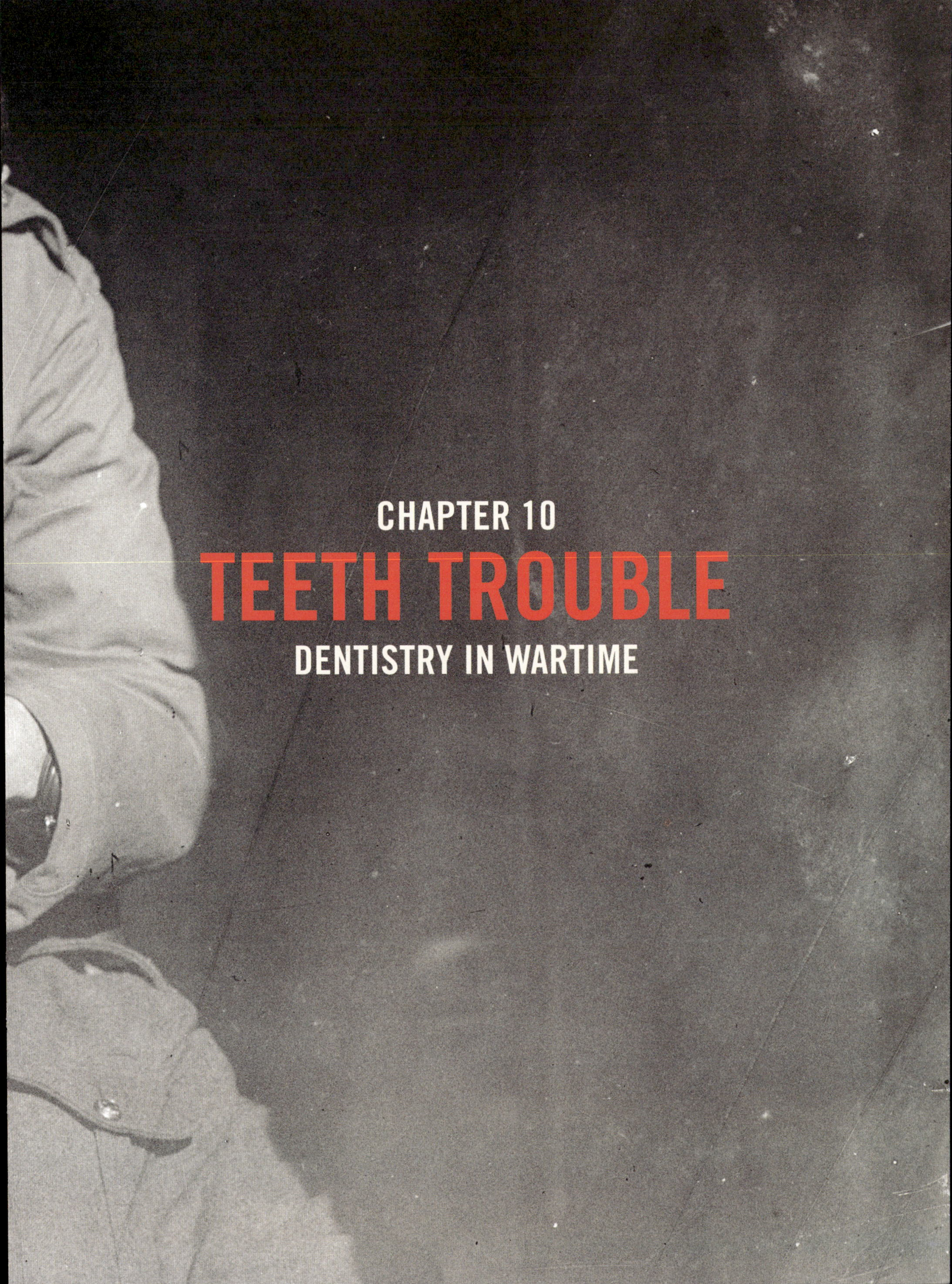

CHAPTER 10

TEETH TROUBLE

DENTISTRY IN WARTIME

previous pages
This is almost certainly a shot staged for the photographer at the New Zealand Dental Hospital in Nielles in northern France, but tooth extractions were also common on transports taking the troops to war — and they could be fairly brutal affairs. ALEXANDER TURNBULL LIBRARY, 1/4-009512-G

The soldier's smile's a winning smile
That carries all before it —
From officer to rank and file,
No lady will ignore it.
— Will Lawson, *Historic Trentham*

On 17 August 1914, less than a fortnight after war was declared, Christchurch's *Sun* newspaper printed a stern article headed, 'WANTED, SOME DENTISTS. TEETH OF THE SOLDIERS'. Troops must be able to 'assimilate their rations . . . to keep them in fighting "trim." But they cannot do that unless their mouths are well filled with sound teeth. A man who is insufficiently provided with teeth or who suffers from toothache, soon becomes unfit for duty.' Many of the 'fine, able-bodied men' already accepted for military service would find it 'impossible to masticate their food'. Yet 'Dental attention would make them splendid soldiers'. After examining the mouths of some 'strapping members of the Expeditionary Forces', the *Sun* reporter was 'surprised at the state of their teeth, and the sparsity of teeth in their upper jaws'.[1]

He was not alone in his concern. Not only did many successful recruits have poor teeth, but also an alarmingly large percentage of those rejected had been turned away for that reason. Of the 39 men examined in Ashburton in mid-August, for example, most of the 13 who failed had 'teeth trouble'.[2] It was the same story in Nelson and in Marlborough, although one hopeful, a South African War veteran known as 'Daring Jack', refused to take no for an answer. '"Do you think I want to eat the Germans? . . . I want to fight them."' He was delighted when, after 'repeated entreaties', he was selected. Some men went from place to place until they found a dentist willing to pass them.[3] Engineer Charles Saunders, who enlisted in London, was concerned that he might miss out owing to the loss of some back teeth. '[S]o I got a friend of mine to make me a plate with three teeth on it and, just before my turn came, I slipped it in . . . I could just speak, but couldn't have bitten an oyster.' After assuring the doctor the plate was comfortable, Saunders was passed. Once outside, he 'pitched the plate into the street and watched a Hammersmith bus run over it'.[4]

This was not a new problem. In 1911, when medical examinations of cadets for the Territorial Force began, a reporter noted that 'most of the lads have teeth missing. Some are very bad in this respect.'[5] There was also widespread general concern about the state of New Zealand children's teeth, and the cost of dental care. Early in August 1914 the socialist *Maoriland Worker* inveighed against the price of visiting a dentist — and even of 'tooth-brushes, pastes or powders' — for working people.[6] Although Geoffrey Wild still had his own teeth when he joined up, his two front crowns were 'a legacy from the bad teeth that were typical of the youth of the day — unless perhaps their parents could afford regular and expensive dentistry'.[7]

Men anxious to serve headed for their nearest dental surgery. In Wanganui, the *Chronicle* noted on 7 August that 'dentists have been particularly busy during the past few days, some of the main occupants of the chairs being "men of war".'[8] Patriotic dentists offered their services free or at reduced rates. In Akaroa, Raymond Dearsly, who would later serve in the New Zealand Dental Corps, was keen 'to supply artificial sets of teeth gratis to any of the [Banks] Peninsula men volunteering for the expeditionary forces'.[9] Trooper Frederick Foote, on final leave in Auckland, called at a dentist's office 'to enquire if by chance he could do a few stoppings for me'. Putting off other patients, the dentist did two hours' work, for which he refused to charge. When Foote left for his train he found that the dental nurses had filled his overcoat pockets with 'very useful presents'.[10]

During the two months before the departure of the Main Body, civilian dentists worked on the men both privately and at the four initial training camps at Alexandra Park in Auckland, Awapuni Racecourse in Palmerston North, Addington (later Sockburn) in Christchurch, and Tahuna Park in Dunedin. The New Zealand Dental Association, too, was quick to make a practical contribution. Early in September, 40 members of the Auckland branch established 'Something like a record in dentistry' when they 'gratuitously attended to the teeth' of some 900 enlisted men. At Alexandra Park a dentist inspected each man, decided what was needed and booked him an appointment with one of the 40. 'If the work done so cheerfully by the Auckland dentists were expressed in hard cash, it would be fully £1500.'[11]

Ten dental surgeons, each with the rank of lieutenant in the New Zealand Medical Corps, sailed with the Main Body, one per

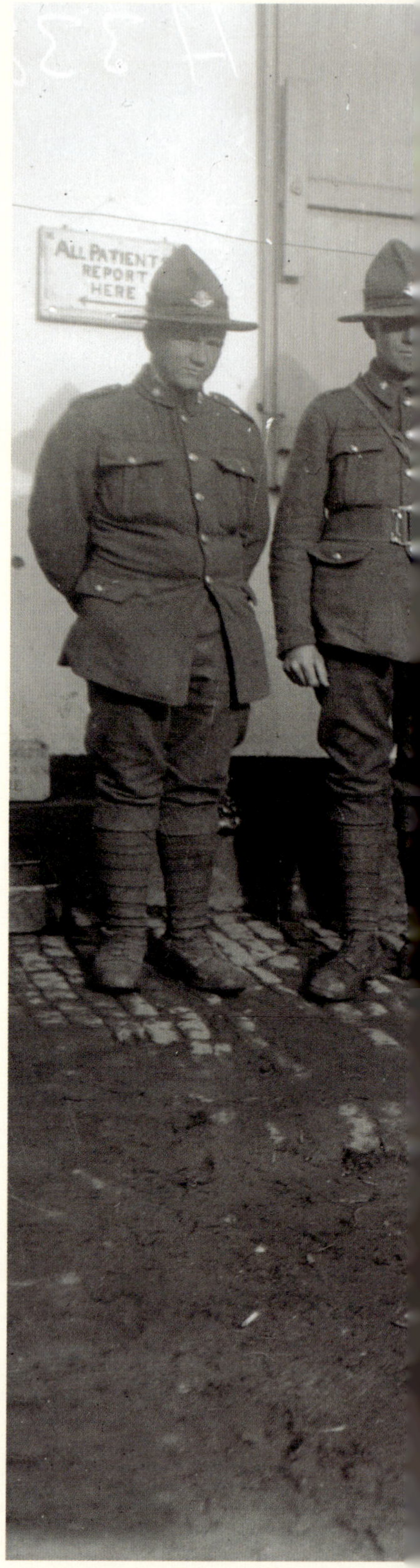

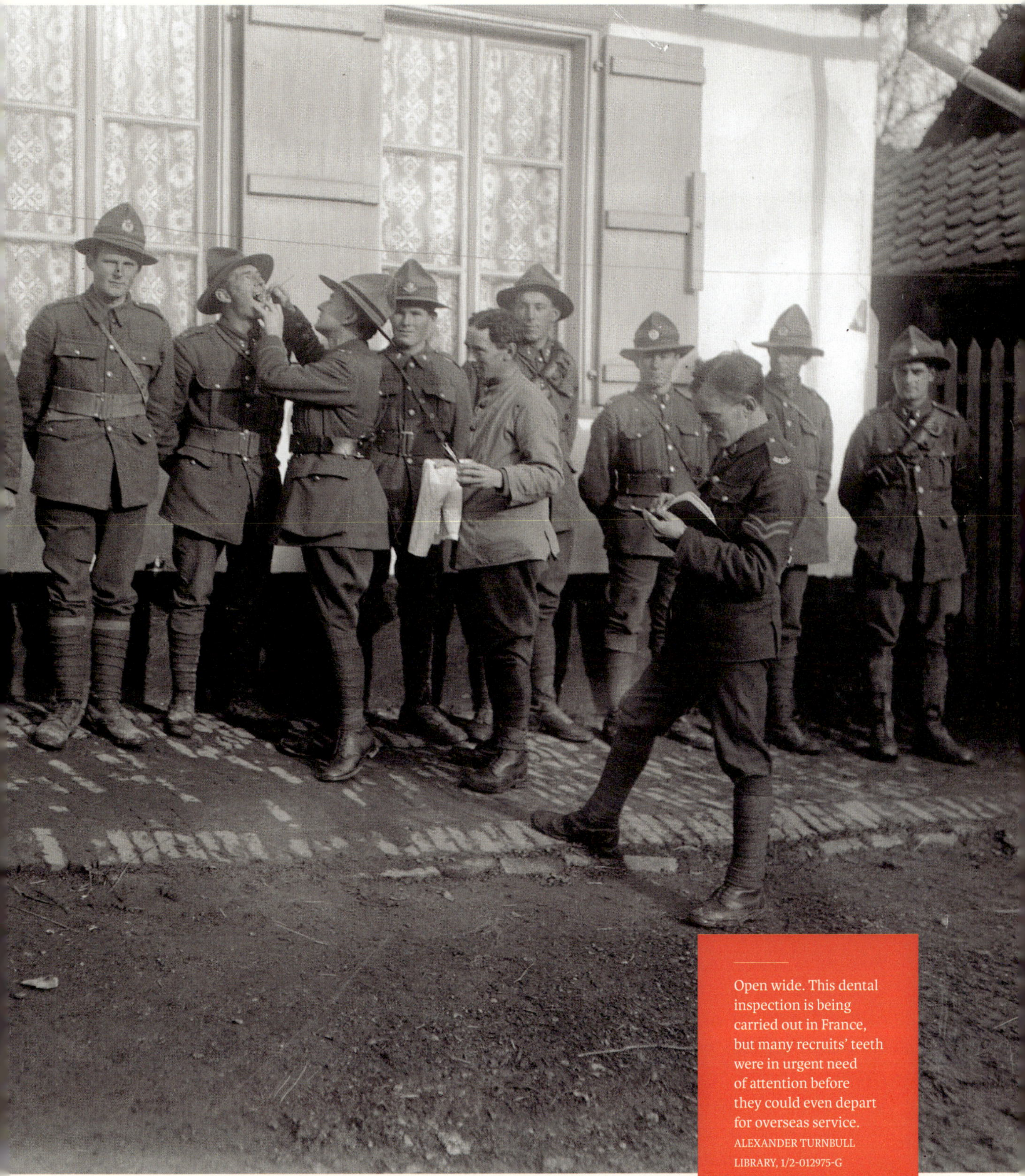

Open wide. This dental inspection is being carried out in France, but many recruits' teeth were in urgent need of attention before they could even depart for overseas service. ALEXANDER TURNBULL LIBRARY, 1/2-012975-G transport, to 'render the men dentally fit to take the line at once'.[12] Douglas Beere and Bertram Finn came from Auckland, and John Fairchild and Ernest Rawson from Wellington. Arthur Logan had a practice in Palmerston North. Representing the South Island were Raymond Dearsly of Akaroa, Francis 'Tiny' Tymons from Christchurch and John Don, Donald Green and William McKenzie from Dunedin. Each dentist had to provide 'his own travelling chair and a foot engine. The army supplied a cabinet of instruments with amalgams, cements, medicaments, etc. At this stage no provision was made for Denture work or repairs to Dentures.'[13]

A dental examination of all ranks revealed serious problems, but a treatment system was soon set up. A later official description of shipboard dentistry was optimistic — 'Fortunately the weather was very good and the sea generally calm, and operator and patients readily adapted themselves to the novel experience of treating and receiving treatment to the roll of the transports'[14] — but the men's experience was rather different. Trooper Claude Pocock reported wholesale extraction — 'some chaps having as many as eleven teeth out, and in spite of my having six out some months ago I had to get as many more out today'. The men dreaded dental parades: 'not painless, this time, but gouge them out like a navvy in a shingle pit'.[15] An 'advertisement' in the *Athenic*'s shipboard newspaper saw the humorous angle: 'Up-to-date dentistry. Mr ______ announces that he will attend daily on this boat-deck to extract teeth absolutely painless. The band will attend to drown the shrieks. No extra charge for drawing the wrong tooth or dragging the patient more than once round the deck.'[16]

And the discomfort was not all on the patients' side. Because so much deck space was needed for horses, the dentists had trouble finding somewhere to work, and on some transports officers were given cabins originally intended to be surgeries. Arthur Logan, on the *Orari*, had 'just a little box in a room. I could touch the walls on all sides without extending my arms to their full length, and I was literally surrounded with horses. In fact, if I were in my surgery when the time came for exercising the horses it was impossible to get out again for perhaps a couple of hours.' He was, however, quite comfortable 'and my chair and equipment fitted in nicely, with enough space for one patient and myself'. The size of the cabin was 'an advantage, in a way, as when the ship rolled the patient and I simply propped our hands against the wall on either side and so kept the chair, patient and dentist on an even keel'.[17]

Egypt, too, brought challenges for the dentists; all 10 were also promoted to captain. One was attached to each infantry battalion, mounted regiment and field ambulance. At Zeitoun camp, near Cairo, where the New Zealanders trained before leaving for Gallipoli, accommodation was once again bothersome, but after persuading the NZEF to recognise their requirements, the dentists swiftly got down to business. Because of the scarcity of timber in the desert, they were forced to work in floorless bell tents. Logan divided his assigned tent into two and used half as his sleeping quarters. It was a long way from 'operating in one's own surgery fitted with modern appliances ensuring asceptic and hygienic conditions'.[18] The heat was punishing and flies a constant irritation. When the hot, dry khamsins blew, the tents had to be laced up, shutting out the light.

William Deans never forgot his desert dental experience. He was having trouble with a wisdom tooth so took his place in 'just an ordinary chair' in a tent under a 'hot blazing sun'.

Although the dentist was 'fairly rough . . . he got the tooth out all right'. But Deans continued to run a temperature and his jaw swelled, so Dr Neil Guthrie had a look. 'I didn't notice he had . . . one hand behind his back and . . . a little knife and he gave me three cuts in the jaw without any hesitation. It was evidently forming an abscess there or something, the conditions being so rough and everything.'[19] This was not the last time a doctor would act as dentist. On the Western Front in April 1917, James Berry 'Pulled a couple of teeth out for [a] Maori who then wanted more out' and in May 'Extracted 2 teeth, some tooth, some soldier & some dentist'.[20] Soldiers sometimes, understandably, preferred to visit a private dentist. In January 1915 William Wilson called at the 'lovely rooms' of an Italian dentist in Alexandria who had a female assistant/interpreter: 'She is a real little gem and us boys are all in love with her. My lower set had to be cut in two and an inch of new plate put in. He made a decent job of it but he also knows how to charge.'[21]

Dentures, and their repair, were a 'vexed problem' for Logan, cropping up 'with disconcerting regularity . . . I was quite helpless. I had no gear what so ever for denture work.' He eventually volunteered to go into Cairo and find a dentist who could do this for the Wellington Mounted Rifles, 'at a much reduced cost to the individual soldier'. He finally located someone suitable but then had to face the fury of his commanding officer when the bills came in.[22] Soon, though, the dentists were given full equipment and dental mechanics were appointed.

New Zealand's dentists assisted other Allied forces who had not brought dental surgeons with them. Australian dental officers did not arrive in Egypt until 12 August 1915, so four New Zealand dentists, including Logan, were temporarily transferred to the Australian hospital and ambulance sections. The Australians may have been late in realising the importance of dentistry, but once they 'sprang into action' they 'did everything on a much more lavish scale', as Logan discovered when he did a second, much longer stint with the No. 1 Australian General Hospital at Heliopolis from early March to mid-August 1915: 'I had only to express a wish for an instrument or piece of equipment and it was immediately ordered.'[23]

British troops camped near Zeitoun also took advantage of New Zealand dental treatment. Their teeth were generally 'in a deplorable condition, and the gratitude of the "Tommy" . . . was no less marked than his astonishment at not having to pay for it. The invariable question was: "Is it true you take teeth out here for nothing?" Previous to our arrival the Egyptian dentists were making quite an income out of the boys from Lancashire, who could ill afford to pay.'[24]

Only four dental surgeons were to go to Gallipoli, two with the New Zealand troops and two with the Australians, and there was considerable speculation about who would be drawn in the ballot. The winners were Beere, Don, Finn and McKenzie. Soon after the Gallipoli landing, William McKenzie 'established a dental chair somewhere in the trenches near Russell's Top'.[25] According to Malcolm Ross, this was 'made by an Australian non-com. It was a rude enough bit of furniture, but it had an adjustable wooden headrest, and was quite a success.'[26] The complexity of getting cumbersome dental equipment to the peninsula meant that each Gallipoli-bound dental officer could take 'such instruments and materials as were required only for the immediate alleviation of pain', although more surgical tools, trained mechanics and a denture-making outfit would arrive later.[27]

According to Ross, the makings for the first dental surgery on the peninsula, not far from the Turkish lines, were 'begged, borrowed, or stolen, and three Turkish prisoners helped to build it'. Initially it had a blanket roof but after this was penetrated by shrapnel pellets, 'timber and iron . . . were sent along to replace the blanket, and the operators worked in less fear of the overhead bursts. Once a shell landed within 10 feet of the surgery, and exploded in the ground without doing any damage, but it was sufficiently close to add a little excitement to the work.'[28]

The day the surgery opened, in mid-June, there were 40 patients waiting. Among them was Yorkshire-born New Zealand signaller Bill Leadley, who had broken his bottom set of dentures on hard biscuits while sailing to Gallipoli. Both these and the loathed bully beef were ruinous for teeth, real and false. According to John Russell, 'the cabinbread-type biscuits were as hard as boards & could only be nibbled around the edges . . . our dental crowns were quite unable to cope with the hard remainder.' Ormond Burton's satirical piece on army biscuits said it all: 'Remember the cracking of your plate, the breaking of this tooth, the splintering of that. Call to mind how your finest gold crown weakened, wobbled and finally shrivelled under the terrific strain of masticating Puntley and Chalmer's [Huntley and Palmers] No. 5's.'[29]

Leadley had lost his upper set of teeth in a bayonet charge just after the landing. By 27 April he was reduced to pounding the biscuits into a powder. By 8 May he was 'feeling the effects of poor feeding, and had to drop out for a spell, as I was so weak'. His request to be sent to Alexandria for teeth was turned down. On 20 May, having heard that a dentist had arrived at Anzac, he found him on the beach and was told that his problem could be remedied as soon as the necessary dental instruments arrived. As May became June, Leadley was 'still persevering with powdered biscuits, but [feeling] awfully weak'. Finally, he had an impression taken on 13 June and received his top teeth a few days later. Although they initially seemed a good fit, they soon made his mouth 'rather sore, but [it] is better than being without any'.[30] The Gallipoli dentures, which lasted for many years, were so tough that Leadley amused his children by bouncing them on the floor and catching them.[31]

Others, too, had mishaps. Cecil Malthus, hospitalised on Mudros in September 1915, lost his plate while swimming, and Sapper Cervantes Bell, with the 6th Wireless Troop in the desert, 'had the misfortune' to mislay his false teeth while washing in a swiftly running stream.[32] Dentures could apparently disappear in other ways. *KoauKoau*, the shipboard magazine of the *Mokoia*, which left for France in August 1916, warned, 'If you wear false teeth don't sleep with your mouth open, as the rats are liable to get away with them.'[33] On the Western Front, at Rossignol Wood, Ormond Burton found Corporal Jim Holst 'dying on a duck board, and everyone standing reverently round to see the last of him. A bit of a wound in his neck, and he was obviously choking to death! On an inspiration I put a finger in his mouth, and fished out his false teeth from the back of his throat. Jim immediately started to take a new interest in life, and departed cheerfully on a stretcher.'[34]

Leadley had expected his new teeth might be 'rather rough', words that could be justly applied to some of the early dental treatment on the peninsula. Foote was horrified by the experience of a Waikato man who was forced to have all his teeth extracted. 'He had to sit on a stump without painless' — the dentist said he had no anaesthetic — and was 'sent

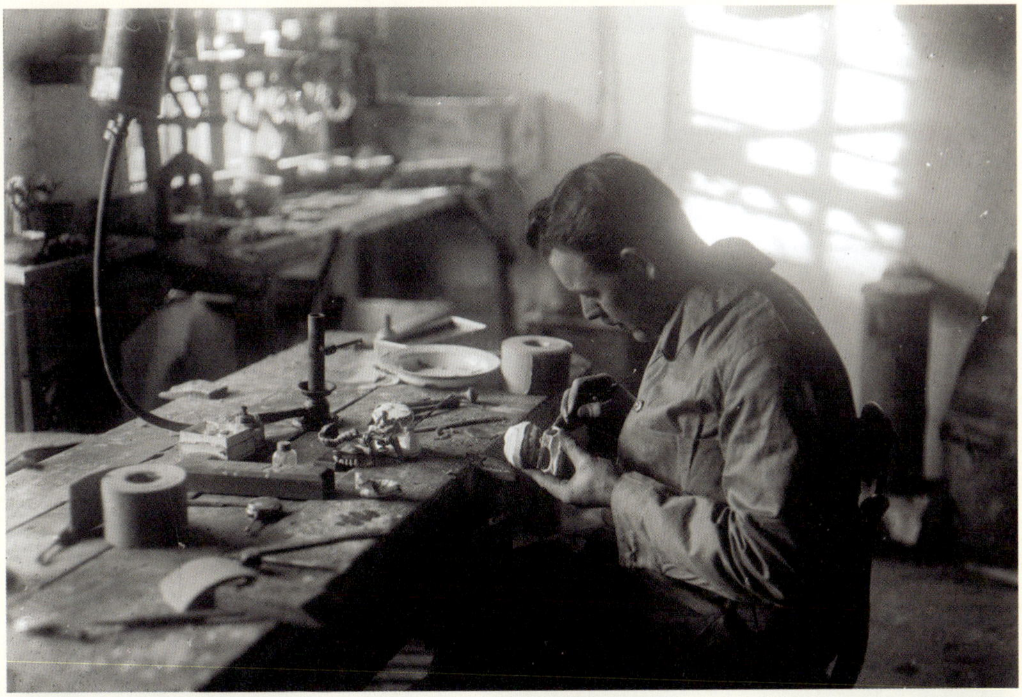

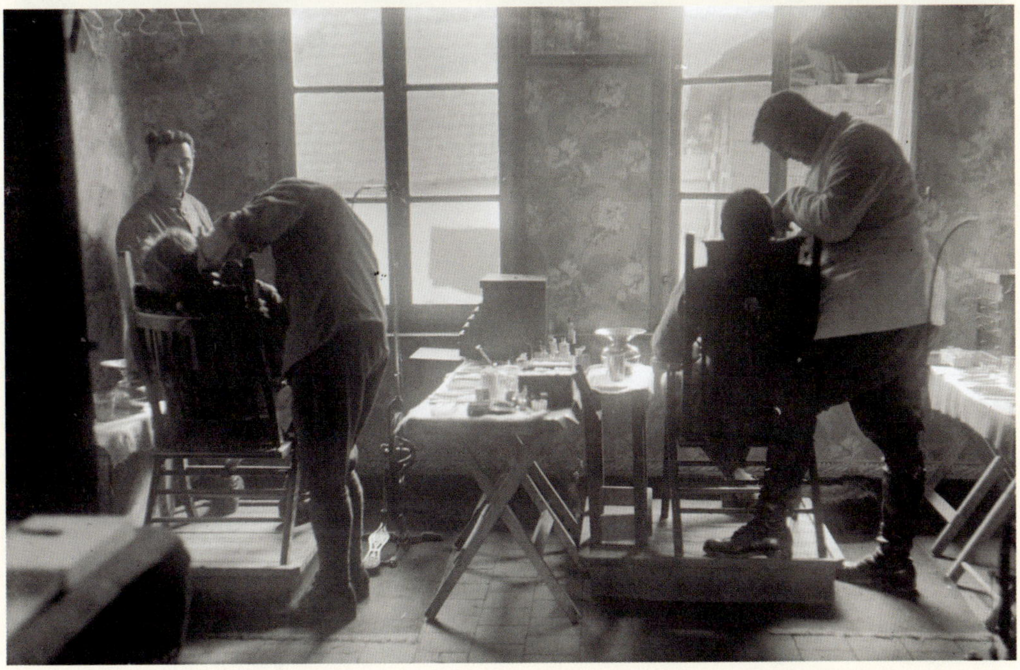

above An army dental mechanic puts the finishing touches to a new set of dentures manufactured at the New Zealand Dental Corps laboratory in Nielles in late 1917. Dentures had also been made on Gallipoli, under extremely challenging conditions. ALEXANDER TURNBULL LIBRARY, 1/2-012970-G

below With their soldier patients seated in ordinary chairs, and taking advantage of the natural light from the windows, two army dentists administer treatment at Nielles in November 1917. ALEXANDER TURNBULL LIBRARY, 1/2-012976-G back to the trenches to live on hard biscuits and tinned meat'.[35] Although no dentists had officially accompanied the Australian troops, a few who had enlisted in fighting or medical units volunteered their services. When Trooper Roderick McCandlish broke a tooth in July, the doctor sent him to an 'Australian Hospital Dentist — he tore my mouth up and did not get the tooth'.[36]

George Thomson, who was on Gallipoli by early August after serving with the Mounted Field Ambulance on various British transports and hospital ships, had been a dental mechanic in Timaru before enlisting. Following Charles Thomas's death on 26 August, he 'could not bear to stay in the ambulance' and on 4 September left for Walker's Ridge to 'start at the Dentistry. I feel confident I can produce the goods.' With Don in charge, there was only one other mechanic but more were expected from Egypt. When Thomson began work about 9 the next morning he found it 'Quite a treat to get back with the teeth and plaster. Things pretty brisk but very decent chaps to work with.' After Don and the sergeant went to Mudros on 10 September for dental supplies and a break, Thomson was 'going the pace': by the time they returned on the 20th he had made 11 new sets of dentures, done 14 repairs and taken several impressions. At the beginning of November the staff moved to 'new dental Parlours' at No. 2 Outpost.

Those working there — more dentists would arrive later — were under almost constant fire and the scarcity of fresh water required frequent visits to the beach for sea water to use in the vulcanisers. As Carbery would write, 'a dental hospital capable of carrying out any form of repair or mechanical work and the making of dentures and provided with cylinders of nitrous oxide gas and dental engines perched on a trenched hill side, cheek by jowl with a very noisy mountain battery, surely reaches the "limit" in front line dentistry'.[37] Sergeant James Downey, who had been a dentist in Hokitika before the war, told a friend back home: 'The firing line is only four miles from where I am, and the artillery a mile away. Death, in the shape of eight-pound armour piercing shells, often smiles at us.' Big guns firing every night about five o'clock 'over my tent where we work compels us to beat a retreat to a dug-out. The night before last, and last night, two of the shells dropped ten yards behind me. No damage was done.' He was now 'tip top' after a fortnight in hospital with a bad attack of dysentery, and had 'plenty of work to do. At present I have about fifty cases of artificial dentures to make. I have two assistants and an orderly, and I will be getting two more assistants next week. I start at nine in the morning and finish about ten at night. It is some going.'[38]

Logan, at Heliopolis, was desperate to get to Gallipoli. He eventually landed at Suvla Bay in the first week of November 1915, accompanied by his trusty assistant Sidney Lumb and 20 cases, seven of them containing dental equipment. The pair 'climbed the hill to the right as instructed and quite by accident came across a little row of dug outs cut into the bank, with a narrow terrace in front. In one of these we found my good friend and fellow dentist, Capt. "Pot" Don,' who was working with Fairchild and Dearsly, though they were away. (Dearsly was probably in hospital: on 24 October MO William McAra had given him castor oil and a tin of cornflour for dysentery, and intended to evacuate him the next morning if he was no better.)[39]

The dental surgery was in a large camouflaged tent just below the dug-outs. Logan and Lumb were soon 'working with the constant noise of shelling, and rifle and machine gun firing'. Some 10 days later, Tymons, Green and Beere arrived unexpectedly from Egypt and 'we were quite a merry band of "gumdiggers"'. Logan thought John Don a 'most remarkable little man', unfailingly 'cool, calm and unperturbed' in the face of heavy fighting and unremitting gunfire.[40] Save for some time between 8 and 17 August with the New Zealand Field Ambulance in Chailak Dere, 'administering A.T.S. [anti-tetanus serum] injections and registering the wounded' at the dressing station,[41] and that reluctantly taken leave at Mudros, Don worked solidly from 25 April until a week before the evacuation in December.

Poor dental health was associated with and could lead to other physical troubles. Sanitary commissioners visiting the peninsula towards the end of 1915 'noted a marked prevalence of gingivitis or pyorrhoea', which they 'believed to be a predisposing cause in gastro-intestinal disorders'.[42] The same connection was being made back in New Zealand: 'Letters from Gallipoli will show you that on any sick parade a considerable proportion of the men have gone under because of their teeth — septic pneumonia, gastro-enteritis, and many other diseases most common to the trenches.'[43]

Like Don, Bertram Finn went beyond the call of duty, and of profession, on Gallipoli. Attached to the No. 4 Australian Field Ambulance from 26 July to 21 August, he was awarded the DSO for his courageous work evacuating wounded from No. 3 pier below Chailak Dere on the night of 7 August. His citation read, 'he worked day and night with unceasing zeal and without rest . . . under continuous fire, on one occasion the dressing station being heavily shelled for an hour, and many assistants and wounded being hit'. He was, in Logan's estimation, 'quick in anger but equally quick in getting over it . . . he never bore a grudge and was a good and loyal friend'.[44]

When the peninsula was evacuated, George Thomson noted that 'dental goods' were among those stored on the beach '& the last party to leave put a match to it, it was an awful shame, but it would have cost too many valuable lives to have attempted to save the stuff'.[45]

Back in New Zealand, civilian dentists were continuing to help in the community and in the camps, but despite their best efforts poor teeth remained ubiquitous. When Bugler Frederick Welsh enlisted in April 1915, a handwritten note on the bottom of his medical examination form read 'Fit if teeth are attended to — stumps to be extracted & carious molars filled'. Improved teeth did not help Welsh when he reached Gallipoli: he was killed in October.[46]

In June 1915 the New Zealand Dental Association, led by chairman Thomas Hunter, told a receptive government that its members would 'treat all recruits free of charge as far as time permitted, between enlistment and being called into camp', provided they were reimbursed for the cost of materials. At every recruiting centre a dental officer appointed by the association would inspect each man's mouth; the 'dentally deficient' would go to an association member for treatment. Men who could afford it would be expected to pay; the government would finance the rest 'at hospital rates'. Every man sent to a dentist would have a chart made of his mouth that could go with him if he was called up for training before the treatment was completed. There would be dentists in the camps, attached to the NZMC. Hunter and Professor Henry

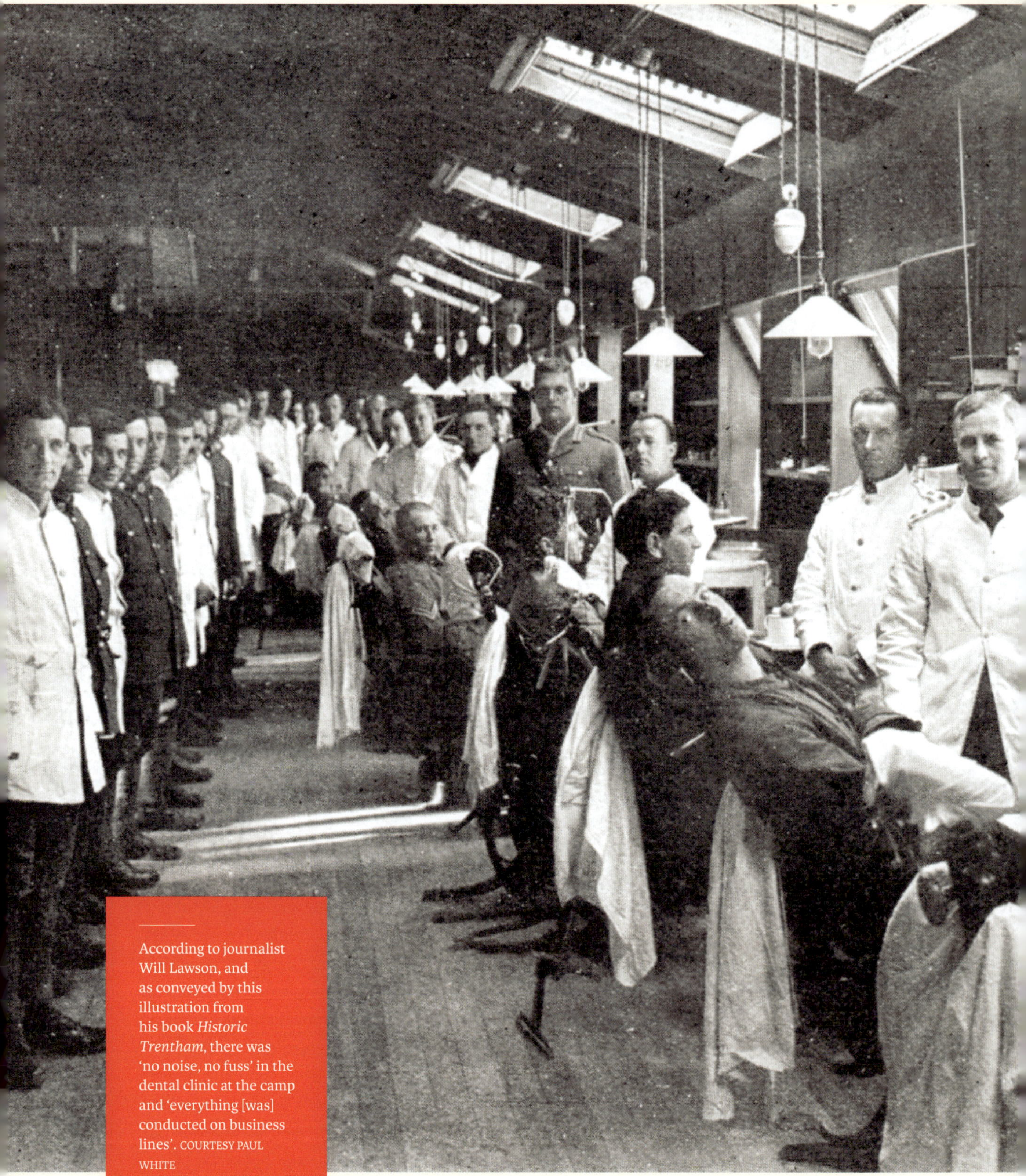

According to journalist Will Lawson, and as conveyed by this illustration from his book *Historic Trentham*, there was 'no noise, no fuss' in the dental clinic at the camp and 'everything [was] conducted on business lines'. COURTESY PAUL WHITE

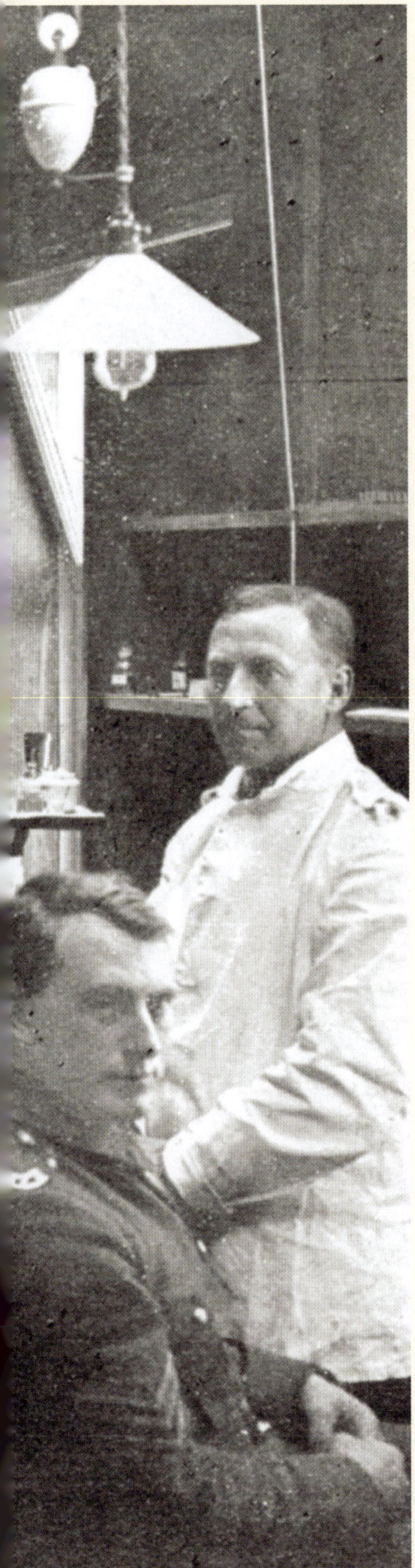

Pickerill of Otago University would be in charge of the 'portion of the scheme outside the camps'.[47]

But more was needed. As Wellington dentist Howard K. Jackson pointed out in a letter to the *Dominion* in October, the many men requiring dental treatment often could not afford it and 'so are lost as recruits . . . "Oh, well! if the Government won't pay it for me, I'm off 'out-back' again."' Jackson suggested the formation of a Dental Corps, 'controlled at the head by a dentist having proper military status, the same as the Canadian Government has established'. Although the camp dentists were lieutenants in the NZMC, 'dentistry is outside the sphere of the doctors, and they do not profess to understand the requirements'.[48] Pressure was also coming from the front. While inspecting Don's 'excellent' establishment on Gallipoli, Godley had been told of complaints 'that the dentistry arrangements at Trentham were not very satisfactory', and of troops going overseas with 'indifferent plates, etc.' which had to be repaired or replaced. According to Don, 'men . . . had been told that they would get their teeth fixed up alright when they got to the front'.[49] Tension between what was being done in New Zealand and at the front would continue even after the corps was formed.

Jackson's was not a lone voice. Hunter, Pickerill and other dentists pressed hard for a corps, and in November 1915 their advocacy paid off with the establishment of a Dental Service Corps, later the New Zealand Dental Corps. Hunter became the director of dental services (DDS) and was later the corps' historian. Papers like the *Dominion* reported the news with due seriousness, but the *Free Lance* took a more frivolous approach: 'a military dental corps has been formed in connection with the New Zealand forces. Their duties presumably will be to fill up the gaps in the front.'[50]

The corps began modestly but it was not long before more dentists were needed at Featherston and Trentham. Suitable buildings such as surgeries and workrooms were required, too, along with mechanics, orderlies and equipment. On 21 January 1916 an advertisement in the *New Zealand Herald* invited applications for 'seven dental orderlies for service at the Trentham, Tauherenikau, Rangiotu [near Palmerston North], Awapuni, and Narrow Neck camps. Applicants must be young men who have returned from the front, and who are, through minor defects, unfit for further active service. No previous dental training is necessary.' The corps grew steadily, but it was only by the end of September 1916 'that it could be said the organisation in New Zealand was coping satisfactorily with the work'.[51]

A year after the corps' formation, journalist Will Lawson produced both a straightforward 'advertorial' description of the dental work in the camps, for the *Sun*, and a more humorous account for his book *Historic Trentham, 1914–1917*. In the newspaper, he described '12 white-coated operators, three of whom are captains and the others lieutenants of the New Zealand Dental Corps, . . . attending to patients in chairs . . . ranged in a row along one side of the surgery. At the other side of the room, nine mechanics, a sergeant-major, and eight sergeants, work at high pressure at benches and braziers, while white-coated orderlies move to and fro.' Once a patient had had an impression taken for much-needed dentures, the mechanic worked up a casting first in wax and then in rubber, which was vulcanised 'to get the requisite toughness and hardness' — for those rocklike biscuits. It was hard, hot work. The heat came from kerosene-guzzling primus stoves, which also boiled the water. According to Lawson, the men went willingly for their treatment, as the dentists had 'an excellent name for care and gentle treatment among the troops'.[52] It was not always so. In November 1917, the *Observer*, describing 'The New City' that was Trentham camp, remembered the old days when 'the farrier sergeant got to work on the rancid molar with a pair of pliers and a farrier private to hold the patient's shoulders'.[53]

Painless or not, the output of dental work in the camps was impressive. Between November 1915 and November 1918, the dentists filled more than 220,000 teeth, did just over 18,000 scaling operations and performed almost 100,000 extractions. They made some 24,000 artificial dentures and repaired 3500. Men sat in their chairs on a total of 270,000 occasions.[54] Dental procedures were not the only focus; the work included 'dental prophylaxis and a vigorous propaganda, a moral tooth brush drill, which had a wide effect in keeping the men alive to the importance of oral cleanliness'.[55] Dentists were also on hand during medical boards for returning troops. 'Waiting for him are the dentists, who examine his mouth with an electric torch, calling out to assistants in technical language, the treatment which the soldier should receive to bring his mouth into a condition as good as when he commenced to serve . . . The State is not willing to make all soldiers dentally perfect at its expense, but it will repair the ravages due to active service.'[56]

Dentists did not travel light, as the NZEF discovered when it reorganised the dental staff, under brave Bertram Finn, following the evacuation of Gallipoli. In Logan's view, the dental component was 'gradually being put on a much more satisfactory basis',[57] but he was less than impressed with the situation in Moascar at the beginning of 1916, when he, Beere, Don, Green and Tymons had only a few pairs of forceps, limited anaesthetic and no gear.[58] Logan and Tymons were forced to go into Cairo to purchase equipment.

It took some weeks, and a considerable amount of confusion, before the dentists in Egypt were informed, in March, about the establishment of the Dental Corps. Two dental sections, each headed by an officer, were attached to each of the three field ambulances, and one to the Mounted Field Ambulance, which remained in Egypt. With each pair of sections went 'nine panniers of equipment containing surgical appliances and prosthetic plant'. Naturally, 'the total weight of the equipment — 7½ cwt [381 kg] — [was] thought to be overmuch for the ambulance transport' and later reduced.[59] There were also two sections for the New Zealand Infantry base depot, which accompanied the division to France, and one for No. 1 New Zealand Stationary Hospital, recently arrived from Salonika, where it had treated 1000 dental cases. The problem of heavy dental gear would re-emerge in France, when No. 2 Field Ambulance moved from L'Estrade to Ebblinghem in mid-August. It was 'rather too much' to add, to already overloaded transport, 800 lb of gear and baggage belonging to two dental officers.[60]

Arthur Logan, in Dental Section No. 2, sailed from Alexandria for France early in April 1916 with No. 1 New Zealand Field Ambulance, which opened its first tent subdivision at the Château de Morbecque, near Hazebrouck. A dental hospital was set up in the town, in a large building at 42 Rue Nationale, only 1¾ miles from the front line, so that the troops could receive treatment without having to travel to the BEF base at Étaples on the coast. Lieutenant-Colonel Donald Murray of No. 2 Field Ambulance was in overall charge, but Tymons (No. 5 Dental Section) controlled the staff, which comprised dentists Don and Green, several mechanics and three orderlies. The hospital, which was open from 8 a.m. to 1 p.m. and 2 to 6 p.m., would do all repair, denture and prosthetic work, leaving extractions and fillings to the other dentists, like Logan, attached to field ambulances. The latter would also attend ADSs at night to deal with urgent cases. On 13 June the No. 2 Field Ambulance diary reported that the dental hospital was 'doing fine work'.[61]

By late July Logan was with No. 1 Field Ambulance at the divisional rest station at Lestrade, between Steenwerk and Armentières, 4 miles behind the line, with his surgery and workroom in a large marquee. Early in August he found himself in Armentières itself, where his billet was adequate but his surgery was 'in a corner of a huge, gloomy room, almost as big as a drill hall, in a desolate and deserted part of town, where all the surrounding buildings had been blown to pieces'.[62] By then he had just one orderly, as his two mechanics had been sent to the Dental Hospital. Soon after this, the dental sections faced 'a big disappointment'. They would not go to the Somme with the troops in September — 'it would be impractical to move us with all our heavy gear along with the constantly advancing Division' — but be sent to base camp.[63]

After the New Zealanders were withdrawn from the Somme and once again took over the Armentières sector, it became clear that the dentists were not coping with the workload. Dental officers on transports were also struggling, there was a shortage of dental personnel at the bases and hospitals in England, and those at Étaples were always busy. The front line, though, had to take priority and the only answer seemed to be to focus on dental work at Sling, where so many reinforcements bound for France were arriving with sub-standard teeth. At this point, in familiar New Zealand bureaucratic fashion, a report was commissioned from Dearsly, the division's senior dental officer. This, to no one's surprise, revealed that 'the dental condition of the division was very bad', and many men were arriving in Europe with 'hurriedly supplied' New Zealand dentures that required remaking 'owing to shrinkage'. It was difficult, too, to get equipment.[64] Dearsly's suggested solution was to call on trained dentists and dental mechanics serving in the NZEF outside the Dental Corps; Finn, as administrative dental officer, could send instruments over from England.

Godley eventually agreed to extra staff and Logan was put in charge of the re-established Dental Hospital, which was now at Sailly-sur-la-Lys. Dearsly was his second in command and they had a staff of 14. Finding a suitable building proved difficult: a deserted schoolhouse was used, but it was 'a cold and draughty building with a stone floor, and all the glass in the windows had been destroyed by shell fire'. There were also some huts. Winter in such a place was an uninviting prospect, but glass was promised, along with repairs to the leaks in the roof, and Logan and Dearsly found themselves a comfortable billet. When they started work on 30 October, they had a great deal to do. 'Patients came from all directions, as during the Somme Battle the dental work had accumulated. They were even coming direct out of the trenches for urgent work and the Battalions out of the line were simply clamouring for attention.'[65] Units had designated days to visit the hospital; officers came on Sundays. In its first two months, the dental corps 'worked hard and well', treating 1700 cases. Because they were only 4 miles from the front line, soldiers could receive 'efficient treatment without being more than a few hours absent'.[66] The dentists faced shelling and bombing — the 'continuous roar of the Artillery and the rattle of machine gun fire would lull us off to sleep'[67] — and a new problem, the contagious trench mouth or Vincent's angina, also called ulcero-membranous gingivitis.

As Malcolm Ross observed, trench mouth, the 'result of the bacillus that causes ulceration and bleeding of the gums', was not 'confined to men who have been in the trenches . . . and is a disease apt to bring other disorders in its train'. Treatment, which involved painting the gums with Salvarsan — the drug used to treat syphilis — 'or an arsenical solution', usually worked in two to three weeks.[68] It was an extremely unpleasant condition. After two weeks' furlough in New Zealand, John Russell 'reported sick because of a disgusting pussey discharge into my mouth, becoming so severe that I had to rinse it thoroughly, pronto, to avoid the urge to vomit on waking . . . I was prescribed a mouth wash & a nasal douche.'[69]

During a hasty visit from New Zealand in November 1916, corps head Thomas Hunter seemed 'reasonably satisfied', in Logan's words, with the dental work in France, but 'did express disapproval at the officers working in their shirt sleeves' and when he found a dentist 'with a lighted cigarette in one hand while he was trying a denture in a patient's mouth with the other'.[70] Having decided that the corps was woefully understaffed, Hunter recommended that every troopship leaving New Zealand from then on carry a dentist and a dental mechanic. A dental surgeon also travelled on the *Marama* and the *Maheno*.

In January 1917, after a cold and snowy Christmas, Logan was given some extra sergeant mechanics and he and his staff 'put through a tremendous amount of necessary denture work for our troops'. The next four months were 'very strenuous, and we were kept hard at it all the day light hours and every day, including Sundays'. Logan, weary and 'browned off', had been given no leave and had several rows with headquarters in London, who seemed to have no understanding of front-line conditions and difficulties. Late in February the hospital moved to Nieppe, near Armentières, where a house was used, with the surgery on the ground floor and the workroom set up in a backyard shed.[71]

As Ross was aware, setting up clinics in sometimes primitive surroundings required extra care with cleanliness: 'every available measure [was] taken to render the clinic generally aseptic', and heating and ventilation were installed. The correspondent understood, too, how the men's teeth were damaged by the hard food and that their inability to clean them had an effect, as did 'the severe mental strain endured by the troops in the trenches'.[72] The presence of dentists could be welcome, as William Habberfield-Short found at Dickebusch in January 1918: 'Went to the dentist & tooth filled & nerve removed. Very good job & much relief.' Writing to his father from France in March 1918, William Smallfield rather snobbishly complained of having to sacrifice 'a good gold filling . . . for a horrible lump of army amalgam!' when his tooth broke. 'However, a serviceable tooth is an asset, even if filled with such a plebian filling.'[73]

In May 1917, the dental section formed in England to accompany the No. 4 Field Ambulance reached France. It was a 'very mobile unit . . . two small panniers, one pack-mule load, now contained sufficient instruments and material for all operations, surgical or prosthetic'.[74] The Dental Hospital, too, was more easily transported: it was allocated a 3-ton lorry. At the end of May, just before the Battle of Messines, the hospital was moved to De Seule Corner, near Bailleul and close to the Reinforcement Camp. In June Logan finally got 10 days' leave in Britain, where he caught up with Doug Beere (who was working at Hornchurch), Finn, Green and Tymons. On 7 July, soon after his return to De Seule, the hospital, now under canvas, was shelled. One bomb landed 20 yards from Logan's tent.

From then until the end of the war, the dentists continued to be fully occupied, following the division as it moved from place to place. On 21 March 1918, just before the New Zealanders were ordered south as the German Spring Offensive began, the Dental Hospital was sent by lorry to the New Zealand Stationary Hospital at Wisques. As usual, the mobile dental sections stayed with the ambulances. At the NZSH the dentists also treated British, French and American soldiers, along with French and Belgian civilians. 'The French soldiers and civilians were greatly surprised, when in answer to the invariable question "Combien s'il vous plaît, Capitaine?", they were informed there was no fee.'[75]

At Sling camp in England, dental officers and mechanics treated the New Zealand soldiers who were leaving for France. Clinics were later opened at headquarters in London and at Brockenhurst, Codford, Hornchurch and Walton-on-Thames. One to benefit from dental treatment at Walton was Clifford Collingwood, who had been badly wounded in France. In July 1917, he asked the sister if he would be given any teeth before returning home, as his top set 'were practically all broken'. Sister Matilda Fricker 'promptly brought the Hospital Dentist in, and she stood by while he took an impression. He took away my top plate for building up, and I received it on the following afternoon. Sister Fricker came along and said in fun, "Will you have thum thou [some soup]."'[76]

It was to Walton-on-Thames that Logan was posted after he left France in August 1917. He then worked at the New Zealand artillery camp at Ewshot, with two other dentists, one of them the unfortunate Charles Ward (see page 263), before returning to Walton and then serving at Codford. From early February 1918 he spent time at Hornchurch, the New Zealand section at Sidcup, and No. 1 New Zealand General.[77] Logan clearly maintained high standards. Just before he sailed for home at the end of 1918, he received a note from Percival Fenwick, then head of Brockenhurst. 'I would like to offer you my sincere thanks for your loyal and conscientious work . . . It has been a great pleasure to have an officer of your character on my staff.' Logan was kept busy during the voyage of the *Ruahine* in 'quite a big and well equipped surgery on one of the upper decks'. Without a dental mechanic, he did all his own prosthetic work.[78]

New Zealand's army dental record in the Great War was a proud one. The Canadians won the race to establish a dental corps, but New Zealand was the 'only country along the entire Allied front' to have a dental hospital in the divisional area. It also provided 'a complete dental chain' from the training camps to the front line, and soldiers no longer fit for service had 'their mouths made normal' before they sailed for home. But lives were lost. In November 1915, for example, George Thomson, on Gallipoli, was 'very sorry to hear of the deaths of 3 of our Dental men': Albert Beswick, Hugh Shrimpton and Charles Warwood had all died of disease.[79]

Four of the 10 dentists who travelled to Egypt with the Main Body later transferred to combat units: Don joined the air force in France and served there until the end of the war; McKenzie joined the infantry and later became a pilot; Rawson went to the artillery. Green, who chose infantry service in September 1917, was killed in France on 5 April 1918. Tymons received an OBE in 1919 and Logan was 'brought to the attention of the Secretary of State for war, for valuable services rendered'.[80] Sergeant Cecil Burke from Gisborne was a qualified dentist who 'did good work at his profession gumdigging soldiers' molars in Egypt'[81] before asking to go into the fighting lines; he was wounded on 4 May 1917.

The legacy of the New Zealand Dental Corps lasted far beyond the war. Soon after the Armistice there were calls for the army's dental equipment to be used at home, particularly for the nation's children. The widely publicised emphasis on the troops' poor teeth had focused public attention and perfectly fitted the strong eugenic drive of the time for healthy, upright citizens. In November 1918 a letter to the *Evening Post* pointed out that in country districts 'children's teeth were in a serious condition . . . Does the Government propose to demobilise the Dental Corps and dispose of all the equipment they must necessarily have?'[82] As the paper suggested soon after, 'Money by the £100,000 was found to fit our best brawn and brains for the firing line, many of whom have laid down their lives for us. Surely money by the £1000 can be found to make the growing children their fit successors.' An Education Department dental scheme was set up, in 1920, using a large quantity of corps equipment and material. After all, as the *Evening Post* had pointed out, 'As our National [coalition] Government found it indispensable to inaugurate free and compulsory dental service for our soldiers, the equipment purchased could not continue to be used better than for free and compulsory dental treatment for our soldiers' children.'[83]

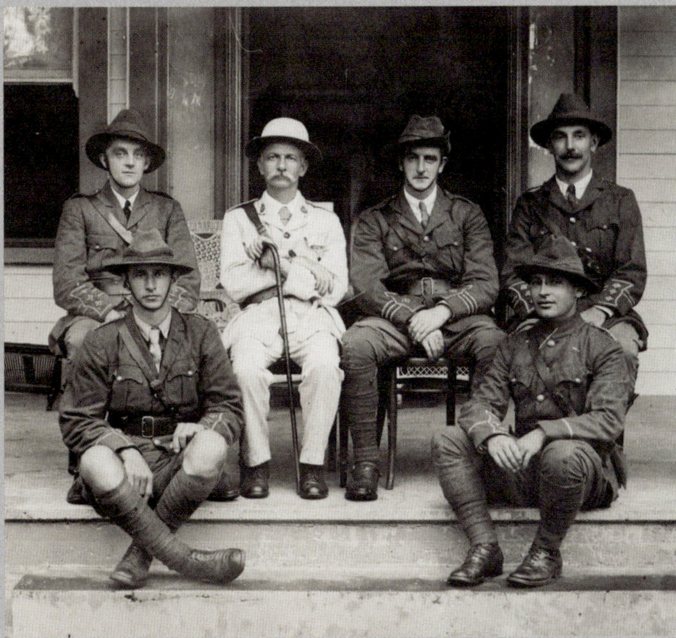

Dentists Lieutenants Charles Ward (left) and David Isaacs sit on the step in this group photograph of NZEF medical staff in Samoa in 1914. Left to right in the chairs are Captain Mick Tapper, Major Henry Kendall, Major Mathew Holmes and Captain Duncan Stout. ALEXANDER TURNBULL LIBRARY, 1/2-148890-F

SERVICE IN SAMOA

Wellington dental surgeons David Isaacs and Charles Ward, who accompanied the Advance Party to Samoa, worked hard during their time in the Pacific, despite being short of equipment. Two months after returning home on 22 March 1915, Isaacs sailed with No. 1 New Zealand Stationary Hospital as dentist and quartermaster. He served his country for five years, in Egypt, Salonika after surviving the sinking of the *Marquette*, and on the Western Front. Awarded an MBE in 1919, he went on to lead a busy life in the capital.[84]

Charles Ward's story did not end so happily. After returning from Samoa, he worked at Trentham and on Somes Island before sailing for Britain at Easter 1917. There he was posted to headquarters and to Sling camp until his admission to Walton-on-Thames on 11 December with trench mouth. After a spell at the Brighton Convalescent home he was back at Walton by 5 January 1918. Then, on the 18th, he went missing. There were rumours that he had been seen after his abandoned bicycle was discovered on the riverbank, but Ward had also left his hat and letters written to his wife Helena that confirmed his intention to commit suicide.[85] A court of inquiry on 15 February declared him missing; a second hearing, the following year, was 'of the opinion' that Ward was dead. The day before his disappearance, he had been given leave to visit his brother, Ivan, who had found him 'very much depressed, would neither smoke nor drink & complained about his health, particularly the condition of his throat, though he seemed reticent as to what was the matter with it'.[86]

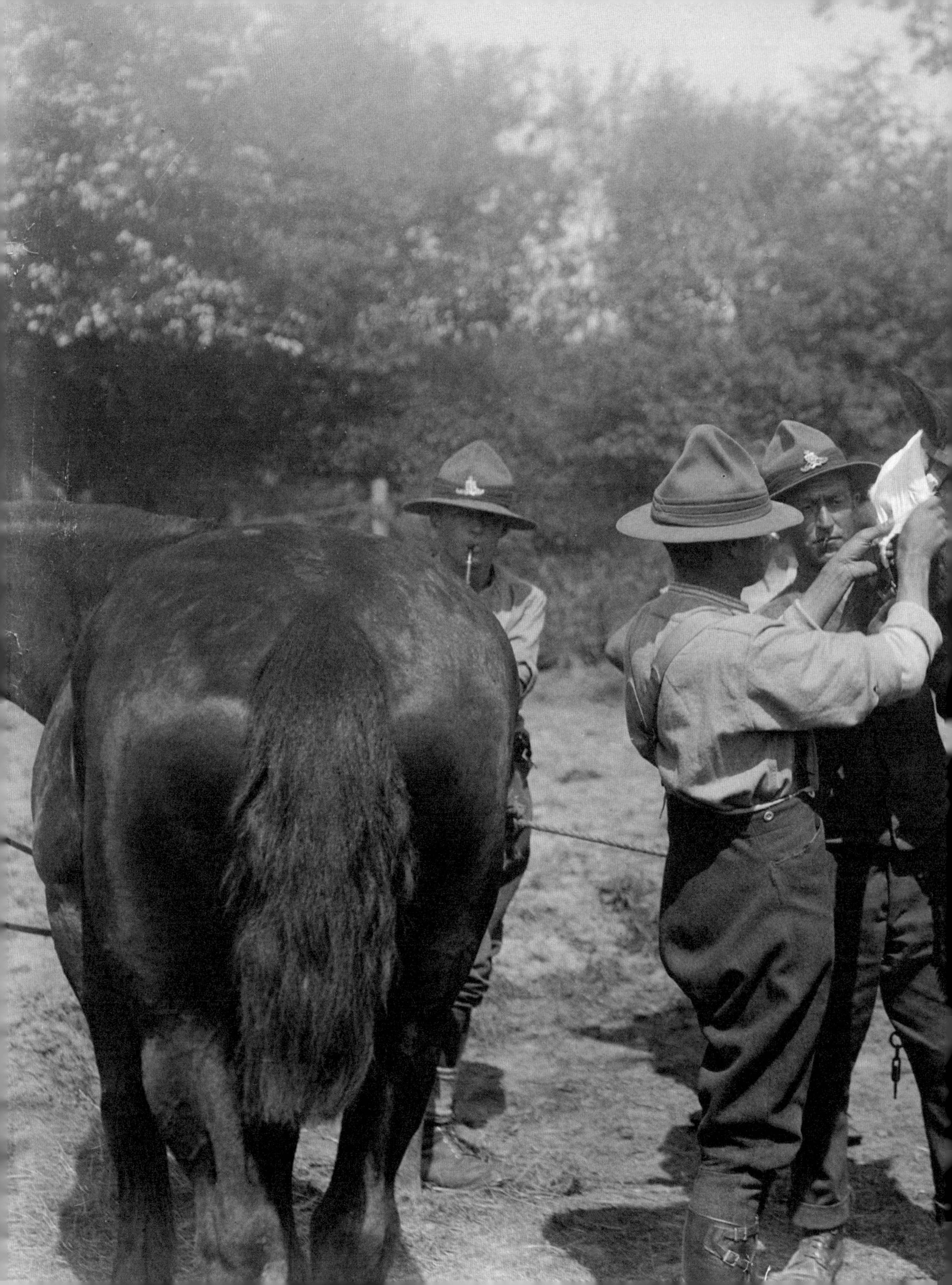

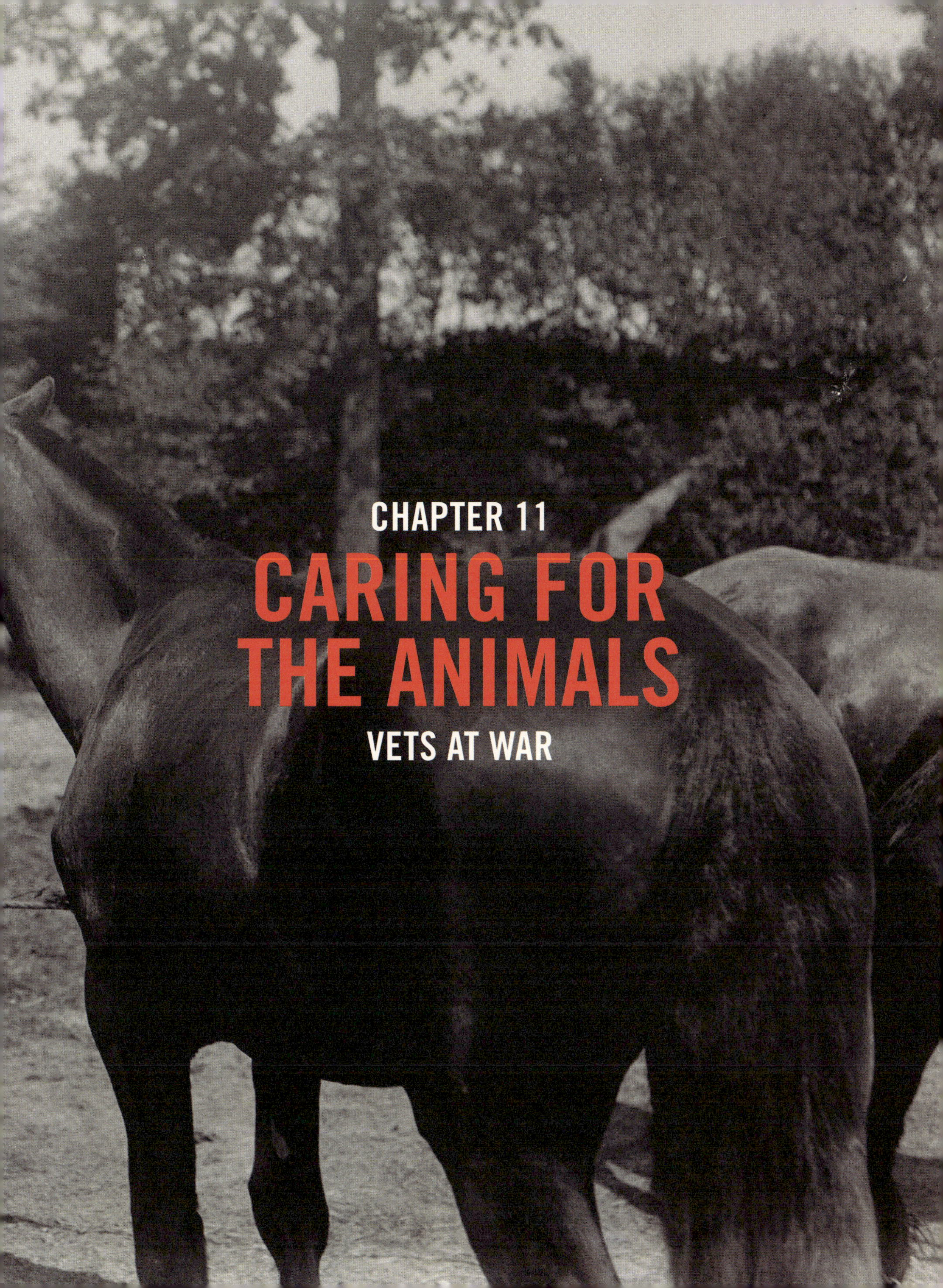

CHAPTER 11

CARING FOR THE ANIMALS

VETS AT WAR

previous pages
Vets were an essential part of New Zealand's medical military establishment. Here, on 22 May 1918 at Louvencourt in France, two members of the New Zealand Veterinary Corps bandage a horse's eye. ALEXANDER TURNBULL LIBRARY, 1/2-013211-G

In four years of war a wonderful improvement has been effected in the various services without which no army is complete. The Veterinary Service is a striking example in this connection.

— 'Taini', *The Kia Ora Coo-ee*

New Zealand sent around 10,000 horses to the First World War.[1] On the Western Front draught horses pulled heavy artillery guns and supply and ambulance wagons; pack horses bore machine guns, ammunition and other supplies. In the Sinai–Palestine campaign horses carried the men of the Mounted Rifles through the sand and heat. Other animals played their part — the indispensable mules and donkeys on Gallipoli, in France and in the Middle East, and, also in the desert, the equally essential camels. Like their human counterparts, these creatures suffered in harsh weather, fell ill, sustained injuries and were wounded or killed.[2] Caring for them were the members of the New Zealand Veterinary Corps (NZVC) — veterinarians, farriers, blacksmiths, saddlers, horse-holders, dispensers — and the men who rode and worked the horses as troopers or drivers.

The corps had been gazetted on 8 February 1906, but despite the appointment of principal veterinary officers (PVOs) in the various districts, and of Lieutenant-Colonel Charles Reakes as director-general and chief veterinarian, by June 1914 it was short of qualified veterinary surgeons.[3] Camps had revealed that there was still 'considerable scope for improvement in the quality of horses' — and in the skills of some troopers. When war broke out, Major Alexander Young, PVO for Wellington, became assistant director of veterinary services and Reakes, now a full colonel, director of veterinary services and remounts (replacement horses). The corps had 23 'active service personnel'.[4]

But not everyone, however keen, could serve overseas. Some had to stay at home to purchase remounts, supervise horse accommodation on the transports carrying the Main Body to war, provide veterinary equipment and train personnel. The NZVC required more than vets at the front. Reakes advertised for blacksmiths, farriers and saddlers: only those who 'proved to be good workmen, steady, and of good character will be accepted'.[5]

A call went out for some 3000 horses and the nation responded enthusiastically. Farmers sold 9347 animals to the government and gifted 1437.[6] Some who had only one suitable horse were happy to give it up; others clubbed together to present a horse. Saddlery, which included saddles, bridles, leather head-stalls, head ropes and horse-covers, had to be 'of a large, strong type, and . . . in thoroughly good order in every way'. Forage was welcome too, though it 'must necessarily be of first-class quality and delivered at the nearest railway station'.[7] Horse-buying was carried out by Department of Agriculture stock inspectors, helped by veterinary surgeons in private practice and the New Zealand Farmers' Union. Any horses with 'the slightest signs of unsoundness' were rejected.[8]

During the war, both on the Western Front and in the Middle East, horse shows and competitions would help to maintain horse quality and care. After a 1916 contest in France, a British officer told Reakes that the New Zealand animals 'were greatly admired' and that 'there were none better in the Army'.[9] There was praise from others, too, though when Eric Catchpole of the Auckland Mounted Rifles arrived in Egypt in December 1914 he thought the Australians had 'a much better class of mounts . . . big lumps of horses more like general utility sorts, and in the best of condition, too'. Carbery, however, considered the 53 heavy and light draught and riding horses brought from New Zealand with the field ambulance 'a good lot and in fine condition'.[10]

Thanks to the Manawatu Agricultural and Pastoral Association,[11] in August 1914 the Palmerston North Showgrounds became a 'concentration camp' where horses arrived at all hours by rail and road. Later the numbers were reduced as animals were sent to Awapuni and other camps, grazed nearby or dispatched to the official Remount Depot established at Upper Hutt in October 1914, handy to the station. At one point, the depot was home to 1000 horses, with about 100 men caring for them, and the lines covered more than 15 acres. The horses were classified for artillery work (pulling gun wagons), as pack animals or as troopers' mounts, and had identification marks branded on their hooves. Each animal's details were entered into a ledger and its progress was tracked. A field hospital at the depot, organised by Captain Harry Reid and run by a veterinary surgeon, dealt with minor problems such as kicks and colds, while more serious issues were handled at the nearby Wallaceville Veterinary Laboratory.[12]

Initially there were some problems in the camps. Unused to being tied up alongside so many other unfamiliar animals, the horses were inclined to kick, and many injuries resulted. Some bit through their halters and got loose, causing several accidents. Leather head-stalls, with light chains to secure the animals to the picket-lines, improved this situation; these would also be used on the transports. There were outbreaks of both strangles, an acute and potentially fatal bacterial condition, and ringworm, which was troublesome rather than dangerous, but very few horses died.[13] In the opinion of future Auckland Mounted Rifles historian Charles Nicol, the AMR horses based at Epsom before the Main Body sailed in October 1914 still had 'a look of roughness about [them], and they were anything but uniform in stamp. Quite a number . . . seemed to have been badly broken, if broken at all.'[14] A lack of shipping meant that, after late 1916, when the final 455 horses reached Egypt, New Zealand stopped sending remounts overseas. From then on, replacements came from imperial depots, which held British, French, American and Argentinian horses, among others.[15]

The horses soon became accustomed to their military life and, because they stayed in camp through draft after draft of new recruits, 'already knew the drill before the men saddled them up'.[16] When future gunner Geoffrey Wild reached Featherston camp in mid-1917, he found the horses 'as quiet as could be, far more familiar with the routine of "stables" and the parade ground than we were'. The animals were certainly well cared for — 'bedded down on straw laid on concrete, fed in mangers on the universal chaff and hay', watered each morning while their bedding 'was forked over and soiled material removed', fed and watered at noon and in the evening, and exercised and groomed daily.[17] Men learnt their new roles, whether as artillerymen, like Wild, dealing with horses and wagons and limbers, or as mounted riflemen, rehearsing their drill manoeuvres on foot before repeating them on horseback.[18]

The first New Zealand horses sent overseas were the 25 that accompanied the Advance Party of the NZEF to Samoa in August 1914. No veterinary officer was included; troops cared for the horses. Most were ridden by officers and men, including the Mounted Patrol, but some pulled wheeled vehicles and served as pack animals for the machine-gunners.[19] It soon became clear, however, as CO Robert Logan wrote on 7 July 1915, that 'few of them are really fit for their work'. A specially convened board had found six horses 'unsuitable for patrol work in this Island, where the journeys are long and the tracks are steep and rough'. Five would be sold at public auction and one shot.[20] Such boards were held regularly during the occupation and several horses were sold or destroyed. Occasional deaths were conscientiously investigated. Local animals did not make adequate replacements.

With 30 horses sent to Samoa in August 1915 went Corporal Nicholas Winders and three other NZVC men. Winders was frank in his brief report: 'In the first place they are too old to climatise and . . . they are the wrong stamp. A smaller and thicker horse would be more suitable for the work.' On 17 September Logan asked for 66 horses, plus equipment, which arrived in three loads, in October, November and December. NZVC Captain Alexander Brodie and two farriers sailed on the final trip. As well as writing a full report, Brodie was to 'make a thorough inspection of all horses, saddlery, and harness, . . . do any Veterinary work . . . make the best arrangements you can, with the men available, for the general care of the horses . . . and generally do all you can to assist the O.C. in all matters coming within the duties of the Veterinary Corps'.[21]

Brodie more than proved his worth. His suggestions greatly improved the horses' health, and he both served on the boards and acted as auctioneer when animals were sold. He also wrote an impressive 22-page report, including photos, covering everything from climatic conditions, water supply, site of horse lines and problems with the work of local farriers ('abominable') to the individual condition of the animals and difficulties with fodder, plus recommendations for building shelters. It had already been realised that a veterinary hospital was needed, and one was opened on Boxing Day 1915 at Vaimea. Brodie found the Samoa horses to be 'remarkably free of disease'.[22]

In response to a request from Logan, another 20 horses were sent to Samoa in September 1916, and a further 20 in November under the care of Brodie, who was returning for a second inspection. The number of horses in Samoa remained around 100 for most of the war: in November 1918 there were 108.[23] When the post-war Samoa garrison force returned to New Zealand from late 1919, they bequeathed their 90-odd horses to the constabulary force that replaced them. Because the animals were by then in poor condition, and owing to strict New Zealand quarantine rules, they were auctioned locally, along with their gear.

Getting the horses to Egypt with the Main Body in October/November 1914 was not easy. Fitting out the vessels was the first challenge. A Wellington reporter permitted to go aboard the *Orari*, which carried 728 horses, considered the arrangements for the animals 'as nearly perfect as human ingenuity could make them'. The horses were placed in 'strong, but narrow, stalls on each side of the boat and a double line running down the centre on the top, second and lower decks, with great feed bins at intervals, stout chains being fixed on each side of the head stalls and attached to rings in the posts, making the divisions between them, thus rendering it impossible for the animals to bite each other'. He had to admit, however, that 'The men at least can lie down in fairly comfortable beds, but not so their four-footed mates'.[24] Godley, himself a horse lover, considered that 'all concerned did their best to ensure that the right thing was done in fitting out ships for the carriage of horses', and that this was reflected in the low mortality among the animals transported overseas.[25] Both he and Reakes cited a figure of 3 per cent. Of the 3817 horses that travelled with the Main Body, 78 (2 per cent) died at sea. This modest number spoke 'volumes for the care and devotion of the men'.[26]

When the NZEF left on 16 October, Young, in overall charge as ADVS, travelled with headquarters staff on the *Maunganui* and an NZVC vet sailed on each of the other transports, with the units to which they were attached. As dentist Arthur Logan discovered, on the *Orari*, 'a horse-boat in the full sense of the word', non-veterinary personnel were expected to help with the animals.

> It fell to the lot of a mere sprinkling of officers and men, including the padre and myself, to do all the feeding out, watering and mucking out necessary . . . On the boat deck to which I was attached there were only three of us . . . to minister to the needs of the several hundred horses stalled there. It was hard work cleaning out the stalls and emptying the refuse through a big hole in the centre of the ship. Incidentally there were a few narrow escapes from kicks, the horses being restless and excited with the rolling of the ship.

Logan even had the 'the unique experience of extracting a tooth for one [horse] at the request of the vet'.[27] This would not be the only occasion on which a medic helped an animal. On Gallipoli in May 1915 NZMC Major Arthur Purchas, watching 14 dead mules and a horse being dragged onto the beach, said, 'You see that brown horse; I removed its eye three days ago and it was doing well. Yesterday it was hit again and died.' The following month Percival Fenwick noted in his diary: 'One poor mule got a piece of . . . shell below the eye. I tried to bandage it, but it would not stand, so I had [to] let it die.'[28]

On the cramped *Waimana*, with 496 horses aboard, the Auckland Mounted Riflemen also had to watch the animals' legs, 'which were very liable to swell owing to the constant standing. Frequent rubbing and hosing with salt water was carried out with wonderful results.' Captain Thomas Blake, who 'lost a remarkably small percentage of horses . . . gained a name for professional zeal by commandeering some of the windsails which were supplying a little ventilation to the suffocating quarters of the men . . . and leading them to the horse stalls on the deck above'.[29]

Thanks to the hard work of Major Peter Edgar and his assistants, only 17 horses on the *Orari* had to be destroyed during the voyage. That sad task fell to Tiny Emerson of the British Army Reserve, who 'would walk up to his victim, point his revolver at a spot in the centre of the forehead, pull the trigger and nonchalantly walk away. There was never any doubt about instant and painless death. The animal just dropped in its tracks.'[30] Such executions did not always go smoothly. On the *Ruapehu*, Trooper William Pyle reported on 14 November, 'Another horse bad today. Our veterinary luminaries engaged it with a revolver & left it for dead with a sack over it. Shortly after they came to heave it overboard and the poor brute was standing up.'[31]

Logan became fascinated by his equine shipmates. 'Every day as feed-time approached they would begin to stamp their feet, it was as good as clock work for the whole ships company. At night time, if orders should come, as sometimes happened, for all lights to be turned off, they would get into a frantic state and would shiver and neigh with terror until they were turned on again.'[32] Before they were fed, the horses were watered, 'taps having been placed at points along the lines. The utter helplessness of the animals makes the men especially careful in their duties and not a single horse is ever missed.'[33] Quality could be a problem. The rolling of the *Waihora* in February 1916 'stirred up the rust in the tanks giving the water the colour and thickness of pea soup. On Tuesday it was particularly bad and several cases of colic made their appearance.'[34] Mucking out was an all-day job: 'In each line of horses they'd have one stall empty. They'd shift a horse along, that stall would be cleaned out, and he'd be shifted along one. You could only do one horse at a time.'[35]

Horses and humans did not always cohabit happily at sea. On the *Maunganui* on 11 November 1914, NZMC Captain Alexander Trotter had 'been sleeping on deck lately as cabins even with port holes open and fans going are rather thick with concentrated essence of horse, superheated'. When Trooper Alfred Philps travelled from Wellington to Hobart with the Second Reinforcements in December 1914, he and his companions were strapped into tiered bunks amidships. 'The bulkhead doors were open at both ends and there were 250 horses at each end of us. Every time the ship tossed all the horse manure and everything else came under the bulkhead and under our bunks and out the other door.'[36]

Norman Hassell of the Field Artillery had a similar experience on the *Knight Templar* the following April. 'The awful stench which arose from these 400 horses beneath us was terrible at times . . . The manure . . . had to be packed in baskets and carried up to the next deck where it could be tipped overboard. This was done night and morning but in the interval it would simply wash about in the stable urine which had no proper outlet.'[37]

Hassell's description of the horses' situation on his ship contrasted sharply with the Wellington journalist's resolutely positive 1914 account:

> Each horse was enclosed in a space just big enough for him to stand in, with a rail at his chest, one at his rump and one on each flank. The rolling motion of the ship caused these poor brutes to sway backwards and forwards unceasingly and in a very short while each poor animal had huge sores on its chest and rump from this continual chafing. To keep them from getting down in their misery each one had a broad belt slung under its belly and suspended from two hooks fastened into the cross-beams above.[38]

Although the animals were rested and exercised at ports along the way while the vessels were being coaled — MO William McAra described the 'Great sight of 40–60 horses rolling in sand' at Albany, 'hard to tear them away'[39] — the journey was long, uncomfortable and restrictive.

Also on the *Knight Templar* in 1915 was John Wintle, a farrier with the Auckland Mounted Rifles. In the 'exceedingly hot' weather, some horses 'simply fell in their stalls, and died in a few minutes'. There were only Major Thomas Lilico of the NZVC, his orderly and Wintle to look after sick animals. 'I think I will soon qualify for a veterinary surgeon. It is a great experience treating the different cases.'[40] As Hassell recalled, despite the men's 'unceasing care and attention', 23 horses died during the six-week voyage. Their condition on arrival was also telling:

> [W]hen we came to [disembark] we found that very few of the horses could walk. Considering that the poor brutes had been penned up for over six weeks without being able to move an inch even, this was not surprising . . . [On] the broad gangway they simply fell down on their fore-legs or noses, and more often than not brought their man down with them. Several of them jumped or fell into the water, and we had to salvage them by the aid of a rowing boat and long tow rope, but even they were all landed safely.[41]

Arrival in Egypt at the beginning of December 1914 was a relief for both the men and the horses of the Main Body. As Nicol noticed, the animals that had experienced 'more airy quarters', such as those on the *Star of India*, were 'well-conditioned and glossy coated', whereas some from the *Waimana* 'had lost their hair in patches through constant sweating'. Once ashore, the horses revelled in their new-found freedom: William Pyle's 'played up sure, as soon as he felt his feet on dry land'.[42] The animals could not be ridden immediately, but required three weeks of exercising and rehabilitation. On 4 December, they were taken out into the desert where 'they absolutely took the upper hand kicking about and rolling like a crowd of lambs. One man was kicked in the stomach and was collapsed for a few minutes; another had a cut on the head, but in the long run we arrived at a high iron picket fence round the race course where we tied the horses up and gave them nosebags.' But then some camels appeared

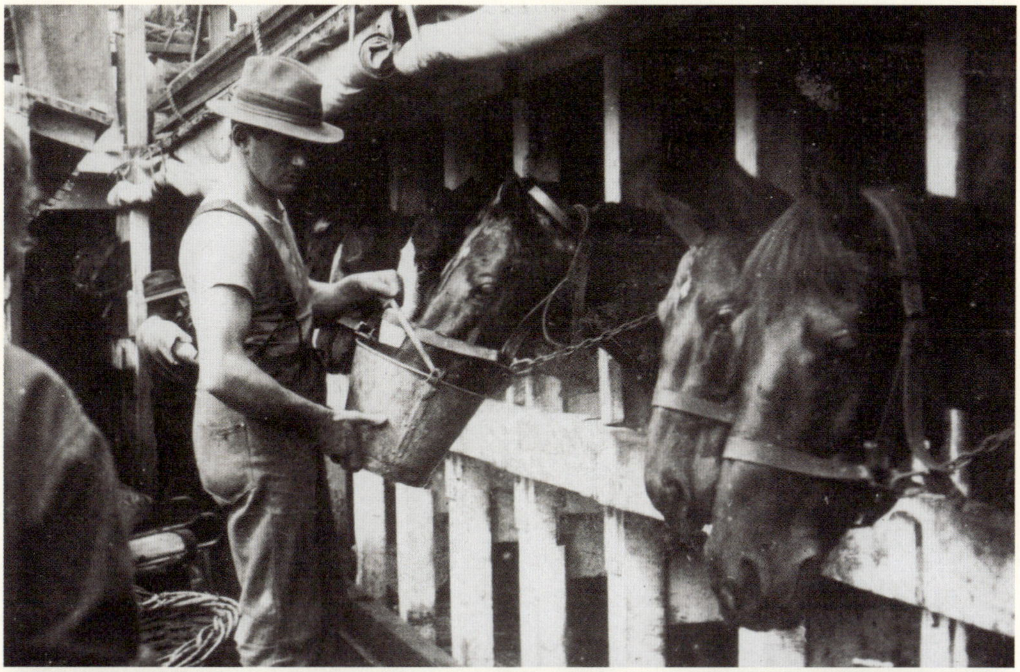

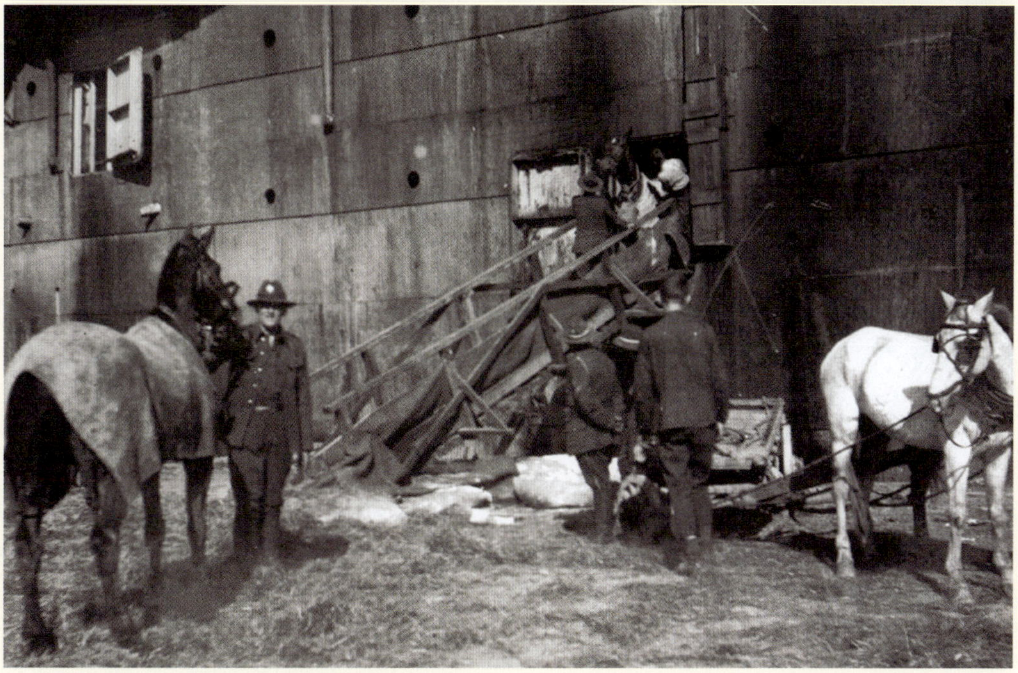

above Sergeant Murphy feeding the horses on board the transport *Knight Templar*, which left New Zealand for Egypt in April 1915. The cramped conditions and securing chains can be clearly seen. Despite the care of men like Murphy, 23 horses died during the voyage. ALEXANDER TURNBULL LIBRARY, A1-O-862-02-5

below After so many cramped weeks on a ship, standing on solid ground once more in Egypt was a huge relief for the horses. Here animals are being unloaded from the *Waimana*. NATIONAL ARMY MUSEUM, 2001.1058

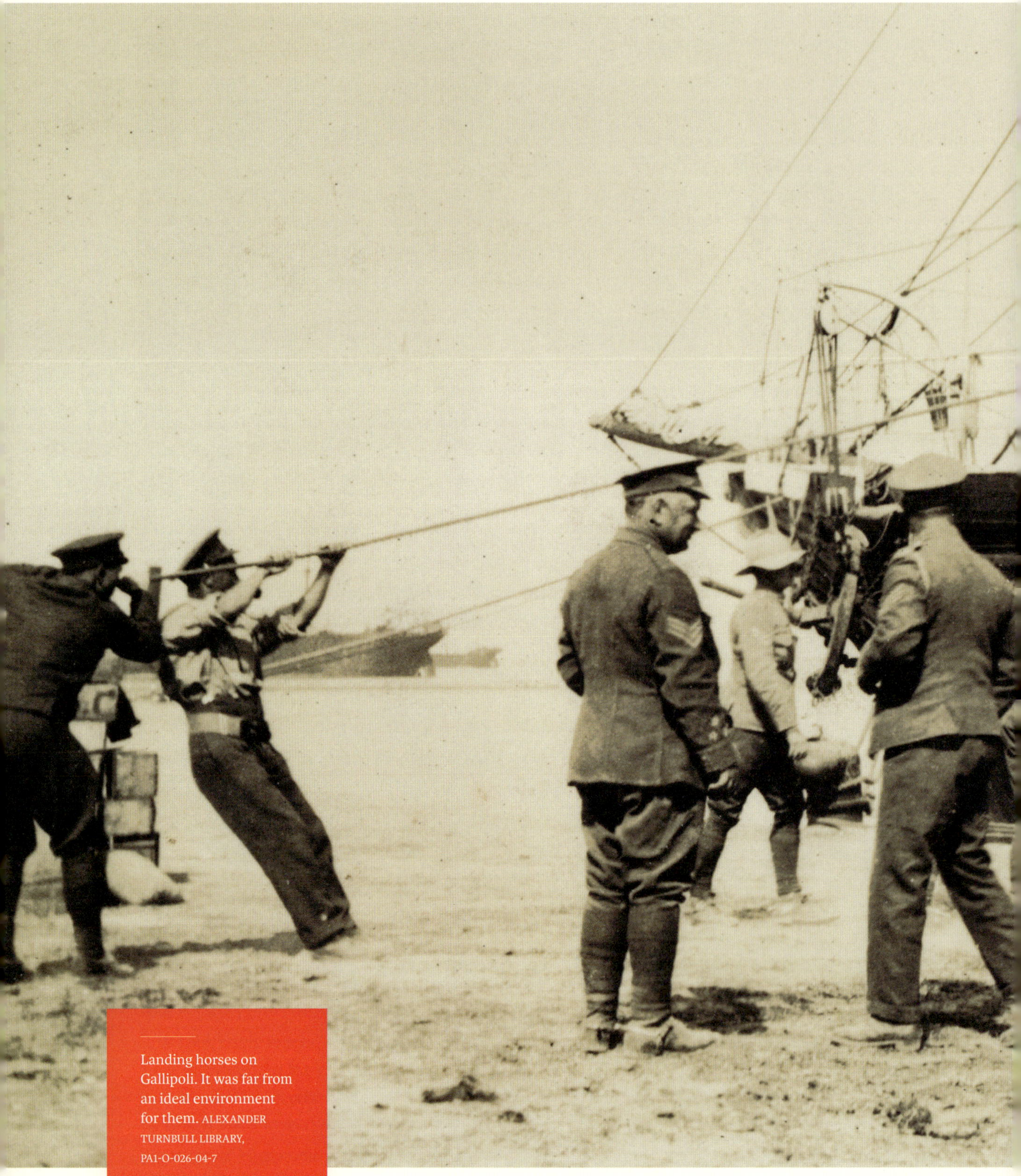

Landing horses on Gallipoli. It was far from an ideal environment for them. ALEXANDER TURNBULL LIBRARY, PA1-O-026-04-7

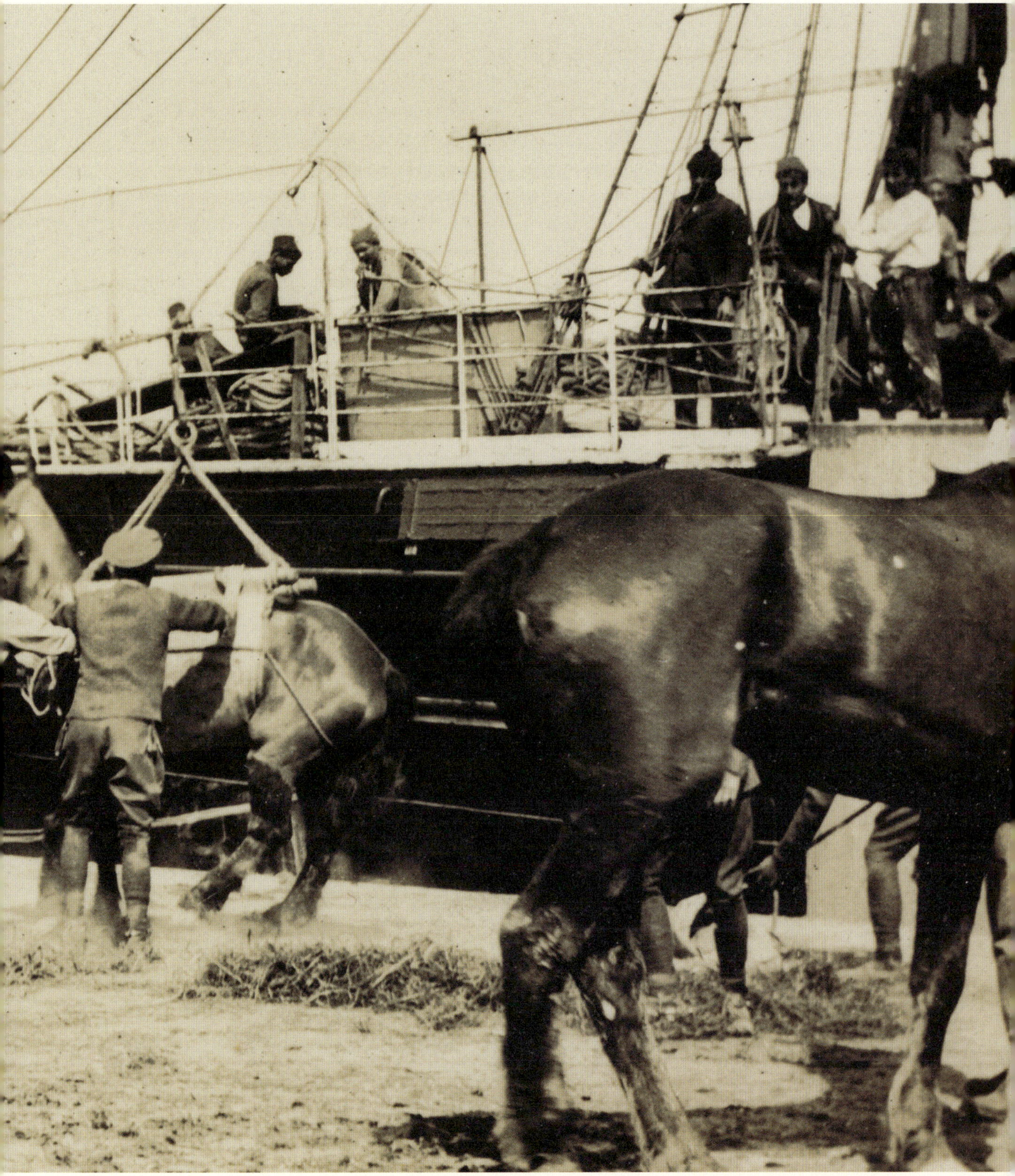

'and there was pandemonium. Horses in all directions.' Apart from the oppressive heat, the horses had to cope with the terrible irritation of the ubiquitous flies. The initial stables, made from rush matting, failed to provide sufficient protection from the sun and had to be rebuilt with wood from the stalls on the transports. A veterinary hospital was also erected.[43]

The NZVC officers, under Major Alexander Young, 'had to make the best shift that they could' in Alexandria, including dealing with 'the tricks of some Egyptian dealers in forage'.[44] After about a week, Eric Catchpole noted that the horses 'could do with some green stuff. Then again, chaff is getting short, and we have been using tibbin . . . it is rice straw just as it is left after threshing, . . . very coarse and dry, and it is almost impossible to mix the oats and bran with it. The bran we are using is some German stuff from a boat which was caught in Alexandria when war was declared.'[45] One soldier remarked that the 'Egyptian fodder . . . is not nearly so good as the feed from New Zealand', but Lilico recalled 'plenty of green feed in Egypt', including locally grown barley and maize.[46] Food would also prove a problem in the Sinai and Palestine. Trooper Bill Owers remembered broken straw mixed with a handful of barley — green food was 'like giving them a dose of medicine'. The Indian hay issued in July 1917 was so poor that the horses refused to eat it.[47]

Most mounted men formed close bonds with their animals, grooming and caring for them assiduously, and were devastated when they had to be taken away or shot because of sickness or injury. 'The poor old chap, my best friend, my companion through many trials and dangers, my good omen and mascot,' wrote Trooper Frederick Foote. 'He was a very sick animal, he had foundered was the Vet's diagnosis. I do not know what happened to him other than that he was sent back to base.'[48] Sergeant Garioch Clunie mourned his loss: 'Poor little chap was hit in one of the recent attacks out here and they destroyed him in Mobile [Veterinary Section]. It's rotten luck . . . and I don't think I am likely to get another one like him for he was the best little pony in this Squadron.'[49] A hospitalised horse could be replaced by a possibly inferior non-New Zealand animal. Foote 'was left with a tiny little remount, game as a mountain goat, but far too small for my weight and signal gear etc'. In the view of Captain Hubert Hatrick of the Auckland Mounted Rifles, 'New Zealand & Australian horses are without a doubt miles better than the Home animals.'[50]

More NZVC personnel, officers and other ranks set sail from New Zealand with the Second Reinforcements on 14 December 1914, arriving in Egypt on 28 January 1915. There were two mobile sections, headed by Captains Charles Simpson and William Smith (to support the mounted brigade), and two veterinary hospital sections, commanded by Captains Daniel Machattie and Donald Rait (one for the infantry and one for the artillery). Each hospital could treat about 250 horses. After receiving their uniforms and basic military training at Trentham, the NZVC farriers, smiths and drivers, many recruited from farms throughout New Zealand, had been trained at the nearby Remount Depot. Like the troops, the horses attended a daily sick parade. Supervised by a veterinary officer, the NZVC men could deal with minor injuries and ailments, but seriously ill or hurt animals were sent away for treatment at hospitals or convalescent depots.[51] The NZVC worked hard at Zeitoun camp, where a six-week influenza epidemic affected almost all of the 5000 horses and killed some 75. Ringworm was also widespread.[52]

'No horses whatever,' wrote Herbert Hart a few days before the Gallipoli landing, '— except those hauling the guns — will disembark for several days after us, it being hoped that we will then have secured enough country to render the landing of the transport and horses possible.'[53] But the peninsula, with its lack of water and difficult terrain, was not suited to horses. Most of the draught animals taken to the Dardanelles were either not landed at all or, before long, returned to Egypt.[54] The big creatures could not drag the heavy guns up the steep slopes — the men did this punishing work — and the mounted troops fought without their horses. 'We are off to the Dardanelles as infantry some time this week,' wrote Pyle on 17 May. 'We are going to leave our horses here. I'll be sorry to see the last of my nag. He is looking very fit just now. Its hard luck after all the months of looking after them to abandon them, but it appears they would be of no use over there.'[55] More artillery horses were landed later.

On 6 May Lieutenant Thomas Ritchie of the NZMC noted that 'No 3 Battery NZFA [New Zealand Field Artillery] went ashore yesterday. The weather was very rough, but they managed to land their horses & guns safely.'[56] The occupation of less challenging terrain made it possible for 5 Battery to take all its horses when it arrived in August. Although more heavy guns, pulled by the horses, were used, by the time of the December evacuation all but three of the gun teams had gone back to Egypt.[57] The last horses departed with the men and their guns when the peninsula was abandoned. As Hart recorded on 15 December, some animals were killed. 'Today the artillery horses were shot. One despatch rider who gallops along the beach daily from Chailak Dere to Walker's Ridge went into hysteria when he was informed that his horse, which had been wounded under him three times, had to be destroyed in that manner.'[58]

There was a veterinary presence on Gallipoli. Alexander Young sailed to the peninsula with other headquarters staff on the *Lutzow*. Major Charles Neale, who had served in South Africa, was the first New Zealand veterinary officer to arrive, attached to the ASC. When he returned to Egypt on 20 August 1915, having been mentioned in despatches for his work, he was relieved by James Stafford, who remained on the peninsula until the evacuation.[59]

The animals that did play a vital part in the Gallipoli campaign were mules and donkeys, which carried water and ammunition — both in small carts and on their backs — and sometimes wounded men. Driver Alfred Stratton encountered many horses and mules during the war, but it was the latter he remembered. 'The mules were all real characters; they were strong, tough, agile, easy to ride, fast walkers, they would eat almost anything and they were alive to all that was going on . . . Yes, the mules took things very calmly.'[60]

The New Zealanders had first encountered large numbers of mules and donkeys in Egypt, and were often appalled to see these creatures, and 'squibs of ponies', pulling top-heavy carts about twelve times their size. 'The mules are the staunchest and most patient beasts I have ever seen,' Eric Catchpole decided, 'and will lay right down to it and pull every time they are asked; it's an absolute outrage the way they are overloaded.' One soldier marvelled that a 'tiny wee donkey pulled 23 bags of donkey chaff . . . each of which weighs 160lb, through the heavy sand . . . a distance of 200 yards, without a single stop'.[61] Although mules could exhibit the stubbornness for which they were legendary, overwhelmingly they were admired for their stamina and stoic service. They also proved invaluable in the Sinai and Palestine.

The mules on Gallipoli were handled by muleteers belonging to the Supply and Transport Corps of the Indian Army. Four mule cart corps, each consisting of some 650 men and almost 2000 mules, originally landed on the peninsula, and more animals arrived in May.[62] As historian Peter Stanley has pointed out, 'the entire invasion force had reason to see their presence as a stroke of luck'. They carried stores, ammunition and water to gun positions, often at night to avoid being shelled, and transported mail.[63] The Indians established their mule lines below Walker's Ridge in what soon became known as Mule Gully, and men and animals worked tirelessly. William Rusden of the Auckland Infantry Battalion saw 'Boxes, tins of water and ammunition . . . strapped on to a hardy little mule and every half hour or so, away they would go, each mule with an Indian bound for the trenches'.[64] It was a dangerous business. 'The number of dead mules on the beach is very large,' Percival Fenwick wrote on 9 May. 'The pinnace tows them off in eights or tens and then sinks them a mile from shore.'[65] Hundreds of mules perished, as did their brave drivers. At Suvla, 11 mules and 15 men were killed in one day when a shell hit the mule lines, and not long afterwards, 225 of a group of 350 animals died within three days.[66]

Donkeys played their part, too. In May ambulance man John Thomson reported that 'A few donkeys are being used for those who can sit on them comfortably'. Charles Begg and his medics had 'managed to capture a dozen little donkeys from the Turks, and most leg wounds come down riding the donkeys. They often ride right . . . alongside the operating table.'[67]

'Coming back to Zeitoun had a home like feeling and we were over-joyed to get our horses back, we loved the creatures and they in their turn gave us a great feeling of security.'[68] Frederick Foote's pleasure at being reunited with his horse after Gallipoli was shared by Godley: 'One of the greatest joys being back here, is to be able once more to gallop about in the desert on my good New Zealand horse.'[69] The troopers of the New Zealand Mounted Brigade fought in the Sinai and later Palestine, and there were also changes in the NZVC. When Young went to France with the division in April 1916, Stafford took charge in Egypt. No. 2 Mobile Veterinary Section became a hospital at Bir-el-Mala, on the eastern side of the Suez Canal, with Machattie in charge. The staff there went to great lengths to avoid sending quality New Zealand animals back to the base, since once they were 'merged in the mass of horses it was usually a case of good-bye'.[70]

The mounteds found that their charges 'had been well fed and under exercised', which made them excitable and sometimes very tricky to mount. 'The horses did not know the camp and were inclined to bolt in directions that were embarrassing.' Most, however, took off and 'ran their energy down' in the desert. A routine was soon re-established, and the training was tough. 'We rode many miles day after day,' Foote recalled, 'galloping into mock action and handing over to horse handlers to take the horses back, and practising again galloping in to pick their riders up. All in the hot sun with equipment on the saddles and rifles and ammunition . . . The horses knew the orders as well as we did.'[71] Mounted riflemen dismounted to fight. Four

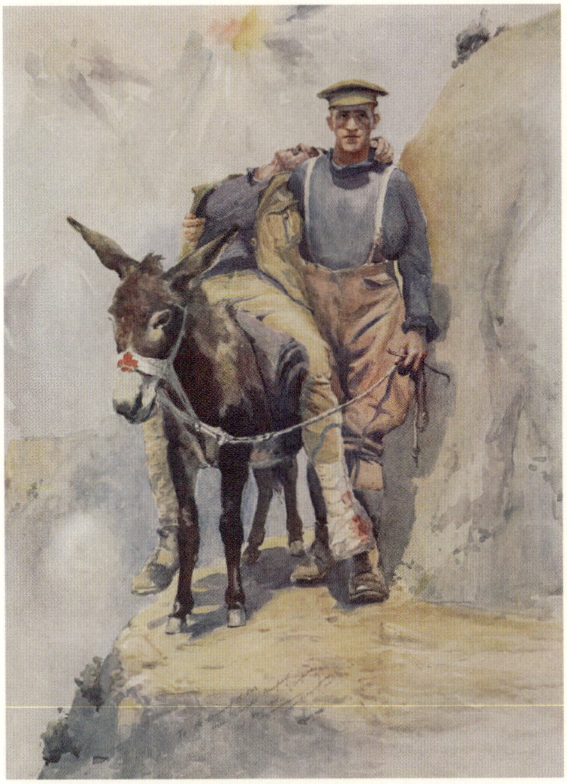

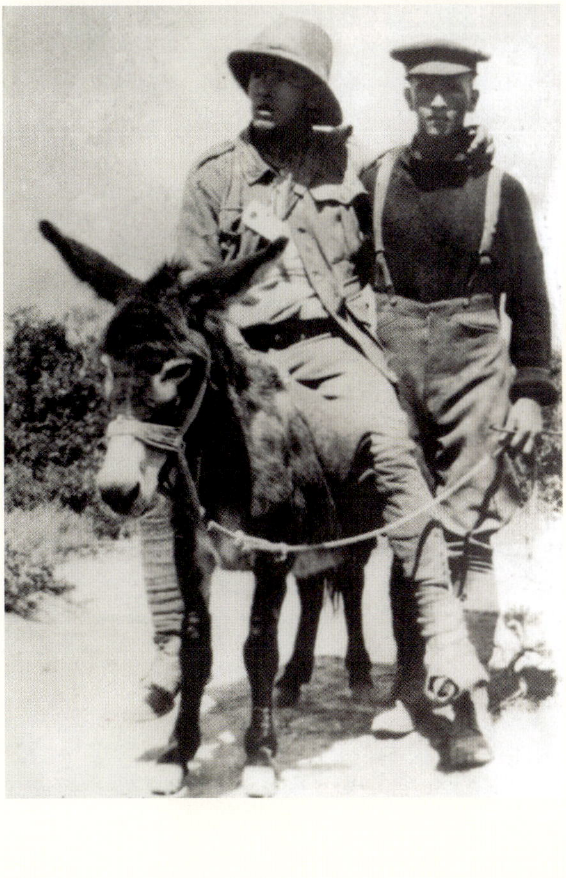

One of the most famous images of the First World War, *Private Simpson, D.C.M., & his Donkey at Anzac*, was painted by Horace Moore-Jones in 1918. The photograph he used, however, was not of Australian stretcher-bearer Private John Simpson Kirkpatrick who, with his donkey, was renowned for his work in carrying the wounded on the peninsula. The model was actually New Zealand stretcher-bearer Richard (Dick) Henderson. After being badly gassed on the Western Front in 1917, Henderson was invalided home in February 1918. There are several versions of Moore-Jones' painting. ALEXANDER TURNBULL LIBRARY, C-057-002 [PAINTING]; NATIONAL ARMY MUSEUM, 1992.760 [PHOTO]

men would ride to the front line, where the horse holder remained with the horses while the other three troopers went forward.

The desert was a harsh place for both men and animals. 'Sand,' Foote wrote, 'was the greatest enemy of the horse. It did not pass through him, but settled in the lower part of the stomach. When this sand gave trouble [a complaint known as sand colic], medicine would relieve the problem temporally, but after a year or so horses were liable to become debilitated and sent to base.'[72] Late in November 1915, a post-mortem on a senior officer's horse 'disclosed sand in its stomach weighing 70lb. Though this was an exceptional case it was . . . quite a common occurrence.' Bill Owers remembered having to muzzle the horses and wondered if they craved the salt in the sand. Bites from flies caused sores at the corners of the animals' mouths and eyes — fringes were attached to their heads to protect the latter — and the insects also retarded the healing of cuts and wounds.[73]

Water was a constant preoccupation. In Palestine, James Rudd of the Canterbury Mounted Rifles 'used to pour a little water in my hand and my horse would just lick and lick as long as I held my hand out. Sometimes we used to sit under our horses bellies to get a little shade.' The horses could be without water for days; dehydration was sometimes fatal. Despite their thirst, the animals remained alert to bad water. One group of troopers, after riding all day, 'arrived at an old well & immediately drew water up . . . & just drank & drank', but the horses would not do so. When the men drew water again the next morning, 'it was dreadful . . . then we realised why our horses would not drink . . . their instinct was better than ours.'[74]

Sickness, injury and death, especially from the sky, were ever-present threats. 'The greatest enemy of the horse is probably aircraft,' wrote 'Taini' in *The Kia Ora Coo-ee*, the magazine for the Australians and New Zealanders in the Middle East. 'Could our dumb friends speak, they would surely wax eloquent upon the manifold inequities of enemy aircraft . . . hurling death and destruction from the skies at unoffending horses.' When he was acting as a horse holder, Owers worried about aeroplanes 'because they always went for the horses — they were the best target'. In the second Battle of Gaza in April 1917, waiting horses, standing in the open, were constantly bombed and shelled: of the 2000 or so mounted brigade horses, over 100 were killed and some 300 wounded.[75] There was often no need for burial: 'The jackals which scour the desert at night in thousands soon make short work of any dead bodies — human or animals.'[76] When a mule with a broken leg had to be shot in August 1917, its carcass was dragged out into the desert; next morning only clean bones remained. Larger animals seem to have been a different matter. Charles Malone of the Imperial Camel Corps reported burying camels in December 1917 and early January 1918.[77]

The first Battle of Gaza in February 1917 had been even harder on the horses. At one point they went for 72 hours without water and, until some chaff was found, had only barley to eat. The result was diarrhoea and deaths. Anthrax made a brief appearance in the hellish Jordan Valley in the opening months of 1918 but was promptly dealt with and only three horses died. There were more deaths later — some 150 altogether, including 28 on one day — from poison thought to be 'tablets of strychnine, arsenic, and other medical materials mixed accidentally or designedly with barley abandoned by the Turks on the roadside'. The troopers had picked this up and fed it to their horses.[78] Snake bite, potentially fatal, was another peril in the Jordan Valley, as were mosquitoes. 'I've seen the horses tethered there, and the only way they could get rid of the mosquito[es] would be to throw themselves on the ground.'[79]

Like many of the New Zealanders, Beet Algar of 15 Camel Corps initially thought camels were 'terrible things', but he came to regard them as 'marvellous animals'.[80] Perfectly adapted to their environment, they could carry impressive quantities of water, equipment and rations, and also transported both wounded soldiers and the men of the Imperial Camel Corps (ICC); the linesmen of the signallers' troop rode camels to reach communication lines in need of repair. Founded early in 1916 to fight the Senussi, an Egyptian Islamist group backed by the Ottoman Turks, and originally manned by Australians, the ICC was expanded in March 1916 and then, in December, reorganised as a brigade of three, later four, battalions. At this point two New Zealand camel companies, 15 and 16 Camel Corps, joined the ICC, which now also included British troops.[81] Each company had a veterinary sergeant in its headquarters group. In 1917 and 1918 between 400 and 500 New Zealand men fought in the Sinai and Palestine as members of the ICC; 41 died. Like the troopers, the cameliers dismounted to fight. Horsemen were not always convinced about camels. 'For patrol work they may be better,' Hatrick decided, 'but give me a good old horse for all round work.'[82]

The NZVC had to extend its skills to deal with these unfamiliar animals. A camel remount depot and hospital were established beside the cameliers' training depot at Abbassia, just outside Cairo. One common complaint was the skin condition called mange, caused by mites, which, if not dealt with, could 'destroy a camel force in the field in from three to six months'.[83] By the end of 1917, after weeks covering long distances on minimal food and with their saddles left on for days at a time, the camels were exhausted and suffering badly from mange. Cold, wet weather did not help. Veterinary treatment at Rafa was ordered, but on the journey south many of the already weakened camels sank up to their fetlocks in the waterlogged ground, often becoming completely bogged. The kindest solution then was usually to shoot them. At Rafa the veterinary staff, with Egyptian help, treated the animals and heavy sacking offered some protection against the cold. Gradually, with food, rest and later regular exercise, they recovered and by March 1918 were again ready for war.

'Probably the worst sight I saw,' wrote William Wilson on the Somme in September 1916, 'was just before we entered the trench. The ground was all quite freshly torn up and 6 horses were lying dead with their harness still on them. Their bodies were frightfully torn. A big shell must have landed on them as the limber was matchwood.'[84] This was not an unusual situation. Particularly for farmers like Wilson, encountering dead and injured horses and mules on the battlefields of the Western Front was a sad and disturbing experience.

More than 3000 horses and mules went with the New Zealand Division from Egypt to France. Some riding horses were taken to Europe, but the largely static trench warfare of the Western Front called chiefly for heavy horses and mules to pull the ammunition wagons and the guns — six-horse teams, in twos with a driver to each pair (riding one horse), were needed to drag a two-wheeled limber with a gun hooked to it — and to act as pack animals for the ASC, carrying rations to the gun pits and fodder to the horse lines. Mules proved their worth yet again.[85]

As in the desert, horses and mules were easy targets for shellfire or aerial bombs, either when negotiating the ruined landscape or when tethered or stabled in open areas. Particularly in the summer of 1917, German aircraft deliberately dropped bombs on the horse lines in an attempt to cripple Allied transport.[86] At Ploegsteert in July 1917, bombs fell around the transport lines of No. 2 Field Ambulance, 'causing 20 casualties amongst ambulance horses and damage to Horse Ambulance wagons'. Bomb-proof walls were built to help protect the horses; in June 1918 orders were given to raise these to 5½ feet.[87] Roads were targeted, too. On 14 November 1917, Herbert Hart saw one 'lined with derelict wagons, limbers, carts and dead horses throughout its whole length. I counted 87 horses or mules and 124 vehicles.'[88] 'It is an awfull sight,' Len Wilton told his future wife, 'to see six or seven horse blowned to pieces on a line beside a lot being wounded & you have got to get in amongst them & get the rest away. Then in some cases a man or two will be wounded & they have to be got out of it.' His friend Lincoln Murray was found semi-buried next to half a horse, a man blown to pieces and one or two others wounded.[89]

The considerable task of burying dead horses and mules was not always practicable, as Gunner Harold Kretschmar told his father in September 1916: 'the horses killed are left unburied and after a few days lime is sprinkled over them to hasten the decomposition. The smell is awful.'[90] That same day men of the New Zealand Sanitary Section were ordered to bury 'large quantities of refuse, dead horses etc which has been deposited in shell holes'. Earlier in the year, 21 animals had been buried at the 'horse cemetery' at Armentières, and in May 1918 there were 53 burials after the section took over an area with 'a considerable number of dead horses & mules lying exposed'.[91] Unburied animals were not always abandoned. At one point, Eric Hames and his mates 'were convinced that the meat in the stew became very dark and tough, and swore that they were feeding us . . . dead mule'. Hart saw 'many signs that the Hun eats all eatable parts of horses slain', and at the end of the war Harry Highet ate 'a marvellous stew of horse' made by local villagers.[92]

Ammunition was usually taken up to the line in wagons, but packing was not uncommon. '[You] saddle up both neddies,' Geoffrey Wild wrote, 'and put a pack, with four pouches on each side, on each donk. [The term 'donk' seems to have been used for donkeys, mules and horses.] While there are no shells in the packs you can ride one donk, but when fully loaded there is no room for a seat.' John Russell recorded 18-pounder shells being delivered to the gunners in wicker baskets on pack horses; each animal carried six.[93] Horses also pulled ambulances, particularly early in the New Zealand Division's time on the Western Front. In April 1917, No. 1 New Zealand Field Ambulance recorded that the horses 'have stood the work well but begin to feel the strain. One heavy draught was killed by shell fire.'[94] Horses also moved field ambulance supplies. In July 1917 No. 2 Field Ambulance lost 18 of their 'valuable animals'.[95]

Drivers like Wild had many duties involving their horses. Finding feed was time-consuming and sometimes risky. In June 1917, Alexander Wilson and his mates filled nine bags with

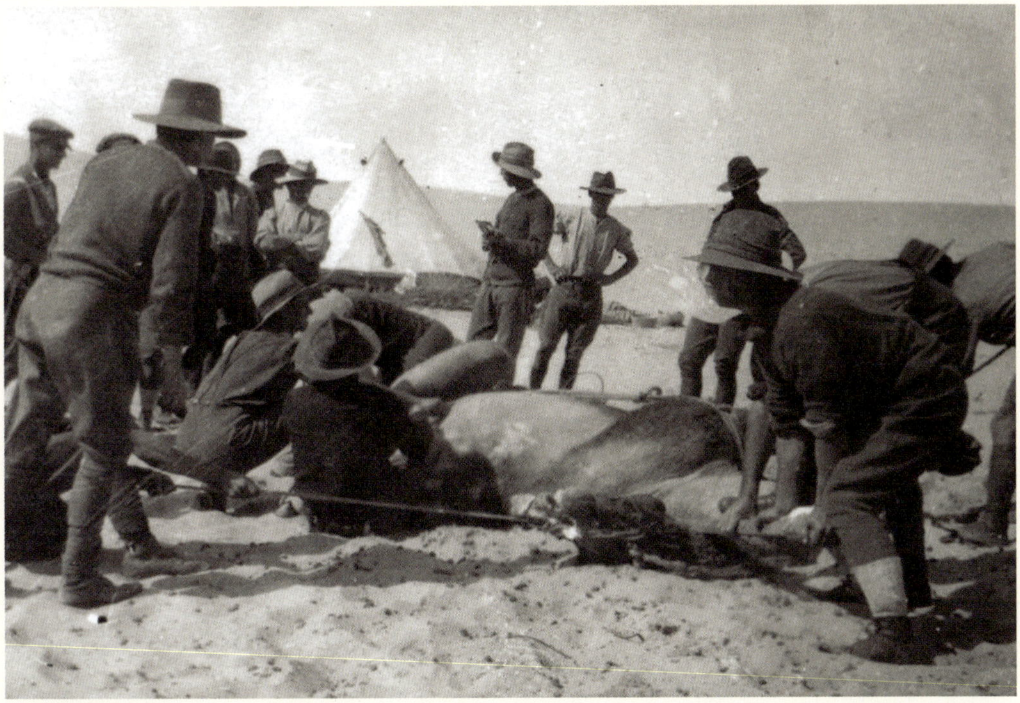

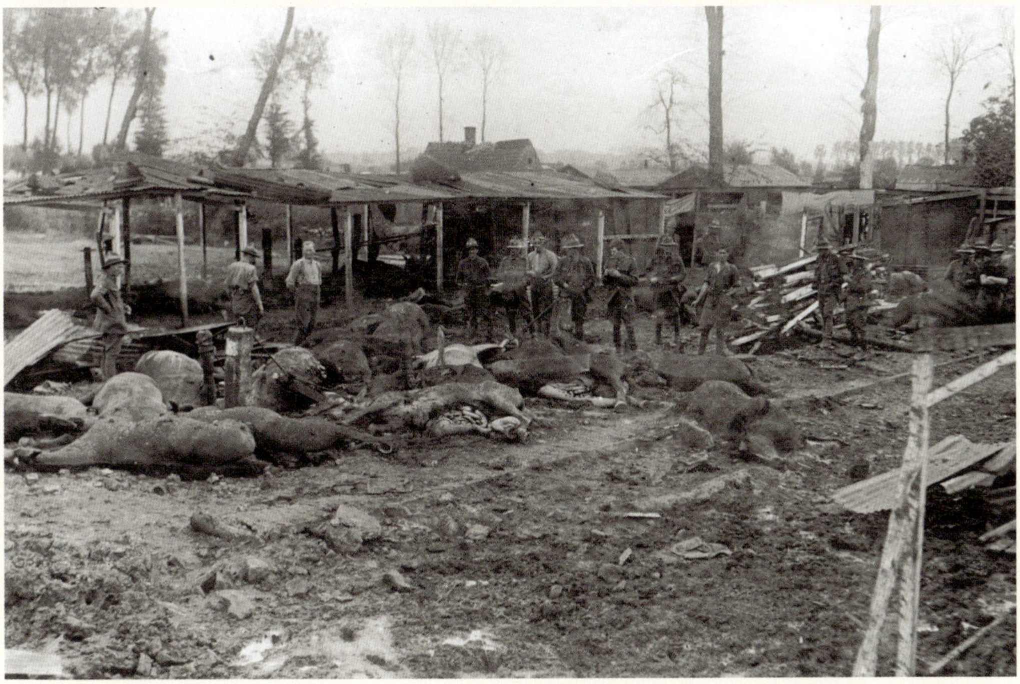

above A veterinary sergeant works on a camel in the Middle East. No one who rode or cared for them had any pre-war experience of these extraordinary but essential animals. NATIONAL ARMY MUSEUM, 1993.1220

below The handwritten caption under this 1917 or 1918 photo of the mutilated carcasses of army horses in France reads 'Dumb victims of the war. 94 horses were destroyed in a German bombing attack.' ALEXANDER TURNBULL LIBRARY, 1/2-013713-G grass which they mixed with the hay, but the next day, while they were 'cutting grass for the "chevaux" . . . the old Frenchy went crook . . . & after various searchings we had to return with empty sacks'. Watering was difficult, too. Sometimes the only liquid available was what lay in shell-holes, or there was the kind of unsupervised chaos Clarence Hankins experienced at Fricourt in late September 1916. 'Thousands & thousands of horses go there & pack up in a heap outside the gate. It is just push through & get water where you can there is no regulation. It is no bon for the horses they get their heels torn to pieces.'[96] When the horses were moved from place to place, sometimes by train, they had to be settled, groomed, picketed, fed and watered before the men could rest.

The weather, especially over the cruel winter of 1916–17, was hard on the horses and those caring for them. At Bois de Grenier in January, thick snow was followed by a brutal frost.

> There was no shelter of any kind for the horses and we had to tether them out on open lines where the poor brutes simply stood and shivered all day and night, the awful cutting wind being a real agony to them . . . The puddles that their hoofs made in the night froze every time the horses stood long enough to go to sleep, so that in the morning . . . each foot brought up a jagged piece of ice with it which had to be broken off before they could move. To untie knots and unfasten buckles was sometimes impossible owing to the intense cold which made our fingers useless to us.[97]

In freezing conditions, as John Russell found at Abeele on Boxing Day 1917, roads became treacherous: 'Horses can't stand on it, all sorts of limbers are lying in ditches, having skidded right off the road.'[98] The constant wetness, added to occasional food shortages, lack of shelter and unreliable rail transport, caused the horses to lose condition and made them prone to such infections as mange.[99] Although the division built hot-water sulphur baths to dip the horses regularly, this process prevented rather than cured the problem. Mange was not, mercifully, a major curse among horses from New Zealand, where the affliction was rare.

Then there was the mud. In October 1916, No. 1 Field Ambulance laid bricks in the horse lines so the animals did not have to stand continually in clammy mud. A year later, at Passchendaele, 'We had to pack the ammunition to the positions, and even then horses often sank to their bellies or slipped into shell holes [which could be 4 to 6 feet deep], became exhausted, and had to be shot to save them a lingering death by drowning or suffocation.' Mules suffered too: 'Many . . . get stuck daily and have to be destroyed.'[100] As future New Zealand lawyer Leonard Leary, serving with an English regiment, wrote, 'Anyone who has seen a horse wounded hopes never to see another. The appeal in the eyes of the prostrate beast as you draw your colt to finish the business, the crying driver as he gives his friend a last hug, are heartrending.'[101] The horses were often exhausted. One night in September 1916 Clarence Hankins left the lines at 6.30 and reached the guns about midnight. 'The horses are just about done & keep laying down in the harness on way home.' Dragging heavy loads through sometimes belly-deep mud and over broken roads frequently strained muscles and injured legs.[102]

Like the fighting men around them, horses were exposed to gas both when working and when stabled near trenches or large groups of troops, and suffered debility and severe eye and skin lesions as a result.[103] In May 1917 Lieutenant-Colonel Harry Reid, who had succeeded Young as ADVS, reported on the use of anti-gas horse respirators: 'The animals appear to take kindly to the new form of apparatus.'[104] Norman Hassell had a different experience at Hébuterne that year. 'Even our horses had to wear gas masks, and as it was almost impossible to adjust them properly . . . once we had our own on, it can readily be imagined what frantic moments we had.' In a sudden barrage of gas shells, the men had to 'dismount, unstrap our horses' bags, and get them adjusted properly before we could look to ourselves. The horses of course hated them worse than we did, and it was exasperating in the extreme when each horse persisted in holding its head as high as possible to prevent us putting them on.'[105]

One of the most serious and common injuries for horses on the Western Front was picked-up-nail. The building of military structures, the destruction of houses and the use of boxes to fuel cooker fires left thousands of nails scattered on the roads, where they all too easily penetrated hooves. Although steel protective plates were tried, these tended to slip on the uneven cobbled streets, buckling and bruising the soles of the horses' feet. 'The inevitable result was a crop of lame animals painfully making their way to hospital.'[106] There the usual treatment was thorough cleaning and iodine dressing; any complication meant evacuation. Tetanus was the big threat but, like the wounded men, the horses were routinely inoculated with anti-tetanic serum.

Then there were caltrops, four-spiked pieces of metal deliberately left in fields and on roads by the Germans to cripple horses. When stood on, these cruel devices pierced the hoof to the joint, carrying bacteria into the wound, which thus became inaccessible to cleaning and could not heal. Horses were also affected in less measurable and treatable ways. For these sensitive, intelligent creatures, accustomed to a routine of regular work, eating and sleep, exposure to 'the horrors of sight and sound that accompany the business of war-making to-day' could cause 'a strange malady' not unlike neurasthenia in humans.[107]

On the Western Front, as with the troops, there was a chain of treatment and evacuation for sick and injured horses. The veterinary officers also oversaw forage, ensured that the stables were kept clean and checked the horse lines. Animals that could not be treated on the spot were collected at the mobile section, sent on to a veterinary CCS and then, for serious cases, to a base hospital, usually the New Zealand Veterinary Section attached to the British No. 4 General Veterinary Hospital at Calais.[108] Although many horses 'did exceedingly well under efficient surgical treatment', they could not return to service unless they were completely sound, and a number had to be destroyed.[109] Initially, evacuation was mostly done by barges, along the canals and rivers of northern France. This worked well and the horses were comfortable. Trains, sometimes harder to come by, were the alternative. Owing to the lack of NZVC personnel, 'suitable assistants were drawn from the ranks, wherever possible, to help in first aid and in the routine veterinary treatment'.[110]

As part of the post-Gallipoli reorganisation, the two veterinary hospital sections in Egypt had been disbanded and most of the staff sent to divisional regiments. Some 26 ORs had sailed for France as a veterinary section, which in June was attached to the British No. 2 Veterinary

Hospital at Le Havre, where the New Zealanders did 'valuable work'. Their next move, in March 1917, was to the Calais hospital, which was still being built; the NZVC men offered practical assistance with its construction. The New Zealand section, which became a base depot where NZVC personnel were trained, was given its own ward, headed by Peter Edgar, with 75 ORs; Edgar later had charge of the whole hospital, as consulting and operating surgeon. During its 23 months at Calais, surgery made up most of the section's work, but it also treated a range of diseases. By the time it was disbanded in February 1919, it had dealt with almost 7000 cases.[111] Godley approved when he visited in late 1917, and the British authorities agreed: 'No better work has been done anywhere . . . it is a model of efficiency and good order.'[112]

Deaths from sickness and injury, exchanges and replacements make it difficult to know exactly how many of the New Zealand horses sent overseas were still with the division when the war ended. At the end of December 1918, the division had 'just under 4500 "animals"'. Famously, of the surviving horses, only four officers' mounts — Beauty, Bess, Dolly and Nigger — made it back to New Zealand in 1920.[113] The reasons for this tiny number were a severe lack of transport and tough quarantine restrictions designed to keep destructive diseases out of a small, vulnerable and heavily farmed nation. Accordingly, the horses, both in Europe and the Middle East, were shot, sold or kept by the British army.

In Egypt, the New Zealand troopers' horses went into the Imperial Remount Depot at Moascar. At first the fittest animals stayed there and others considered suitable for work were sold locally. Those regarded as unfit were killed. (Later, unable to use such a large number of horses in Egypt, or to transport them home, the British were forced to sell or shoot more.) Concerns about mistreatment or neglect by what Reakes called 'the callous Egyptians' led some men to have their horses declared unfit, convinced that 'a merciful death was a better fate for a faithful horse than bondage to a pitiless taskmaster'.[114] This practice has sometimes been sensationalised and inflated, leading to the misapprehension that the Australian and New Zealand horsemen 'shot their horses in significant numbers'. There was certainly, though, 'many a sad parting between man and horse — mates in the hard years of war'.[115]

A similar process — joining other British army horses, then selling, keeping or killing — was followed with the New Zealand horses in France. When Private Leslie Marfell helped to look after the Allied horses in Germany in 1919, the animals 'had to be fed the whole time — they didn't have any pastures. They were inspected and those that were 100 per cent were being sent back to England. Those that weren't, we took up to the abattoirs.'[116] But some 100,000 of the 400,000 imperial horses in France, including many from New Zealand, eventually crossed the Channel.[117]

Wartime vets worked under great strain in trying conditions. At the end of December 1916, after the Battle of Magdhaba in the Sinai, 'the doctors decided' that Captain Donald Rait, on detachment to the New Zealand Mounted Rifle Brigade, should have a rest and be treated for chronic blepharitis, an inflammation of the eyelids exacerbated by desert dust. 'I have been an honest faithful worker,' he told his wife, Blanche, 'so I feel I deserve

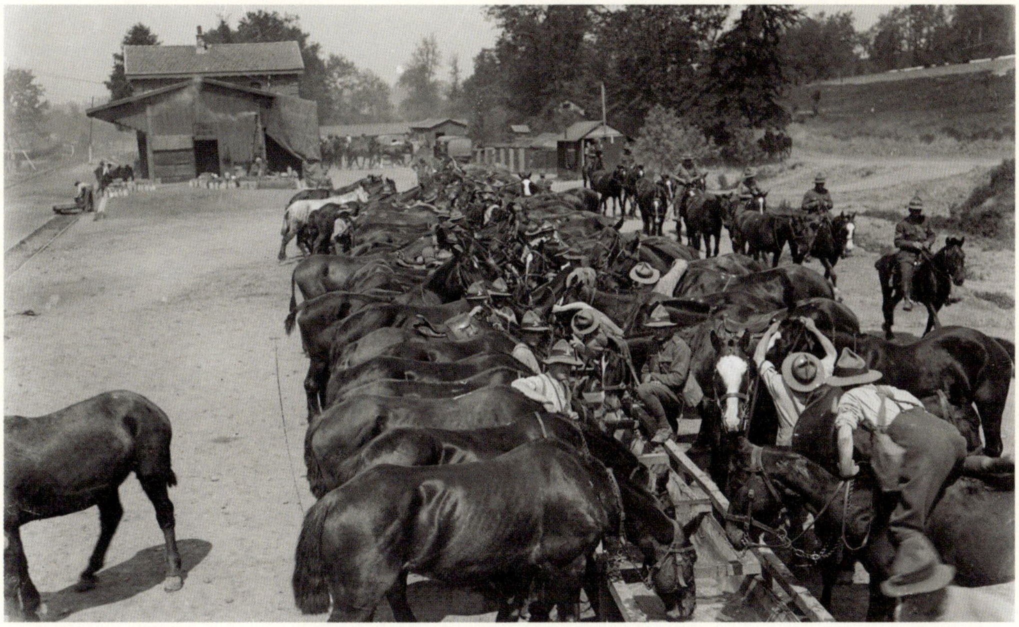

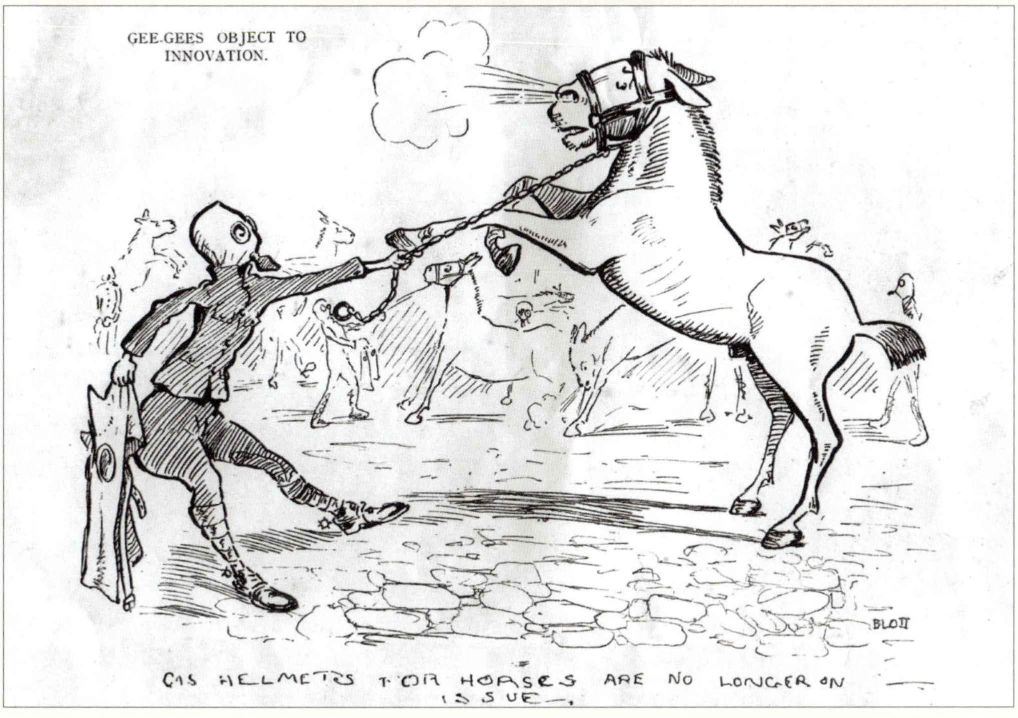
GEE-GEES OBJECT TO INNOVATION.
BLOTT
GAS HELMETS FOR HORSES ARE NO LONGER ON ISSUE.

above Horses drinking from troughs in rows at a watering point in Louvencourt, France, on 1 June 1918. This orderly approach was not always the norm. ALEXANDER TURNBULL LIBRARY, 1/2-013735-G

below Under this cartoon in *Shell-Shocks: New Zealanders in France*, sent to his wife at home in the Hokianga in 1917, New Zealand Divisional Ammunition Column driver William White wrote: 'We had a few goes like this but do not bother about gas masks for our animals now. They have to take their chance.' COURTESY PAUL WHITE the spell . . . I expect I am run down. The constant work and night rides must of necessity be rather trying.' There had been no sleep for two nights during the battle. On the second, Rait saw 'aeroplanes with wings as big as the sky' and took shelter as bombs fell only yards away. He relished the 'feeling of peace' at the hospital: 'a bed to sleep on after months of being down on the sand under a blanket is delightful'.[118] Rait, who served for two years in Egypt, died on 26 November 1917 in Palmerston North after being kicked in the chest by a horse he was treating.

As well as Charles Neale, who was later also given an OBE, several NZVC members were decorated for their work during the war. Charles Reakes, the head of the corps, received a CBE in 1919, Thomas Blake was given a Croix de Guerre for his work as an interpreter in France, both Peter Edgar and Harry Reid were mentioned in despatches (Edgar twice) and awarded OBEs, and James Stafford received the DSO for gallantry in the field in the Middle East after being mentioned in despatches in July 1917.[119] Sergeant Spencer Barnes, who was attached to the New Zealand Field Artillery, won the Military Medal.

A number of NZVC men lost their lives. Eight NZVC other ranks had died by 3 January 1916, and more would follow, both killed in action and as victims of disease.[120] Three veterinary officers died under unusual circumstances. After serving in Egypt, Scottish-born NZVC vet Daniel Machattie was hospitalised in London in 1915, then admitted several times in Egypt for anaemia and cardiac debility. In September that year, he was sent to the Australian Remount Depot at Heliopolis. There, on 20 December 1916, 37-year-old Machattie shot himself in the head with a Webley Mk VI revolver. He left behind two letters, one for a colleague and one for his sister Bessie: 'I hope mother and yourself are well, tell her I am very sorry to do this, and that she must not let it worry her, too much. But I have suffered from sleeplessness for a good many years now, and it seems to me this is the only way to get some rest.'[121]

Captain George Waugh, like Machattie a Scot, had also served in Egypt before returning to work in New Zealand and then sailing back to Europe. He was 'of an argumentative nature, irascible . . . in his dealing with men'. Following a drunken dinner, he rode up to a checkpoint late on 25 May 1917, seeking directions to his billet. After refusing to provide identification he galloped off, but soon returned and repeated the performance. When he appeared for a third time, young Private Arthur Connolly, having decided he must be a spy, again requested ID. Waugh replied, 'I am a New Zealand officer,' and demanded to speak to someone senior. He then struck Connolly, who was holding his horse, and took off. After his three shouted warnings were ignored, Connolly fired, hitting Waugh in the lung. He died the next morning and a court of inquiry found the death to be accidental.[122] In Reid's estimation, Waugh was 'an excellent veterinarian, possessing knowledge & sound judgement on all matters pertaining to the subject of horsemanship'.[123]

Perhaps the most bizarre death was that of Captain Jacob Primmer, who was killed in France on 12 June 1917 when struck by lightning while sheltering from heavy rain in a cookhouse beneath a large tree. All the men with him were injured. 'The veterinary surgeon was much liked and respected by us all,' said Gunner W. J. Wilson, 'and his case was rendered particularly sad by the fact that his wife [Melanie] was in Paris expecting him to go and see her.'[124]

The First World War was a gruelling experience for the animals who served in it and the men who cared for them. Although horses were not used as expected on Gallipoli or on the Western Front, where only the Otago mounted riflemen participated in a limited cavalry capacity,[125] they, and mules, camels and donkeys, were essential to New Zealand's war effort. As was so often the case, praise from 'Home' was regarded as the ultimate compliment for the NZVC. On Anzac Day 1919, the *Dominion* proudly printed the words of Major-General John Moore, Director of Veterinary Services for the British Expeditionary Force in France: 'I am glad that the New Zealand Veterinary Corps . . . has proved its mettle. Without question it has justly merited the goodwill and high regard of the Dominion to which it belongs . . . there remains a deep sense of gratitude for all the splendid assistance it has rendered.'[126]

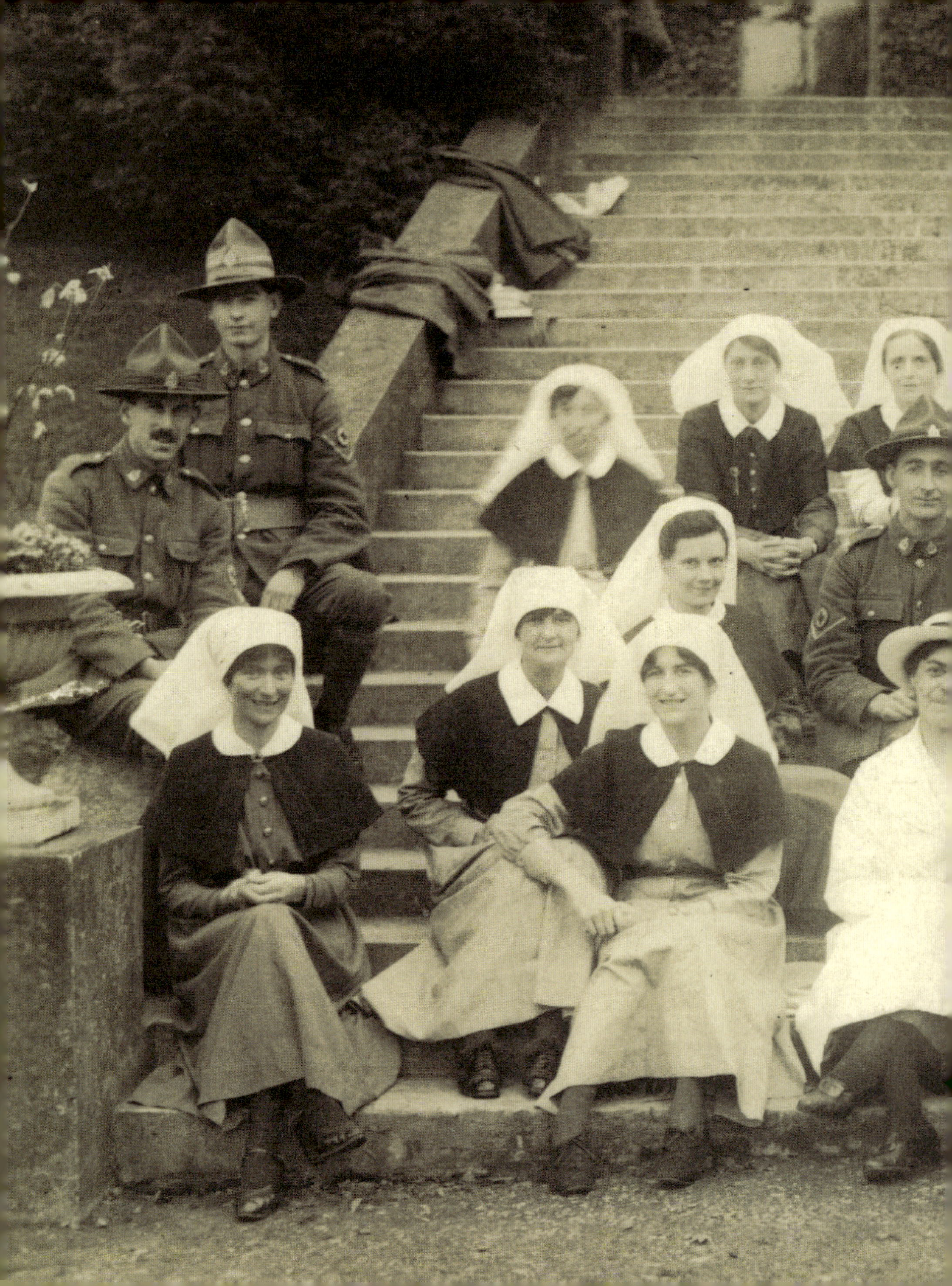

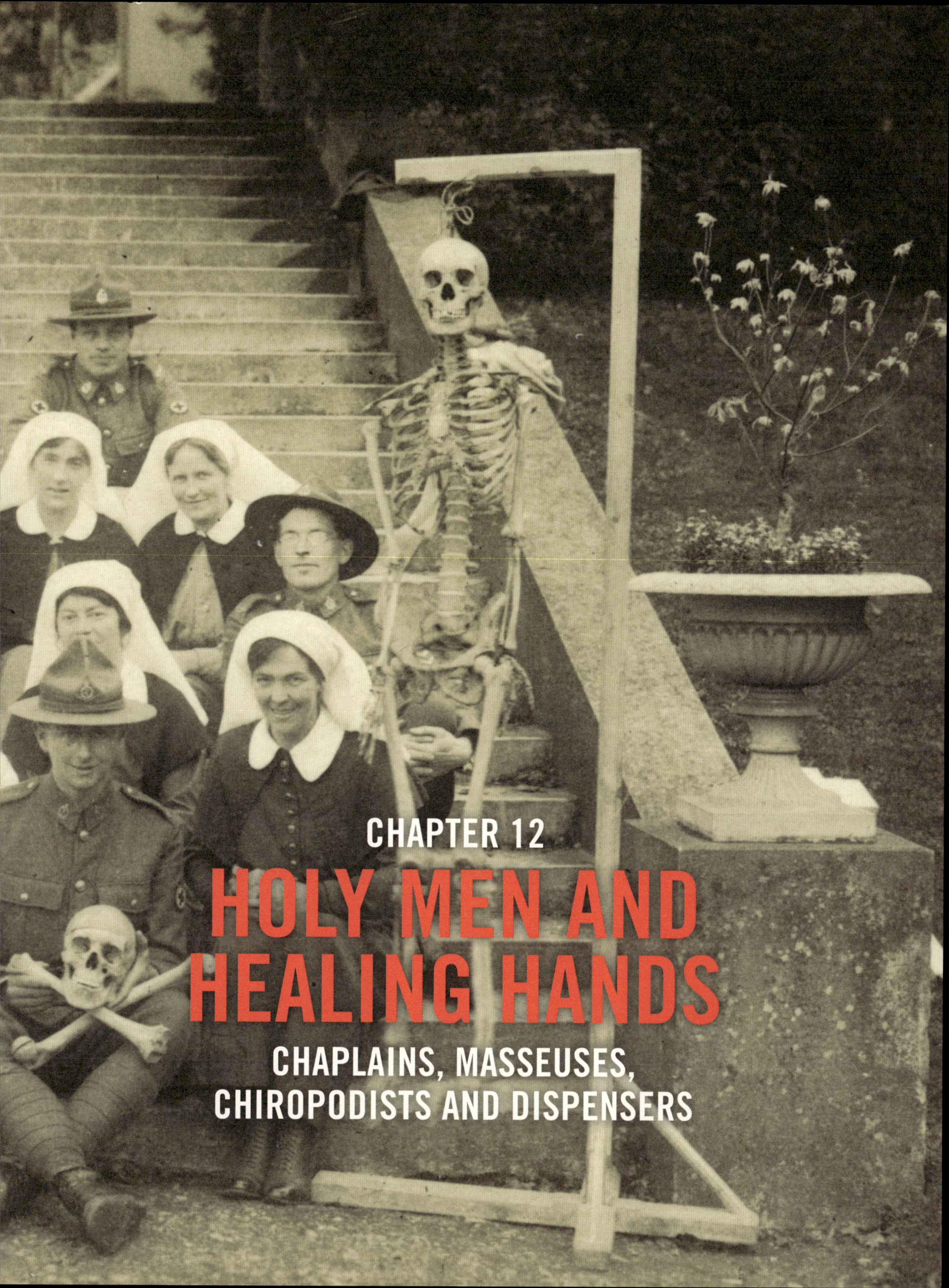

CHAPTER 12

HOLY MEN AND HEALING HANDS

CHAPLAINS, MASSEUSES, CHIROPODISTS AND DISPENSERS

previous pages
Humour was not forgotten by wartime healers. In September 1918, nurses and medical staff at Hornchurch Convalescent Hospital pose for the photographer with a skull and crossbones and a skeleton on a wooden frame.
AUCKLAND WAR MEMORIAL MUSEUM, PH-TECH-925-264

Please don't expect too much in the way of letters. I find so very much to do these days, time is not nearly sufficient.

— Chaplain Ronald Watson, 9 April 1918

'Into the ward came a chaplain. The man of God in the uniform of Mars.'[1] John A. Lee's words are a reminder that, although they were not officially medical personnel, many New Zealand padres worked tirelessly and courageously alongside doctors, orderlies and bearers in the front line, and in hospitals. Of the 13 who left with the Main Body, four were wounded and two killed in action; they all faced illnesses of various kinds.[2] Chaplains also served on hospital ships. On her first charter the *Maheno* carried Anglican William Gillam, Presbyterian Daniel Dutton and Catholic Thomas Segrief, who had served in Samoa.[3] All three men later sailed on the *Marama*. Alongside their usual duties, seagoing chaplains helped to make beds, assisted with serving meals and dressed wounds. They also 'did much to publicise the work of the white [hospital] ships, offering lantern-lectures back home between voyages and writing open letters to their congregations'.[4]

Even the chaplains' non-medical tasks could be dangerous. Burials were particularly risky. On Gallipoli these were carried out at night, supposedly for greater safety, but as Methodist John Luxford found, despite the darkness, 'the snipers kept up fire, and spent bullets fell, hence every precaution was necessary'.[5] Henare Te Wainohu (Ngāti Kahungunu and Ngāti Pāhauwera), who landed at Anzac as chaplain to the Maori Contingent on 3 July 1915, went to work immediately with MO Te Rangi Hīroa and his stretcher-bearers, digging out 'a capacious aid post. He was in [the] thick of the action at Sari Bair, risking his life to go out with the medics.' Te Wainohu, who would be awarded the Serbian Order of the White Eagle and mentioned in despatches in 1918, 'sustained the spirit' of the Māori unit in the Dardanelles and on the Western Front.[6] There was peril there, too, for the men of God. 'Day and night,' wrote Malcolm Ross after the Somme, 'often under fire, they administered to the wants of the living and the dying, and, wherever possible, gave the dead decent burial.'[7]

The padres were not always young men. Luxford had served in South Africa and was 60

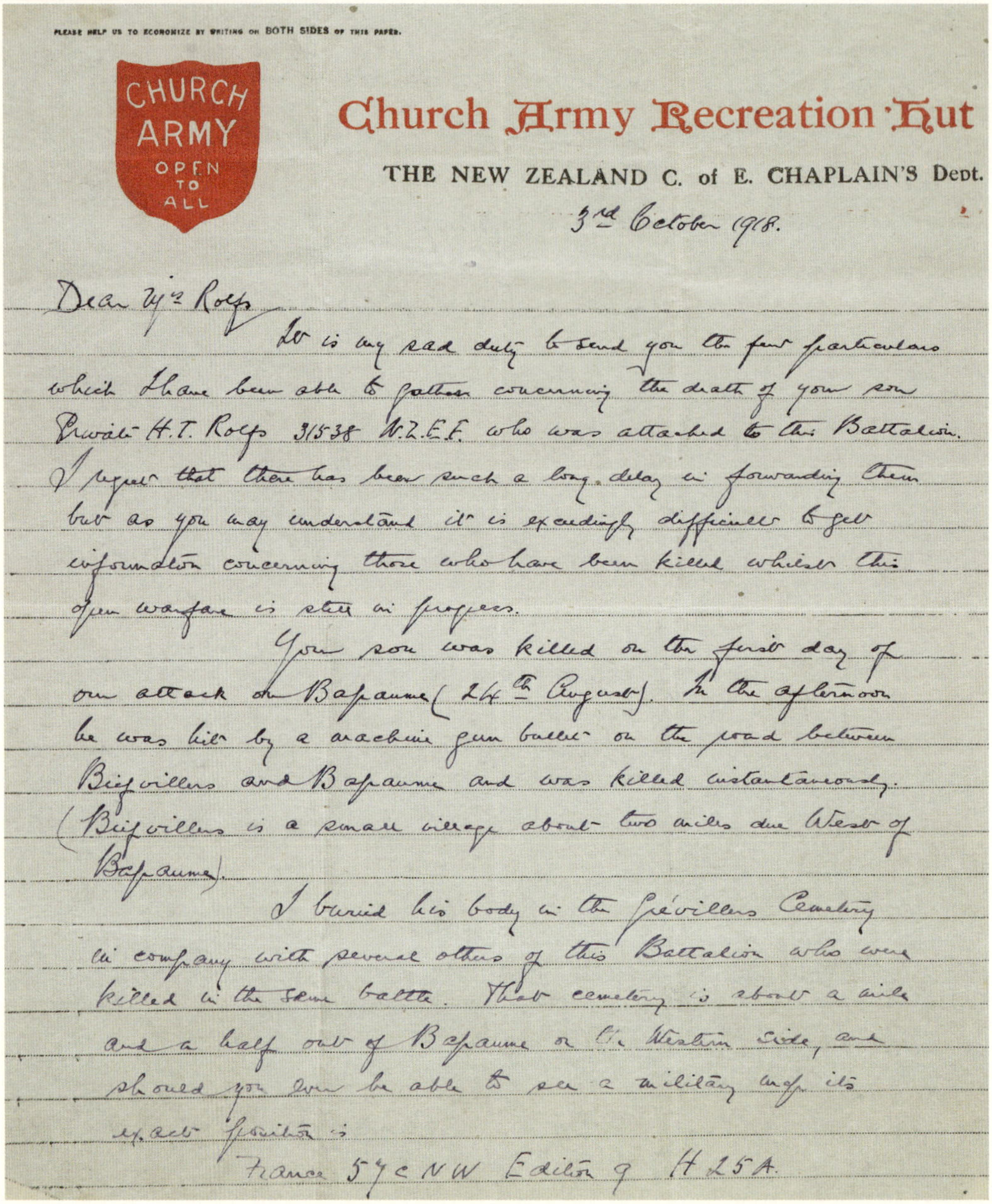
PLEASE HELP US TO ECONOMIZE BY WRITING ON BOTH SIDES OF THIS PAPER.

CHURCH ARMY OPEN TO ALL

Church Army Recreation Hut

THE NEW ZEALAND C. of E. CHAPLAIN'S Dept.

3rd October 1918.

Dear Mrs Rolfs

It is my sad duty to send you the few particulars which I have been able to gather concerning the death of your son Private H.T. Rolfs 31538 N.Z.E.F. who was attached to this Battalion. I regret that there has been such a long delay in forwarding them but as you may understand it is exceedingly difficult to get information concerning those who have been killed whilst this open warfare is still in progress.

Your son was killed on the first day of our attack on Bapaume (24th August). In the afternoon he was hit by a machine gun bullet on the road between Biefvillers and Bapaume and was killed instantaneously. (Biefvillers is a small village about two miles due West of Bapaume).

I buried his body in the Grévillers Cemetery in company with several others of this Battalion who were killed in the same battle. That cemetery is about a mile and a half out of Bapaume on the Western side, and should you ever be able to see a military map its exact position is

France 57c NW Edition 9 H 25A.

Writing to bereaved families and, if possible, explaining how their men died and where they were buried was an endless task for busy wartime chaplains. Herman Rolfes from Kaikōura was killed on 24 August 1918 but Chaplain George Cruickshank was only able to write to his mother, Frances, on 3 October. TE PAPA, GH011681/1 years old when he was working at a relentless pace on Gallipoli. On 8 August 1915, at Chunuk Bair, a bullet struck his right thigh, severing an artery; the leg had to be amputated in Britain. He was mentioned in despatches and then made a CMG for outstanding service on the peninsula. 'During the August Offensive, he occupied a dressing station near to the firing line . . . and did the work of more than one man of half his age. Minus his coat, his sleeves rolled up, he dressed and bandaged for hours at a stretch.'[8] After he had recovered sufficiently, Luxford, with an artificial leg and leaning on 'a stout walking stick',[9] was, at his own request, transferred to Walton. While there he was diagnosed with prostate cancer, of which he died at his Auckland home in January 1921.

'I am now part and parcel of the New Zealand Stationary Hospital,' wrote Presbyterian chaplain Ronald Watson from Amiens on 1 April 1917. Three days later he told the 'Folks at Home', 'I have been going at top, endeavouring to get to know all the ins and outs of the hospital buildings . . . I have been picking up things medical in most rapid style.' He had longed to be on the front line, 'where things are being done, rather than where broken men are to be found', but now considered this posting 'one of the best things that could happen in many ways'. A few months later a sick and muddy New Zealander in an ambulance told Watson, much to his amusement, 'When I saw you coming, I knew you were a padre. Your smile has done me as much good as a hot cup of coffee. It is as useful as sunlight soap.'

Watson was hospitalised twice himself, the second time after being ordered out of an RAP with a temperature of 101°F. In early April 1918 he staggered through knee-deep mud, under fire, to deliver YMCA gifts: 'I am getting my nerve very much improved, I am glad to say.' The work was wearing, though. 'I am often fed [up] to the teeth with the sight of maiming and blood and the handling of dead bodies,' he wrote at the beginning of May. 'For the last six weeks I have gone with the [1st Otago] Bn. wherever it has gone. I sleep in the R.A.P, with the Doctor [Harold] (Gibson).' For his brave work in bringing in the wounded near Bapaume on 25 August and 5 September, Watson was awarded the MC. After 11 months with the Otagos, his 'narrow escapes' came to an end on 8 October 1918 when he was wounded while helping a young soldier with a badly broken thigh. He ended up in Walton and wrote home from hospital on 8 November, 'Lately, I have been receiving numerous letters of hearty congratulations on my getting the Military Cross. So I am wearing the ribbon and quite proud of it too.'[10]

Another chaplain to receive the MC, for his heroic work with the wounded during a German attack on 5 April 1918, was Clarence Seton from Raglan. As fellow Anglican padre Clive Mortimer Jones told his parishioners, 'I am so glad that the work of the chaplains in general and the courage of Mr Seton is thus recognised. Please don't expect to hear similar news of me. I am much too "windy" under shellfire and am not looking for medals, which means going into great danger! I think I'm ten years too old for this life and get more nervous every time I hear a shell, even if it is a mile away.'[11] Jones was no coward, however. When the headquarters cook was hit at Le Quesnoy, the chaplain 'picked him up and got the "Doc" [Captain Richard Barron] . . . [O]ur temporary aid-post (a newly made shell-hole which we quickly enlarged) was kept busy. We had to get the cases away as quickly as possible, as the whole of that paddock was being heavily shelled.'[12] The Reverend Clement Houchen, from Te Kuiti, also an Anglican, was awarded the MC in November 1916 for his work at the Somme: 'he tended and dressed the wounded under very heavy fire with great courage and determination.' Houchen lost the sight in his left eye as a result of a gunshot wound at Passchendaele. Seven of the 13 Main Body chaplains were honoured.[13]

Sickness was always a threat. Former West Coast and Nelson Anglican vicar Thomas Fielden Taylor, who had brought in wounded from the Daisy Patch in May 1915 and been shot in the back soon afterwards, was mentioned in despatches in April 1916. He felt it a 'great come-down' when he was forced to leave his regiment in France on 25 August that year, because of illness. When he reached the NZSH, he had 'six pints of pleural effusion pumped off me'. After time at Brockenhurst, and a spell at a stately convalescent home in the vain hope of improving 'creeping' rheumatism that meant he could not use his arms, wrists or legs, he was invalided home on the *Maheno* at the end of October.[14]

Presbyterian chaplain John Lopdell, attached temporarily to the Canadian Tunnellers, spent the Christmas and New Year of 1917–18 'in a Hun pill box, not many hundred yards from Mr Fritz's front line'. He admitted that his health had 'not been too good': his heart was 'affected' and his throat was 'still suffering from the effects of the gassing I got in October. If I had not been as strong as a horse I would have had to give in then. Gas is a beastly thing.' He added, 'I am sure a rest or even an ease off is all that is necessary to set me going again.' He was too optimistic. On 13 March 1918 Lopdell was admitted to the Brighton Convalescent Home suffering from disordered action of the heart. He sailed for New Zealand in August.[15]

A number of chaplains lost their lives, among them 56-year-old Scots-born Presbyterian minister William Grant, chaplain to the Otago Mounted Rifles. On Gallipoli, Grant wandered 'up and down the beach all day long helping the wounded', taking 'absolutely no notice of the shrapnel and the bullets'. Without an orderly or his own dug-out, he slept 'where he dropped'.[16] On 28 August 1915, 'A wounded man was lying outside a trench. The Padre went out to try and bring him [in] under heavy fire. He never came back.'[17] Grant left behind a widow and five children, two of whom were serving at the front.

Catholic padre Major James McMenamin, who landed on Gallipoli on 25 April and was evacuated, sick, in September, returned to New Zealand to convalesce but, despite his frail health, insisted on going back to Britain, where he was at Walton before serving in France and Belgium. 'Father Mac' was 43 years old when he was killed in action near Messines on 9 June 1917. Irish-born Catholic chaplain Patrick Dore was 'the friend and counsellor of everyone . . . His presence was a better tonic than any the doctor could give.'[18] On Gallipoli, as chaplain to the Auckland Mounted Rifles, he worked alongside the Medical Corps until he was wounded near the spine on 28 August, resulting in partial paralysis of his right leg.[19] After treatment in England, where he was awarded the MC, he was invalided back to New Zealand late in 1916. His wound became infected and he died of surgical complications on 15 July 1918. At his funeral in Palmerston North, the Awapuni Medical Corps band was part of the procession.[20]

Captain Guy Bryan-Brown, who had been chaplain and a schoolmaster at the Anglican Christ's College in Christchurch, was only 32 when he lost his life. He reached France on 29 May 1917 and was wounded on 12 June but remained on duty. On 4 October that year he

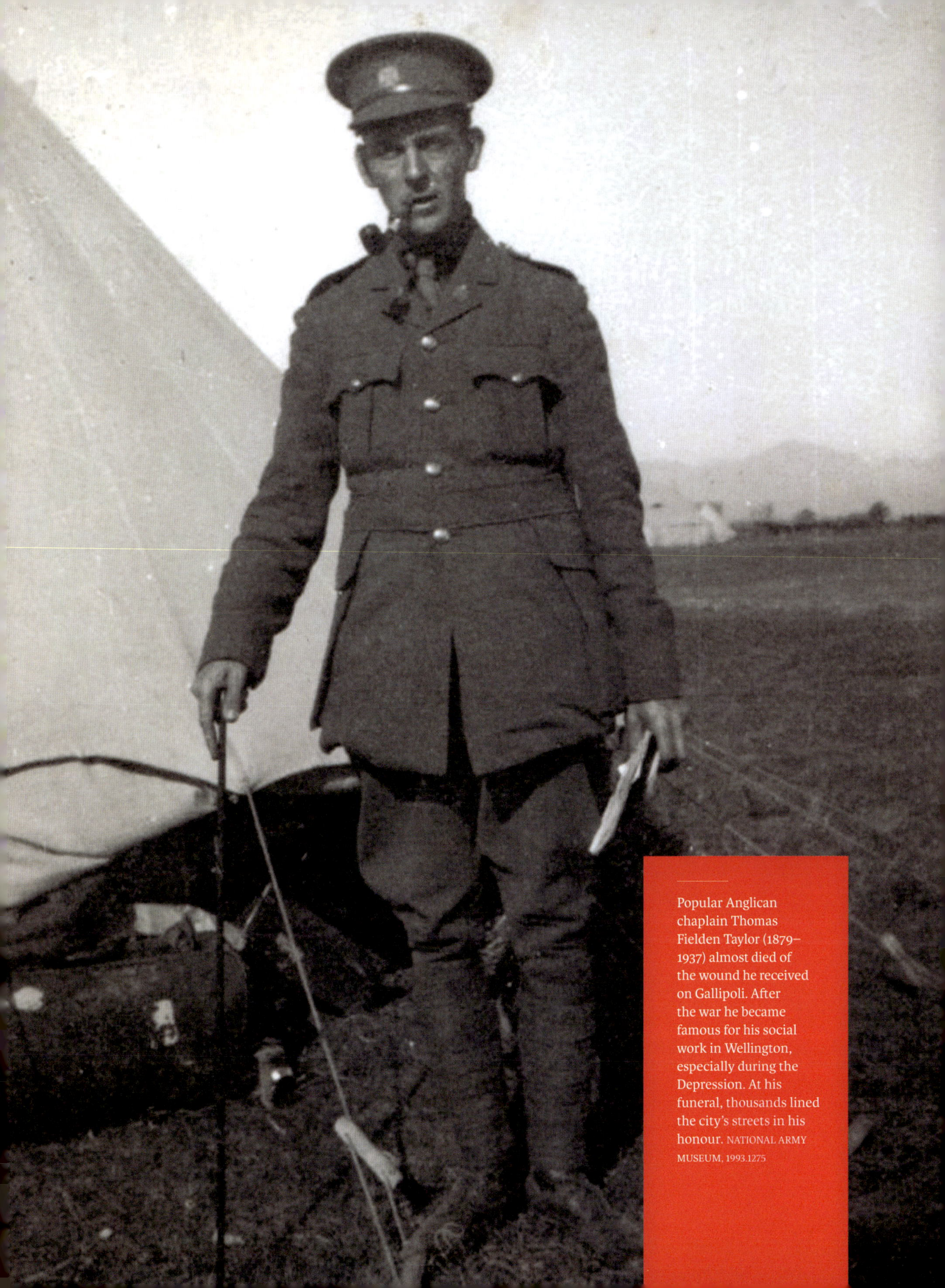

Popular Anglican chaplain Thomas Fielden Taylor (1879–1937) almost died of the wound he received on Gallipoli. After the war he became famous for his social work in Wellington, especially during the Depression. At his funeral, thousands lined the city's streets in his honour. NATIONAL ARMY MUSEUM, 1993.1275

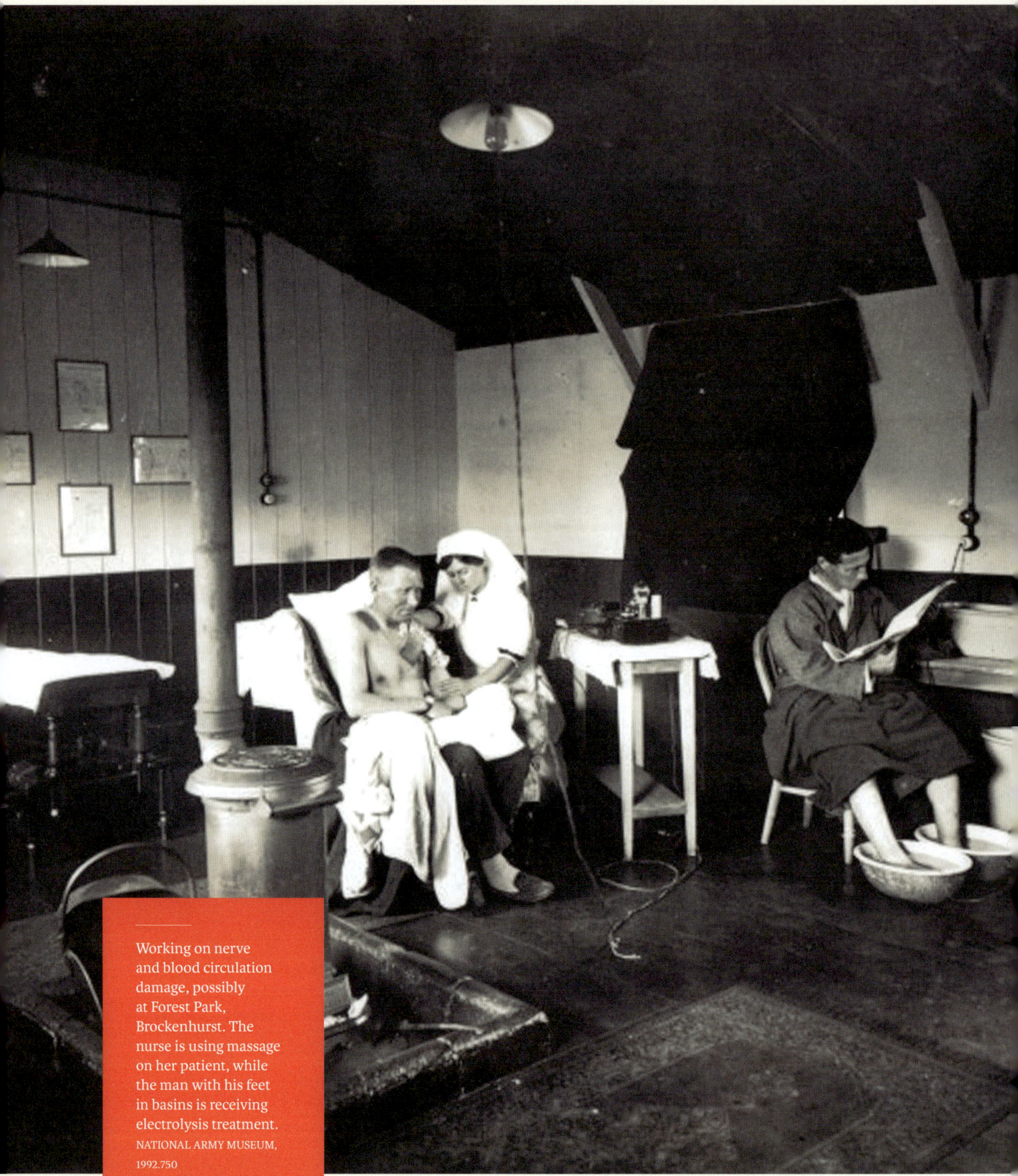

Working on nerve and blood circulation damage, possibly at Forest Park, Brockenhurst. The nurse is using massage on her patient, while the man with his feet in basins is receiving electrolysis treatment. NATIONAL ARMY MUSEUM, 1992.750

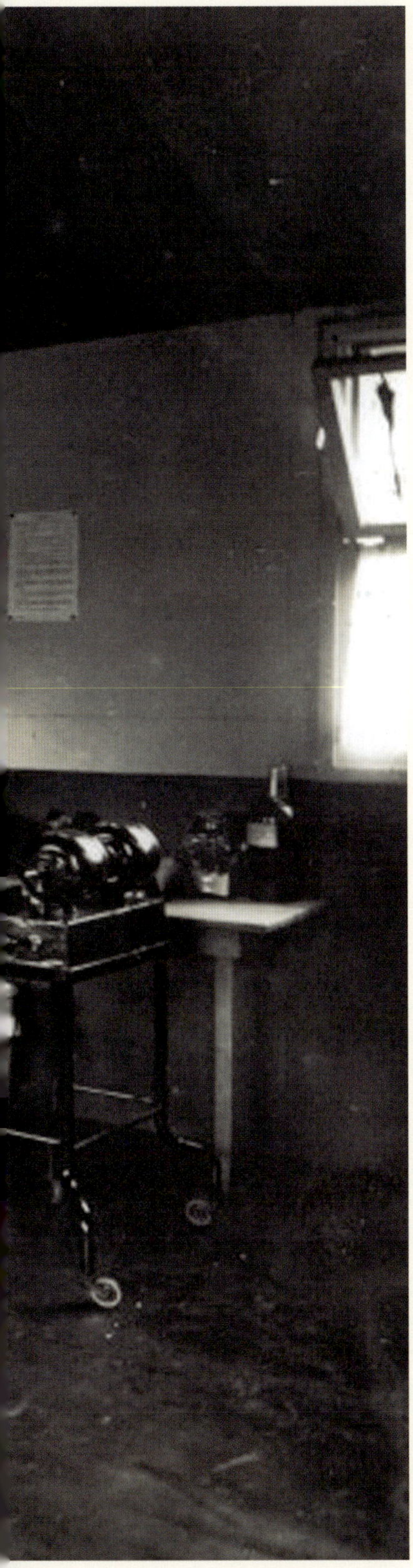

and two bearers were killed while trying to bring a stretcher case into a pillbox RAP during the attack at Gravenstafel. Methodist chaplain Alexander Allen was assigned to Walton after leaving New Zealand on 14 March 1917, but crossed the Channel on 15 September, where he worked at an RAP receiving casualties from the Third Battle of Ypres. He was killed in May 1918 while caring for the wounded. As Watson wrote, 'Allen was a great chap and ever so lovable.'[21] After Anglican John Burgin, the chaplain to the 3rd and 4th battalions of the New Zealand Rifle Brigade, was gassed at the Somme, he was sent to Brockenhurst, where he served for six months before being invalided home in 1917. On 2 December 1920, aged 51, he died of a heart attack that was directly attributable to his wartime injury.

'Do not think of the wound,' wrote British surgeon Lieutenant-Colonel A. W. Sheen in *The Lancet* of January 1915, 'think of the limb below it. Endeavour to minimise the crop of cripples which this war will bring forth.' He continued: 'Everything possible must be done to prevent stiff joints, atrophied, paralysed, glued-together muscles, lengthened tendons, loss of grasp, dropped hands, and dropped feet.' The patient must be 'carefully and methodically put through different movements and exercises', with the explanation that 'all this painful exertion is for his own good, and to give him a useful limb later'.[22] Massage — what would now be referred to as physiotherapy — played a significant role in treating the wounded during the First World War, and the New Zealand medical services were no exception.

In the late nineteenth century, the word 'massage' covered a multitude of practitioners and levels of experience; many doctors were, rightly, wary of untrained quack 'therapists'. Massage also suffered, in some quarters, from scandalous accusations that it was no more than prostitution by another name.[23] For such reasons, in 1894 a quartet of British masseuses had established the Society of Trained Masseuses which, by 1900, had become the Incorporated Society of Trained Masseuses (ISTM). A small group of Australian massage therapists had made a similar move in 1906. Both countries had instituted proper training and standards for their profession, and several New Zealand masseurs and masseuses had studied overseas. Future NZANS sister Bertha Nurse achieved an ISTM qualification in Britain in 1909.[24] A School of Massage was opened at Otago University's Medical School in July 1913. Although the inaugural course was beset by problems, five women did graduate the following year.[25]

By 1915, massage was proving helpful to the growing numbers of wounded. When Hester Maclean visited the Royal Herbert Hospital at Woolwich in London, she found it being used 'fairly extensively and the treatment is arranged for without expense to the War Office, by Sir Almeric Paget's Fund for massage'.[26] The British government had welcomed the prompt offer by the aristocratic Paget and his wife of 50 trained masseuses, who became the Almeric Paget Military Massage Corps. New Zealanders trained and served with this group,[27] and Kiwi soldiers received Almeric massages. While Harry Kitson was recovering at Woodcote camp, Surrey, in late 1915, he had 'a dear little Irish girl to massage me every day at 11 o'clock. She belongs to Lady Paget's massage voluntary aid society. I get massaged on the back & neck every day & arms & legs alternate days. They tried light vibration but it shook the nerves up too much.' The treatment took nearly two hours.[28]

As Kitson intimated, massage was more than purely a hands-on business. It also involved hot-air and whirlpool baths, and all manner of electrical devices. 'I began a new treatment today,' he told his sisters in January 1916, 'descending galvanism, might do some good . . . Rather funny for this new treatment I have to have all the hair off the back of my head, looks decidedly odd.' At Oatlands in November 1918, amputee Alec Hutton had daily massage 'to improve the circulation [in the stump] and remove the scars which are more or less weak. It is quite wonderful what is done . . . Of course they have the latest appliances here but at present I have only the hand variety, the electricity is to come later.'[29]

Massage was also one of the earlier treatments for shell shock. 'Why I work so late,' wrote masseuse Ruby Millar from the *Maheno* in 1917, 'is that after supper I massage two men and leave them asleep usually. One a Lieutenant (20 years) was blown up on 24th Dec and his nerves have all gone to pieces. The other, the Colonel I have mentioned before, only sleeps if drugged, and then only for a couple of hours. They are both improving but usually walk the deck at some time during the early hours or play cards.' One night, a doctor in the Indian Medical Service watched her at work, then questioned her about the techniques and offered 'some very good advice about these neurasthenic cases. I was told afterwards that [he thought] I had done the work "beautifully", leaving the boy asleep.'[30]

Also in the massage and physiotherapy arsenal, both overseas and at home, was mechanotherapy, which, as the *Evening Star* explained to its readers in November 1916, was 'a new development' particularly suited to 'those suffering from muscular and nervous ailments'. Unlike orthodox methods, it involved 'the exercise of a patient's will-power in co-operation with medical and mechanical treatment'; its name was 'the only terrible thing about it'. Practised successfully overseas for some time, it had been introduced to New Zealand by Marshall Macdonald, who would later head the neurological section at Balmer Lawn. During his voyage home from working in France, he had performed several experiments on wounded soldiers with 'most excellent effects. Men who had thought that they were permanently paralysed were induced to make the necessary effort of will as a means of recovery, and within a very short time their wasted powers returned to them in a remarkable manner. Accompanying this Auto-suggestion treatment is the use of special instruments.'[31]

The New Zealand medical military hierarchy soon appreciated the recuperative potential of massage, and it was used in training camps and overseas hospitals, on hospital ships and transports carrying the wounded, at convalescent homes such as the one for officers in Brighton, and in hospitals for returned soldiers in New Zealand. As early as mid-January 1916, when the *Marama* took extra staff to Egypt for Pont de Koubbeh, also on board was Danish-born masseuse Louise Petersen. In June 1916 the *New Zealand Herald* reported on the great benefits of electric massage and baths at the Rotorua Sanatorium, given by the six male masseurs to the many patients 'suffering from bullet wounds, causing partial paralysis, and other injuries, which only time and unremitting care can heal'.[32] When a deputation of returned soldiers had approached outspoken Christchurch MP Dr Henry Thacker earlier that year with grievances regarding their treatment, he had recommended 'up-to-date hydrotherapeutic treatment and deep massage' for Sydney Phillips, who had come home with five bullet wounds in his legs. Twenty-five-year-old Charles Angrove, wounded in the right knee on Gallipoli, required hot packs and massage 'to prevent contraction of the muscles above the knee. If such injuries do not receive prompt treatment limbs are likely to suffer permanent injury.'[33]

The NZMC never had a massage unit, though some men who had been masseurs before 1914 continued to use their expertise during the war as members of the corps. Among them was self-employed masseur Alfred Steed-Roberts, who plied his skill at Awapuni and Featherston camps and on the third charter of the *Marama*, and Harry Croker, who had been a masseur at the Government Baths in Rotorua, and also served in the camps and on the *Marama*. The best known was larger-than-life Fred Hornibrook, who described himself on his attestation form as a 'Physical Culturist & Masseur'. The longtime companion and later husband of Ettie Rout, he took months to convince the army to accept his services, then travelled from Britain to New Zealand and back again on the *Marama* in 1917, 'massaging his way through dozens of patients a day, singing favourites like "The Bells of Hell go Ting-a-ling-a-ling for you, but not for me", at the top of his lungs'.[34]

Although, in her contribution to *The War Effort of New Zealand*, Hester Maclean gave no date for its establishment, a Massage Corps was set up as a branch of the NZANS, 'when the need for such treatment was demonstrated'. An initial 31 masseuses, including two from that first trained Dunedin quintet, Flora Gray and Edith Thomson, 'performed splendid and valuable work in aiding the recovery and restoration of the men to normal life'.[35] Another corps member was Ruby Millar from Seacliff in Otago, the youngest of four women who took the second massage course in Dunedin, from 7 April 1915 to 7 December 1916. 'We were supposed to work only four hours a day,' she remembered, 'but it was more often six or seven. Our first patients were men wounded at Gallipoli.' After joining the NZANS in Wellington, Millar sailed on the third charter of the *Maheno* in January 1917. Also on board was fellow corps member Dorothy Miller, who had been working as a masseuse in Christchurch, and trained masseuse Janet Knox Anderson. The women were given the rank of staff nurse. Although Millar was not 'the most miserable person on the boat', she took a while to find her sea legs, but was soon enjoying her mostly English patients. 'I shall be very sorry when many of them go off in Egypt for we all like the "Tommies". DM and I are doing twenty cases a day, starting at seven am and I do not finish until 10 pm. We take an hour off for lunch and dinner and a little less for breakfast. It is hard going but the boys are nice.'[36]

The masseuses, and masseurs, on the hospital ships quickly proved their worth. On the *Maheno* trip that included Millar, Miller and Knox Anderson, the ship's massage and electrical department administered more than 1000 treatments. When nurses were banned from serving on the *Maheno* and *Marama* for fear of submarine attacks, male staff had trouble keeping up with demand. When the *Marama* returned to New Zealand in May 1918, after Passchendaele, 'The electric massage apparatus which was shipped in England proved of great value on the voyage, and many men owe their present condition to the treatment received on the way. Over 7000 treatments were given.'[37]

'Massage treatment becomes more and more necessary,' William Parkes told Allen in December 1916, 'and is a special feature of the electro-massage department of the Convalescent Hospital at Hornchurch.' By this time, the 'very complete Physio-Therapy Department' was headed by two medical officers and staffed by 18 masseuses and masseurs. Besides 30 massage couches, there were 'whirlpool baths, mechanotherapy apparatus, radiant heat and light baths, all accommodated in suitable quarters where 400 cases could receive treatment daily'.[38] By 1917 masseuses were desperately needed at the other New Zealand hospitals. 'We are so very short of masseuses here,' Mabel Thurston told Hester Maclean in August, 'I shall be very glad when the others arrive.'[39] Once six masseuses landed on 17 September they were quickly put to work, three at Brockenhurst and three at Walton. When the *Corinthic* left New Zealand for England in early 1918, she carried another half-dozen.[40]

One man to benefit from the treatment at Hornchurch was Bill Malcolm, whose wounded jaw and lower lip had been successfully operated on at Walton before he was moved, on 1 October 1918, for special treatment and dental care. He described the 'ionisation' process, which utilised a battery attached to two sheets of lead, one placed over the scar and the other on his arm. 'I must say I can't stand it too strong on my chin. The Sister who manages my old chops says they will be able to bring it back to normal after awhile. When she is finished with me for the morning she makes me twist my jaw all roads, but I am afraid she has a good laugh when I try to whistle although it won't be long before I can do that.'[41]

When Henry Drew visited Hornchurch in March 1918, he found that men were treated at the massage hut or, if they could not be moved, in their beds. 'The average number of massages each week is 800, but as many as 2000 have been done in that period, which shows that the masseuses have no easy time.'[42] About 20 Almeric Paget masseuses were on the staff, but NZANS nurses Louise Brandon and Daphne Commons, under the aegis of the New Zealand Public Health Department, had started a massage course that would fit them 'for top positions in New Zealand'. By the end of the year they would be 'fully trained & certificated in massage and electricity & Swedish remedial exercises, together with special training for treatment of Infantile Paralysis'.[43]

Thurston was so impressed with the success of the treatment that she pushed for the establishment of a massage school at Hornchurch, which opened on 1 March 1918. When the first six-month course began in mid-September, four sisters and seven staff nurses were enrolled.[44]

In Thurston's view, 'Every trained Nurse should be made to take her massage, electric, remedial exercise course and in the interests and for the future success of our N.Z. Sisters every effort should be made to give them the necessary training, and to endeavor to give all vacant posts to our own women.' Thurston gave 'no encouragement' to the 'very many inquiries' she had received from English 'masseuses who are anxious to come to N.Z. for work'. She would replace the Almeric staff at Hornchurch once the New Zealanders were trained.[45] Although Hornchurch was the acknowledged massage centre, masseuses worked at other hospitals, and trained women like Dorothy Miller and Knox Anderson also brought their skills back home.[46]

Hester Maclean championed massage, both during and after the war. 'The well qualified masseuse will now find her opportunity,' she wrote in April 1918, and massage will 'take its place side by side with the trained nursing of serious medical cases'.[47] She was a prime mover in the establishment of a massage training course in 1918 for 'a number of young men not fit for active service and a number of young women'. By October that year the 30 future masseuses were attending classes at Otago University arranged by the Defence Department, which paid their fees. They would be obliged to serve for the rest of the war 'and two years after if required'. The 30 young male trainees attended lectures at Tauherenikau camp, then went to Rotorua's King George V Hospital or elsewhere to work as medical orderlies and masseurs, 'but they are for military service only, and not qualifying for the purpose of carrying on the profession of massage after the war'.[48] Maclean was determined, too, as massage training continued in Dunedin, that the practice be properly registered in New Zealand, and the Masseurs Registration Act was passed in 1920.

After the war, massage expertise was desperately needed in New Zealand — and was indispensable on the home-coming vessels. On 1 January 1919 Thurston reassured Maclean that the *Ruapehu*, about to leave for New Zealand, would be bringing Sister Ina Bennett; 'the proud possessor of both the I.S.T.M. and Medical Electricity certificates, she should be of great value to you'. On 3 April she wrote, 'On each transport now I hope to send you Sisters who have taken their massage course, as I fully realise they are much needed.'[49] As well as the massage facilities in the various military hospitals, there was an outpatient massage department in central Wellington's Brandon Street medical headquarters where, suitably, Sister Louise Brandon was assisting in April 1920 after having been charge sister of the massage department at King George V Hospital. Not long after that, however, she and Sister Maud Haste were demobilised in order to start their own massage practice in the capital. Sisters Ruby Makeig and Grace Ward, of the Chalmers massage staff, did the same in Christchurch: they 'have secured rooms and obtained necessary equipment from Defence, and intend to commence their work at once'.[50]

Just as the troops needed to be able to chew their food, so they had to be able to march, sometimes for long distances, in boots that were often far from comfortable or properly fitted. After six hours of picket duty on the *Athenic* on his way to war in October 1914, Cecil Mathus had a skinned heel. Although this 'healed nicely', he was afraid he would 'never get reconciled to those beastly misfit boots'. When stretcher-bearer Norman Gray received his boots at Awapuni in July 1915, they were 'like nothing you have ever seen. I haven't tried mine yet. I am waiting for the assistance of a crane to get them on.' The French roads did not help. 'Talk about dead beat,' Harry Hall told his sister Vera after marching with a 'full pack for 13 miles. I had new boots on — a size too big & so I suffered in consequence. Now I have 2 pairs of socks on to fill up the gaps.'[51]

Too many men were being treated for lameness, and some commanding officers were not being sufficiently careful about foot inspections. Something had to be done. At its formation in early 1916, the New Zealand Division had no trained chiropodists. When the Eighth Reinforcements were undergoing training at Trentham in 1915, a professional chiropodist, R. H. Taylor from Christchurch, was in camp training army chiropodists, who were given pouches of instruments, but no certificates, when they qualified.[52] Irish-born former grocer Robert Poots, of the Wellington Infantry regiment, was taught by Taylor and 'acted as chiropodist unofficially . . . At Armentieres carried on as chiropodist and had plenty to do.'[53]

The *Dominion* reported in September 1915 that there was to be a chiropodist at Trentham throughout the war. 'In addition to his professional duties, the officer will be required to give a certain amount of instruction.'[54] Following the appointment of Sapper, later Sergeant, Robert Seymour as a full-time chiropodist to the 2nd Brigade, and his departure with the Ninth Reinforcements along with two men 'for instruction in chiropody', the decision was taken to train one chiropodist for each battalion. Starting with the Tenth and Eleventh, each reinforcement draft would train two men per 1000, who would then sail with their draft, giving lectures to the men during the voyage.[55]

As well as teaching and lecturing on foot care, the conscientious and hard-working Taylor, who had been appointed chief chiropodist at Trentham, was responsible, with others, for attending to the feet of the men in camp. This was no small task. During the week ending 7 October 1916, for example, 185 soldiers needed treatment for everything from flat feet to hammer toes.[56] In a February 1917 article, a *Dominion* reporter paid tribute to the busy Trentham chiropodists' hut, under the trees. 'Blisters which, to the civilian mind, would seem to debar further marching, were treated and bandaged skilfully, so that the soldier could walk without feeling them at all, and every man was made fit for the road, and was keen for the moment to arrive to be off again.'[57] Dutch-born Corneles Zeven, who had been a surgical chiropodist in Auckland before the war, would serve at Trentham. Featherston, too, had a camp chiropodist, with, from 1916, his own purpose-built office.[58]

There was also on-the-spot chiropody teaching in France. The first three-week school was run at Armentières, in the chemical lab of the technical school, from the end of June 1916, with Captain Neil Guthrie of No. 3 Field Ambulance in charge and Seymour working as his assistant. Eighteen men, sent from each battalion, were taught the basic principles of antisepsis and surgical cleanliness along with 'some elementary knowledge of the various deformities of the feet that lead to bad marching, and the modification in the boot necessary to relieve such conditions as flat foot, metatarsalgia [a painful inflammation of the ball of the foot] and other deformities'.[59] Attached to the school were boot menders and cobblers, plus a clinic that offered 'ample teaching material' in the form of some 400 men with bad feet. Each of the 14 students who made the grade returned to their battalions with a box of instruments 'and did some good work during the marches to the Somme'. Such skills were definitely needed — in just one week in early September 1916, 45 men were sent to the CCS with foot injuries caused by marching — and specialists were appreciated. As a private wrote late in 1916, 'The dentists are experts, and the chiropodists are absolutely out on their own.'[60]

A second chiropody school held at No. 3 New Zealand Field Ambulance in Estaires, for three weeks from 12 December 1916, was motivated by the increasing occurrence of trench foot. William Smallfield was selected for the third course in January 1917, at which Poots was an instructor. Along with men like Smallfield, chosen from various battalions, two NZMC nursing orderlies from each field ambulance attended. Their 'marked aptitude for the work' made them an asset when they returned to their usual roles. 'We receive lectures every morning, and have to take enormous notes,' Smallfield recorded on 15 January 1917. 'The first part of the course is the general physiology of the body, and the second specialises in feet.' The afternoons brought interesting 'practical demonstrations when patients are being treated by the M.O. . . . My slight knowledge of physiology has been already of great service in helping me to follow the Major, and it is quite a treat to listen to an educated man lecturing.' As well as the long and 'fairly stiff' exam, there was a practical test in diagnosing and treating a patient. Back in the trenches, Smallfield was delighted to be handed, on 10 February, a certificate of efficiency in chiropody, and to learn that he was the only man in the brigade who had passed, with 82 per cent. He was keen for chiropody work 'when there is an opening'.[61] Another divisional chiropody school was held in September 1917.

A chiropodist could not always help, however. 'Underside of heels very sore,' wrote Jim Currie at Armentières in June 1916. 'Got some Condy's crystals and bathed feet. A medical chap painted them with iodine. Will have to go sick to-morrow with them.' Currie's feet were dressed next day by the battalion chiropodist, but when he reported sick again the following morning, the verdict was, 'I am afraid that you will have to make the best of a bad job.' With his feet well wrapped in bandages, Currie found the last part of the day's march, on cobblestone roads, 'very trying'. A 20-mile march after 'months in the slush and mud' caused blisters for Ormond Burton and his companions in March 1918. 'I went over all the feet of my platoon that night with boracic, iodine and in many cases applied bandages and cotton wool.'[62]

The biggest challenge on the Western Front, however, was trench foot. In this ubiquitous affliction, which the French christened pieds gêlés — frozen feet — 'Feet first went numb, then started to burn, turned red and blue and swelled up, making the wearing of boots more intolerable than ever.'[63] Along with volatile temperature changes and badly fitting boots, wet socks were the chief cause, and the men had strict orders to remove these daily and replace them with dry socks after rubbing their feet with odorous whale oil. Claude Weston recalled the 'familiar sight [of] the "sock men" trudging down the communication trenches with their sacks on their backs'.[64] But the rules could not always be followed: 'On the Somme they didn't take their socks off, for 21 days, some of them.' By September 1917 Sergeant Tom Lane of the New Zealand Rifle Brigade, who had missed out on fresh socks during 10 days on the front line, had no feeling at all in his feet. He was eventually taken to an English hospital in Rouen

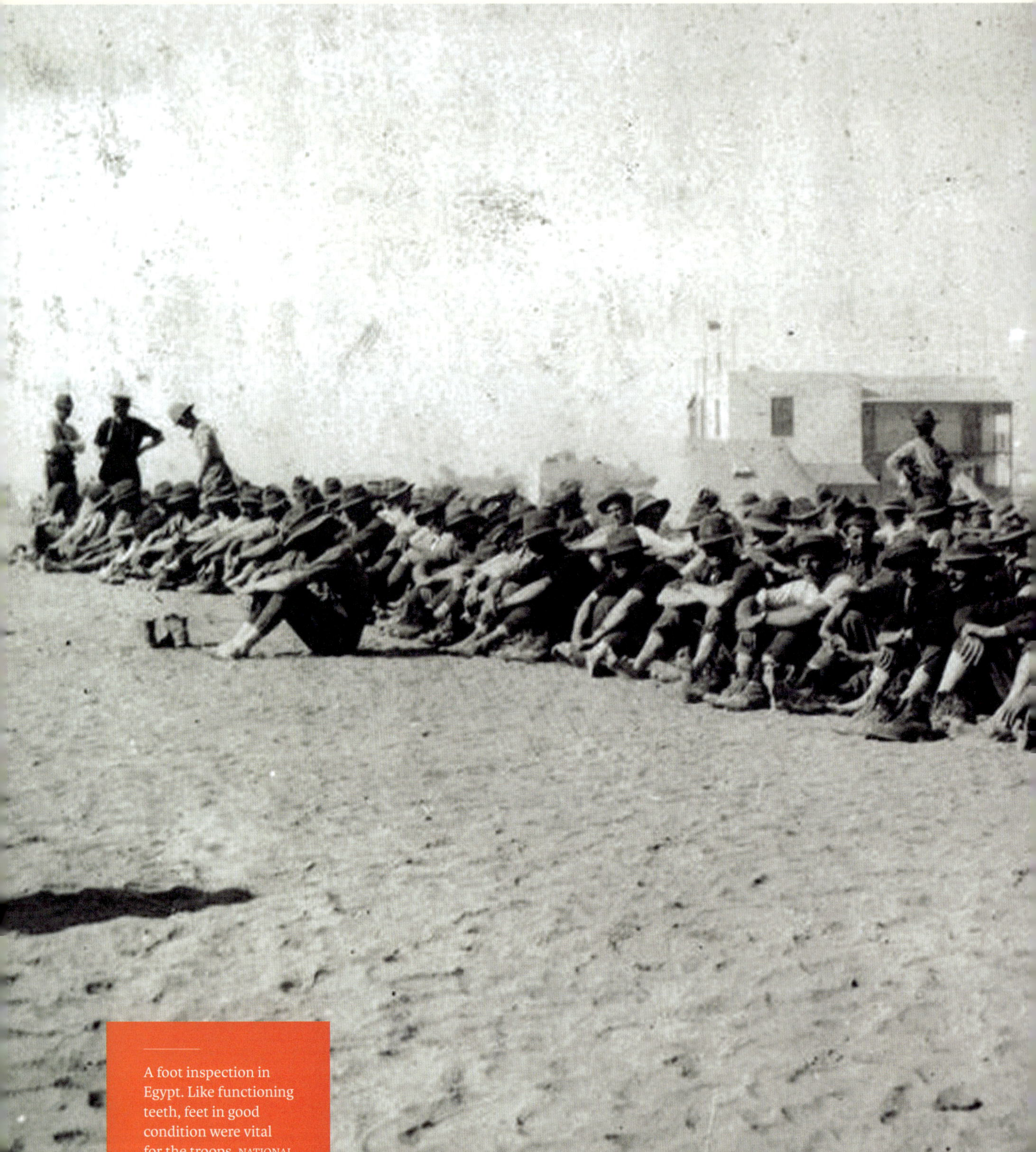

A foot inspection in Egypt. Like functioning teeth, feet in good condition were vital for the troops. NATIONAL ARMY MUSEUM, 1992.1149

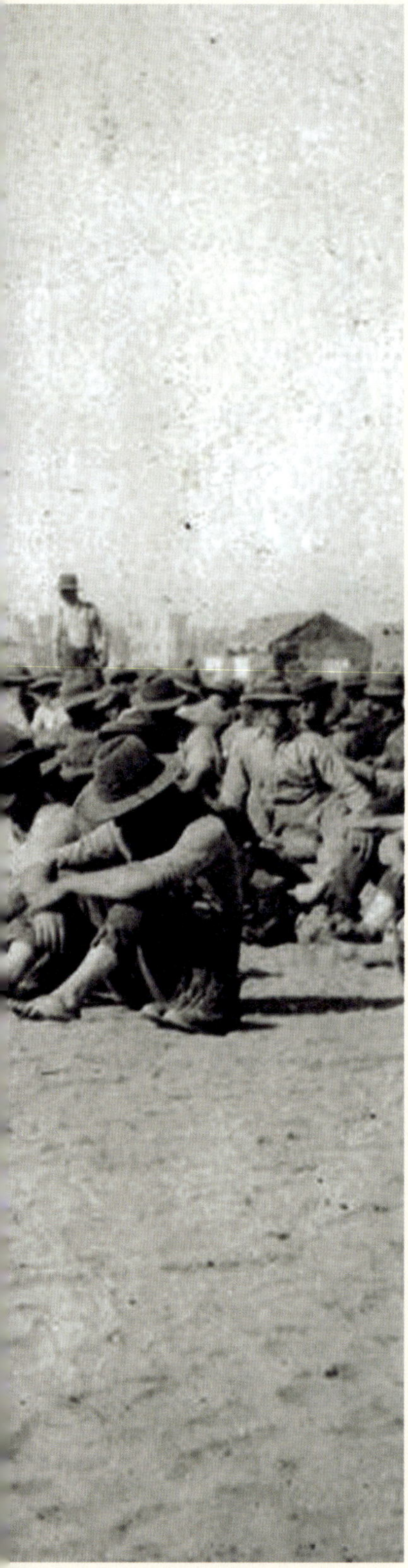

where they were bandaged with boiling hot boracic lint every two hours. 'Then the pus broke out at the ankles [by now black]. The swelling went down as the pus came out. The smell was terrible. The nurses always came with a mask on.'[65] Precautions such as duckboards over the treacherous mud and water, better drainage and the issuing of rubber thigh-boots did help, but the ghastly conditions at Passchendaele caused a resurgence of trench foot. Late in 1917, at Charles Begg's urging, the method used by the French army was instituted: washing the feet with camphor soap and dusting them with camphor borax powder before putting on fresh socks.[66]

It also became clear at Passchendaele that the wet, constricting puttees wound around the men's lower legs were not helping — an order on 11 October asked officers to ensure that medics removed the wounded's puttees and loosened their bootlaces.[67] There had already been concern. In August 1916 the *Evening Post* had described the puttee as 'in some respects a dangerous article of wear for the trenches, since it is apt to restrict the circulation, and this renders the feet cold, with consequent liability to chilblains, frostbite, and the pedal infirmity known as trench foot'. But putting on a puttee loosely meant 'the warmth of the roll is reduced, and damp strikes through and is liable to cause rheumatism'. Should puttees even be worn in the line? 'It was frequently observed in advanced medical posts that the puttees of the wounded were very tight and that the feet were visibly swollen, even with the boots on.'[68]

Military chiropodists did not necessarily have an easy life. Their work was voluntary, done in their own time — their British army counterparts were paid extra — 'and in no way absolved them from other duties in the trenches'. Because it made no economic sense to train men working in this manner, the best that could be offered was to avoid, if possible, 'repeated losses by battle casualty of the trained chiropodists employed on other work'. Nor did the New Zealand regulations allow for chiropodists to be promoted. Later, the battalion chiropodist, with defined duties, became a 'whole time member of the regimental medical detachment', but until then he had in some cases acted as corporal medical orderly.[69] Robert Poots was filling such a role at Messines on 8 June 1917 when, 'under particularly heavy shell fire' and with 'unflagging energy', he 'rendered most valuable assistance' at his battalion's RAP at Boyle's Farm. The next night, when six soldiers were wounded at the crossroads near Blauwe Molen, and again with shells falling all around him, Poots headed out to tend to them. When the fire proved too intense, 'he removed each of these men to a place of safety and dressed their wounds'.[70] His bravery earned him a Military Medal.

Chiropodists were injured and killed. At Messines, in 1917, one had a very close call when an RAP was hit by a German HE shell and four of the seven men there were killed. The doctor and the other survivors, who seized shovels in the hope that some men had been buried alive, came upon a steel helmet and heard a faint voice calling, 'I can't breathe; don't trouble; I'm all in.' They dug vigorously, scraping the earth away from his head and allowing him to breathe properly, and 'presently recognised the Chiropodist! There had very nearly been a slump in chiropody.'[71] Rifleman John Barrett was killed in action on 4 October 1918, not long after being trained at Sling as a chiropodist.

The wounded and sick needed drugs and the NZMC needed men with a reasonable level of literacy and numeracy, if not pharmaceutical knowledge, to supply these safely and responsibly. Dispensers, as the military called them, served with field ambulances, on hospital ships, in headquarters and in hospitals. Four hundred and ninety men with a pharmacy qualification or background enlisted — their absence caused some New Zealand pharmacies to close for lack of expertise — but only some made use of their skills during the war.[72] Chemist's apprentice Leslie Butler, who served with No. 4 Field Ambulance, recalled that one wartime dispensary in France was 'in the charge of a staff-sergeant whose assistant had been a plumber in civilian life, while apprentices and assistant-pharmacists were the stretcher-bearers'.[73] Terminology was problematical. The terms chemist, pharmacist, pharmaceutical chemist and dispenser (sometimes prefixed by 'qualified') were all used, often loosely and/or interchangeably. There was confusion about roles and qualifications, and dissatisfaction regarding rank.

As Wanganui pharmacy manager Bromley Hill explained in a letter to the *Dominion* in June 1916, a civilian dispenser was qualified only after a three-year apprenticeship under a registered pharmaceutical chemist. 'That is according to the law.'[74] He, and other pharmacists, were unconvinced that the authorities and the defence minister understood the need for proper training in this specialist role, or were aware of the subtleties of the different terms. On 22 July 1915, 'Chemist' of Wellington had complained that the dispenser role on the *Maheno*'s recent maiden voyage had gone to 'a man without any qualifications whatever' rather than 'a young man who left a good position to enlist,

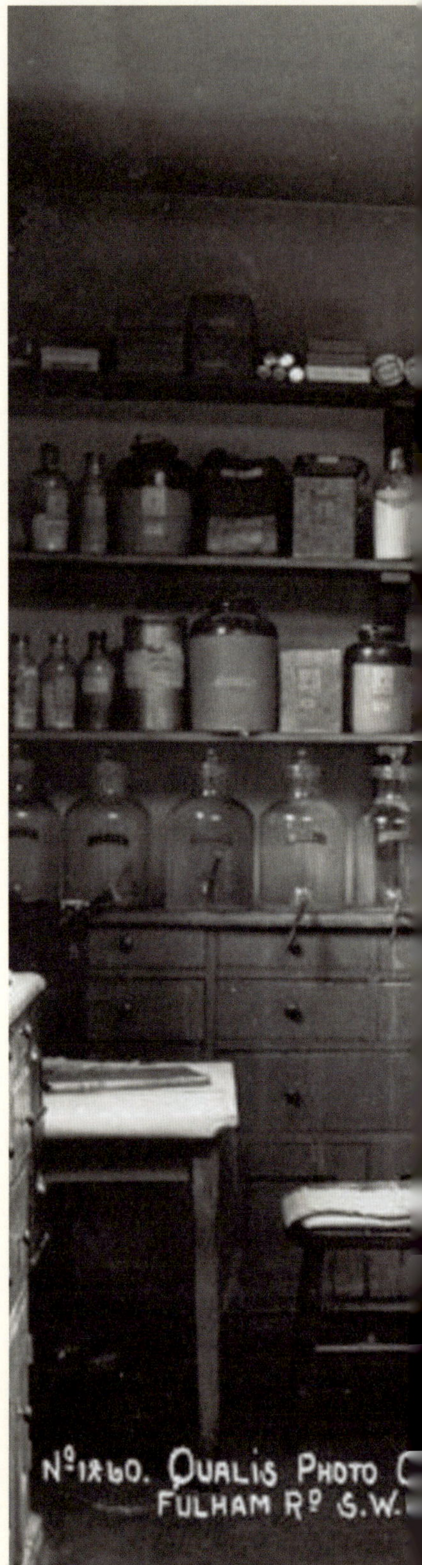

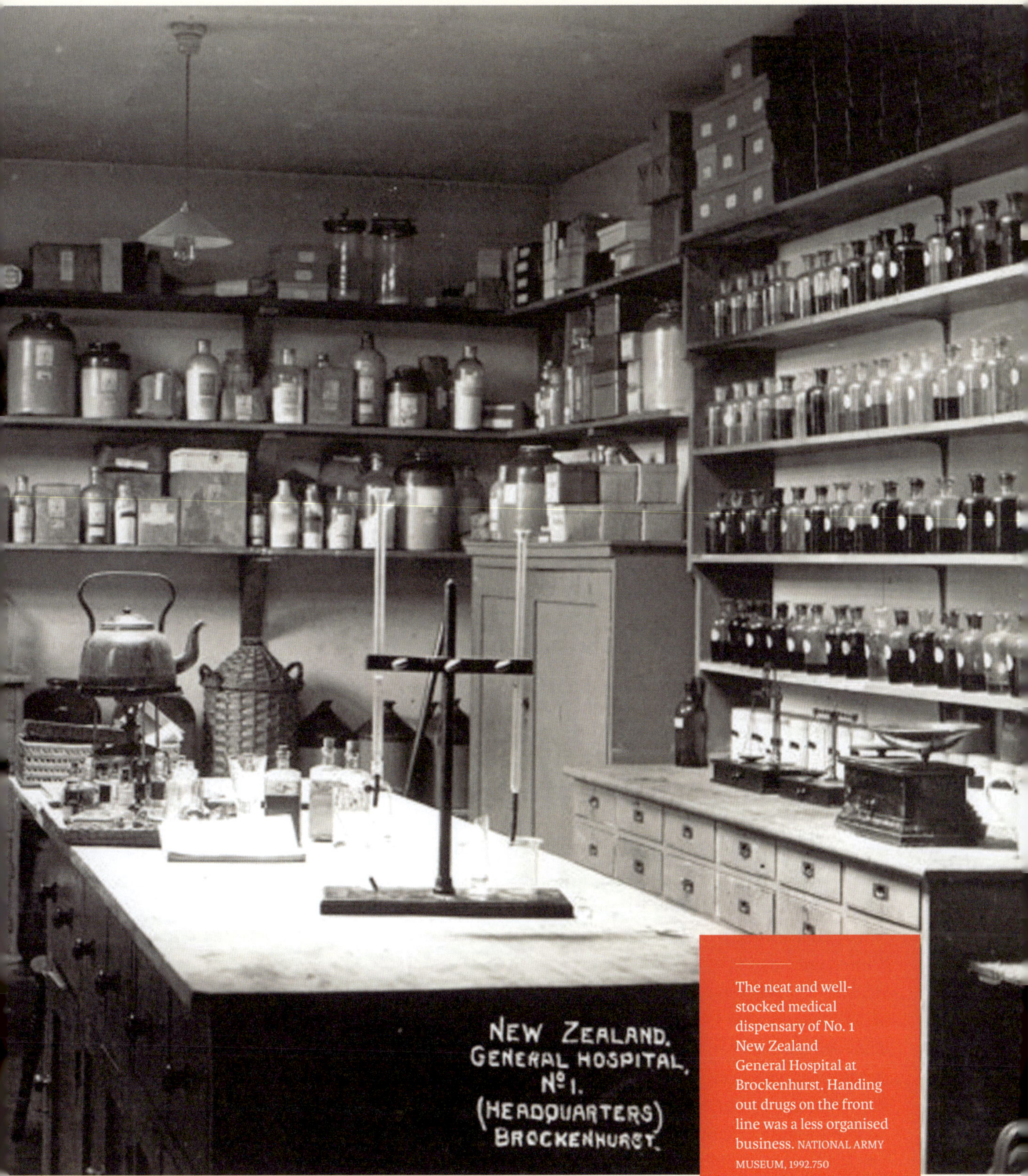

The neat and well-stocked medical dispensary of No. 1 New Zealand General Hospital at Brockenhurst. Handing out drugs on the front line was a less organised business. NATIONAL ARMY MUSEUM, 1992.750

being led to believe by the authorities that he would be appointed'. The editor assured readers that, according to James Allen, a qualified dispenser had been chosen. In fact, two dispensers travelled on the ship.[75] In Hill's view, Allen's mention of the 'medical training' provided at Awapuni for future NZMC dispensers confirmed the minister's misapprehension: 'all the experience they gain at Palmerston is very, very harmless'.[76] As historian Lea Doughty has noted, the Defence Department, basing its approach on the much less testing British model, failed to understand the degree of education pharmacists required in order to attain qualification and, therefore, registration.[77]

Rank was a problem too: sergeant was the highest available for dispensers in the NZMC. At Pont de Koubbeh, with its 1000 beds, qualified pharmacists, acting as dispensers, were only corporals or sergeants, which made them subordinate to both dentists and nurses. As another correspondent, 'Pharmacist', wrote, 'The position of a dispenser in a large hospital is highly important . . . [He] is capable of relieving doctors of much routine work in hospitals, and his services are being increasingly used for this purpose. Why, then should all New Zealand pharmacists on active service be refused commissions?'[78]

As far as the military was concerned, dispensers did not need to be qualified pharmacists; they merely had to 'pass a basic exam showing they could dispense medicines out of the right bottle'.[79] Such minimally trained men might have no idea what was in the tablets they were handing out, since these were supplied ready-made, numbered for different uses and kept in a compartmentalised tin 'to discourage theft and self-medication'.[80] The most infamous was the ubiquitous No. 9 Pill, a compound of rhubarb, colocynth and calomel that was used as a laxative but also widely dispensed for a variety of ills. In Douglas Stark's view, 'Number nines were used to cure the troops of headaches, heartache, stomach-ache, malingering, laziness, cuts, scabies, shell-shock, and dysentery, and on the whole acted fairly well.'[81] These cure-alls bequeathed their name to the bingo call, 'Number nine, doctor's orders.'

There was also the risk of mistakes, which could have fatal consequences. 'Vigil', writing to the *Dominion* in September 1916, was concerned about 'our soldiers' well-being and protection from misadventure . . . The handling of drugs and chemicals, compounded or otherwise, in permanent military hospitals would certainly be best left to the responsibility of a properly qualified pharmacist, and not to an incompetent, inexperienced lance-jack [lance-corporal].'[82] Doughty has evidence of deaths caused by unqualified men dispensing the wrong drugs. One soldier died when given strychnine instead of quinine.[83]

Dispensers worked both at home, in the military camps, and overseas. Former Timaru UFS [United Friendly Society] Dispensary manager and partner in the Ashburton Drug Company, William Chappell, was appointed to take charge of the new dispensary at Trentham camp late in 1915.[84] He later sailed as a sergeant dispenser on the fifth charter of the *Maheno*. George Hards, who worked for a chemist and then at the internment camp on Somes Island for the Defence Department, was made dispenser to the New Zealand auxiliary base hospital in Alexandria in December 1915 and left on the *Marama* that month to take up his new role.[85] Service in the Middle East often caused sickness. Douglas McKenzie, who had started his apprenticeship in 1911 but was not qualified, became a dispenser at the ANZAC sick quarters at Moascar in Egypt before serving with the Mounted Field Ambulance. He was plagued by illness. Eventually, in July 1918, a medical board decreed 'debility foll. neurasthenia': 'Patient has lost great deal of Condition. From 9st 2lbs to 7 st 6lbs. Shaking hands tremulous . . . heart rapid 120 per min.' A 'Change to New Zealand' was recommended and McKenzie came home.[86]

The New Zealand hospitals in Britain had NZMC dispensers on their staffs. They included James Watson, formerly of Wellington Hospital, who took charge of the dispensary at Hornchurch, and Frederick Dolphin from Palmerston North, who served in France with No. 2 New Zealand Field Ambulance before doing dispenser duty at Codford 'in connection with venereal patients'.[87]

The *Maheno* embarked on her first voyage in July 1915 with two dispensers among her medical staff: Staff Sergeant Walter Hall and Corporal Bertrand Donaldson, who would also travel on the third charter.[88] The former had been working for a chemist in the capital before he enlisted and served in Samoa. He was dispenser on the *Marama*'s second charter and by the end of 1917 a member of the medical section of the Thirty-third Reinforcements. Hall committed suicide in June 1923. He had been drinking for years and had become addicted to drugs. As the coroner said, the case was 'a very sad one'.[89]

When the *Tahiti* left New Zealand in October 1915, her sergeant dispenser was Adolph McLennan, who was perhaps understandably better known as Barney. Fellow field ambulance man Norman Gray shared his cabin. McLennan, who had been working for a Wanganui chemist before the war, would go on to win the Military Medal and bar. When he enlisted, his superior in the Territorials described him as 'a first rate ambulance man and also very good in drill', but McLennan had other talents. On the *Tahiti* he proved to be 'on very good terms with some of the Bakers and we manage to get pastry, shortbread and sponge cake for supper sometimes'.[90]

Working as a dispenser on a hospital ship or a transport was no sinecure. As one man explained, 'I . . . have had to do nursing and dressing as well. We are kept busy at times 20 hours out of the 24. Still, it is a labour of love, and I know I am doing my little bit to alleviate suffering.'[91] When influenza notoriously struck the Fortieth Reinforcements on the *Tahiti* in 1918, the dispenser was 'a non-commissioned officer with two years' experience of transport work, and very efficient'. He, too, succumbed, 'through fever and overwork'.[92]

Extra duties for seagoing dispensers could sometimes be unexpected. Reginald Fear, who had run his own chemist/optician business in Wellington, left with the Main Body as a sergeant dispenser, but, owing to a shortage of doctors, was ordered to take temporary charge as acting medical officer of 'a big transport in the Mediterranean'. 'I don't know how many men there are to assist me,' he told his family. 'I don't think it altogether fitting that I should take over so many different responsible positions as I have done since leaving New Zealand on a sergeant's rank and pay, do you? However, I don't mind, as it is a great experience, and it's war time, you know. I suppose I am to consider myself honoured in being given such responsible duties. I guess it's the first instance on record of such a step being taken.'[93]

When Sam McWilliams, who had worked for pharmaceutical manufacturer Kempthorne Prosser in Wellington before the war, wrote home to friends from Gallipoli on 15 July 1915, he was 'dispensing strong medicine for the Turks'. After the 25 April landing he had been on hospital ship duty for a few weeks. 'By Jove, we put through a few cases, and some nasty ones at that.' On one trip to Alexandria he was assistant dispenser. Back on the peninsula, he had been at the beach dressing station and clearing hospital, and then the ADS next to the firing line. 'We work right to the trenches.' He had also discovered that pharmaceutical knowledge could have surprising benefits.

> We do our own cooking, and one chemist's assistant here made some scones the other day. Asked what he used for baking powder, he told me in confidence he used 20 grains soda bicarb, and 20 grains of bismuth subnit. (a mixture that would have much the same effect as a seidlitz powder [a laxative and digestion medication]). It would certainly cause an effervescence. The scones rose all right. Rather ingenious, eh? If the scones were indigestible, he gave 3½ grains of bismuth to digest them.[94]

Lance-Corporal George (Sonny) Skerrett (Ngāi Tahu), who left with the Main Body, had begun a chemist apprenticeship but was a labourer in Bluff when he joined the Otago Infantry Battalion in August 1914. When Jack Gilchrist died on the *Ruapehu*, Skerrett took over as dispenser.[95] He landed on Gallipoli on 25 April and was 'at his post continually' until falling dangerously ill in September. 'We are having a sorry time of it,' he had told his parents, 'and if this lasts much longer I am afraid we shall all be knocked out as the strain and want of sleep is terrible.' A friend who had returned to New Zealand told of last seeing Skerrett 'in the field bare headed and his sleeves rolled up to the armpits assisting Captain Baigent . . . to attend to the wounded and dying on the Gallipoli Peninsula'.[96] Also on Gallipoli was Private Frank Histed, who had been working as an apprentice for a Queen Street chemist in Auckland. After a month at the Egyptian Army Hospital in Cairo as assistant dispenser, 'he was picked to go to Ismailia, after the Suez fight, to assist in the nursing of the wounded Turks'. Histed landed on the peninsula on the third day and 'had many narrow escapes' during his four months in a dressing station 200 yards behind the firing line.[97]

Lance-Corporal Thomas Hill, the son of a Cambridge chemist, was working in his father's shop when the war broke out. He was dispenser to surgeon George Craig on Gallipoli where, after several months in the firing line, he was struck by a bomb on the back of the neck. He then had an appendectomy, followed by an attack of pneumonia. After some time in hospital, he returned to New Zealand in April 1916.[98] Also wounded on the peninsula, in October, was Hamilton chemist's assistant Corporal John Kelly, with the Wellington Infantry Battalion, who had been a dispenser at Lady Godley's Convalescent Home in Cairo.[99]

Some NZMC dispensers later chose more active service. Neale Eagar, who was a sergeant dispenser at Pont de Koubbeh and served on the *Willochra* and the *Maheno*, joined the Royal Flying Corps in April 1917. He would die of exposure in the Sinai in 1920 while serving with 14 Squadron RAF. After working as a dispenser in Cairo for some time, Richard Wade from Invercargill asked to be transferred to the Otago Infantry Battalion;[100] he was shot twice in the right hand. Cyril McHardie from Palmerston North served as a sergeant dispenser at the Luxor Convalescent Home from February to June 1916, when he began officer training. He joined the Wellington Infantry Battalion and died at the Somme on 22 May 1918.[101]

Some trained men returned to their pre-war role after being wounded. Qualified chemist Sergeant Richard Dowling suffered from sickness in Egypt and was then wounded twice on Gallipoli. When apparently recovered, he became a dispenser at Hornchurch, then Codford, before being invalided home on the *Maheno* in 1916, suffering from 'neurasthenia and vertigo'. A sadder story lay behind the bare facts, as the findings of a September 1916 medical board at Codford revealed. Under the heading 'Present Condition' were these words: 'Is very nervous and melancholic. Unable to concentrate his mind on his duties. He gets very nervous about the smallest detail and is frightened about dispensing drugs wrongly. Is lethargic and sleeps very easily but has troubled dreams.'[102] Dowling made it home, but some NZMC dispensers did not. Jack Gilchrist lost his life on the *Ruapehu* in 1914 and Private Frederick Bowell died at sea on 13 February 1917 while returning as an invalid on the *Marama*.

Because Defence personnel records usually lack any details about a man's role within the NZMC, it can be difficult to ascertain whether qualified chemists served as such in wartime. For instance, James Bird and Victor Charles Rhodes, two of the 22 NZMC men who drowned when the *Marquette* was torpedoed on 23 October 1915, were chemists before enlisting, but it is not certain if they were dispensers for No. 1 New Zealand Stationary Hospital.[103] Of the nine members of the Pharmaceutical Society killed in the First World War, only one, Cyril McHardie, is definitely known to have been an NZMC dispenser.[104]

Although several women were employed in hospital pharmacies in New Zealand during the war, hardly any managed to serve their country overseas.[105] One exception was the wife of surgeon William Porteous, who was serving in France with the NZMC. A qualified dispenser, Edith Porteous was appointed to a position at Walton-on-Thames.[106] Ever since she and her two little daughters had arrived in England, the Association of Women Pharmacists had repeatedly asked her to take on such a task, but the long hours and need to leave the children had deterred her. 'The urgency for women taking up men's jobs has so increased, and the need for chemists is so great, that on being asked to become the dispenser at this hospital, I felt I must try.' A soldier's wife was looking after the girls and Porteous was 'hoping that the plan will work well. There seems little likelihood of Dr. Porteous being free for some time, so that I shall be glad to do my little "bit" while he is doing his.'[107]

One 26-year-old Auckland woman tried very hard to serve her country, offering herself three times as either an assistant dispenser on a hospital ship or an ambulance driver. As well as being 'physically strong and well', she had six years' experience as a dispenser, a certificate with honours in first-aid work and 'considerable practical experience in dressing wounds'. She was also 'used to driving a 20-horse-power motor-car, and had done repairs and vulcanising'. If she was unsuccessful again, she requested 'an exemption badge', as many friends asked why she had not enlisted, 'and she felt very keenly about it'. In reply, the authorities referred to 'regulations not permitting the enlistment of women' and expressed 'much regret . . . that the lady's exceptional qualifications could not be availed of'. To add patronising salt to the wound, they suggested that 'ladies in the same position as the applicant could help the recruiting campaign by influencing eligible men to enlist'.[108]

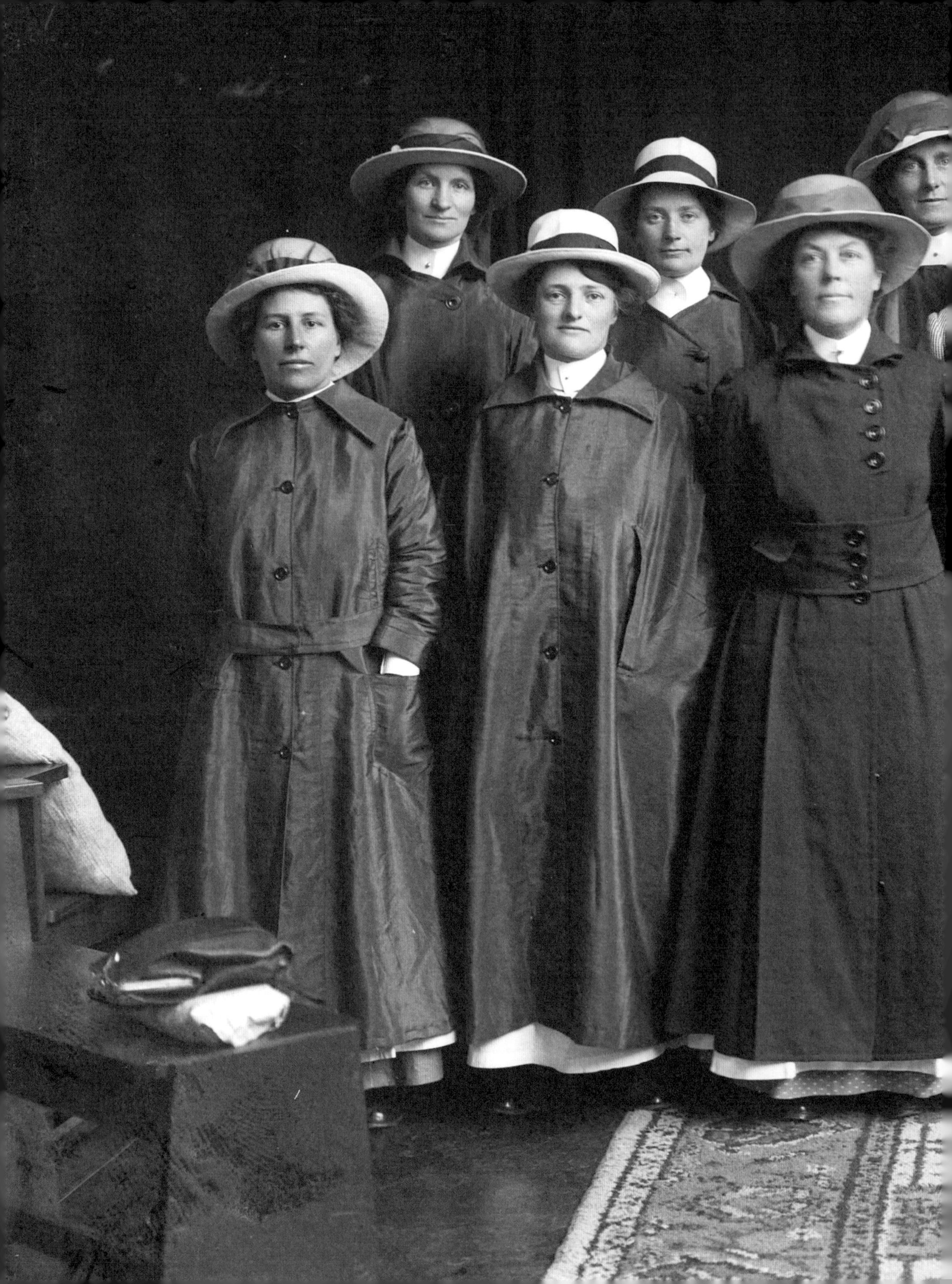

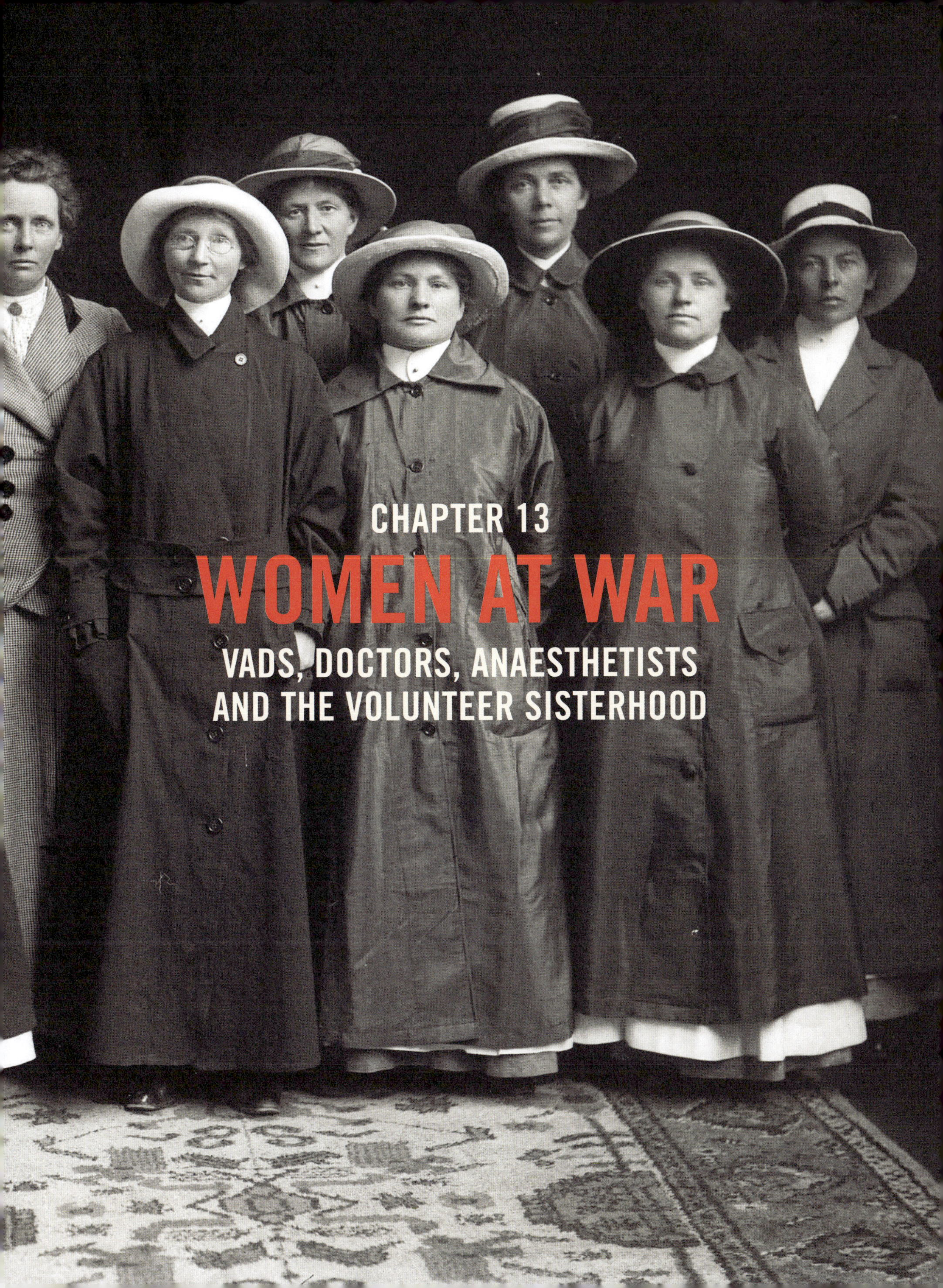

CHAPTER 13

WOMEN AT WAR

VADS, DOCTORS, ANAESTHETISTS AND THE VOLUNTEER SISTERHOOD

previous pages
A hatless Ettie Rout is surrounded by panamas when she is photographed with the first New Zealand Volunteer Sisters to go overseas in October 1915. On either side of her are Marion Higgens and Agnes Kerr (with glasses); Dora Murch is at the far right of the front row. The third, fourth and fifth women from the left in the back row are Emily Leggatt, Ada Ballantine and Eileen Neilson.
ALEXANDER TURNBULL LIBRARY, 1/1-014727-G

The women in war must hold nothing back.

— *Press*, 17 October 1914

'Hitherto, the untrained voluntary aid has been the eleventh plague in Egypt . . . [T]hey are not, as a body, a brilliant success. Individuals are beyond praise in their unselfish, unpaid work in convalescent hospitals. But girls are girls!' These words appeared in the gossip column of the *Free Lance* in April 1916. In August that year, Godley wrote to ADMS William Parkes in England: 'I see that you are talking of taking on V.A.D.s. If you do, be sure that they are good ones, and be careful that they do not get mixed up with the officers in any way.'[1] These statements reveal the all too frequent attitudes to female VADs — members of the British Voluntary Aid Detachment — who served in a variety of roles during the war. The Voluntary Aid scheme had been established by the War Office in 1909, and because of the nature of the work, such as performing domestic duties in hospitals, most recruits were female. When war broke out, assisting with nursing work appealed to large numbers of young British women not at all suited to the horrors of military medicine. There were many extremely competent exceptions, most famously Vera Brittain, but because VADs were untrained, and because some proved less than serious about their work, they were often patronised by men, who bestowed such nicknames as 'Very Adorable Darlings'.[2]

Enthusiastic society ladies could indeed be a liability. As MO Alexander Trotter observed on 7 May 1915, while 'every trained nurse in Egypt is being worked overtime . . . a lot of fashionable women with low necked dresses, earrings etc, are doing an hour or so a day. Many of these are quite useless and many have got tired of it already.'[3] Even serious and dedicated VADs could initially find medical work a shock. On her first day, the woman who did Eric Burnett's dressings at Pont de Koubbeh 'was either very excited or frightfully nervous . . . her hands were shaking so much that she could hardly hold the bandages. She told me afterwards that in the hospital at Alexandria . . . she used to do only orderly work such as looking after gift stuff, sorting clothing, mending and things like that.'[4]

Both British and New Zealand VADs worked in the New Zealand hospitals, and sometimes individuals let the side down. In August 1917, the acting matron of No. 1 New Zealand General Hospital was forced to dismiss two VADs for 'unsatisfactory behaviour'. One was 'seen embracing a patient in hospital clothes in the street' while the other, despite a warning, had 'been reported for coming in late and for unseemly behaviour with men . . . when in her uniform'. As David Wylie, Brockenhurst's OC, pointed out, 'Conduct of this kind cannot but reflect adversely upon V.A.D.s and is felt very keenly by many . . . doing duty here.'[5] Occasionally the work was just too much, despite the best of intentions. In May 1918 E. Hanson begged to resign from VAD work at Brockenhurst 'owing to attacks of nausea . . . Having tried in three consecutive hospitals I find it impossible to continue nursing.'[6]

Perhaps inevitably, trained nurses were cautious about VADs. They could represent a challenge or a threat, and their sometimes more frivolous image could cause exasperation and invite scorn.[7] They were often criticised in letters and could face unkindness and impatience in the wards. In her *Kai Tiaki* editorial for October 1915, Hester Maclean noted that in some British military hospitals VADs were doing 'excellent work', acting as probationers — 'being frequently women of high intelligence, [they] very quickly become of the greatest service'. There was a qualification, however: 'It is only when the women . . . wish to take the work which nurses only should do, that they are not an advantage.'[8]

New Zealand nurse Clare Jordan, running a small British Red Cross hospital early in the war, concurred. She and another sister were 'wholly and solely in charge of the patients', but VADs from the local village came in to do housework and other domestic duties. 'We are most fortunate to have fallen in with sensible people who don't imagine that . . . they understand all about nursing. They never even venture a suggestion about the patients, and never grant any requests without consulting us.'[9] As they proved their worth, though, many VADs won the nurses' admiration. Bertha Taylor decided that those 'who do nothing but scrub floors and general cleaning' deserved recognition, 'for they are quite often gifted women who have not been used to doing such work'. At Brockenhurst in 1916 Edna Pengelly was willing to give praise where it was due for Otago sisters Elizabeth Stewart and Agnes Herbert: 'they do so much for the men and are a real help in every way'.[10] VADs made a significant wartime contribution, often performing tasks as testing, and as skilled, as those done by the nurses.

As the war ground on, and patient numbers increased, more VADs were required to replace male orderlies sent to work at the front.[11] In its October 1916 editorial, *Kai Tiaki* noted an appeal from the British VAD 'for selected women from the Colonies and Dominions'. Because New Zealand did not have its own VAD scheme, any response would have to be private, by women already living in Britain or able to travel there independently. If any 'suitable women' wished to go, they would probably 'obtain work as orderlies and ward workers'.[12] Mabel Thurston was not, however, short of VADs for the New Zealand hospitals. 'So far,' she noted in January 1917, 'I have had no trouble finding all the V.A.D. help I require and this principally from N.Z. girls already in this country with their parents or friends and the wives of officers who gladly fill in [for] the few months that their husbands are away.'[13] As she wrote at the end of the year, with these women, 'ladies [who] have arrived during the war' and others from the VAD headquarters at Devonshire House in London, 'to whom we can apply to fill any vacancies', she had plenty of help. 'I therefore suggest that no more ladies be sent from N.Z.'[14]

A New Zealand woman wishing to work as a 'VAD nursing assistant' had to sign a contract for 12 months or the duration of the war, whichever was the lesser: 'I offer and agree to serve at home [Britain] in any Military Hospital to which I may be posted.' There was a one-month probation period. The pay was 20s a week and there was an allowance of £4 towards the regulation VAD uniform. This contract could be renewed for six months at a time.[15]

Among the New Zealanders who worked as VADs in Britain were Ethel Hirst and Gladys Luxford. Hirst went to England with her mother Marion in 1916 so they could be closer to her brother Ben, who was serving in France. Ethel Hirst worked hard for the New Zealand War Contingent canteen at Hornchurch before transferring to the Kia Ora Club at Brockenhurst and then taking on ward duties at Walton. When Ben Hirst died of pleurisy in May 1918, mother and daughter returned to Auckland, where Ethel toiled at a convalescent home during the November flu epidemic.[16] When John Luxford went to Walton-on-Thames as chaplain, he sent for his wife and daughter, who was desperate to become 'a very small cog in the big military machine that was functioning to win World War One'. Gladys Luxford began by waiting on tables in the nurses' mess room, but was, against her parents' objections, promoted to work for Sister Emily Nutsey in Ward 5. (Each 36-bed ward was staffed by three sisters and five VADs.) Two deaths on her first morning, and three on her second, were a harsh initiation, but Luxford was eager to learn and quickly became practised, and gentle, at dressing wounds. Like many VADs and nurses, she also contributed in her spare time: half a day off per week and one and a half days once a month. When a convoy was due, she would hitch a ride to the station in an ambulance and help to distribute cups of cocoa to the arriving wounded. English VADs also offered hospitality in their own homes.[17]

VADs were needed not only in the wards, but also as cooks, dispensers, clerks and drivers. Females behind the wheel were still a novelty. 'We have a woman driver for the ambulance, Miss Pearce,' Edna Pengelly recorded at Brockenhurst on 26 July 1916.[18] This was Agnes Pearce, from Wellington, who would later marry NZMC surgeon Duncan Stout. 'The Misses Agnes Pearce and [Violet] Bell [also from Wellington] are driving motors in connection with hospitals, and doing splendid work,' the *Evening Post* reported in September 1916. 'Apparently their hours on duty are very considerable, as they may be called out at any time, early or late.'[19] Pengelly was less sure about the 'two lady ambulance drivers thrust upon us' at Codford in May 1917, though she had to admit that one of them, a Mrs Mathias from Wellington, was 'a very nice woman'.[20]

Twenty-two-year-old Deborah Taylor was employed at Brockenhurst as a 'Chaffeuse, New Zealand Voluntary Aid Detachment/New Zealand Army Service Corps, Mechanical Transport' — in other words an ambulance driver — from August 1916 until her return to New Zealand in May 1918. She transported hundreds of wounded men to and from the hospital in vehicles that she maintained herself.[21] On 31 January 1917 she noted in her diary: 'We went to the station & then I went to Balmer Lawn & worked on the Ford . . . I tightened up the steering & cleaned the sparking plug.' She also collected food orders, ferried padres and medical staff, and took patients and nurses for drives. But the wounded were her top priority. 'We were up all last night,' she wrote on 10 June, 'about 198 came in in two convoys. One at 11.30, & one at 4 AM . . .

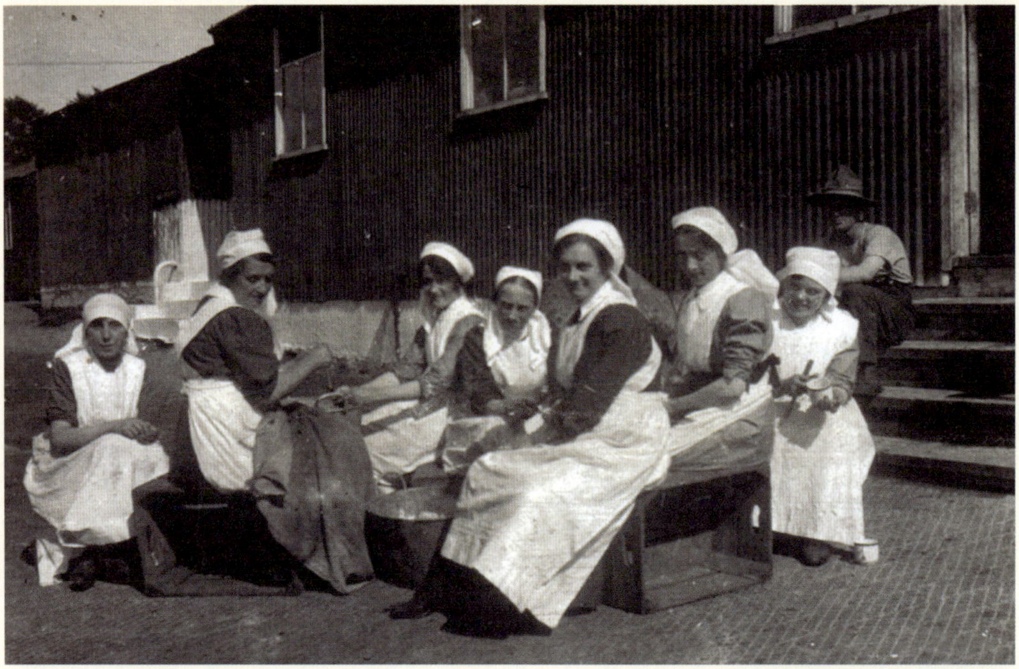

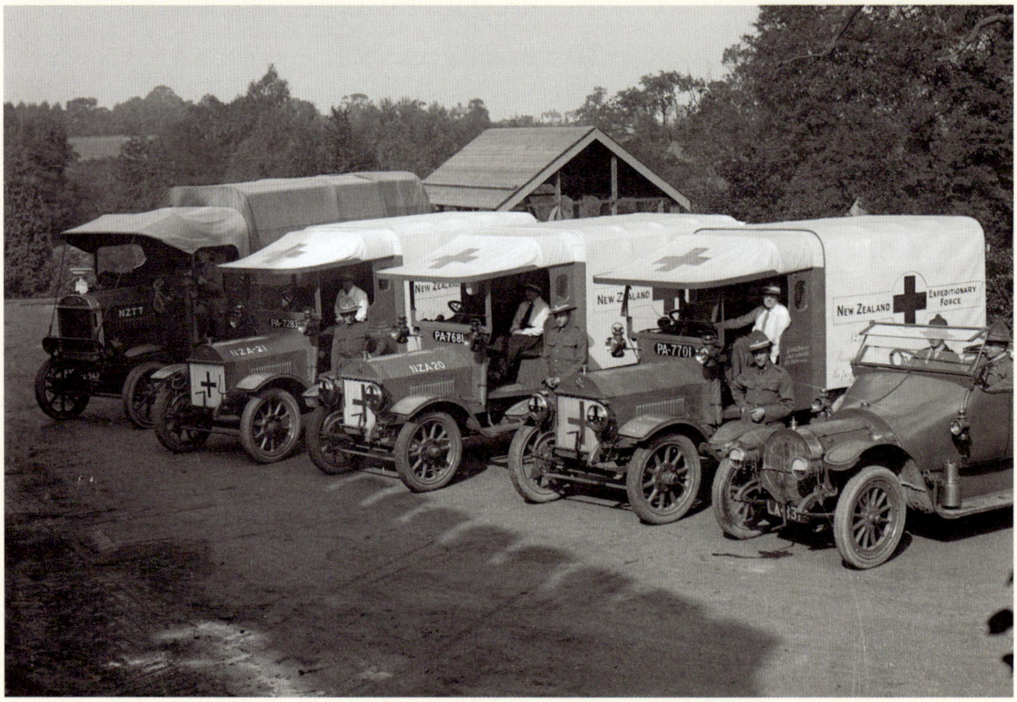

above Much VAD work was far from glamorous. These young women at Hornchurch are peeling potatoes. NATIONAL ARMY MUSEUM, 1993.1214

below The white-shirted women ambulance drivers of the Motor Transport Section at Hornchurch sit in their vehicles for this photo. Females driving, let alone servicing, cars were a novelty in these years. ALEXANDER TURNBULL LIBRARY, 1/2-013953-G

To stand on the platform & see the hospital train steam in out of the darkness is quite a sight.'[22] Taylor, who lost two brothers in the war, was awarded an MBE in 1920.

For close to two years, the women ambulance drivers at Hornchurch were headed by Gladys Henning, who had gone to England in April 1917 after working for Ettie Rout's Volunteer Sisterhood in Egypt. Like Taylor, she was cruelly affected by the war. Her brother was killed at Messines and she bravely continued working after her husband, Lieutenant William Henning, MC, died of wounds received at Bapaume in September 1918. Henning returned home on the *Ruahine* in January 1919.[23]

When Agnes Pearce and Violet Bell were made MBEs in 1917, along with a cook at Walton and two nursing VADs at both New Zealand hospitals, *Kai Tiaki* was generous in its praise. This recently created civilian honour was 'well earned by the women who have so cheerfully undertaken tasks which are so monotonous and uninteresting, though . . . so necessary'.[24] It was a different matter, however, when Aucklander Bessie Ernest received the Royal Red Cross in the 1918 New Year's Honours. Other VADs were also given the prestigious award, the first time it had gone to untrained nurses. Ernest had certainly done her bit, having worked at British military hospitals on the Western Front since 1915 and been mentioned in despatches in June 1917, but Maclean, always protective of her qualified nurses, was not amused. 'This young lady, excellent as her services undoubtedly have been, is not a nurse, and it is not certain that she has been doing nursing work at all. Nurses do not grudge recognition of service in the V.A.D. workers, but it certainly is a sore point that so many of these have latterly been awarded the decoration which . . . has been regarded as the special prerogative of the trained nurses.'[25] Kate Fulton, who was a VAD at Walton in 1917 before joining the Scottish Women's Hospital as an ambulance driver, received 'a somewhat unique decoration for a woman' when she was awarded the Croix de Guerre for her bravery and sangfroid under shellfire at Soissons.[26]

Although it was not compulsory for them to do so — the matter of marriage remained a vexed issue throughout the war[27] — some NZANS nurses became VADs when they married. Once Sister Myrtle Galloway wed Captain Herbert Hutson of the NZMC at Hornchurch in February 1918, she 'retired' after two years' active service and took up VAD work. Women not considered fit enough for full nursing or rigorous overseas service sometimes had to be content with a VAD role. Erica Hoby wanted to go to Serbia with Dr Agnes Bennett in 1916, but her last-minute failure of a medical consigned her to VAD duties at Codford instead.[28]

The wartime contribution of female doctors from New Zealand is often unacknowledged, or unknown, however, recent research by historian Jane Tolerton has revealed much more about their work.[29] They included a remarkable quartet — Agnes Bennett, Mary Blair and Jessie Scott, who worked overseas with the Scottish Women's Hospitals for Foreign Service (SWH), and Dr Elizabeth Gunn, who fought hard to serve her country.

The SWH, intended to provide mobile hospital units for the treatment of the wounded, was the idea of Edinburgh doctor Elsie Inglis. Very soon after war was declared, she and the SWH committee offered both the War Office and the British Red Cross two 100-bed units staffed by women. Perhaps inevitably, the male military hierarchy was not interested. The French and Belgian Red Cross, however, were happy to accept, and the SWH established its first hospital in France at Royaumont Abbey. Throughout the war this extraordinary organisation, via 14 medical units and the voluntary commitment of some 1000 female doctors, nurses, drivers and orderlies, served in Corsica, mainland France, Malta, Romania, Russia, Salonika and Serbia.[30] Blair, Scott and Bennett turned to the SWH because female doctors were no more welcomed by the New Zealand military than the nurses had initially been.[31]

Born in Dunedin, Mary Blair graduated with a BSc from Auckland University College in 1902 before studying at the London School of Medicine for Women. (At this time only some half-dozen New Zealand women had medical degrees.) She achieved her MB BS in 1907 and an MD in 1910, and by 1914 she held several roles, including that of honorary anaesthetist at a hospital in Plaistow. As was common, she earned a living from her private practice.[32] When war was declared, Blair was keen to use her skills. After working briefly in France,[33] in August 1915 she led an SWH unit to Serbia. The original destination was Valjevo, but when Blair's group reached the Greek port of Salonika in October it was overflowing with refugees who had been forced out of Serbia after the invasion by German, Austro-Hungarian and Bulgarian troops. Some 240,000 Serbian army men and civilians had perished in the retreat through Albania. Blair worked in Salonika before taking up a new SWH challenge: leading a group of sick and exhausted refugees to Corsica.[34]

Blair had her work cut out for her. The arrivals were 'all destitute, and no provision had been made for housing them', so until proper infrastructure could be built, she and her team had to put typhoid fever, pneumonia, appendicitis and maternity cases together. Her efficiency in establishing separate wards for men, women and children, and for rehabilitation, made her 'the most honoured person here. She is saluted by everyone, and no end of gratitude is lavished on her and Dr. Blair's mother, who is with her, has her hand kissed many times a day in token of respect for "Mademoiselle votre fille".' Her achievements were 'the talk of the place . . . Outside and inside she directs and plans.'[35] The desperate need for medical officers at the front propelled Blair's next move. In September 1916, following a call earlier that year for women doctors to replace men in Maltese hospitals, Blair worked on the island under the auspices of the RAMC.[36] She was mentioned in despatches late in 1917 and received other decorations, including the Serbian Order of St Sava.

On 3 July 1915 the *Oamaru Mail* reported that Dr Jessie Scott had agreed to act as the medical officer for the first group of Ettie Rout's Volunteer Sisterhood to leave New Zealand.[37] Just six days later, however, the *Star* in Christchurch had a new story to tell. Scott had telegraphed the secretary of the Volunteer Sisterhood to say 'Edinburgh cables offer me surgical post Scottish Women's Military Hospital. Serbia, salary and fare one way. Will accept if you release me.' The secretary had replied: 'Very sorry to lose your services, but I certainly think you ought to accept Edinburgh offer.'[38]

Born near Christchurch in 1883, the youngest of nine children, Scott had graduated MB and ChB from Edinburgh in 1909. She achieved her MD in 1912 while working as assistant medical officer for the London County Council. Back in New Zealand in 1913, Scott headed a

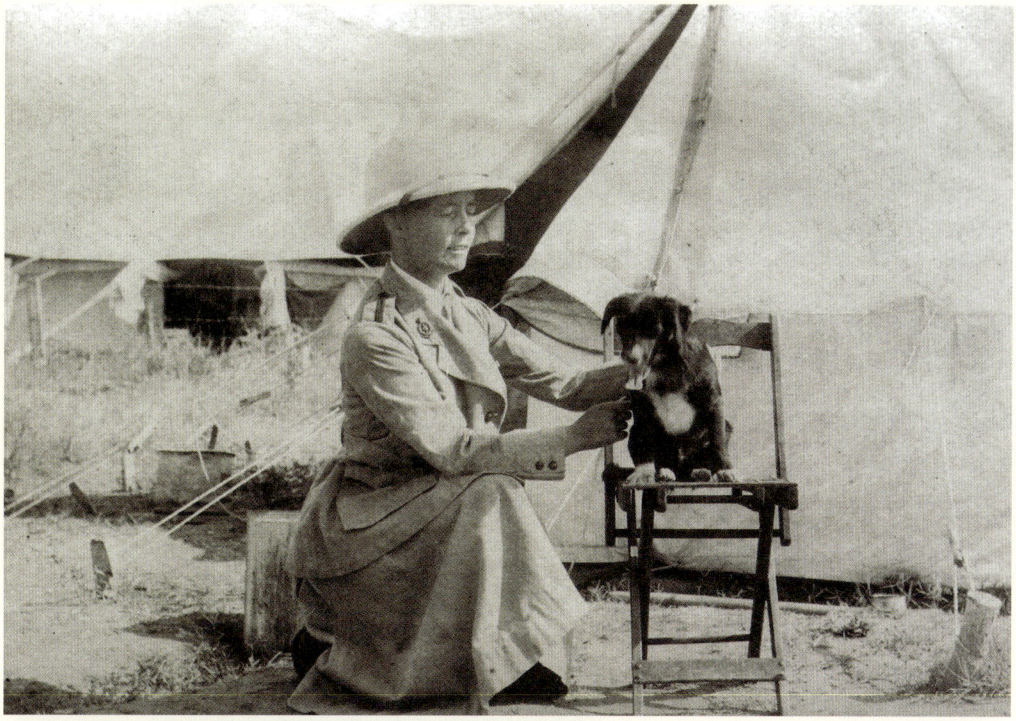

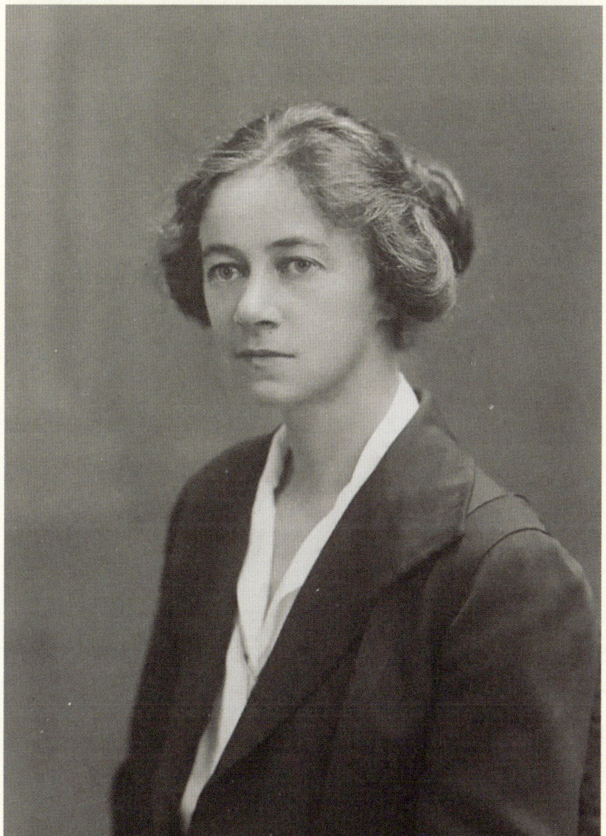

above New Zealand doctor Mary Blair poses with her beloved dog Muggins, who accompanied her to Salonika. AUCKLAND WAR MEMORIAL MUSEUM, KINDLY DONATED BY FAMILY

below As aletter to the *Auckland Star* noted in 1915, Jessie Scott 'had a (comparatively) easier and far safer and pleasanter billet offered her, but, with the heroism of a Joan of Arc, she has chosen the difficult and most unpleasant task of doctoring those plague stricken people, victim of the cruel war raging in Europe. Medical men in Auckland who know what she is going to face, are warmly praising her courage.' ROYAL NEW ZEALAND ARMY MEDICAL CORPS HISTORY COLLECTION big isolation hospital in Auckland during that year's smallpox epidemic.[39] When she reached Serbia at the beginning of September 1915 she went to a unit at Lazarevac, where they dealt with many medical cases, mainly typhoid and malaria. 'We doctors (three), the administrator and two others of the staff, are sleeping in tents. It is getting very cold now.' The worsening weather soon made the roads impassable for motor vehicles and only bullock wagons were useful. 'One must wear top-boots and a skirt which is very short, or not at all if it is dark. At nights in wet weather we plough about from one place to the other with lanterns.'[40]

By 31 October, Scott and her colleagues were having 'a fairly hot time' at Kruševac following the invasion of Serbia. When the Austrians were just hours from Lazarevac, the local hospitals had been evacuated. Scott and the other doctors and nurses left on the last train for Kruševac, crammed into cattle trucks for a miserable three-day journey. Most of them ended up sleeping and cooking in a single room of a hospital where they treated over 500 surgical cases in three weeks. 'The wounded [Serbians] are pouring into the place in hundreds daily.' With food short, the women were advised to head for Montenegro. Most of the nurses did so, but several doctors, including Scott and Elsie Inglis, who had joined them with her unit, decided to stay.[41] The Germans, who arrived 'very quietly' on 6 November, 'were quite nice and polite', and the 40 SWH women and three other doctors were allowed to carry on with their work. Kruševac became 'a big prison centre' and as the Germans rounded up Serbians from the surrounding villages, 'many of our old patients were brought back again'. Then the Austrians took over for six weeks, until, with most of the hospital's patients recovered, evacuation was ordered.

After a long, comfortless train journey, which began on 13 February, the now 52 women — another SWH unit had arrived — reached Vienna, where they were cared for by the American consul. They were sent on to Zurich some 10 days later and finally made it to London on 29 February. 'We had an exceedingly interesting experience,' Scott decided, 'not accompanied by great hardship.' They had been short of food and subjected to shellfire, and faced 'other excitements', but had not experienced 'the actual discomforts' of the nurses who had walked across Albania. The unit, though, had lost everything.[42] This was not the end of Scott's war service. She continued her SWH contribution with the Serbian army until 1918: on 12 February 1917 she was in London after six grim and testing months of mainly surgical work at the 200-bed hospital in Ostrovo, 'within the sound of the guns at Monastir'.[43] Like Blair, she was decorated by the Serbians.

When Scott was working in Ostrovo, the doctor heading her unit, No. 7 of the SWH, was Sydney-born Agnes Bennett. After graduating MB, ChM in 1899 from the Edinburgh Medical College for Women, founded by Inglis and two others,[44] she worked at a Scottish asylum. She returned to Sydney in 1901 to establish a medical practice, but was forced by prejudice against female doctors to return to mental health work. When she was 33, the chance to purchase a Wellington practice was providential. Bennett became medical officer at St Helen's Hospital in 1908 and honorary physician to the children's ward at Wellington Hospital two years later.[45]

Early in March 1915, newspapers reported that Bennett would soon leave New Zealand to join the French Red Cross, a decision she made after the government turned down her offer to serve overseas. She left on the *Ulimaroa* on 1 April, but when she reached Cairo, the

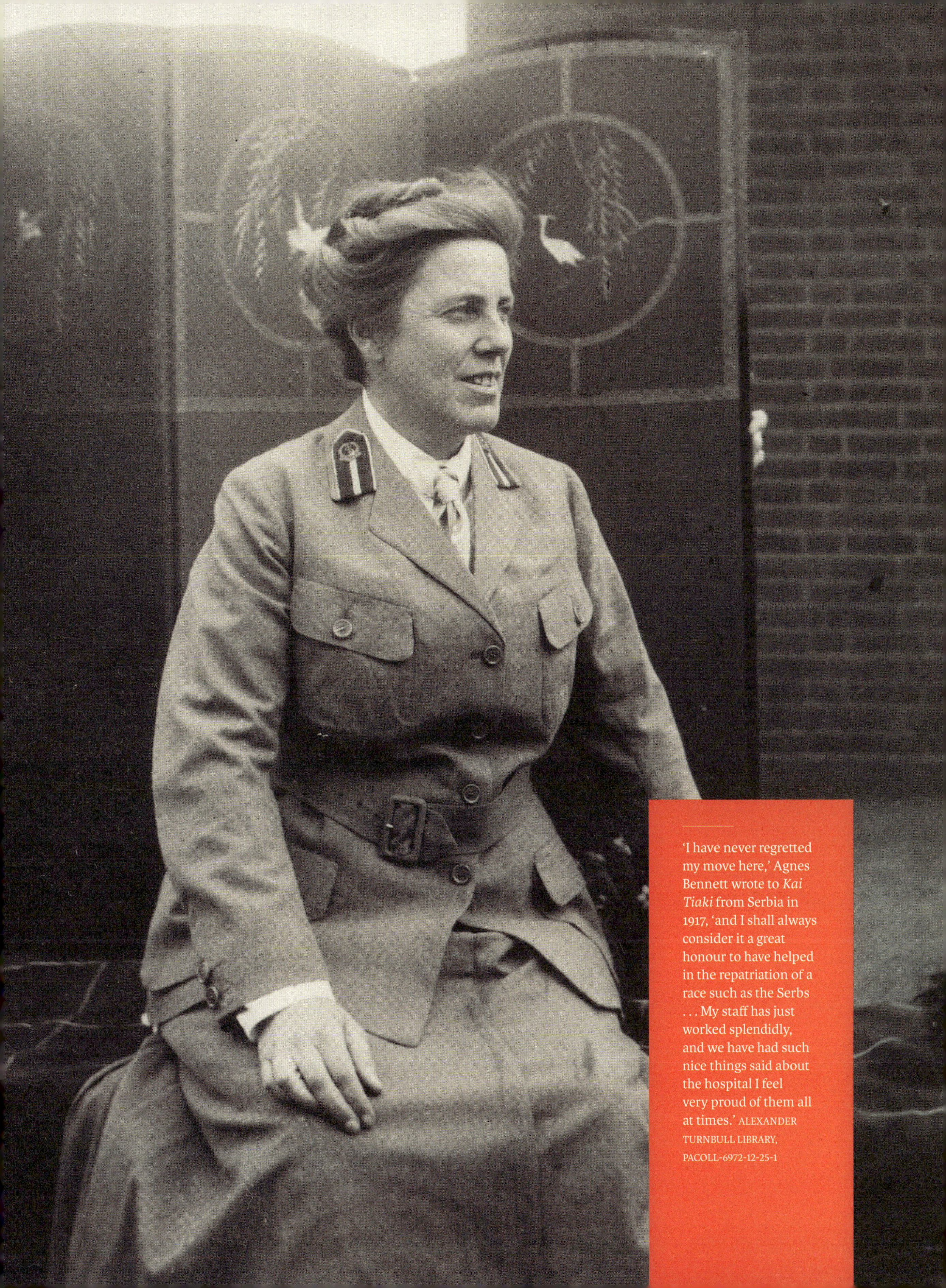

'I have never regretted my move here,' Agnes Bennett wrote to *Kai Tiaki* from Serbia in 1917, 'and I shall always consider it a great honour to have helped in the repatriation of a race such as the Serbs . . . My staff has just worked splendidly, and we have had such nice things said about the hospital I feel very proud of them all at times.' ALEXANDER TURNBULL LIBRARY, PACOLL-6972-12-25-1

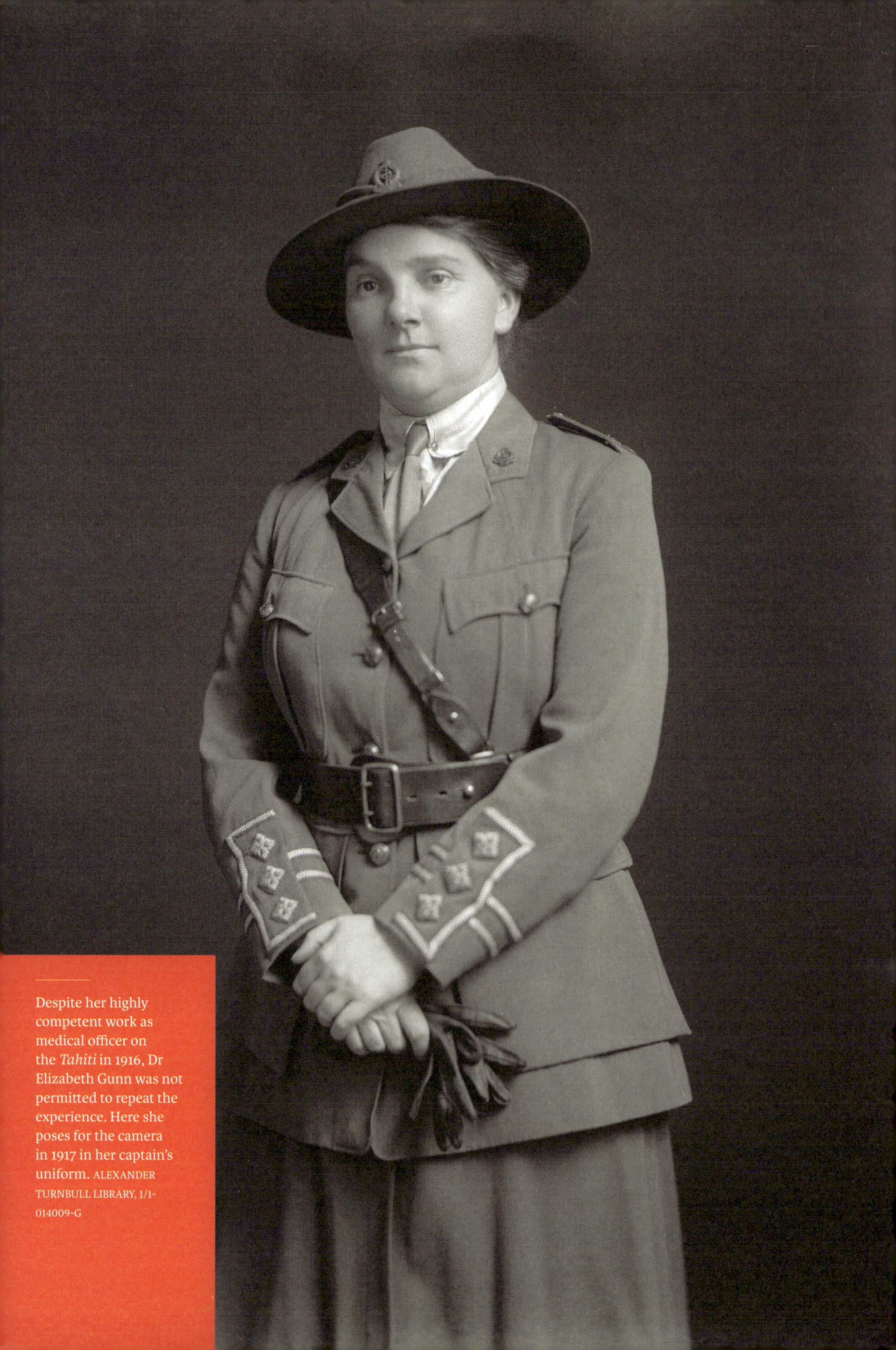

Despite her highly competent work as medical officer on the *Tahiti* in 1916, Dr Elizabeth Gunn was not permitted to repeat the experience. Here she poses for the camera in 1917 in her captain's uniform. ALEXANDER TURNBULL LIBRARY, 1/1-014009-G

New Zealand Medical Corps, via her former Wellington medical colleague, Mathew Holmes, offered her a post. Bennett was 'not actually commissioned, although graded as a Captain for the purpose of pay, allowances and status generally'.[46] She was attested on 19 May at the Egyptian Army Hospital at Pont de Koubbeh, where she worked with Drs Hugh Acland, the chief surgeon, Hugh Widdowson and John Campbell, taking charge of the isolation ward with her friend Dr Grace Russell, a civilian doctor who had been sent to the hospital by the British medical authorities.[47] Bennett later moved to the Imperial Infectious Diseases Hospital at Choubra. Practical and energetic, she was not shy about asking for help from home. 'The things we want are really things for the trip out to New Zealand: soft shirts, "slacks" (for hot weather), singlets, socks, and well-made pyjamas that would do for deck wear . . . They would also immensely appreciate some good boiled sweets . . . and money for tobacco for the voyage.'[48]

Bennett worked in Egypt for nearly a year before resigning and returning to England. By May 1916 she was back in London, purportedly for a rest. In late July, however, the *Herald* reported that she was to command 'a woman's unit, to be sent for work in Servia [Serbia] . . . her work will have heavy responsibilities attached to it.'[49] The SWH unit, which included Jessie Scott and Australian doctor Lilian Cooper, as well as some 20 nurses and about 16 orderlies, reached Salonika on 13 August. By the time Bennett was writing from their Ostrovo camp at the end of October, appalling weather was preventing ambulances from going out, so that 'patients were left up on hills in dressing stations with the very minimum of attention . . . to-night have come just horrible cases. To-morrow we shall be just as busy as we can possibly be all day in operating theatre.'[50]

Even the indefatigable Bennett was not impervious to illness. She was forced to resign in October 1917 after a bout of malaria and, having been honoured by the Serbians, she was back in New Zealand in February 1918, giving talks about her work. But she was soon back in Britain, working in the Royal Infirmary, Glasgow, during the influenza epidemic, then at Netley military hospital near Southampton. She fell ill again and was forced to convalesce 'in the country' before sailing for New Zealand on 1 April 1919 aboard the *Paparoa*, on which she assisted the medical officer, Captain George Adams.[51]

Bennett's great friend and fellow doctor Kate Hogg studied in Sydney and Edinburgh and also struggled to establish a private practice in Australia. She eventually moved to Wellington, 'apparently as a locum' for Bennett, who gave her away when she married James Neill in 1913.[52] She joined her husband overseas during the war and on the *Ruapehu* returning to Wellington early in 1919, she was 'in sole charge of health of soldiers' wives and children — the latter have been treated skillfully, — the former tactfully at all times by Dr. Neill'.[53]

On 25 September 1915, Dunedin-born Dr Elizabeth Gunn, who had qualified in Edinburgh and was working for the school medical service, talked to Surgeon-General Robert Henderson about serving her country. He accepted her offer, and immediately appointed her to the NZMC 'for employment on a hospital ship'.[54] His 15 October staff recommendations for the *Marama* included Gunn as a 'supernumerary' with the temporary rank of captain, but this suggestion was turned down. Henderson then offered to send her on a transport to Egypt, but his cable — 'Have you vacancies for one good surgeon and one young capable lady doctor in

New Zealand General Hospital' — produced no joy. By 15 November, Gunn, understandably fed up, had decided to call on James Allen. He was away, so she saw William Massey instead. 'She seems to be very upset,' the prime minister reported, 'over the turn affairs have taken . . . what has happened has done her much injury professionally, as people want to know, after her appointment had practically been made, what has happened to prevent her being sent to Egypt for medical work there.' When, in December, Allen asked if Henderson could use Gunn's services, he answered that she could take charge of the Izard Measles Hospital at Trentham.

Not until the end of March 1916 did Gunn get her wish, sailing to Egypt and back on the *Tahiti* as permanent MO. Her fellow doctor, William Little, had only praise: 'This lady has at all times and in all circumstances proved a loyal and effective colleague.' The *Tahiti*'s captain, F. P. Evans, in a letter to Henderson, who seemingly had 'lingering doubts of the suitableness of women for the medical duties of such an environment', decided that Gunn, being 'possessed of unusual force of character [was] therefore an exceptional case'. Despite being 'very glad indeed' that Gunn had 'done so well on the voyage', Henderson returned her to Trentham, 'as I think her services will be more usefully employed there'. Coping with an outbreak of pneumonia and cerebro-spinal meningitis at the camp was too much for Gunn's health — she suffered from rheumatism — and she was given long leave to recover. She went on to have a distinguished career as a school doctor and founder of the children's health camps movement.[55]

Other New Zealand women who served in Serbia during the war were Dr Ada McLaren, who worked for the Anglo-Serbian Hospital, better known as the Berry Mission after its husband and wife founders, James and May Berry, and former Otaki native health nurse Ethel Lewis, who was in England when war was declared. Within a few days Lewis was nursing in a Belgian field hospital, then spent nine weeks in an Antwerp hospital until it was evacuated when the Germans arrived and she returned to England. She then departed for Serbia. In the trenches on the Bulgarian frontier, she received a slight shrapnel wound to the shoulder and saved the life of a Serbian officer. During the great retreat, Lewis and another nurse took 400 patients, none of whom survived, through the mountain passes of Albania, on foot, in knee-deep snow, eating a single slice of bread a day and often sleeping in pigsties. Lewis carried one man on her back for 2 miles and was suffering from a frostbitten knee when the exhausted hospital staff finally reached safety. King Peter himself would honour her brave contribution in Serbia. After recuperating at Brockenhurst, Lewis 'unfortunately broke her arm, causing some amazement amongst the staff by appearing for duty in that condition'.[56] She returned to New Zealand on the *Willochra* in 1916 and joined the NZANS the following year. In 1918 she sailed back to Britain to work at Codford.

Also in Serbia were New Zealanders Sister Agnes Kerr, who had led the initial group of Volunteer Sisters to Egypt and worked in Alexandria, and Mildred Stephens, who had been in charge of Lady Carnarvon's military canteen on the Alexandria docks, set up principally for Anzac soldiers, for six months from February 1916.[57] In August that year the two women joined Bennett's SWH unit. Having reached Salonika early, they helped out at the hospital's Trench

Unit, which was 'overcrowded with French and Serbs, ill with malaria and dysentery, and understaffed'. When their own group arrived, they went upcountry to nurse wounded Serbian soldiers at a field hospital 'within sight and sound of the shell fire'.[58] Late that year, Stephens spent six freezing weeks at a dressing station as an orderly. In February 1917 Bennett lent the two women to the Serbian Relief Fund (SRF) to establish a small camp in the ruined village of Brod, very close to the front line. 'The other day,' Stephens recorded, 'a big unexploded shell fell quite close to us. I heard it come whizzing past my ear, and it fell about ten yards away.'[59] They fed some 140 children each morning and between 50 and 90 in the evening, and did their best for the many people suffering from 'malaria, tuberculosis, rheumatism and some sort of fever, which may be paratyphoid complicated by malaria'. The work was 'heart-breaking . . . nursing them is impossible — we can only dose them, feed them, and do sort of first-aid dressing. The dreadful hovels they live in!'[60] The women eventually, with the assistance of the SRF, established a small hospital and dispensary in the village. Kerr went on to join the Scottish Women's Transport Column. After suffering from malaria for two or three months, Stephens was forced to return to London before undertaking welfare work in France. Both women received the Croix de la Miséricorde, a Serbian decoration, for their SWH work.

'Just when things were getting quiet with us again,' wrote Sister Margaret Davies of the NZANS from No. 10 British CCS, about 10 miles south of Dunkerque in France in April 1918, 'I left our hospital and went to No. 2 Stationary (British) to take a course in anaesthetics, and am still at it. I expect that you have heard that . . . many sisters are being trained in this work, so as to release some of the medical officers.'[61] Davies, Jean Porteous and Ellen Schaw were the second NZANS group to take the course, which consisted of two or three months at a base hospital, followed by four weeks at a CCS. The first trio, Maud Atkinson, Blanche Huddlestone and Susan Nicholas, had studied at No. 13 American General Hospital in Boulogne. Davies, Porteous and Schaw had arrived only recently, after three months at the British hospital at Abbeville. 'We did not have much work during the first two months, but we made up for it in the third, when the fighting commenced down there.' All the German wounded were taken to that hospital and, because the women's instructor was on leave, 'we gave all the anaesthetics; the surgeons seemed quite satisfied, and we gained confidence with so much work.'[62]

Huddlestone, who had trained in Wellington, was almost certainly the anonymous author of 'Nurses as Anaesthetists' in the July 1919 issue of *Kai Tiaki*. She wrote of the two months' training at the American hospital, 'our instructor being a woman, who was a professional anaesthetist of 6 or 7 years' experience'. As well as daily practical work, lectures and a final exam, there was study and 'reading anything and everything relative to anaesthesia'. The surgical team worked long hours, 'the wounded coming in almost faster than one could cope with them. One lived in a constant state of "moving on," and at one casualty clearing station we stayed 3½ days, our admissions during that time being 3,600 casualties. At another place in ten days the admissions were 23,000.' She added, 'We were frequently told by our surgeons that our work was more satisfactory than that of many a male anaesthetist, who was much more interested in watching the operation than in paying attention to the anaesthetic.'[63]

After her month at No. 10 CCS, Davies was attached as anaesthetist to a surgical team, which headed north to work at another CCS for 'a strenuous ten days', before returning to No. 10, now joined by a Canadian and a British CCS. Following the battle for Kemmel, the wounded arrived in 'a continuous stream, each CCS would fill up in a few hours'. In bad weather, 'the place became a sea of mud' and at night 'not a glimmer of light could be shown as the German planes were over . . . The stretcher-bearers had to carry their burdens along the muddy, slippery duckboards as best they could in the dark.'[64]

Both Davies and Huddlestone loved their anaesthetic work, but their hard-won expertise, and that of the other trained women, would prove a hindrance when they sought such work in New Zealand civilian hospitals after the war. Anaesthetics had become a specialised area for doctors, and nurses could not break into a male domain. Huddlestone concluded, rather wistfully, 'I found the work very interesting, and was most anxious to be a success at it, and am truly sorry that one cannot go on with it in this country; however, it helped one to do one's "bit," even if it was only a temporary war arrangement.'[65]

In early July 1915 outspoken socialist, journalist and labour activist Ettie Rout launched the Volunteer Sisterhood in her home town of Christchurch. The scheme lacked ministerial approval but, as Rout explained in an article printed in both the *Lyttelton Times* and the *Sun*, 'the originators [were] going ahead with it all the same'. She made an 'urgent call' for 20 'competent and intelligent' women 'between the ages of 30 and 50, preferably between 35 and 40',[66] to 'submit themselves to a month's special training, for preference at Trentham, under the supervision of the New Zealand Medical Corps', before leaving for Egypt. They would have to 'give up one year of their life on the claims of humanity alone for practically no payment at all', though they would receive a uniform, free transport to Egypt or elsewhere, insurance against illness, accident and death and an allowance of 10s a week. A summary of costs and a plea for donations followed. Applicants would have to be pronounced 'physically and organically sound by a duly qualified medical practitioner', and have their 'character, capacity, good temper, and suitability for the work . . . certified to by three independent persons'.[67] At this stage Rout was promising Jessie Scott as the inaugural medical officer. Not everyone was impressed, least of all Christchurch's morning paper, the *Press*. '"It would be madness to send them to Egypt," declared Mrs _____ in a tone of horror. "They do not know what the situation is . . . They would simply be in the way. Moreover, they could not stand the climate. It would be an act of criminal folly to allow those women to go to the country."'[68]

Rout, however, was well aware of public unease over the recent serious outbreak of illness at Trentham, and saw her chance. Unwilling to risk further possible scandal, Thomas Valintine, as head of military hospitals, accepted Rout's offer of help at the camp, though her suggested 20 volunteers were trimmed to 10, plus a trained nurse. Rout fulfilled her confident promise to meet the deadline, despite then having no actual volunteers, when 200 women contacted her on the day her article appeared. As with VADs, some trained nurses were chary of Rout's initiative, particularly as she was inconsistent in her characterisation of what the Volunteer Sisters would do — nurse themselves, or help nurses. Interestingly, however, Samoa veteran Louise Brandon, who had been sent to Trentham in late June to establish a hospital, welcomed the women and put them straight to work.[69]

Rout continued to attract overwhelming support as she recruited in Wellington and Auckland and, despite unyielding government opposition and public disapproval, partly whipped up by the *Press*, she gathered enough money to dispatch the first group of Volunteer Sisters to Egypt in October 1915. At the end of December she departed for Egypt with a second contingent. The women, clad in specially ordered blue dresses, white aprons and caps — with panama hats and blue capes for outdoors — worked mainly in the YMCA at Cairo's Ezbekieh Gardens, where they produced meals for the men and served tea and coffee. John Moloney saw 'the redoubtable Ettie Rout' at Ezbekieh late in February 1916. 'She is doing great work.'[70] When the New Zealand Division left Egypt for France, Rout and some of her sisters stayed on to provide much-needed recreation, and non-army food, for the mounted troops fighting in the Sinai. With the support of the formidable Louisa Godley, Rout opened the Tel-el-Kebir Soldiers' Club near the Suez Canal. 'We are getting on splendidly here,' she soon reported. 'We have five large marquees up now, and have surrounded the only group of decent trees in the place. It is an oasis for the boys, in every way. They throng the place now.'[71]

When the New Zealanders moved on, Rout followed, to places such as Moascar and Kantara. Like Brandon, and like Jessie Scott, Agnes Bennett formed a favourable opinion of the sisterhood's work in Egypt. 'Without their help . . . they would have lost more lives, and many nurses would have broken down under the strain. The volunteer helpers saved the nurses many little jobs which must be done for the patients, and for which it is not necessary to have a fully trained nurse.' They got the trained medical staff 'through the strain of the big rushes, which is the time when their help is needed'. Godley was also an admirer: 'I saw a great deal of her work in Egypt, and think very highly of it, and so does my wife.'[72]

The Volunteer Sisters also worked in British hospitals. At the end of September 1916, the YMCA offered Clara Rogers and others, including Ada Ballantine and Dora Murch, 'the sole charge and management' of a hut at Codford. After viewing the land, 'we at once decided it was where we were needed'. The 150 by 30ft building would be 'furnished according to our own taste and made as comfortable as possible, for the huts in the Salisbury Plains are the only places where the boys can find amusement or break the monotony of camp life'. Keen to give the troops 'a New Zealand Christmas away from New Zealand', they were asking for 'socks, mittens, handkerchiefs, gloves, mufflers, cigarettes, pipes, and all such things'.[73] By July 1917 Rogers and Ballantine were, Rout reported, 'giving large numbers of the New Zealanders in Oatlands Park and Walton-on-Thames hospitals very fine outings'.[74]

Rout is, of course, best known for her campaign to reduce the high incidence of VD in the NZEF by issuing the men with prophylactic kits and setting up properly inspected brothels. Unlike most of the military hierarchy, and zealots such as William Pettit, she took the clear-sighted view that VD was an inevitable and purely medical matter: soldiers would

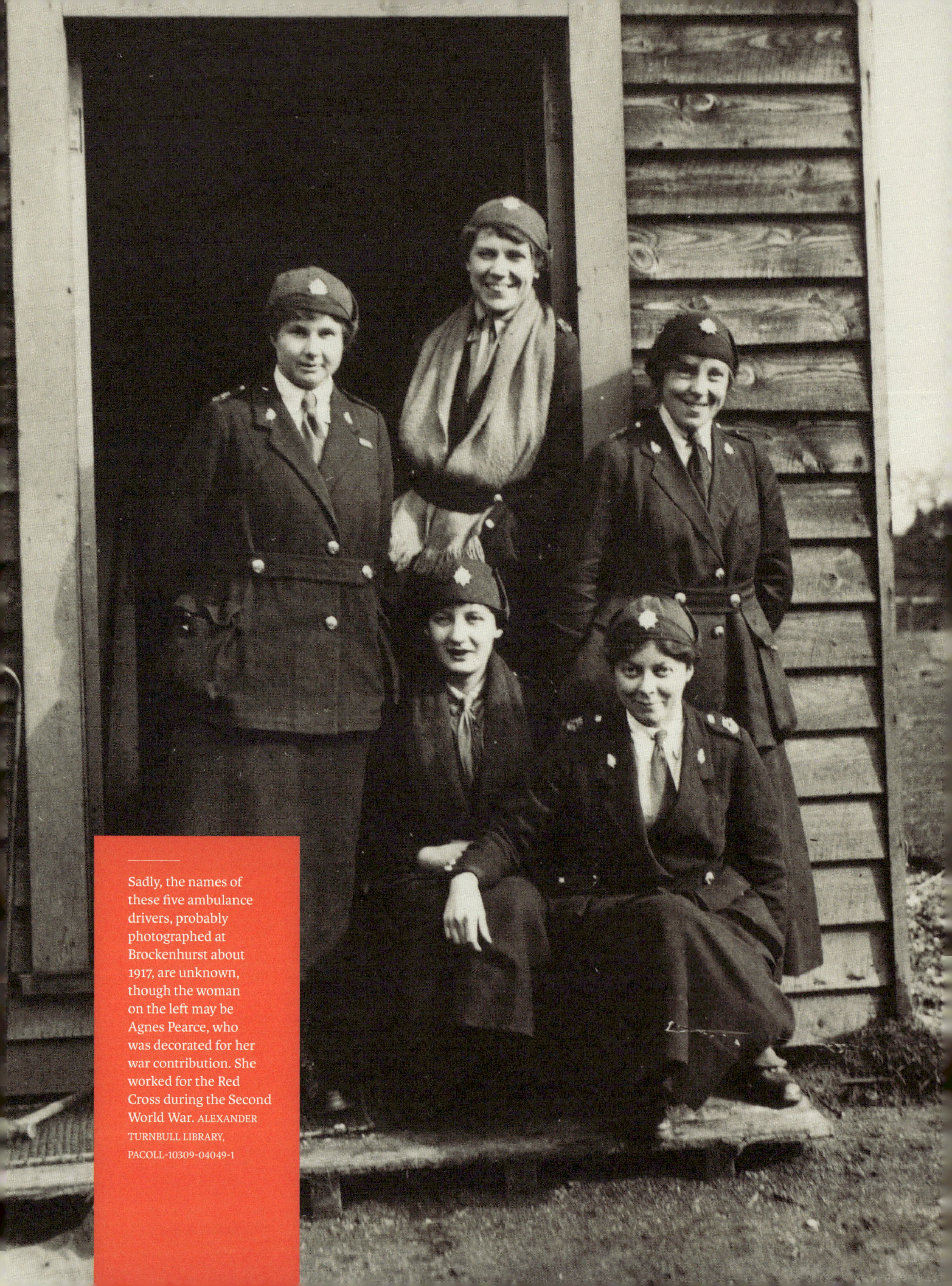

Sadly, the names of these five ambulance drivers, probably photographed at Brockenhurst about 1917, are unknown, though the woman on the left may be Agnes Pearce, who was decorated for her war contribution. She worked for the Red Cross during the Second World War. ALEXANDER TURNBULL LIBRARY, PACOLL-10309-04049-1 sleep with prostitutes and, without sensible protection, would be infected with sexually transmitted diseases.

Having failed to convince the NZMC to follow this approach, she took her campaign to London, arriving there at the beginning of May 1917. She had Lady Godley and High Commissioner Thomas Mackenzie on her side; her new quarry was the head of the NZEF in Britain, Brigadier-General George Richardson, with whom she eventually formed a helpful alliance. With typical verve and determination, she amassed as much information as she could from leading doctors, visited the Codford VD hospital and found out how the Australians and Canadians were dealing with the problem. At Richardson's suggestion, she chose Hornchurch as the site for her New Zealand Medical Soldiers' Club, where the prophylactic kit she had designed herself went on sale. James Allen had been resolutely opposed to Rout, but the support of Richardson and Henderson changed his mind, and at the end of 1917 the NZEF made Rout's kit freely and compulsorily available — without crediting the hard work she had put into its creation.

Rout's next destination, in April 1918, was the French capital, where she established 'a one-woman social and sexual welfare service for soldiers',[75] meeting them as they arrived by train on leave and distributing signed cards with the address of a clean brothel that she had found and regularly checked: 'I have visited Madam______'s house on several occasions during the last two months in company with medical officers and we are all convinced that at the present time it makes safe and suitable provision for the sexual needs of the troops.'[76] She had real success, even allowing for her characteristic boosterism: 'The Australians and Maorilanders . . . are now the cleanest troops that have ever come to Paris.'[77]

After the war Rout ran a Red Cross depot in France. She was mentioned in despatches for her Egyptian work, and decorated by the French, but still little supported at home. Noting that 'No New Zealand paper has dared to say the same thing', the *Observer* quoted from Melbourne's *Punch* at the end of 1919: 'in the esteem of the Diggers, none ranks higher than Miss Ettie Rout . . . Prophylactics, advice in pamphlet form, and sensible motherly talks, were dispensed . . . and the good which resulted would surprise many a whiskered one who would raise sanctimonious hands against such service.' The 'mutterings' of her critics were 'drowned in a chorus of thankfulness from the men who know. The plucky New Zealand girl is as much entitled to a Royal Red Cross as any Army nurse.'[78]

PART 4

Maimed and Mended

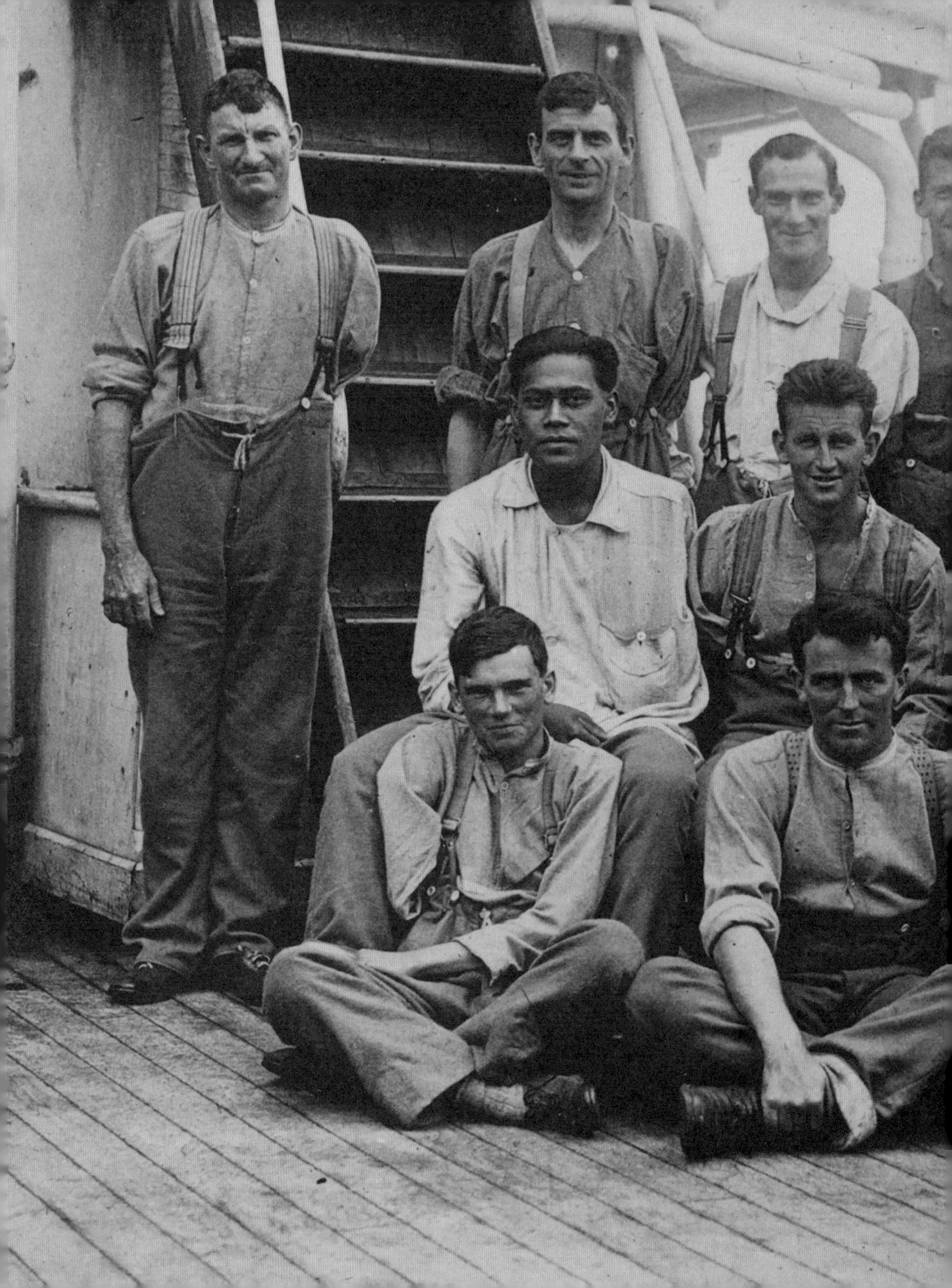

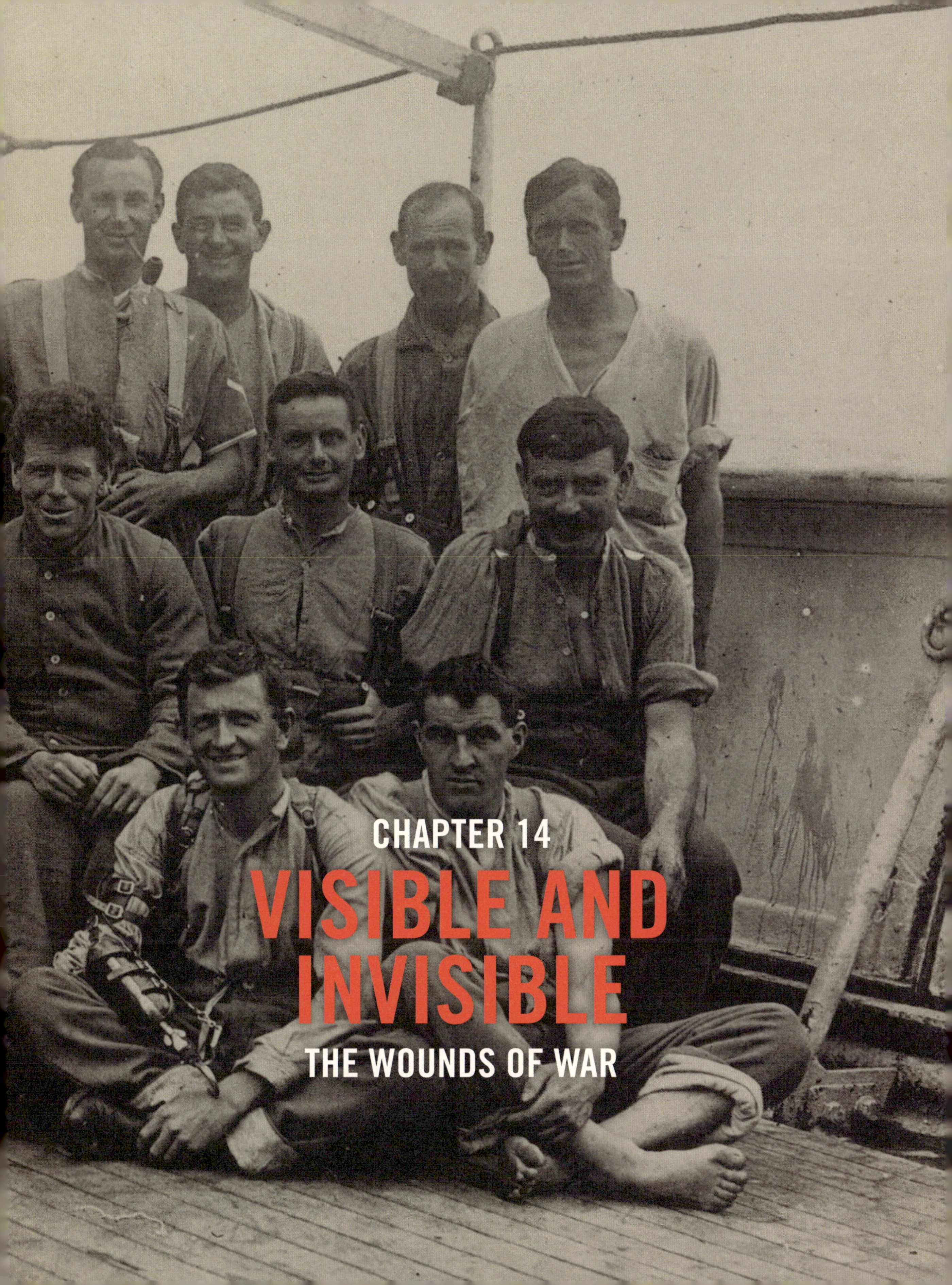

CHAPTER 14

VISIBLE AND INVISIBLE

THE WOUNDS OF WAR

previous pages
All but one of the men in this photograph, taken on the *Marama* by Bill Yates, are missing an arm. They were far from unusual. WILLIAM YATES ALBUM, COURTESY WILLIAM YATES FAMILY, FEILDING LIBRARY

> The weapons of destruction . . . are immeasurably more powerful, more accurate, and more deadly than was ever the case before; they are more plentiful and more varied, and the devilish ingenuities of chemistry as applied to ballistic science have reinforced lawful with unlawful weapons of the most terrible character.
>
> — *Dominion*, 14 February 1916

In her little eight-man ward at the American Ambulance in Neuilly-sur-Seine early in October 1914, a New Zealand nurse was dealing with wounds that would reappear thousands of times over the coming years:

> one amputation of leg, thigh terribly shattered, two cases of bullets in jaw, one with . . . holes right through each cheek, and lower maxilla fractured, the other with bullet lodged in the right side of neck; two more with bullets and shrapnel in legs and feet, and two shoulder cases; also one with no wounds of any kind, blown seventy yards by a [lyddite] shell, general concussion and later, neuritis and rheumatism, having been wet to the skin for a whole week.[1]

The more sophisticated and powerful weapons used during the First World War could hurt, maim and kill with terrible, unprecedented accuracy. The often multiple wounds they inflicted were far worse than anything seen before.

Although when it entered, and sometimes left, the body, a rifle or machine-gun bullet often left only a small hole, this might conceal a very severe wound. When Ormond Burton was wounded at Bellevue Spur on 4 October 1917, he felt a stab in his chest and saw the front of his tunic turned to rags. 'Nothing was visible except a small round hole more or less over the heart.'[2] This type of wound was noticed by NZMC doctors even before Gallipoli. While treating wounded Turkish prisoners at Ismailia in February 1915, Major Donald Murray observed 'the "explosive" effect of the modern pointed [rifle] bullet fired at close quarters with the great destruction of tissue and multiple shattering of bone produced'.[3] If a bullet entered the body undamaged, there was usually little bleeding, just a bluish hole. At a Gallipoli roll-call a soldier who appeared to have fainted was turned onto his back: 'Right between his eyes there was a little blue mark, like a dot made with a slate-pencil.'[4] But when, as often happened, there was a ricochet, the tumbling bullet 'did not enter the flesh point first but made a huge hole and could easily smash a bone'.[5]

Men struck by a bullet from a sniper's rifle often likened the sensation to being thumped by a heavy weight. On Gallipoli, Private John O'Neill 'suddenly . . . felt as if someone had hit me on the thigh with a sledge hammer and over I went. There was no pain then, my leg was quite dead. The bullet went clean through the bone and out again.' As Lieutenant James Macfarlane, shot five times during the fighting on Sari Bair, told a reporter, 'The bullet lands with the violence of a blow from a sledge hammer. It leaves a numb feeling, but does not begin to hurt for an hour or more.'[6]

Most casualties in this war, though, were the result of artillery fire: 'The power of a bursting shell or mortar bomb was virtually inconceivable . . . in that pre-atomic era.'[7] 'Although I was carrying 80 lbs of signalling equipment,' wrote Clifford Collingwood in June 1917, 'I felt myself turning over and over in the air, and then struck the paved road. I found myself in a sitting position with my left leg lying at a right angle to its normal position. As I was unable to move, I realised [it] was fractured.'[8] Most wounds from shellfire, however, perhaps 70 per cent on the Western Front,[9] were caused not by the blast itself, but by shell fragments and shrapnel. (The latter term strictly referred to the lead shrapnel balls but was generally also used to describe the splinters from the casing of the shells containing them.) Although these vicious pieces of spinning, jagged metal had a low velocity compared with bullets, their weight and tendency to fly in groups meant they could cause multiple wounds. Even a single shell fragment was capable of 'transversing the abdomen, ripping through the chest, perforating the intestines, and causing other damage needing very complex and dangerous surgery'.[10]

The earth thrown up when shells hit often buried and suffocated men, leaving them with bad concussion. 'In our work,' wrote John Thomson of No. 1 Field Ambulance on Gallipoli, 'we find the worst wounds are from the sharpnosed Mauser bullets or the burst case of a shell . . . Have seen some poor beggars hit with shell casing & don't want to see any more.' Engineer Charles Saunders noted, as many did, the 'most peculiar' sound of a shell case, or a piece of one, 'hurling through the air . . . It whines and hums just like a lost soul.'[11] An apparently minor shell injury could have a disproportionate effect. As John A. Lee put it, 'a very small pellet of steel could play hell with a very large heart'.[12] And realisation of injury was not always immediate. When Arthur Field was wounded in 1916, he had the impression that 'I had been merely bruised on the hip and my leg stunned for the time being by a bit of flying brick, of which cataracts were falling, whereas in reality a piece of shrapnel or shell had gone in through my thigh and was lodged in the centre of my pelvis'.[13]

Shrapnel also carried scraps of germ-laden uniform or equipment, which it drove into the body. In an era without antibiotics, this increased the likelihood of infection, particularly in the richly manured French and Belgian farmland, where gas gangrene and tetanus were always a threat. Lee described one young man: 'High explosive had blown big bits of flesh out of his body and sewer-mud into bare flesh ... [It was] as if some giant appetite had bitten huge portions away and what remained was rotting.'[14] The risk of such an outcome was exacerbated when injuries were left untreated during long journeys from the battlefield. By the time William Taylor reached hospital, his wounded arm was 'swollen beyond belief ... After much probing the doctor finally removed two-and-a-half ounces of steel shell, a piece of khaki, a rag of shirt, a tatter of singlet, and a flood of pus.'[15]

The blast wave accompanying a shell explosion could pass over obstructions and through bodies, rupturing eardrums and lungs and causing brain and spinal cord haemorrhages. 'Fellow soldiers would be often unsettled when they saw pressure wave victims dead with no obvious signs of external injury.'[16] The air displaced by the explosion could blow men over, propel them for several metres or remove their limbs. In 1917, one captain had 'the extraordinary experience of being blown from one end of a trench to the other by a Jack Johnson [shell] and then blown along again by another, with the result that the nerves of his throat became affected and he lost his voice.' At Messines, William Anderson saw a man who 'was buried to his shins [in a shell explosion] and his boots were all the clothing remaining on him'.[17] The blast wind could even mean total disintegration. In the Sinai campaign, a trooper was leading his horse, 'when a shell burst right on him, there was a cloud of black smoke ... in a minute he staggered out into vision, but as the smoke cleared the horse was gone, a small piece of saddle was found but that was all'.[18]

Hand grenades, too, could create serious injuries. On Gallipoli, Private Percival Toms was wounded in 13 places by a Turkish grenade, '1 in the chin, which fractured my lower jaw and smashed my teeth, 9 in the arm, 2 in the side, and 1 in the foot'.[19] It was a German ball grenade or *Kugelhandgranate*, commonly known as a pineapple, that wounded Lee in France. 'I heard a whining something falling, swishing through the air. I ducked, and because the trench was full of slime I grasped the parapet, such as it was, to prevent myself falling into a mudbath ... It must have fallen close to my extended holding arm.'[20]

There was often nerve damage. When ambulance man Alfred East was wounded in the head by shrapnel in August 1915, he ended up in a Maltese hospital. 'I am able to sit up and write, but my left arm and leg seem as heavy as lead, and when the doctor rubbed a nail brush across my foot I could not tell what it was.' Writing from Brockenhurst in September 1916, Cuthbert Free told his mother about the 'awkward cut in the left hand [where] a piece of shrapnel tried to take my thumb off ... Fortunately, no bones are broken, no sinews cut — but the thing scooped up the nerves and the thumb feels neither hot nor cold now.'[21] The degree of pain felt was governed by the number of nerve endings at the wound site. Those in 'nerve-rich places like heads, hands, and feet were extremely painful'.[22]

Multiple, and far more complex, injuries were common in this war. Private William Arcus was shot in the face on Gallipoli. A machine-gun bullet smashed through his left cheekbone, then 'parted in two pieces', both of which were still in his head when he came home in July 1915, despite two operations. 'He was also shot in the middle of the back and also lower down.'[23] James Macfarlane described his five Sari Bair wounds: 'First a bullet caught me in the face; next I got a bullet through the right arm, which smashed the bone. A third shot found its way through the fleshy part of the back below the left shoulder blade. I received that little lot all within the space of five minutes.' He was then shot twice more, in each wrist.[24]

As well as being hit in the upper right arm by high explosive, William Taylor gashed his hand on revetting wire, suffered an abscess on his arm and was wounded again when machine-gun fire blasted his rifle from his hands. 'Fortunately it was across my stomach, protecting my vital organs, but the bullet travelled along it and caught two of my fingers.' Lawrence Sarten of the Canterbury Infantry Battalion was wounded 22 times during the war.[25] Wounds were not always received in battle. As Henry Winter recorded on Gallipoli on 7 June 1915, 'Two men squatting at the Latrines were shot this morning, one through the hand and stomach and the other through the leg, hard lines to get shot there.' A couple of weeks later, he reported on a man who 'got his arm shattered with a cap from a shell while bathing in the sea and as I came back I see them cutting his arm off at the hospital'.[26] Many were wounded in this way while chancing a desperately needed swim.

Compound fractures, where the damaged bone protrudes through an open wound, were common and those of the thigh (femoral) were particularly risky. At Helles in May 1915, one MO noted 'a large percentage' of such wounds, 'and many of them were terrible smashes. Small entrance holes, bone in splinters and exit of bullet had stripped away nearly all the muscle on other side of limb right away. — Holes you could put two fists into.' Douglas Stark's Gallipoli wound 'wasn't bad for a beginner — in the left leg, a hole through which he could have put three fingers'.[27]

Head injuries were common too, especially before the New Zealand troops were issued with steel helmets in 1916. Soft caps offered no protection. Soldiers on lookout or spotting duties in the trenches were frequently injured in the face and head, and eyes were lost when hit by fragments from the broken mirrors on periscopes.[28] On the Western Front, enemy fire also came from above, and although deep trenches gave some protection against small-arms fire, head and face injuries from airborne shrapnel and metal shards were frequent. When front-line helmets came into use in France, they were the British-designed Brodie inverted bowl style, which, 'although cheap and simple to manufacture, gave good protection from falling shrapnel and secondary, low-velocity fragments'.[29] In William Wilson's opinion, the Brodies 'are like soup plates and we look like a lot of chinamen with them on . . . We are a hard lot of cases. What with gas helmets, goggles, iron lids and sundry other articles we should take a lot of killing.'[30] Although it did not cover as much of the back of the head and neck as the stronger, heavier German Stahlhelm, the Brodie prevented many deaths.[31] There were attempts, too, to provide front-line medics with body protection. After a nearby ammunition dump was hit, imperilling No. 1 Field Ambulance before Messines, the men were issued with steel waistcoats but, as MO William Aitken reported, 'They were very uncomfortable and soon discarded.'[32]

A minimising laconicism marked the soldiers' descriptions of being wounded. This was born partly of the understated male antipodean style and partly of a desire not to unduly alarm anxious family and friends, especially as a condition or prognosis might alter

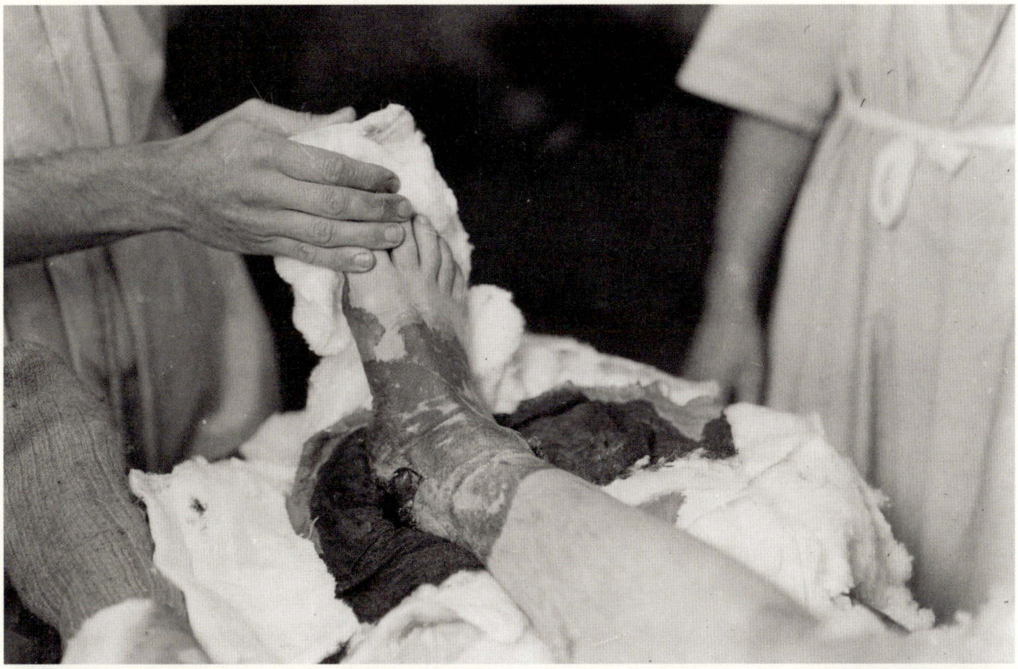

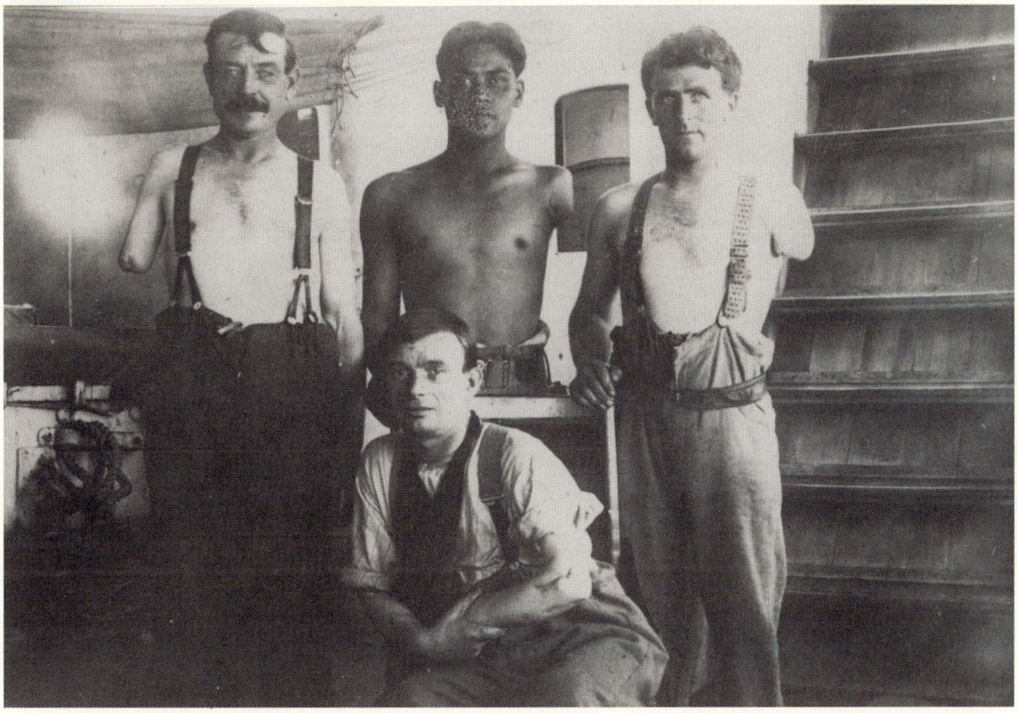

above The blood-soaked dressings tell the tale of the damage done to this soldier's ankle by a gunshot wound. The photograph was taken at a No. 2 New Zealand Field Ambulance dressing station. ALEXANDER TURNBULL LIBRARY, 1/1-002077-G

below A sobering group portrait of wounded New Zealanders taken on the *Marama*. WILLIAM YATES ALBUM, COURTESY WILLIAM YATES FAMILY, FEILDING LIBRARY during a letter's long journey to the southern hemisphere.[33] 'I got it' was a popular phrase. 'I got it in the hip,' wrote Wanganui man Phil Bennett when he was wounded on Gallipoli on 8 May; 'I got my little lot through both legs,' reported Private Walter Tindale on the same day. Like Private A. W. McNeill, hit on 7 August, many said that they had 'stopped a bullet'.[34] It was all about euphemism. 'Something of a muggins, aren't I?' Lieutenant Frank Turnbull told his mother. 'Have really only been in two fights and in both of them I have been silly enough to get winged shortly after the start of the affair.'[35] The newspapers employed similar language. When the *Willochra* arrived in July 1915 with the first wounded from Gallipoli, a *Dominion* reporter recorded that 'Private W. H. Keats . . . met his bit of trouble [a bullet to the right side of his foot] on April 28, only three days after landing'. He also, like the soldiers, used the word 'luck'. William Arcus had 'experienced more than the ordinary run of bad luck', while Private William Treseder 'had the ill-luck to run his eye against one of his comrade's bayonets'.[36] Comparison was useful. When Corporal Jack Cardwell 'got a crack during the big advance on the Somme', he was keen to reassure those at home that 'there is nothing to worry about, as my wound is nothing compared with the wounds of the majority of the poor fellows'.[37] 'When you see boys with both legs off at the thighs or both feet off & an arm off at the [shoulder],' Alec Hutton told his sister in 1918, 'you understand that I have received very mild treatment at the hand of the Hun.'[38] Hutton had lost his left foot and been badly wounded in the right leg at Bapaume. Some men did not reveal the extent of their injuries until they got home.

Black humour could sometimes help, at least after the event. Joseph Cody, who would be awarded a Military Medal at Gravenstafel in October 1917, was wounded by a sniper on Gallipoli while digging a trench.

> I was scratching away good-oh . . . when thump, and I gave a yell and a wriggle. I was under the impression that the Main Trunk Express had hit me, or Halley's Comet or something of the sort. As no bearers were in sight I began to feel about and see what was left out of the wreck of the 'appy 'ome, and found a lump out of first finger and a hole clean through second finger and left hand smashing foresaid second finger to blazes. Also discovered pair of neat little holes in right side, one just in middle of thigh, the other just above the kidneys. It made things very uncomfortable as I couldn't move, and I particularly wanted to get out of that vicinity and get myself fixed up as I didn't overmuch like the idea of pouring good Colonial gore over the hill side.[39]

That *Dominion* reporter who met the *Willochra* did his best to paint a positive picture for the public, but the reality could be difficult to avoid. NZMC man Cyril Wallace 'looked ill, he went on crutches, because he was slowly recovering from paralysis, his nerves were shattered, but he was wondrously cheerful'. Although he was 'getting all right now' and said he would be 'doing the hundred in ten and a fifth again',[40] Wallace had been before a medical board in December 1914, 'very depressed' and 'melancholic', and assessed as neurasthenic. He would be discharged as unfit in February 1916 — someone wrote on the form, 'partly simulated & malingerer' — and in October 1922 would commit suicide in Switzerland.[41]

As was all too clear from the patients hobbling or being stretchered off the *Willochra*, the doctors and orderlies on Gallipoli, and the nurses on hospital ships and in the Egyptian wards, were dealing with seriously wounded men. There would be thousands more on the Western Front. At the Daisy Patch in early May 1915, Dr George Home 'was never so thankful to have lots of morphia on hand'. Most with light wounds, such as a bullet graze, were dressed and returned immediately to the firing line. Frank O'Connor, with the Wellington Infantry Battalion, 'had a piece taken out of his scalp' at Gaba Tepe, got a dressing and went back to the fight, only to end up 'with a bullet through the skin at the root of his neck'. With 'two unhealed wounds', he then lost the sight of his right eye. Home noted, too, that 'a great many of our casualties occur because men go through a machine gun stream of bullets to bring in one who has just been hit'.[42] When Clutha Mackenzie, son of High Commissioner Thomas Mackenzie, was blinded on Gallipoli, Roy Dalrymple was close by. 'A moment after the concussion shell had exploded in our trench I heard him say something and looked down, and there he was trying to get past me. Both his eyes were blown out by the concussion. He was crawling along the trench . . . Apparently he did not have much pain but it was the most pitiful sight I have seen.'[43]

Dalrymple himself was wounded in the buttock that day. His vivid account reveals the mental and psychological stress of being injured.

> Was it going off, surely the dam thing had been there about two hours! I'll have a look at it! No! Look out there is a fuse fizzing, just about off. Where will it hit me, what will it feel like, Ugh! And I screwed up my face and all possible portions of my anatomy. Why does it not go off? When the deu . . . Bang — biff, something hit me as a whack on the side, and along my leg. 'I'm done! No I'm not! Let's have a look.' All my pants torn and bloody and I think I had better get out while I can. I suppose the bomb only took about a second to explode, but during my wait for it I went through all those thoughts and a good many more.[44]

Although injury meant pain and potential disability, even death, many men yearned for what they called a Blighty, a backsheesh or a buckshee — a wound bad enough to take them to hospital, or even home, without guilt about leaving the fighting, and their mates, behind. Wounded twice on Gallipoli, Private Raymond Ward told his father in May 1915: 'In spite of the painfulness of wounds, and the unpleasantness of hot fomentations and the like, my heart is already softening to that sniper for having given me such a respite.' When future Second World War commander Howard Kippenberger got a 'smack on the arm' in November 1916, his mate Frank Hanly was 'almost speechless with admiration'. As they went down the sap, 'Frank led the way . . . explaining to all and sundry "Old Kip's got a buckshee". I came next, wearing the pleased and happy expression of so fortunate a person.'[45] Not everyone was eager for a such an escape, however. 'I don't want any of these blighties,' Len Wilton concluded. 'I have seen to[o] much of that sort of thing. I seen a boy not long ago going down to the dressing station as happy as a sand boy with a piece of iron in his leg but he finished up with having his leg taken off.'[46]

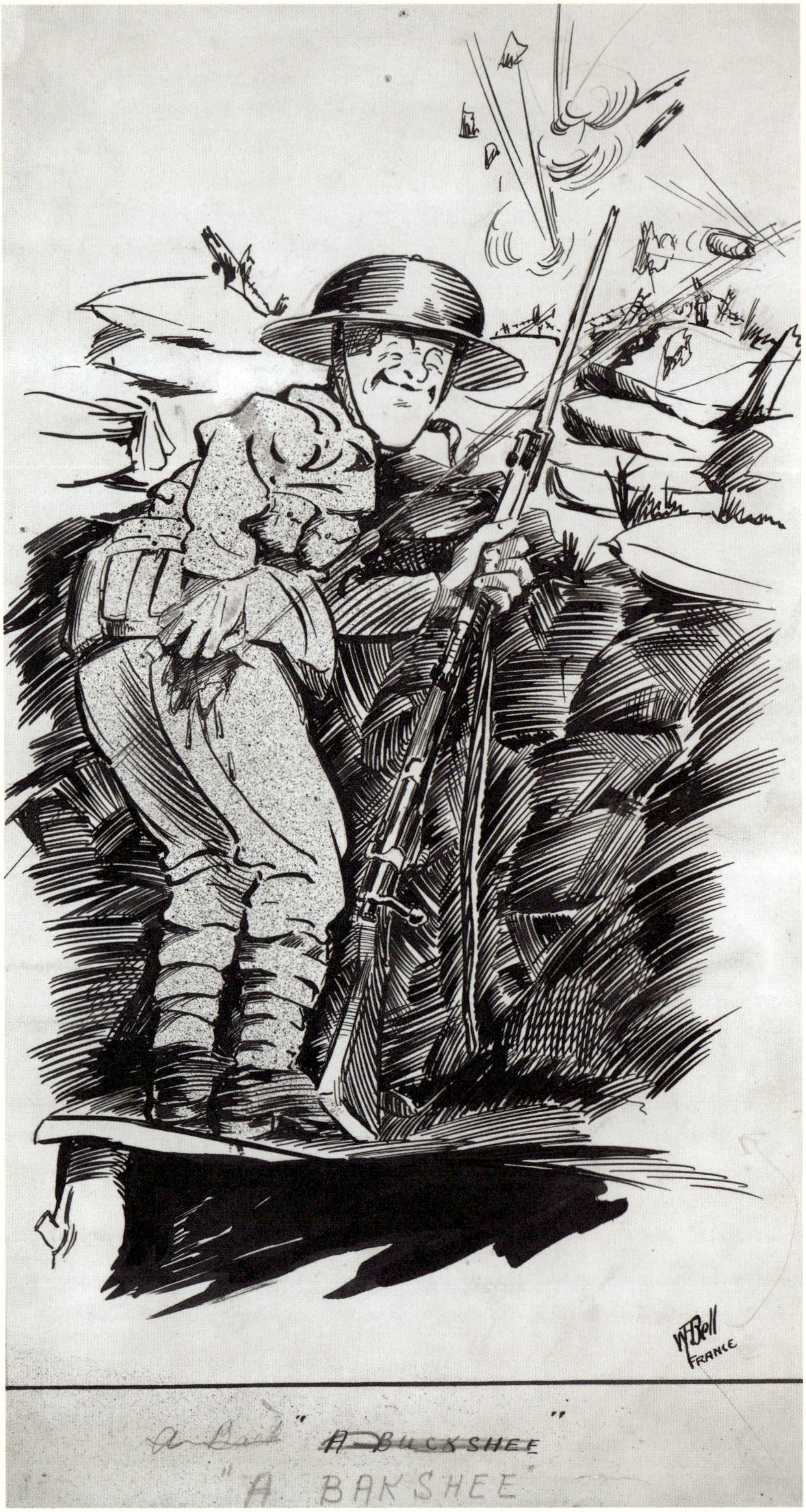

A flesh wound like the one delighting this soldier was a Blighty (or buckshee) that guaranteed a trip to hospital, or maybe across the Channel. An original drawing by W. F. Bell for the 1916 publication *Shell-Shocks: New Zealanders in France*. ALEXANDER TURNBULL LIBRARY, A-222-011

The adjustment to being wounded could be considerable. 'I was no longer a soldier,' wrote Claude Weston, 'but some other person; still an individual perhaps, and yet not quite. I became a patient.' Weston, a barrister in civilian life, was awarded a DSO in 1917 after being badly wounded in October that year. 'It is an opinion generally held,' he continued, 'that the moment a patient is undressed and snuggles in between the cool white sheets of his ward bed, his troubles are ended . . . Of a truth his duties have only begun, and no one has more need of coolness, judgment and a sound philosophy than the sick man entering the gates of a Hospital.' Unlike disease, wounds did not run 'the same definite course; a wounded man has his ups and downs, and must simply face each day as it comes . . . "Don't worry, and keep quiet," are not bad instructions.'[47] There was indignity, too, as Clifford Collingwood found. 'I could not lift myself on to a bed-pan, or fix myself up, so an orderly had to lift me up on to a pan and later clean me. I felt very sensitive about this, but the extreme weakness and the severe pain I was in, helped me to accept the . . . assistance. Many others in that huge ward were in a similar condition.'[48]

Weston noticed differences in how men endured pain and confinement. '[T]he more highly-strung find it hard, very hard, but the great majority of those I met were brave, patient philosophers.' Attitudes could alter, too, as Alec Hutton observed among the amputees at Brockenhurst. Men 'arrive feeling themselves terribly badly wounded but after a time when the fellows have told them that they are not wounded at all unless they have something wrong besides a leg off they begin to think things are not so frightful after all.'[49] Many, of course, were facing 'a maimed and dislocated future'. Weston pitied men 'who feel a dull ache in the lost part for weeks after the amputation — a harsh reminder of their loss'.[50] Among those forced to adjust to life as a 'limbie' was John A. Lee who, in his novel *Soldier*, left a searing description of the wounding in France that cost him his left arm.

> Agony unbelievable. The fingers of my arm seemed a tangled mess. I reached with my right arm and felt a tacky something. I staggered to the bivvy . . . I held the pulpy end of the arm up and took notice. I had no hand, no forearm. Two jagged bones protruded from a tangled mass of flesh . . . What had been an arm looked like a bloody chrysanthemum. I know I was groaning in agony. But from the confused arm end streams of blood started to leap into the air, at each heartbeat pulsing my life into the bloody ditch.

After Lee's companions fashioned tourniquets from bootlaces, two stretcher-bearers arrived. At the dressing station, the MO gave him first one and then a second opium pellet. 'It's more painful than a lot more dangerous wounds,' he explained. 'Every nerve between your hand and brain is yelling in protest . . . Lucky it didn't get you in the guts or chest as well. You'd never have made it.'[51]

Accidents accounted for wounds such as William Treseder's bayonet injury and the one Ormond Burton suffered when his knee 'connected with' the point of a fixed bayonet left on a fire step.[52] On Gallipoli, at the beginning of August 1915, William Malone noted 'a bad accident in the trenches' when the fuse of a mortar bomb misfired. The resulting explosion blew off the hand and forearm of Sergeant Robert Nairn, who died soon after.[53] In France in

June 1916 Herbert Hart recorded a 'frightfully depressing accident' during live bomb practice which killed two men and wounded two, one seriously.[54] There were similar occurrences in the camps at home.

Self-inflicted wounds were not uncommon, particularly as New Zealanders faced their 'first prolonged experience of trench warfare' on the Western Front. 'For men pushed to the limit of physical and mental endurance', an SIW, as it was known, provided 'a certain way out, one where the risk of future punishment was immaterial compared to the pressures they were escaping'.[55] By May 1918, Len Coley remembered, men were 'willingly exposing themselves to machine-gun bullets to get injured'. This usually involved arms and legs. 'I even saw one man stand on his hands in the trench with both legs pushed over the top. No matter how hard some tried, very few were injured in this way. A few men even injured each other deliberately. German rifles and ammunition were plentiful for this task.'[56] The official view was clear. Regardless of whether the SIW was accidental or intentional, a court-martial would be required. 'The M.O. will, therefore, particularly note the position, direction, etc., of the wound, and especially if there is any blackening of the skin or burning of clothing, showing proximity of the weapon. He will note anything the man volunteers about it.'[57]

Malingering, or 'swinging the lead', was widespread and its manifestations were 'staggering in their variety and inventiveness'. The men faked an impressive range of medical conditions, from shell shock to appendicitis to epilepsy.[58] At the less serious end, the aim was often to avoid parades or fatigue duties, as Douglas Stark managed to do at Suez. When he described 'exactly' how he felt, the MO 'looked pretty serious, and said, "You've got the symptoms of sunstroke, old man. You lie down and keep quiet." He gives me a chit and when I hand it over to the Colonel I'm excused fourteen days. I didn't mention I'd read up about sunstroke in a book the night before.'[59] More extreme attempts were both bizarre and dangerous, as historian Ashley Ekins recounts. 'They took drugs to simulate respiratory and circulatory system disorders; they ingested picric acid to imitate jaundice; they put irritants in their eyes to simulate conjunctivitis; they deliberately infected slight injuries; and they injected petrol, paraffin or turpentine into knee joints to induce synovitis and abscesses.' There were even attempts to become infected with venereal disease.[60]

On Gallipoli, William McAra 'examined a man with suspected insanity; forgets coat when appearing before General or any officer; couldn't learn drill, at least said so. Laid down on road when guard bringing him to see me — said no strength to walk — couldn't find lunacy about him. Sent him to Ear Hospital — got out wax each ear.'[61] Not all the troops approved of such behaviour — in Lee's words, 'honest illness stifled among the unmanly subterfuges of the few rotters'[62] — and the military machine had no time for what it saw as cowardice, but these elaborate stratagems were often born of genuine desperation. A young Australian on Gallipoli told McAra 'where one can go & get a bullet through an arm or leg for [£?]5. Also can have a bone broken "in a safe place" for a higher price. It seems incredible but when men are here for months, anything is tried by some so as to get away.'[63] Doctors, expected to watch for and expose malingerers, were frequently put in an invidious position.

The myth of sacrifice and heroism promoted in the newspapers and by the government required tales of stoicism and courage, and sufficient unbiased accounts show that many badly hurt men were indeed brave and uncomplaining. 'Our boys are magnificent in battle,' wrote George Home at Helles, 'but even more so, when they are wounded. They stood grievous and painful bodily damage . . . in a way that I marvelled at.' William Malone described the 'strings of wounded men' passing him on Gallipoli: 'No cries or groans, not a whimper or complaint. The only cry I heard was from one poor chap who was shot up most ghastily, and his wasn't a cry, it was a repeated "oh Daddy" "oh Daddy".'[64]

Kippenberger was touched by the courage of one man in France. His right wrist and hand had been smashed, there was a big gash in his right thigh and he had a flesh wound in his neck. 'Huddled on his knees, and his face sweating with his agony, he yet smiles . . . Put on field dressings, "Sorry old chap, not a drop of water myself", and work him into a more comfortable position. Whatever his pain, he won't make your job harder by showing it, thanks you in a pleasant voice, and settles down to wait, hours probably, for the stretcher-bearers. You feel like choking to see their gameness.'[65]

But many injuries were too agonising for stoic silence and such ordeals as an ambulance journey or frequent dressing of wounds tried men cruelly. When Clifford Collingwood had to endure a new type of splint on his shattered leg, 'The pain which followed was very severe, for although I did not cry out or make any noise, I had to bite the pillow and tears were being wrung out of me. I wished my leg was right off.' When a replacement splint was fitted later that day, 'I had an interesting few minutes, and had to keep my face buried in my pillow . . . for I wanted to keep quiet, if possible.' He wrote of 'Men in pain groaning all night, sudden screams of severe pain'.[66]

Of course the effects of wounds did not end with the Armistice. Many hundreds of men went home with significant disabilities that limited their ability to earn a living, ruined their private lives and sometimes left them struggling with chronic pain and disfigurement. After Bill Dyer was wounded at Passchendaele, the field hospital staff were 'unable [to] remove all the shrapnel and merely stitched him up as best they could. The shrapnel stayed with him for the rest of his life.' His son saw the wounds just once: 'from the top of his right shoulder to his buttocks was one big scar . . . one buttock was smaller than the other because of the wound. In addition . . . he was wounded in the hand and gassed.'[67]

Not all wounds were visible. On the morning of 26 April 1915, the day after the Gallipoli landing, MO Cyril Tewsley encountered an officer 'suffering from very nervous upset'.

> He was a big, powerful man, but reduced to the condition of a child, breaking into tears at the least provocation, and absolutely minus self-control. He was unwounded and we made him comfortable in a sheltered and safe corner. After several hours sleep he woke up a different man. I am satisfied now that he should have been evacuated, but it was my first experience of such a case — later on to become only too familiar — and we let him have his way, and return to his unit. I never heard any more about him.[68]

Some months later, at Hill 60, another MO treated an 18-year-old private whose condition was later 'recognisable as a typical picture of War Neurosis, a term as yet unknown at Anzac'.[69] On 26 August the man went forward with his platoon but when commanded to fire 'could not discharge his rifle, nor even put it to his shoulder; he was told by his officer to crawl back'. By the evening of the 28th his pulse was 120 and his temperature 100°F. 'He could not walk in a straight line. He had violent trembling of the whole body with twitching. He was holding both hands tightly clenched together, and on making him loosen them they both shook violently. He can not sleep; every shot makes him jump or twitch; he says he can never face fire again.' As the doctor noted, the lad was no coward, advancing under heavy machine-gun fire and retiring only when ordered: 'I believe his nervous system, probably like his body, weak in the first place, has been permanently shattered.'[70] As one man hit in the arm on Gallipoli said, 'This nerve trouble is far worse. Even yet when a door bangs I feel as if I had had an electric shock.' MO Alexander Trotter encountered one man who 'fainted several times at the sound of the guns'.[71]

As Australian medical historian Graham Butler would later write, in a chapter entitled 'Moral and Mental Disorders', such cases came as a surprise to the MOs on the peninsula, who were 'called on to diagnose the condition and decide the disposal of men who, as the result (as it often seemed) of some "shocking" physical experience, were unable to control tremblings, or were "struck" paralytic, blind or speechless; or . . . who had hitherto deported themselves after the manner of men, but now became unable to face the situation, relapsing into a condition of mental anguish, and impotence'.[72] But these symptoms had been familiar to the staff of British hospitals and CCSs on the Western Front since the northern winter of 1914–15. The soldiers themselves had christened such behaviour shell shock, a term that neatly fitted the pre-war belief that mental illness was caused by disease or physical injury. When soldiers injured in, or close to, shell explosions displayed the behaviour and symptoms that Butler pinpointed, along with loss of sight, speech and hearing, amnesia, nightmares, insomnia and extraordinary gaits, it made sense to believe such experiences were to blame.[73] Shell shock was being used in the casualty lists of New Zealand newspapers by September 1915 and was certainly known to New Zealand troops: a fund-raising magazine published in 1916 was entitled *Shell-Shocks: New Zealanders in France.*

Cambridge psychologist Charles S. Myers, who became 'Specialist in Nervous Shock' to the British army in France, used the expression in a February 1915 *Lancet* article when describing three cases in which soldiers had been 'blown up'.[74] But he, and other specialists, were soon aware of inconsistencies in the organic approach. Sufferers included men who had not been close to shellfire, were out of the front line or had not even experienced an attack,[75] and their numbers were growing. There was vigorous debate, but by mid-1916 many doctors had concluded that the 'bursting shell' was not the sole cause. 'Wartime "shell-shock" was in fact very similar to peacetime "hysteria" and "neurasthenia".'[76] It became evident, too, that the variety of physical symptoms constituting possible shell shock was dauntingly wide, and that some could denote other conditions. For example, shortness of breath could mean 'heart problems, tuberculosis, the effect of poison gas, gas neurosis, respiratory infection or a stress reaction'.[77]

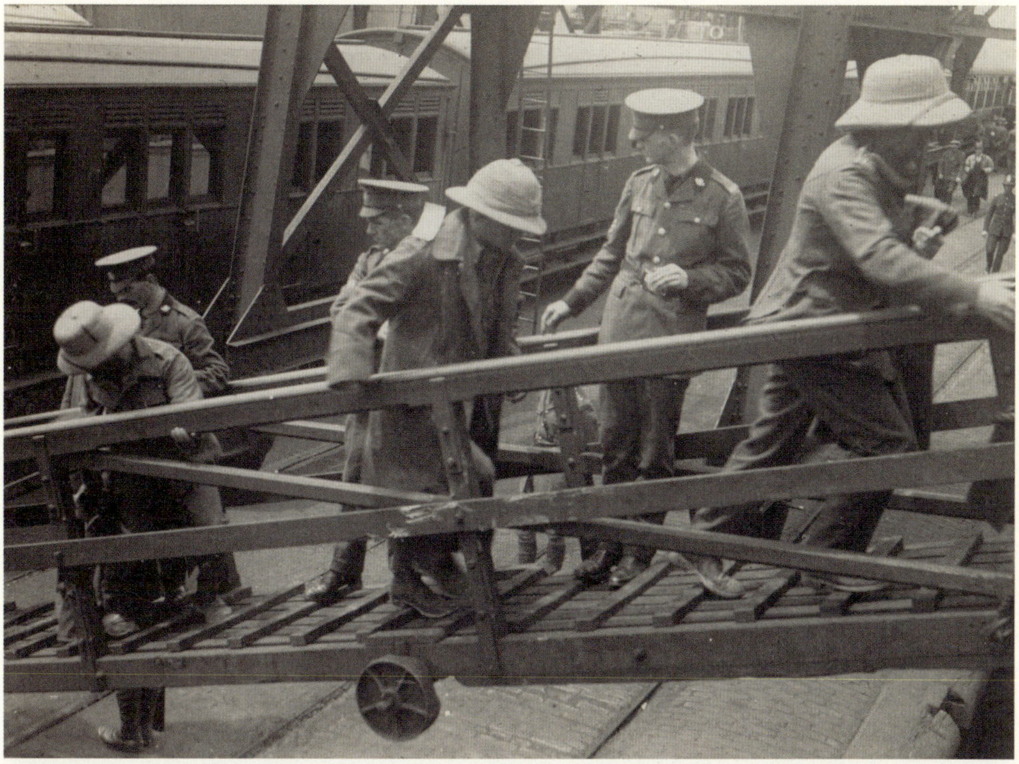

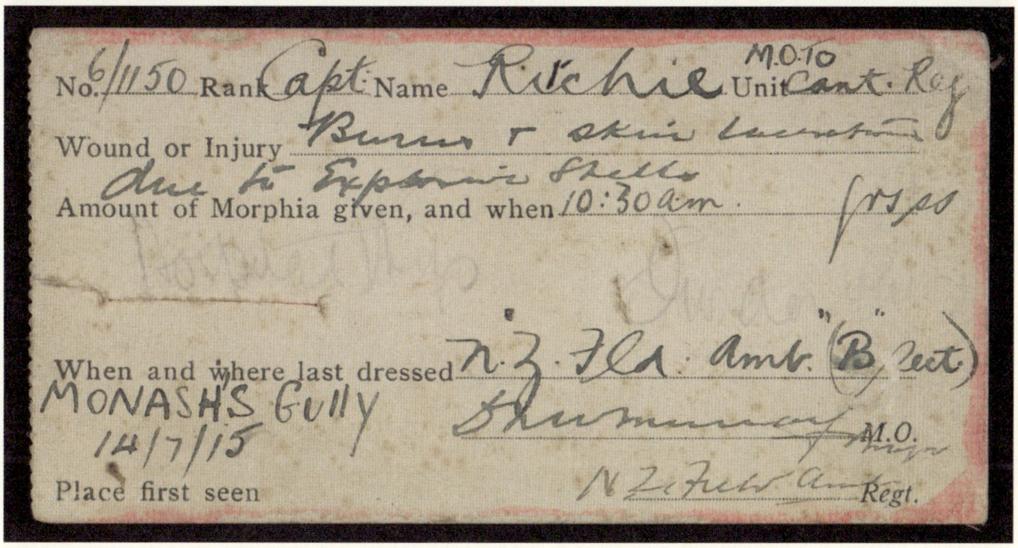

No. 6/1150 Rank Capt. Name Ritchie Unit Cant. Reg
M.O. to
Wound or Injury Burns & skin lacerations
due to Explosive Shells
Amount of Morphia given, and when 10:30 am.

When and where last dressed N.Z. Fld. Amb. (B. Sect)
MONASH'S Gully
14/7/15
M.O.
Place first seen N.Z. Field Amb. Regt.

above Not all wounds were visible. In the parlance of the day, Bill Yates labelled this image, 'Mental patients embarking at Cape Town, S. A.'. WILLIAM YATES ALBUM, COURTESY WILLIAM YATES FAMILY, FEILDING LIBRARY

below The details of Captain Thomas Ritchie's Gallipoli wounds — burns and skin lacerations caused by explosive shells — and treatment are set out on the card that would accompany him when he was evacuated. ALEXANDER TURNBULL LIBRARY, MS-PAPERS-3705-1

Experiencing high explosive close at hand could certainly provoke an immediate breakdown, as Harry Kitson discovered on Gallipoli in June 1915. 'I don't remember much until I woke up in the hospital, but they told me I went quite dotty & was going to rush back with a rifle & take on all hands. I was grabbed & rushed away.' He assured his sisters that he 'soon got alright except for a rotten headache & a bit numb in the arms & legs', but in fact he would continue to suffer, and a medical board held after he was sent home diagnosed 'Neurasthenia H.E. Shell'.[78] Kitson did recover, but he was not alone in his reaction. As William Wilson noted, 'Really nobody who has not been through it knows what the awful sensation of a bursting HE is at close quarters. No wonder men's nerves are ruined for life.'[79] Things were worse on the Western Front. By the time the *Marama* was on the cross-Channel run in mid-1916, taking wounded New Zealanders and other Allied soldiers from France to England, 'Shell shock was a very frequent trouble, and many of those received on board had lost their reason.'[80]

Being buried by an explosion was particularly terrifying. 'BANG,' wrote 21-year-old Sergeant Cyril Coxhead at the end of September 1916, 'I'm thrown down and partly buried.' He extricated himself and found 'superhuman strength' to lift out a badly wounded mate, but then 'seemed to "crack up". I shook like a leaf and my back crumpled up. Some one . . . took us down to the dressing station and set me on the road back but I must have been wandering as it was daylight when I found the Ambulance.' He spent time at a rest camp and was soon back in the line, but at Ploegsteert Wood in mid-March 1917, he wrote, 'I shudder as each gun fires. I have lost my nerve completely and feel like giving in when the shells fly around. It is an awful feeling, but no one seems to notice it on me and thank goodness my men don't.' By May, however, while instructing at a Lewis gun school, he had no choice but to go: 'Was sorry to leave the boys, but as my nerves were getting worse I was unable to stand up to the shell-fire any longer.'[81] When Harry Luckman was buried by an exploding shell in October 1917, he was, according to a medical board, 'demented' when dug out and had to be carried. He endured 30 fits and remained 'very nervous, stammers badly over closed consonants . . . Tremor of hands which are always cold.'[82]

And the strain of constant bombardment and the anticipation of wounding or death had a cumulative effect. 'It was not our first shelling that frightened us so much,' Norman Hassell remembered, 'as the . . . ones three or four years afterwards . . . I could stand up to anything in the way of shell fire for the first couple of years, but the last year or so was my undoing. Every burst used to set me all quivering, and if the Armistice had been delayed much longer, I would probably have been a "shell-shock" case.' As Len Wilton told his fiancée in December 1918, 'If I had not come into hospital when I did I would have broken down in France. I just managed to hang on until I got over here on leave & by reporting to hospital I reckon I have saved my self from a general break down.'[83] In France, Lee wrote, men 'twitched at sounds that were dangerous and at sounds that were harmless' and found themselves 'listening at the silences'. Former Wanganui journalist Sergeant Roland Armit experienced this awful anticipation: 'My ears are atingle with expectancy all the time — expectant of the screech, of one of the hundreds of shells that come our way. This deplorable state of "nerves" has been brought about by what is known as shell-shock: it should be called, "hell-shock".'[84]

Some front-line treatment could be less than sensitive, albeit necessary. At Gommecourt Wood, Charles Carrington witnessed 'a man in a state of hysterics who was not only unable to do his work but was preventing others from doing their work. So my friend . . . just lifted his fist and . . . gave him a bloody great clout in the face and knocked him out and that settled him.'[85] Peer sympathy could be lacking, too, when a sufferer was hospitalised. As Leonard Leary recalled, 'they'd soon pick the bloke who had shellshock . . . you'd be asleep at night and the other blokes [would] imitate the hiss of a coming shell', then bang down a stone hot water bottle and switch the light on and off. 'And if you were still in bed you'd been on the staff. If you were under the bed then you'd been in the war.'[86]

Some men should never have been allowed into the NZEF, let alone sent into battle. They had had problems, but 'falsely confident of their mental and emotional stability, would, suppressing their past history, enlist'.[87] On 5 February 1915, Private Dan Bardsley was found in the Egyptian desert with a jagged wound in his throat and cuts on his left wrist, 'which he stated were self-inflicted'. When he returned to his unit in March an obviously sympathetic Cyril Baigent investigated Bardsley's case — 'his troubles began when he was 11 yrs of age' and he had wanted to throw himself off the transport taking him to war — and recommended a medical board.[88] This, held by Charles Thomas the next day, decided that Bardsley was 'suffering from melancholia with suicidal & homicidal tendencies'. As Thomas told his wife, Milly, 'He will be returning to N.Z. in a few days poor chap . . . He is off his head . . . he is under a guard day and night.'[89] This arrangement did not prevent Bardsley from jumping off the *Tahiti* on 29 April 1915; his mother committed suicide soon afterwards. Trooper Horace Haycock left New Zealand with the Main Body but was sent home in May 1915. As two medical boards in Wellington noted in July, 'He is a confirmed neurasthenic who should never have enlisted, he must have concealed his condition at the preliminary medical examination.'[90]

In *A War of Nerves*, Ben Shephard suggests that the term shell shock was 'an early example of a common modern phenomenon: a medical debate, hedged with scientific qualifications, taken up by the public and the media in an oversimplified way'. The 'image of the shell itself — a violent, concussive *deus ex machina* . . . took root in the public imagination', although it could be argued, at least initially, that the expression passed from laypeople to the medical profession.[91] It also allowed many men and their families to avoid the stigma associated with words such as 'hysteria' and 'neurasthenia': '"Shell-shock" was a vehicle . . . of consolation and legitimation.'[92]

What did the military make of shell shock? In its view, especially among the rank and file, mental illness equalled weakness, something to be dealt with by severe discipline unless committal to an asylum became necessary. Eventually there was reluctant official recognition that this was a genuine medical problem and should be treated as such, but concerns about morale and malingering remained widespread. The military also, of course, relied on doctors to manage the phenomenon.[93] From late 1915 the British army distinguished between shell shock and concussion patients, harmed by enemy action and to be labelled 'Shell-shock W' (wound), and those whose breakdown was not considered directly attributable to such causes; they were marked 'Shell-shock S' (sickness). This decision meant that some men, genuinely suffering but labelled 'S', continued to fight when they should have been treated, while those designated 'W' could legitimately be evacuated. As one returned Christchurch soldier pointed out in early 1917, 'such misfortunes as "shell shock" . . . do not entitle a man to the honour [of wearing a wound stripe], although the victim may have seen a good deal more fighting than many of those wounded'.[94] And someone labelled 'W' could even, without 'any overt intent [of] malingering . . . start to develop symptoms previously absent. The disease followed the diagnosis.'[95]

For hard-pressed New Zealand MOs on the Western Front, particularly those at dressing stations, controversies about terminology were largely irrelevant. They needed rules to follow. On the Somme in September 1916, ADMS Charles Begg directed that 'Cases of unconsciousness following the bursting of a shell in close proximity, injured eardrums, paralysis or paresis, aphasia, etc., will be evacuated as "wounded shell shock." Cases of hysteria, neurasthenia, debility, etc., will be cleared as sick.' ('Debility' is a common term in the medical history sections of First World War personnel records.) Front-line officers were not always particularly sympathetic, though others, in Charles Carrington's view, accepted 'a genuine breakdown by a man who had . . . done his best and . . . couldn't take any more'.[96]

The official military line was made abundantly clear in 'Instructions to Field Ambulances. Shell Shock, Neurasthenia Disposal', issued on 14 October 1916. Those who had not maintained 'mental equilibrium' because they lacked the required 'nerve stability' could not 'be allowed to escape disciplinary action on the ground of a medical diagnosis of "Shell Shock" or "Neurasthenia" or "Inability to Withstand Shell Fire"'. Officers and men who had 'failed in their duty' had too often used such expressions as excuses, and MOs, without considering the 'military issues at stake', had put such cases 'in the same category as ordinary illness'. As with suspected SIWs, only a court-martial could decide whether an offender should escape punishment.[97]

By Messines, in June 1917, field ambulances had new instructions. Those who had 'obvious shell shock' were to go to a CCS with the diagnosis 'NYD (not yet diagnosed) shell shock'; 'doubtful cases', including exhaustion, nervousness and possible malingering, were to be labelled 'exhaustion' and dispatched to a divisional rest station.[98] Further refinements soon followed. Neither the RMO nor the ambulance officer was to record any diagnosis, but merely write 'NYDN' — not yet diagnosed, non-efficient — on a soldier's field medical card and 'note any definite known facts as to the true origin of the case. The term "Shell Shock" will on no account be used.'[99] In his *Notes for R.M.Os. of the New Zealand Division*, published in August 1917, ADMS Colonel Donald McGavin stressed that the terms 'shell shock', 'shell concussion', 'neurasthenia' and 'inability to stand shell fire' were '*not* to be used under any circumstances. The diagnosis will be written "N.Y.D.N."' The MO should find out as much as he could about what had happened, note the man's physical condition and 'state his own opinion' in a closed communication. He 'must not express his opinion to the patient, but should assume an air of optimism and encouragement'.[100] The proscription of shell shock followed British precedent, though the 'N' there stood for 'Nervous'. But the term persisted, not least, perhaps, because it was 'concise, alliterative, powerful, not only suggestive of . . . but sounding like war'.[101]

When Andrew Carbery, in his history, came to summarise the types of therapy in vogue for 'war neuroses', he likened the list to 'a page from Rabelais'. It included cerebro-spinal galvanism, disciplinary measures, torpillage ('painstaking, indefatigable, masterful, relentless pertinacity on the part of the operator, fortified by a powerful sinsusoidal current'), suggestion, hypnosis, massage, Faradism (electric shock), lumbar puncture and psychoanalysis.[102] But many of these were last-resort options; suggestion and persuasion, with some use of electricity, were more frequently employed. Auckland neurologist James Boyd, who spent 15 months with the RAMC, worked at a London hospital treating nervous cases. There various methods were used to show patients that their symptoms 'meant that they had merely lost their control. Persuasion succeeded in some cases, and hypnotic suggestion in others,' though the latter could be uncertain. Fresh air and diversion were also important.[103]

Being sent home was often the response. Richard Dowling was working as a dispenser at Codford when he was admitted to the hospital. As CO Percival Fenwick reported on 7 October 1916, Dowling had been boarded some weeks before 'and the Disability was stated to be Melancholia'. In the last few days, it had been decided that neurasthenia was the 'correct diagnosis'. After 'great improvement', Dowling had 'become nervous again. Personally after having the man under my special notice for several weeks, I believe that a sea voyage and the prospect of seeing his family again will have the most beneficial effect.'[104] One afflicted Kiwi was treated in the United States. After being half-buried when he was 'blown in' at Quinn's Post in 1915, Sapper Frank Leyland was left with 'seriously affected' speech, 'and unfortunately the impediment was increased by some violent shell "shock" a little later'. Thanks to the intervention of Thomas Mackenzie and others, Leyland was permitted to travel, at his own expense, to the Bogue Institute for Stammerers in Indianapolis. After four months there he returned to Auckland, 'able to speak slowly, but quite clearly'.[105]

By mid-1917, a New Zealand neurological section had been established at Brockenhurst, in the Balmer Lawn part of the hospital, under the charge of Dunedin's Major Marshall Macdonald, and all New Zealand 'functional' cases, including shell shock and neurasthenia, were sent here. By April 1918, William Parkes could report to Godley that 'exceedingly good results are obtained not only in ordinary functional cases but in hysterical gaits characterised by high stepping; these have proved very amenable to muscle re-education. Neurasthenics have benefited very markedly by isolation treatment which can be carried out very effectively amid the quiet surroundings of Balmer Lawn.'[106]

Shell-shocked British officers were treated differently from the other ranks,[107] and something of this demarcation was evident in Godley's attitude. Assiduous in rooting out any possible malingering in the ranks, he was more forgiving when it came to officers. As he wrote to James Allen from France in June 1916,

> The conditions here, though in most ways easier than at Gallipoli, are more trying to anyone whose nerves are not quite right, on account of the intensity and weight of the enemy's shelling when it comes, and a certain number of officers, especially comparatively senior and oldish ones, are breaking down under the strain and will have to be sent back to New Zealand, I hope you understand that these men are only sent back with the greatest reluctance, and that there is no reflection, except that they are not physically fit enough to stand the strain.[108]

Medical personnel were hit hard psychologically. Constantly exposed to often terrible wounds, to pain and death, and to danger, they were forced to develop a hard shell, an essential insensitivity — a contradictory requirement for people in a caring profession. When the New Zealand hospital in France came under aerial attack in 1917, Nurse Elsie Grey wrote, 'I am sure I would have got shell shock if I had stayed out there much longer.'[109] The correspondence between Hester Maclean and Mabel Thurston reveals how frequently nurses 'broke down' and had to be rested or sent home. On 15 January 1917, for example, Thurston was 'really worried over the worn out condition of many of our nurses . . . Particularly those nurses who were in the "Marquette" seem to be showing bad effects. They suffer from sleeplessness and frequent small illnesses.' On 15 May she reported that Margaret Nixon, just back from Bombay, 'is looking desperately ill and is just a shadow of her former self, her nerves in such a condition that she could not speak without crying'.[110]

The cost for doctors could also be very high. Arthur Evans from Dunedin, who left New Zealand in November 1914, served with the RAMC and then the NZMC until June 1919. He was a senior physician at a London hospital when, on 19 October that year, he went missing and was later believed dead. As the verdict of 'Death due to war service' revealed, his impressive CV masked a troubled history. In May 1917 Evans had been admitted to Brockenhurst, 'suffering from Neurasthenia as follows — Insomnia, Mental Depression, Loss of appetite, Loss of weight, Tremor, Inability to concentrate his mind on any subject and lack of energy'. Six months later he was still 'occasionally depressed'. The original cause of the neurasthenia was noted as 'overstrain'. When Evans was at Codford, Percival Fenwick thought he 'did his work excellently' but later 'noticed that he was becoming extremely nervous and . . . managed to get him short sick leave at Brighton'. He was certain that Evans's neurasthenia ultimately caused his death.[111]

On 31 July 1927, 34-year-old Dr Angus Marshall, also from Dunedin, committed suicide by drinking hyacin, 'self administered while in a state of depression'. One of the 21 Otago medical students who enlisted in 1914, he had worked at Trentham, then gone overseas in November 1915 and served at the NZSH, with frequent stints at CCSs in France. In the last year of the war he was an anaesthetist at Sidcup. Back in New Zealand, he continued this specialist and expert role at Henry Pickerill's Facial and Jaw Department, later part time, while working at Dunedin Hospital. In August 1928 his wife Grace enquired if any medals were due to her late husband, 'as I am sure our small son would appreciate some later on'.[112]

Field ambulance men and stretcher-bearers, too, were under constant pressure. In October 1916, Private L. J. (Tod) Anderson described how 'a certain friend in Southland' had told him he was 'very fortunate to be a member of an ambulance unit. I told the boys about it, and they didn't seem to think so just at the time. We had all been working solid for about 48 hours and were all completely done up with the long carries in the mud, and the strain on our nerves was beginning to tell also. No man can honestly say he is not a bit nervy while under heavy fire.'[113] In October 1917, ambulance man Reginald Napier, who had been wounded on Gallipoli, killed himself in Belgium by drinking chloroform. 'I'm feeling horribly fed up and far from well,' he wrote in his suicide note. 'Where am I going? Well to where so many of the Main Body have gone . . . Au revoir.'[114]

Captain George Sandham, who was singled out for conspicuous gallantry in July 1915 and given an MC in January 1917, was diagnosed with neurasthenia in May 1918. 'He is shaky & nervous. His memory is poor. He misses out words when writing. He cannot apply himself. Suffers from headaches & sleeps badly. He is unduly breathless on exertion & easily fatigued.' Sandham was sent home but in March 1919, though improved, still had occasional headaches and 'muscular twitching of face'. He was hospitalised with neurasthenia in February 1921 and died of tuberculosis in Palmerston North Hospital in August.[115]

Views vary on whether shell shock can be equated with or contributed to post-traumatic stress disorder, but in the end, perhaps, names and definitions matter less than experience, in wartime and often for a lifetime. Frederick Foote's was just one story among many. For three or four years after he came home, shell shock was 'a great handicap . . . and some of the effects lasted much longer than that'.

> I had great difficulty in mixing socially with people and they often thought me unusual and were often justified in thinking so . . . If I went with a party to a dance I might be all right for the evening, I might be all right for half the evening or less. Suddenly, for no apparent reason, the feet slipping on the floor would upset me . . . I would feel wretched and agitated. I would have to get out, get away by myself and I would go. I did not understand it myself and those I was with understood it less.

Foote later applied successfully for two jobs but 'never turned up for either. I was still very weak, sick and restless, and felt I did not have the stability the positions would require.' Without a confidante or an understanding doctor, 'I made a mistake in my decision — I should have studied, and by improving my education, found lifes support and interest in a field more adapted to my physical condition.' Instead he ended up working the land. 'I was only moderately successful, and my progress was slow and hard.'[116]

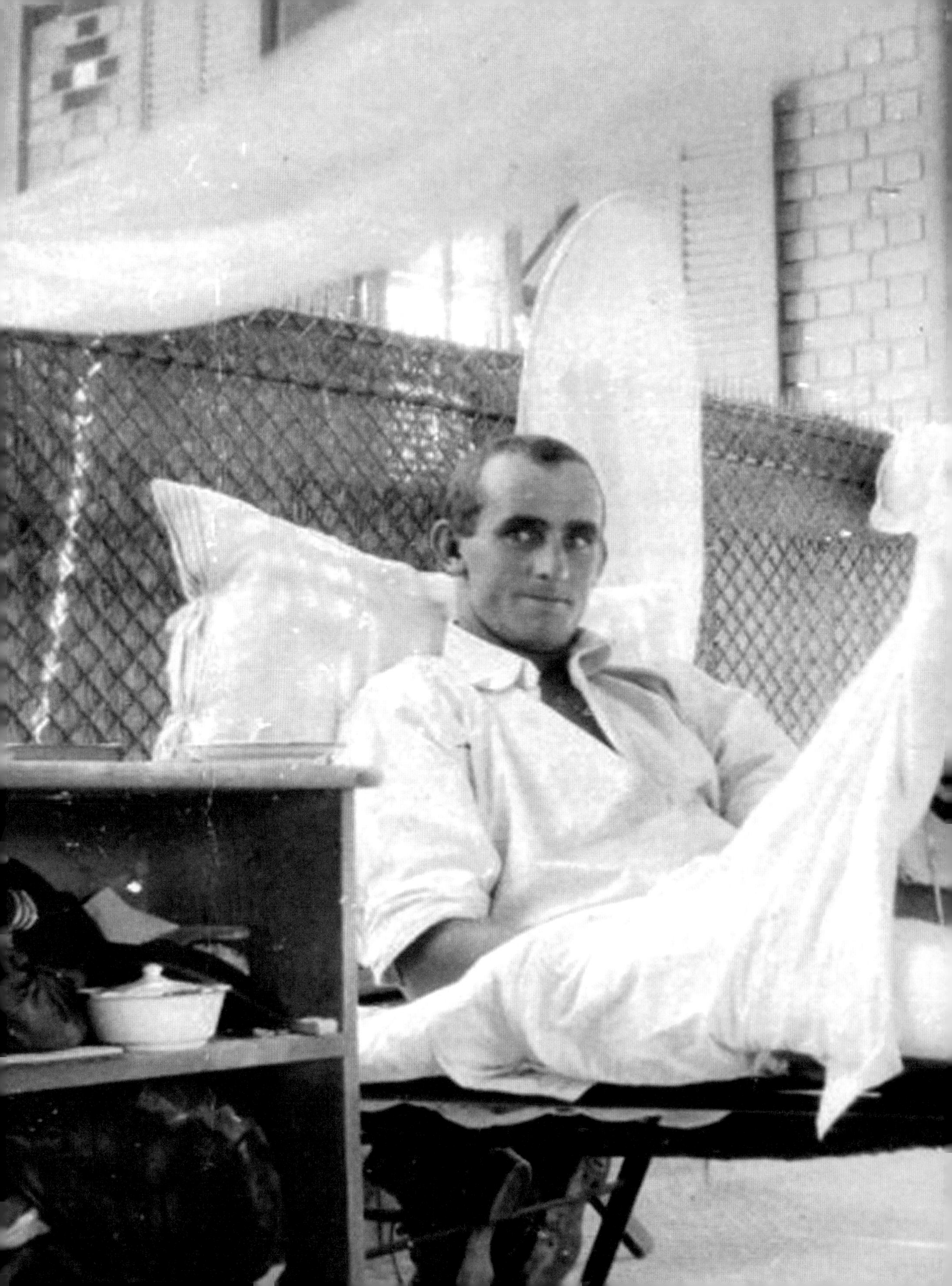

CHAPTER 15

MAKING IT BETTER?

TREATING WOUNDS AND SICKNESS

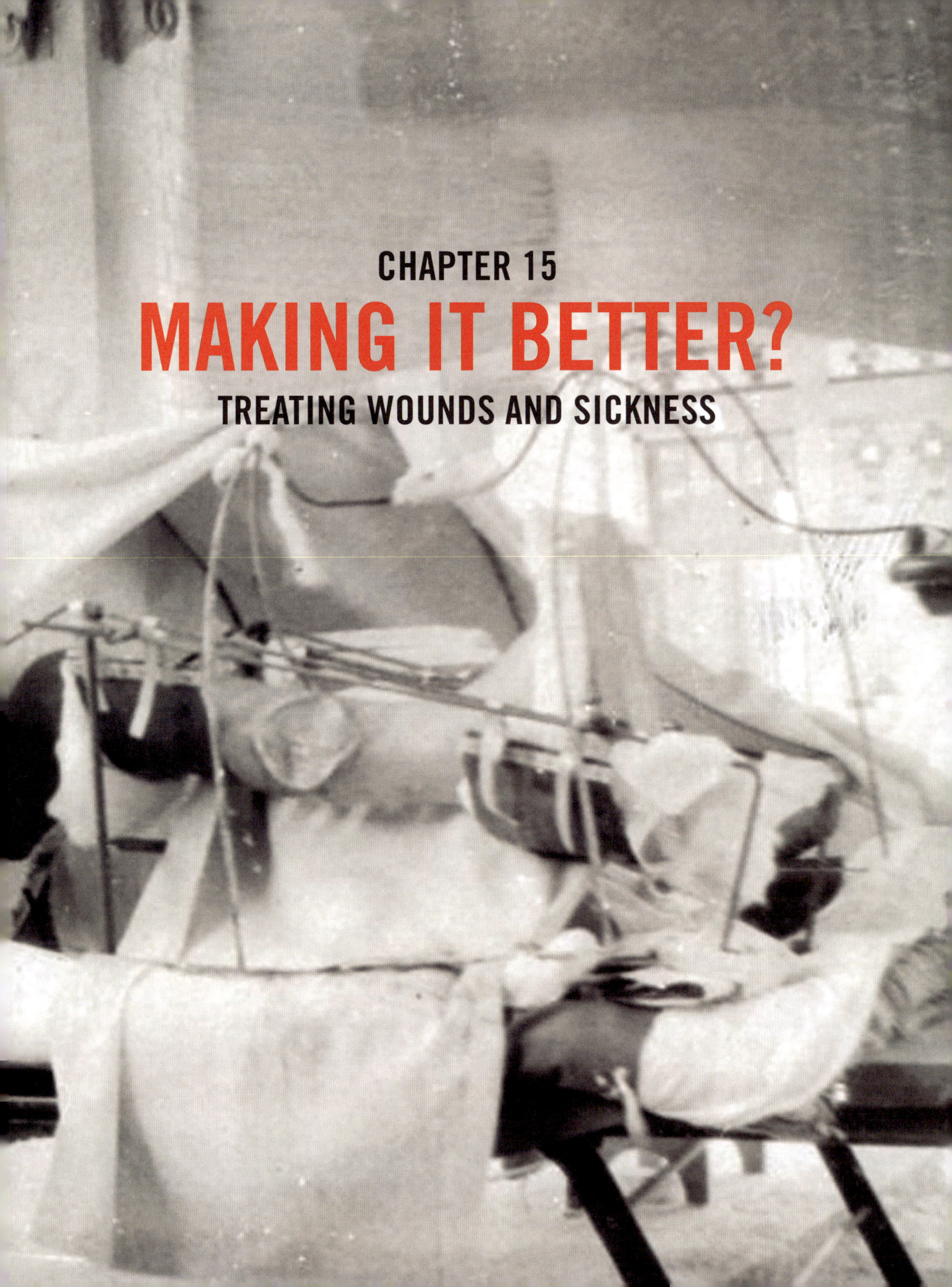

previous pages
Contraptions for treating wounded legs could be dauntingly complex. Trooper Keast of the Australian Light Horse, pictured here at No. 31 General Hospital in Port Said, may have been one of New Zealand nurse Alice Searrell's patients.
NATIONAL ARMY MUSEUM, 1992.1156.2

> Little stiff rattle of wheels as the white trolley comes along bearing trays with white surgical dressings, gauze, cotton-wool, needles plunged into jars of hot water, forceps wrapped in sterile gauze, pots marked with red and blue poison labels . . . What's the name of that blinking little coffin on wheels, anyhow? You'll find out soldier. That's the agony-waggon.
>
> — Robin Hyde, *Passport to Hell*

Some lessons had been learnt in the Crimea and, more recently, in South Africa, but the medical men and women of the First World War faced many alarming new challenges that forced them to innovate and adapt. To modern eyes, some of their methods may seem rather quaint, but it is vital to see these in their contemporary context, and to recognise how many ground-breaking methods were introduced or used more extensively between 1914 and 1918.

The approach to dysentery, for example, with its emphasis on milk, flour and arrowroot, as well as drugs, was different then. MO William McAra, recovering at Pont de Koubbeh, decided that 'the amount of milk & egg I consume would cause me to turn into an omelette if I were shaken'.[1] Tonics were popular too, though not always appreciated. The one ordered for William Smallfield in September 1917 he thought 'the vilest stuff ever made, mostly composed of Quinine and "Ferre" [iron] . . . It is a good job I am in a military hospital for if I was not it would take very great force to compel me to swallow the stuff.'[2] What were termed 'stimulants' — brandy especially, but also champagne and stout — were widely used. On Gallipoli, when the weather worsened, alcohol was employed to combat hypothermia. Over 56 days one ANZAC unit dispensed an impressive 14 bottles of brandy, 18 of port wine and 46 of stout. Frederick Foote's Cairo hospital care included a midday bottle of stout. After George Tierney was gassed at Passchendaele, his treatment included 'having champagne and brandy alternately every two hours'.[3] Hot fomentations — heat packs or poultices to draw out infection — were often employed. 'But for the poisoning setting in,' wrote Gerald Barton, wounded on Gallipoli, 'I would have been fit for service again. At present [in Egypt] I am having hot fomentations on my arm every hour.' After he was wounded for a second time on 8 August 1915, Wanganui solicitor

Frank Turnbull was put on a hospital ship where he was 'indulging in hot fomentations and getting along splendidly'.[4] But, as William Wilson discovered, they could be less benign. After he arrived at Walton-on-Thames in September 1916, for two days his badly wounded and infected leg was put in 'hot packs day and night and twice a day they squeezed the pus out. But this was too much for me. I used to go off as soon as they started.'[5]

The First World War medical arsenal also included drugs, though not antibiotics. Together with diet, the favoured treatment for amoebic dysentery was emetine hydrochloride. Results could vary, as MO Alexander Trotter noted on Gallipoli. 'In some cases emetine seems to have absolutely no effect though in others it produces at least much temporary improvement. Have almost used all we have and more is not obtainable.'[6] Combining emetine and 'powdered ipecacuanha by the mouth' was also recommended by some. Both emetine and the plant-based ipecacuanha induced vomiting.[7] Trench fever, the bane of the Western Front, was difficult to treat. 'The pain caused is very hard to bear,' Smallfield told his mother. 'In bad cases morphia has been resorted to.' More usual were 'Antypirin [antipyrine, an analgesic], Rhenaticin [probably Renacidin, used to irrigate], Aspirin and Caffeine'.[8]

In wounds, infection, especially gas gangrene, was the greatest enemy and various preventative methods were used. As Carbery would write, 'Had the laboratory succeeded in giving us a sure prophylactic against gas gangrene most of the danger from battle wounds would have vanished.'[9] Iodine was popular on Gallipoli, and remained so, but it was not always applied with discrimination. The large hole left in Joe Gasparich's arm after the Second Battle of Krithia was 'dressed' by RAMC men, who 'had a great big pot full of iodine, and a whole lot of brushes of different sizes . . . They grabbed one of these and stuck it in the wound and wobbled it around.'[10]

When Colonel Hugh Acland gave a 'very interesting' but unscripted talk to the nurses at Walton on 22 July 1917, with Violet Barker doing her best to take notes for *Kai Tiaki* readers, he spoke of 'hypotonic saline, and salt packs', and later adaptations, which drew fluid to the wound and retarded the development of sepsis. Acland also named other antiseptics. 'Boracic acid and chloride of lime (Eusol) [short for Edinburgh University Solution of Lime] has been most successfully used,' though it rapidly lost effectiveness, while Flavine, 'a new coal-tar product', looked promising.[11]

What really succeeded was a system devised by French surgeon Alexis Carrel and English chemist Henry Dakin, which became the standard treatment throughout the British army and the NZEF. As Isabel Stevens Lathrop, a Red Cross worker in Paris, wrote, 'It has been the study of years to find the antiseptic that will destroy microbes and not destroy tissues.' She observed the process carried out by Carrel himself at the Compiègne military hospital, on men 'with one or . . . a dozen hideous wounds filled with shrapnel'. After an X-ray, 'the first vitally important step is to clear away every particle of foreign matter [debridement]. The wound must be perfectly clean, and to insure this, the surgeon cuts away the flesh unsparingly.'[12] Small rubber tubes with holes were then inserted into the wound, which was 'left like an open trough so that the Dakin's sodium hypochlorite solution could lie . . . and get longer contact with the tissues'.[13] The liquid was syringed into the tubes every two hours and allowed to be absorbed into the dressings. Later, continuous slow drip irrigation was made possible by suspending large glass containers above the patient's bed on stands, with rubber tubes leading to the small wound tubes. Lathrop was astonished by the results. 'Imagine a man looking fairly well with gashes and slashes ten inches long and perhaps six inches wide; and not one wound, but three or four. The hand of one man was such a mass of shrapnel that the X-ray picture of it was like a case of smallpox . . . We didn't find a soul with a particle of temperature.' And there was another advantage. 'No gangrene, no suppurations, no decay or tissue! Do you know one thing this means? No bad odours when you enter the hospital.'[14]

When Clifford Collingwood reached a CCS after being wounded in June 1917, his fractured leg was 'opened up by removing a strip of flesh 6 inches long and one inch wide, to the depth of the femur. The artery was tied, the wound excised, Carrel tubes inserted, passing through my leg from the front surface to the large hole in the back of my thigh, for drainage.' When he was on the train to Boulogne, 'At regular intervals the Sisters syringed Daken's solution through the tubes in our wounds. They never disturbed our dressings or removed any bandages, for the tubes protruded slightly between the bandages, and were covered lightly with a guard.'[15]

The magic solution was certainly life-changing for ambulance man Colin Gordon, who was taken to Brockenhurst in 1916 with shell splinters in his arm and leg. Because the arm was 'just a gash', the medics decided to leave it alone, but then gangrene set in. 'God's truth! I nearly lost my arm! It looked very inflamed, and pus was forming.' Amputation was considered but after Gordon protested, chief surgeon Dr Louis Barnett said, '"Well, we could try this Dakin's Solution" — which had just come on the market. So they put a big bottle on the stand beside me and had a tube dripping . . . into the wound 24 hours a day. And it got better.' Although the Carrel–Dakin method decreased the number of amputations and reduced the dressing time for overworked nurses, it 'was not always practicable in the face of an inrush of fresh casualties'. As Acland commented, BIPP and Eusol could 'give pretty good results with less paraphernalia and difficulty'.[16]

BIPP was the universal name for a widely used antiseptic called bismuth iodoform paraffin paste — 'intolerable stuff with a smell', according to Starkie — developed by Professor Rutherford Morison of Newcastle. Under anaesthetic, the patient's wound was thoroughly cleaned, mopped with methylated spirits and then filled with BIPP paste. 'Dress the wound with sterile gauze, and cover all with an absorbent pad, which is held in position by sticking-plaster and a bandage. This dressing requires no changing for days or weeks if the patient is free from pain and constitutional disturbance.'[17] Major George Home used Morison's technique extensively over 14 months at Balmer Lawn, treating or supervising its application to 42 fractures and 270 other wounds. For Sister Jeanne Sinclair and her fellow nurses at the hospital, 'the Bipped wounds reduce the work by half, and on night duty even more, because after the first twenty-four hours there is no pain, or practically none . . . and so the patients sleep all night'.[18] In the words of another unnamed nurse, 'If any one had told me a dirty pus wound could be left for days (after having been cleaned up) without needing to be dressed, I should have thought it was a tall romance.'[19]

By contrast, traditional dressings could be an appalling experience for patients. 'For about two weeks,' Foote remembered, 'the agony of the dressing for my arms was beyond belief. The great raw wound was as big as a large dinner plate. They gave me a glass of brandy, orderlies held my arms, it took four pieces of gauze to cover the wound. The nurse would hold the gauze half an inch above the wound and drop it on. I could not help screaming out with the pain, as the nerves were shattered and exposed.' When the dressing team, with the agony-wagon, was two beds away, he would see 'beads of perspiration stand out on a patient's face, when [it] was one bed away they would start appealing to be left in peace, appealing most dramatically, convincingly, and sincerely'.[20]

For the all too common compound fractures of femurs and tibias, the key to successful irrigation of the wound, and knitting of the bones, was a suitable splint. On Gallipoli, where equipment was scarce, although some stretchers had a cradle for slinging a leg, bearers often had to improvise, using sticks and rifles for splints, and sandbags and coats to immobilise fractured limbs. The early splints on the Western Front were not a success. The *Official History of the New Zealand Rifle Brigade* 'found it distressing to record that in the first Somme battle 75 per cent. of cases of fractured thighs died. They were prepared for transport by means of Liston's splint, which consists of long laths of wood stretching from the arm-pit to the ankle and secured by bandages to the body and leg.' This system failed to prevent the bone ends from rubbing against one another, and there was often excessive blood loss, leading to shock and death. The Liston also obscured open wounds. The mortality rate dropped to 20, and sometimes even 15, per cent at Messines and Bapaume, thanks largely to the Thomas splint.[21]

Although this was originally designed by eccentric Welsh orthopaedic surgeon Hugh Owen Thomas, it was his nephew, Robert (later Sir Robert) Jones, who fully realised and championed the splint's wartime use. It consisted of a ring at one end that fitted snugly around the thigh, and two light iron shafts that extended down each side of the leg in a long U; a cross-piece at the bottom meant longitudinal traction could be applied by attaching cords. This arrangement, which could also be used on an arm, immobilised the fracture and stopped the broken bone ends from moving when a patient was being carried, thus reducing tissue and nerve damage as well as bleeding. The 'efficient and simple' splint also allowed 'easy and painless access to the wound'.[22] New Zealand medics on the front line soon saw the advantages of the Thomas splint and championed its use; by 1918 each motor ambulance carried a set.[23]

Even this advance gave no guarantee of complete comfort. After Clifford Collingwood had Carrel tubes inserted in his leg, 'a Thomas knee splint was fitted on to enable a continuous extension to be maintained on my thigh'. He 'awoke suddenly to severe pain caused by cramp in the leg . . . while each spasm lasted the whole leg would be rigid and quivering'. He did, however, feel that the Thomas splint generally made his pain more tolerable. At the beginning of July, in order to keep the leg straight while the bone was mending, 'Cords were fastened to the ceiling and then attached to the end of my [splint], thus raising the leg . . . There was such a strong pull on my leg that the Doctor had to pad my armpits and then bind my shoulders to the head of the bed. This kept me stationary, and I found that . . . I could move my body about slightly, but . . . sufficient to prevent feeling cramped.'[24]

Another popular type of splint advocated by pioneering British orthopaedic surgeon and RAMC captain Ernest Hey Groves involved 'the passing of steel pins through the bone attaching them to supports outside the skin'.[25] New Zealand nurse Clara Cherry, who had her own surgical ward at No. 21 British Hospital in Alexandria, worked under Hey Groves. 'We use splints that I have never seen or heard of,' she wrote late in 1915. 'I am thankful to say our work has brought forth every possible success. We have lost only one femur case and one only had to be amputated. Considering the dozens and dozens that have passed through our hands, I think it more than wonderful.'[26]

Compound fractures were not confined to limbs. At Messines, when US Medical Corps surgeon Harvey Cushing was assisting at the NZSH, most of the head cases 'had compound fractures of the skull without penetration of the dura [the outermost layer of membrane covering the brain]'. After an X-ray, the scalp wound was excised, then enlarged to remove 'depressed fragments of bone and foreign bodies where accessible'. This was followed by arrest of haemorrhage, application of the trusty BIPP and 'closure of the wound without drainage'.[27]

Along with fractures to the femur, penetrating wounds of the abdomen were the most dangerous. When William McAra was binding up a man's profusely bleeding arm after a Gallipoli shell explosion, he was 'sorry to find, after he told me he felt stinging over abdomen, the hole of a bullet entry — it was near region of umbilicus & below its level. These wounds have proved invariably fatal as so much bowel is usually cut.'[28] Initially, on the peninsula, those with such wounds were 'rested, given nothing by mouth, and moved only if necessary. Because the only chance of survival . . . lay in speedy evacuation, their prognosis was almost always bad.' Opium was given for severe pain. Even when abdominal surgery was possible, infection was a danger. Sometimes such wounds contained the contents of pockets or even cartridge clips.[29] When Richard Dowling was shot in the abdomen on 1 September, the wound became septic '& he was opened later by a central incision above the symphysis pubis & and other incision in the appendix region. From the latter, the bullet was removed, but the wounds discharged pus for four weeks after.'[30] On the Western Front, those with abdominal wounds were moved to a CCS as rapidly as possible.

Gangrene caused by loss of blood supply was another problem facing medical staff. After Frank Fougere was wounded in both arms on Gallipoli, his right, with a clean hole, healed quickly, but gangrene developed in his left forearm. 'The nurses used to rub the flesh with powdered bluestone and that burnt it off, and they gave me hot saline baths. They killed the gangrene after a while, but it used to come again. There'd be chips off the piece of bone that was left. They'd form abscesses and I'd have to go into hospital and get them cut out.'[31]

Pain relief was a vital aspect of wartime medical treatment. Sometimes this was all that could be offered, especially in the field and especially on Gallipoli. William Malone knew how vital morphine would be. Before the landing, he arranged:

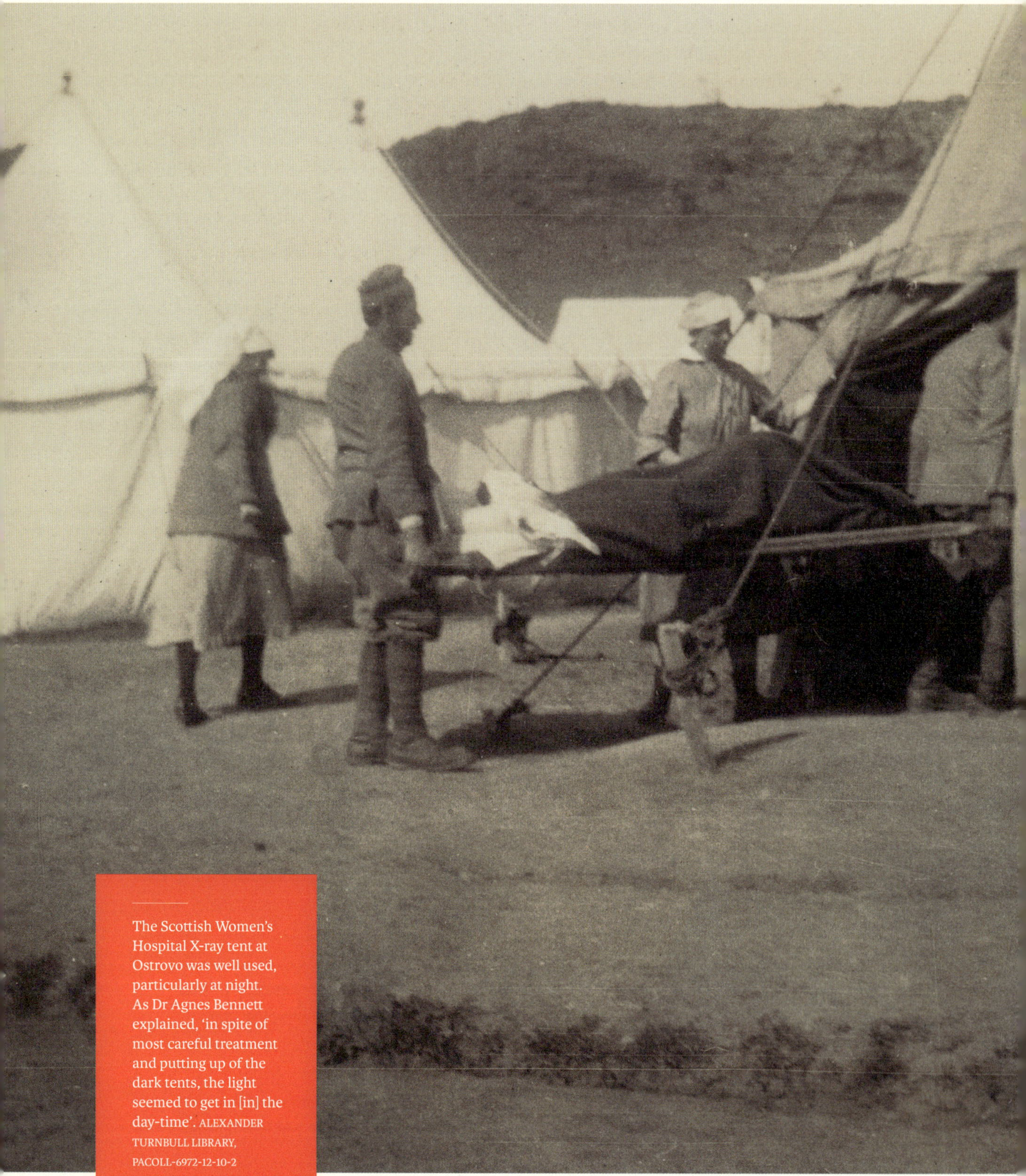

The Scottish Women's Hospital X-ray tent at Ostrovo was well used, particularly at night. As Dr Agnes Bennett explained, 'in spite of most careful treatment and putting up of the dark tents, the light seemed to get in [in] the day-time'. ALEXANDER TURNBULL LIBRARY, PACOLL-6972-12-10-2

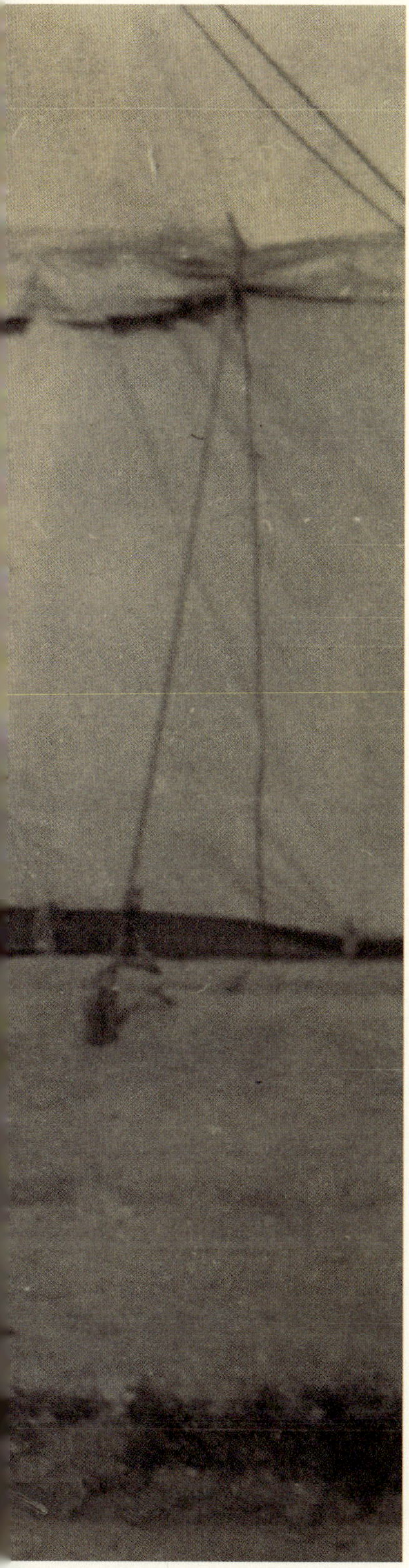

> to issue to every Platoon Commander a phial of morphia tabloids so that any wounded men can be at once given by the nearest man, a tabloid or two to put under his tongue and thus get relief from pain. The tabloid will take from 10 to 15 minutes to dissolve and to work, but it will be a great blessing to the wounded men and a great help to the nerves of their mates who will be saved quickly the hearing of the wounded men's cries.[32]

When Douglas Stark was wounded in June 1918, he was given the drug straight away. 'Morphine starts from the prick in the arm and works upwards in waves of drowsy, heavy gold. First the crushing, tearing pain in back and lungs was beaten down and numbed, then his eyelids were weighted with a sweet drowsiness that made him want to cry. His breath laboured a little less painfully . . . He was drifting out fast on a tide of sleep.' There was more relief soon. 'Dab of iodine, a little tiny prick . . . sleep, drawn up in buckets from the pit of death, and dropped into you through the hollow fang of a tiny needle.'[33]

It was realised later that, early in the war, the dosage of morphine had often been excessive. '[S]ome of the wounded dosed themselves from private stores, and half a grain by the mouth was not infrequently given at the R.A.P.; if hypodermic injection of a further dose was administered at the A.D.S. or M.D.S. the patient was dangerously drugged by the time of his arrival at C.C.S.' Too much morphine could also cause death after operations. The medical instructions for Messines in 1917 made it clear that, in dressing stations, 'morphine was to be withheld or at least given in very small doses', with the time of administration and the dose recorded.[34] When John A. Lee was given his second opium pellet in 1918, the MO told the orderly to 'Make a note on his card . . . If he gets another he mightn't wake up.'[35] With compassion and without official sanction, morphine was often used to hasten the death of appallingly wounded men.

Stark was X-rayed after being wounded:

> 'We're only going to take X-ray plates, we'd like to see just what the bullet's done with your inside. Can't go swallowing lead like you did, soldier, and not expect to have a stomach-ache. There's the big, solemn lights, waiting to fizz and crackle with the power that can see through to your bones. It's all dark except for the white-coated men with the shades on their eyes. Straighten him up, Sister. Get those sandbags alongside his arms, I want him perfectly still.'[36]

His experience was not unusual. Although X-rays had been discovered only in 1895, the technology was well understood and widely used by 1914, and played a crucial role during the war. New Zealand was up with the play. Ferdinand Batchelor, who had made a special study of the subject, sailed with the Main Body and oversaw X-ray work for the NZEF in Egypt. Later Joseph Frazerhurst, who survived the *Marquette* disaster, acted as X-ray specialist with the New Zealand forces.[37] There was no X-ray equipment on Gallipoli, though the Australian stationary hospitals on Lemnos did have such facilities. Both the *Maheno* and the *Marama* had X-ray rooms and there was X-ray apparatus at New Zealand hospitals in Egypt, France and England.[38] X-rays played a vital role in the diagnosis and treatment of severe facial injuries.

New Zealand's nurses also had X-ray training. Fanny Speedy, a member of the first NZANS contingent, had been X-ray and outpatient sister at Wellington Hospital and was disappointed when promised X-ray work at No. 19 General Hospital in Alexandria did not eventuate. Sister Cora Turnbull was more fortunate. She headed the X-ray department of No. 1 Australian General at Heliopolis, where she received 'no end of praise for her exceptional ability and talent in the work'.[39] Even in the tough environment of war-torn Serbia, Dr Agnes Bennett reported that 'our X-Ray apparatus was in great demand, and far into every night we were developing plates'. They screened about 250 cases. 'There was not a great deal of localising done as we found the track of the bullet so patent in most cases . . . The valuable information was in the fact that a foreign body was present.'[40]

But all too often the location of the bullet was not obvious, or there was a need to check for potentially deadly metal. As Malcolm Ross put it, 'Bullets and bits of shell and bombs and shrapnel are located with wonderful and uncanny accuracy. By this means not only is the patient saved a great deal of exploratory cutting . . . but he is even, in some cases, saved the necessity for operation altogether. The deeper in the bullet is the harder it is to locate, and the outer wound is often no index as to the exact locality.' When Trooper H. W. White was hit on the left shoulder by a piece of bomb, the metal was removed 'after a lot of probing and X-ray work, about eight inches from where it went in'. Private Walter North, at Brockenhurst, told his parents, 'I have to get the X-ray on to me one of these days to see where that bit of shrapnel of mine went to; then I expect the knife will come into action and hook it out.'[41]

Sometimes surgery was too difficult or dangerous, or seen as unnecessary. On 17 August 1915, an X-ray revealed a bullet in Garioch Clunie's thigh, 'But Doctor says no need to extract it as it won't trouble me.' Lance-Corporal Kennedy of Dunedin returned on the *Turakina* in April 1916 with a 'shocking depression of the temple, as big as a five-shilling piece. A shrapnel bullet shattered the bone, traversed the entire length of the head, and now still rests at the base of the skull, defying the ability of surgical skill to remove it.'[42] George Rotherham, left with a 'large chunk of metal' in his groin after Gallipoli, was told by doctors, 'If they ever want to cut you open to take that thing out, don't let them because you will be worse off if they do.' The risks were damage to major blood vessels and nerves, and infection.[43]

More often, however, an operation was the answer, even if it was delayed. In July 1915 Trooper William Lewis suffered a compound fracture of his right forearm and a perforated right thigh. 'The piece . . . that hit the thigh is still in. I was under the X-ray yesterday and they have located the shell, but are not going to operate on me to take it out until the arm has healed up.'[44] After reaching Heliopolis, Herbert Hart, wounded on Gallipoli, was X-rayed twice, the films revealing the bullet and three other pieces of metal in his leg, 'which the medicos decided to leave there unless they caused trouble'. Three weeks later, however, at Zeitoun, Major Henry McLean thought otherwise, 'and extracted from the seat of the wound a jagged piece of nickel casing off the bullet'. Rotherham's shrapnel — 'a piece of flat metal as big around as a half crown with seven jagged corners' — was removed 11 years later.[45] The X-ray images, also known as shadowgraphs or skiagrams, could become objects of interest and fascination. When NZMC Major Charles Maguire returned from Egypt in April 1916, he brought with him 'a set of wonderful X-ray photographs, showing bullets, shrapnel and fractures in all parts of the human frame'.[46]

There were some downsides to X-rays. Although protection was recommended for the radiographers, including wearing heavy aprons and gloves and using screens, accidents could happen. In May 1918 the *Evening Post* reported that Aucklander R. G. Applegarth, who was now working for the American Red Cross in Paris, had been 'obliged, last year, to give up his X-ray work at one of the French hospitals, his fingers having been affected'.[47] In June 1917, returned serviceman Private C. Hill was awarded £1300 in damages 'for injuries allegedly received while undergoing X-ray treatment in the Dannevirke Public Hospital' for Gallipoli wounds.[48] The actual process, in which the patient stayed on the table for a few minutes while the plate was developed, and then went back to his ward, could be alarming. When Frederick Foote was taken for X-rays in Cairo, 'the big machine swung over me, it sparked, crackled and banged. I seemed to be frightened of it and was in a collapsed state by the time I was put back to bed.'[49]

At the beginning of the war, anaesthesia methods were not radically different from those of the mid-nineteenth century. Nitrous oxide ('laughing gas') had been used as an inhalation anaesthetic since 1844. It could be given half in half with oxygen to achieve anaesthesia without loss of consciousness, particularly when new equipment allowed for precise measurements. However, because nitrous oxide was usually stored in glass bottles, it was unsuited to the battlefield and used only at base hospitals. Ether had been popular for about the same length of time. Although 'safer than chloroform and more effective than nitrous oxide', it had such side-effects as 'coughing, sore throat, painful red eyes, a headache, drowsiness, laboured breathing and nausea'. During the war it was the preferred anaesthetic at CCSs, often administered via the Clover method, the first portable ether inhaler, or a Flagg's can, a tin can with multiple perforations on its top.[50] Chloroform, a sweet-smelling liquid, was administered by being dropped onto a mask held an inch above the patient's face. Although chloroform was most frequently used on Gallipoli, open ether was favoured for amputations, since those with septic infections were thought to be at more risk with chloroform.[51]

Approaches varied. When NZMC orderly Eric Bardell had 'a little operation' on the *Maheno* in July 1918, 'They decided to give me gas instead of chloroform. Was in theatre from 9:45 to

10:15 . . . I just seemed to have a decent sleep, and woke up immediately they had finished.'[52] After catching influenza in mid-1918, Len Coley developed such badly ulcerated tonsils that he was finding breathing difficult. 'I was given a choice of sitting in a chair or being chloroformed. I did not fancy the idea of choking and perhaps dying while under chloroform. I was sat in a chair, my tonsils were painted with cocaine, and out they came. I coughed frequently and blood spurted everywhere. They stood a Red Cross man beside me to paint the cuts and stop the bleeding when I coughed.'[53]

Before 1914 specialist anaesthetists were rare outside medical teaching establishments: GPs gave anaesthesia, but medical training was not a prerequisite. It would be the same, initially, in wartime, when the role was also filled by chaplains, stretcher-bearers and nurses (several of the last, as we have seen, were later trained as anaesthetists). For Bardell's operation, the ship's dentist administered the anaesthetic. But when the unprecedented number of wounded led to the establishment of CCSs, specialist anaesthetists were appointed. Early in 1918, each CCS was ordered to have at least one on its staff. Improved training followed the arrival, in April 1917, of American anaesthetist Arthur Guedel, who established a training school to teach nurses and orderlies how to administer anaesthesia.

The effect of anaesthetics on severely injured and shocked patients was another area that needed attention; 'wound shock', as it was known, was poorly understood in 1914. Based on his research and observations during war service, British respiratory physician Geoffrey Marshall advocated the use of nitrous oxide and oxygen 'for safety, speed and convenience'. The equipment, though, was heavy and expensive, at least until better alternatives became available — a revolutionary but simple machine was invented in 1917 by English anaesthetist Captain Henry Boyle.[54] The nitrous oxide–oxygen combination, 'given with a good machine' — Blanche Huddlestone considered Boyle's 'one of the best' — could last for as long as four or five hours, 'even for complicated abdominal cases. The patient is got under very quickly, and is awake and apparently none the worse for a long operation the minute the anaesthetic is discontinued.'

As Marshall had found, the nitrous oxide–oxygen mixture was 'invaluable' for operations on men in shock. 'Our patients,' Huddlestone wrote, 'were brought straight in from the "line", pale and cold, and practically pulseless for probably a major operation . . . and it was very necessary that not only should the operation be a success, but that they should be none the worse for having had it, or the anaesthetic.' Huddlestone also mentioned Shipway's, the 'much-used and very excellent apparatus for chloroform and ether', which, because it warmed the vapour, reduced possible bronchial complications. She learnt that 'for the first five minutes an anaesthetic must be given slowly so that the mucous membranes of the throat got gradually accustomed to the more or less irritation of the fumes; after that, one could "speed up" in getting the patient "under".'[55]

Although most soldiers were young, fit men, many of them smoked, often heavily, and lung disease was not uncommon. This increased the danger of anaesthesia. Those suffering from shell shock or nervous exhaustion could require more anaesthesia than other patients.[56] Sometimes things went wrong. Foote 'was told to take a deep breath, my breath caught and would not come in, I tried to breathe, but could not, I choked . . . I never remember getting my breath and the memory was very unpleasant.'[57] As Claude Weston observed, some men 'had to undergo operation after operation, and often they were the ones whom the anaesthetic upset so much for days after'.[58]

Sometimes, there was no anaesthetic. As Beet Algar, shot in the buttock and arm, recalled, 'They never used to bother about anaesthetic; they used to come and roll me over, and the doctor put his fingers in and worked round the wound to try and find this foreign body that was causing the trouble.' When Ethel Lewis was working in Serbia in March 1915, 'At first there was very little chloroform, and deep incision-probing for bullets, etc., was all done without an anaesthetic.'[59]

The medical men themselves could be affected by anaesthetics. The surgeon who examined William Taylor's swollen wounded arm could feel something, but added, 'Listen, son, I've been operating all afternoon and I'm sick with the ether. Do you think you could let me remove this thing without going to the theatre?'[60] In maxillo-facial operations, too, if the method of pumping the vapour electrically through a catheter down the trachea was used, the surgeon was often 'semi-anaesthetised by the patient's exhalations'. The other common method for such surgery, blowing ether vapour into a funnel connected to the patient's face by a rubber tube, could badly stress, and occasionally even kill, the man on the table.[61] In lengthy operations on the nose, mouth and face, the whole airway sometimes had to be completely blocked with gauze so blood would not enter the lungs. Harold Gillies' first anaesthetist, the talented Rubens Wade, often delivered anaesthesia to maxillo-facial patients while they were sitting up, so their airways were less likely be obstructed. The revolutionary technique that became known as endotracheal intubation — in which a rubber tube was inserted through the nose or mouth directly into the patient's lungs — was invented at Sidcup after the war by Irish anaesthetist Ivan Magill, who also worked with Gillies.[62]

After Vincent Jervis was wounded in August 1918, he was taken to No. 3 CCS at Gézaincourt, near Doullens. 'About 12 noon they asked for volunteers for blood transfusion so I put in for that — had my blood tested and found all right and was told to stay here until needed.' He soon reported, 'Had a bit over a pint of blood taken this morning. I do not feel any weaker for it though perhaps I might notice it if I did any exercise.'[63] Blood transfusion had its origins in Alexis Carrel's ground-breaking 1902 work in anastomosis, the sewing together of arteries and veins. American surgeon George Crile built on this, developing a procedure that could attach a donor's artery directly to a recipient's vein; other transfusion methods followed, though incompatibility of blood remained a problem until the identification of the blood types we know today. In wartime, however, matching these was 'too difficult and time-consuming . . . and often impossible in emergency conditions', and the Carrel–Crile technique, which required the donor and recipient to lie side by side, was frustratingly inexact in high-pressure situations — there could be too little blood or too much.[64]

Clotting was often a problem, but early in 1915 the Americans had discovered how to

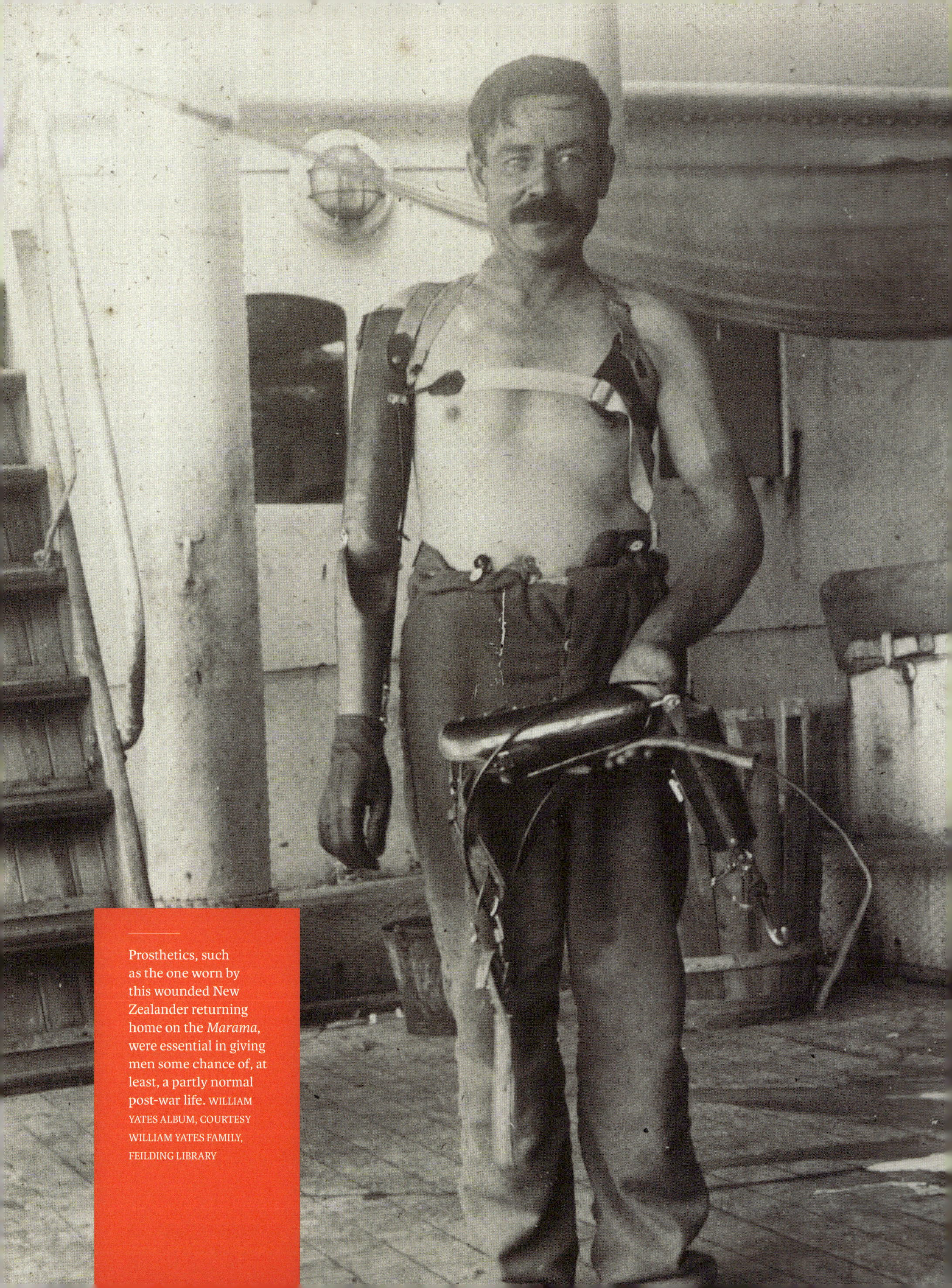

Prosthetics, such as the one worn by this wounded New Zealander returning home on the *Marama*, were essential in giving men some chance of, at least, a partly normal post-war life. WILLIAM YATES ALBUM, COURTESY WILLIAM YATES FAMILY, FEILDING LIBRARY prevent coagulation in the donor's blood, and this expertise was taken to Europe in July that year by the Harvard Medical Unit.[65] In 1918, the 2nd Canadian Division fitted up an advanced resuscitation room not far from the front line. 'Both preserved blood and fresh citrated [treated to prevent coagulation] whole blood infusions were practised with the happiest results . . . the soldiers talked with wonder of the cellars where "the dead men were brought to life by having blood pumped into them".'[66]

Person-to-person transfusion, available from 1916, was popular, though not entirely for altruistic reasons. As Sister Margaret Davies recalled, 'There was always a list of names at a C.C.S. of men — usually stretcher-bearers — who were willing to give blood for transfusion. And it was quite a common sight to see a great strong man on one table, with his arm bared, ready to give the blood that would probably save the life of an almost dead man beside him. The "Donors" as they were called, used to get leave to Blighty [England] after this operation.'[67] Only selflessness was mentioned, however, when the *Observer* reported on 'yet another of our fine lads' who gave blood 'to save the life of a comrade' — in this case a Grenadier guardsman. This 'brave boy' was Private Thomas O'Carroll, who had written to his father: 'Suppose I told you I gave a chap a quart of blood. He was dying of hemorrhage. Anyway he lived and the loss did not affect me much.'[68] It was only later in the war that the collection and storage of blood for transfusion was possible and practised.

In operations, asepsis — the complete absence of bacteria, viruses and other micro-organisms — could be hard to achieve, particularly on Gallipoli, where water for boiling to sterilise instruments was frequently unavailable, and iodine or hot Eusol were used instead.[69] Total sterility could be a challenge, too, in the white-hot speed of CCS surgery on the Western Front, and with sometimes limited supplies. As Ida Willis explained, 'The instrument tables have to do for perhaps fifty or sixty patients, sometimes even more, all soiled instruments being received into a bowl of lotion and taken off to sterilise, these being replaced by a fresh set from the steriliser.' If there was 'much gas gangrene gloves were changed as often as possible . . . but for the general run of cases it was found necessary to wear a pair of gloves sometimes for five or six cases unless punctured. This saved time and wear and tear on gloves, and in a big rush the supply was not unlimited. A bowl of weak Lysol solution stood always ready, and the gloves were scrubbed like the hands before going into . . . whatever lotion the surgeons preferred.' During operations the bowls had 'to be burnt out with methylated spirits, the boiling space being limited'.[70]

Just as the dangers of too much morphine had been revealed, so other medical practices altered during the war. For instance, thinking on the use of the tourniquet to stem severe bleeding was revised. On Gallipoli, where so many wounded were crowded together, often in darkness, it was all too easy for tourniquets to be missed and left on for too long, leading to gangrene. Applying direct pressure was soon favoured instead.[71] In practice, however, as with John A. Lee's 1918 wound, emergency tourniquets continued to be employed on the front line.

Repeated surgery was required for maxillo-facial wounds, but other injuries also called for several operations. After Victor Middlemass was wounded in the face on 8 July 1916, he was operated on in London on 10 August, then taken to Walton where, on 2 November, Louis Barnett 'operated & repaired cleft Pallet of mouth'. On 15 December Middlemass returned to London, where he was operated on six times in the first half of 1917.[72] Some remarkable recoveries were seized upon by reporters. After being wounded at Armentières, and despite being advised that 'the possibilities of recovery by operation were remote', Alfred Sewell risked surgery to remove shrapnel from his spine — and immediately regained the use of his arm and leg.[73] MOs, too, witnessed some extraordinary successes. While on hospital ship duty in 1915, Alexander Trotter noted an operation performed by Charles Hand-Newton on a man whose brain was visible through his skull wound: 'Depressed portion of bone removed and incision closed. Case walks into dispensary next afternoon for his dressing.'[74]

Not all wartime operations were for wounds. Appendicitis was a common reason for surgery. In July 1915, as senior medical officer with the Fifth Reinforcements on the *Tahiti*, William McAra was forced to perform an urgent appendectomy. 'Had to operate — short of instruments and had to use forks and spoons — fortunate in two pairs of gloves. Got vet to give [chloroform] & [Kenneth] Tapper to assist. Large abscess, foul smelling & bowel ruptured — put in two drains & sorry that they were so small. Patient doing well.'[75]

'They would in time brood over their future disability,' wrote John A. Lee in *Soldier*, 'but at present if men lost a limb they had regained life. For a moment the price was not heavy. There was hope to sustain agony. Even the double leg amp metaphorically had his feet on earth.'[76] But the future could be grim. Work prospects were severely reduced and intimate relationships changed, perhaps for ever. Just getting home was not always easy for limbies. When the *Zealandic* left London on 18 January 1919 she was carrying 55 amputees, who, often 'with difficulty', had to 'climb down temporary stairways to the bunks on the lower deck and up to the mess deck'. A 'double amputation and one with the loss of a leg and an arm . . . were made permanent hospital cases to give them beds on the same deck as the mess deck.'[77]

There were very few amputations on Gallipoli itself, 'unless the limbs were hopelessly shattered', but initially there may have been too many hasty operations by overeager and overwhelmed junior doctors on hospital ships. Ambulance man George Thomson could testify to 'Operating rooms like butchers shops. Arms and legs coming off wholesale', while Nurse Mary Grigor remembered 'thirteen amputations in the short trip from Mudros to Alexandria'.[78] On the Western Front, gas gangrene forced doctors to perform far more amputations than they would have wished, and terrible conditions could leave front-line medics with no alternative.

Artificial limbs were needed in abundance and Roehampton was the place to go. As New Zealand journalist Guy Scholefield noted when he visited in November 1917, before 1914 'not half a dozen surgeons in Great Britain knew anything about the development of stumps . . . But the war has changed all that. Roehampton alone has passed about 10,000 limbless men through, and has acquired a whole science from actual practice and observation.' Scholefield warned that thought must be given to 'men whose stumps change after they have returned to their own countries'; dominions unable to maintain limb factories would 'be in a quandary'.[79]

New Zealand had some initial difficulties with 'securing a satisfactory supply of artificial limbs', but from mid-1917 many were being made for the Defence Department at a Wellington factory built up by Gerald Tolhurst, himself an amputee, originally without pay.[80] Some limbs were still imported. By late January 1918 the two staff members, both Roehampton-trained returned men with artificial legs, were 'turning out highclass limbs [and] re-fitting limbs provided for soldiers in England'.[81] The factory remained a Defence facility after the war, but the workshops set up in the other three main centres were later handed over to private firms often staffed by limbless returned soldiers trained under the vocational schemes. The splint shops attached to the four major hospitals became the responsibility of the respective hospital boards.[82]

New Zealand had its own prosthetic invention. In June 1917, J. Wiseman & Sons Ltd in Auckland was sure that 'Disabled soldiers who have returned from the front, and their relatives will be interested in the demonstrations of the McKay Artificial Arm that are to be given at the Surgical Appliance Department'.[83] When Peter McKay of Collingwood near Nelson had had his left hand blown off by gelignite some three and a half years earlier, the expensive American artificial arm he ordered proved useless, so he invented, and patented, his own. Made of aluminium, the arm was operated by a strap attachment to the shoulder. A 'simple movement' of the shoulder muscles made the fingers of the artificial hand open and close, allowing the wearer to write, light and smoke a cigarette, hold a knife and fork, and drink 'almost gracefully' from a glass of any size. Other attachments enabled the wearer to 'drive nails, [and] use an axe, a brace and bit, and other tools in a thoroughly effective manner'.[84] As the Wiseman advertisement explained, McKay was shortly leaving for England 'at the instigation of the Dominion Government, to demonstrate his invention to the Home authorities'.[85] The McKay arm became widely known and used; Lee received one in April 1919.

In July 1916, as machine-gunner Peter Finlayson was turning a corner, 'a bullet hit him just on the shoulder, then passed through his cheek, ripping it open from ear to nose. It was an awful wound to look at.' The following year, also in France, Gunner Norman Hassell saw a man who was 'hit . . . fair in the mouth' with a piece of shell casing, 'making the most hideous wound one could imagine. His nose, jaws and chin were mangled and pulped out of all recognition . . . and his eyes seemed to be the only things left.'[86]

Wounds like these were all too common. Although steel helmets offered protection from skull and brain injuries, faces were exposed as men went 'over the top' of the trench and as they plunged across the battlefield. Both shell fragments and shrapnel, and bullets fired from low-velocity rifles at close range, left men without jaws and noses, or blinded, particularly if they were hit from the side. Also potentially fatal, until facial wounds were better understood, was the well-intentioned injunction for such men to lie down in ambulances or trains. This often 'resulted in the soldier's tongue rolling back in his throat, or blood and mucus blocking his airways'. Damaged mouths and throats could mean that food or water were withheld, sometimes for days.[87] Beyond the physical pain and trauma, severe disfigurement dealt an incalculable psychological blow, leaving men depressed, aggressive and, often, suicidal.

Before maxillo-facial surgery improved, thanks largely to two remarkable New Zealanders, the best solution for such cases was to conceal them. American sculptor Anna Coleman Ladd, in Paris, and former Royal Academy sculpture professor Francis Derwent Wood, in the 'Tin Noses Shop' at No. 3 London General Hospital in Wandsworth, fashioned masks to give these soldiers a face to show the world. Using photographs and 'artistic guesswork', they created partial and complete facial masks, the features meticulously and realistically painted in the finest detail. Made of paper-thin galvanised copper, silvered over, the prostheses were usually held in place with spectacles.[88] But, as New Zealand plastic surgeon Henry Pickerill would note in 1919, although Wood's creations were 'beautiful models', they were 'immobile — they did not move with facial play, they did not fit absolutely level with the skin, and the paint quickly discolored'.[89] The masks were also uncomfortable, insufficiently robust and had to be removed for eating and drinking. Their eerily changeless expression could be deeply disturbing.

It was to Wandsworth that Nelson orchardist George Nuttall went in September 1917 after losing his right eye in June. He had been told by a specialist that 'it would take 7 or 8 operations before my eye socket could be patched up and it is doubtful if ever a glass eye could be fitted', but on 18 September he reported a facial fitting at Wandsworth. By October, however, the eye socket was giving him trouble: 'NZ sons Black day,' he wrote on the 12th. 'After a night of agony, the socket broke down again and bandages are the order of the day.' Eventually he recovered sufficiently to be fitted for glasses and a mask early in December, but once again the socket became inflamed. Nuttall did finally get a glass eye after 'a few more months in blue'.[90]

Masks, however clever, were not a panacea — and they were not conducive to romance. One who realised this was New Zealand ear, nose and throat surgeon Harold Gillies: 'One can appreciate a sweetheart's repugnance at being expected to kiss shapely but unresponsive lips composed of enameled phosphor-bronze.'[91] When war broke out, Gillies, who had been working in London, served with the Red Cross in France — he subsequently joined the RAMC — where he encountered the remarkable French-American dentist Charles Auguste (or sometimes Auguste Charles) Valadier.[92] After recognising the need for special treatment of face and jaw injuries, Valadier had established a jaw ward at No. 13 Stationary Hospital in Boulogne.[93] Although not surgically qualified, he seems to have done all the maxillo-facial operating, but it was decided that he should be assisted by a trained surgeon, and Gillies stepped into that role early in 1915. Gillies also visited Europe's most famous plastic surgeon, Hippolyte Morestin, and saw his superb technical skills in action. Fascinated and inspired, Gillies convinced the British military authorities to open a face and jaw unit at Cambridge Military Hospital in Aldershot in January 1916, and a treatment revolution began that would lay the foundations of modern plastic surgery.[94]

Gillies was as efficient and unorthodox as he was determined. To ensure that he received severe facial cases immediately, he paid for casualty labels, printed with the hospital's address, to be tied to the patients' arms so they would be sent directly to Aldershot. But all too soon, especially after the Somme, it was obvious that, even with more allocated beds,

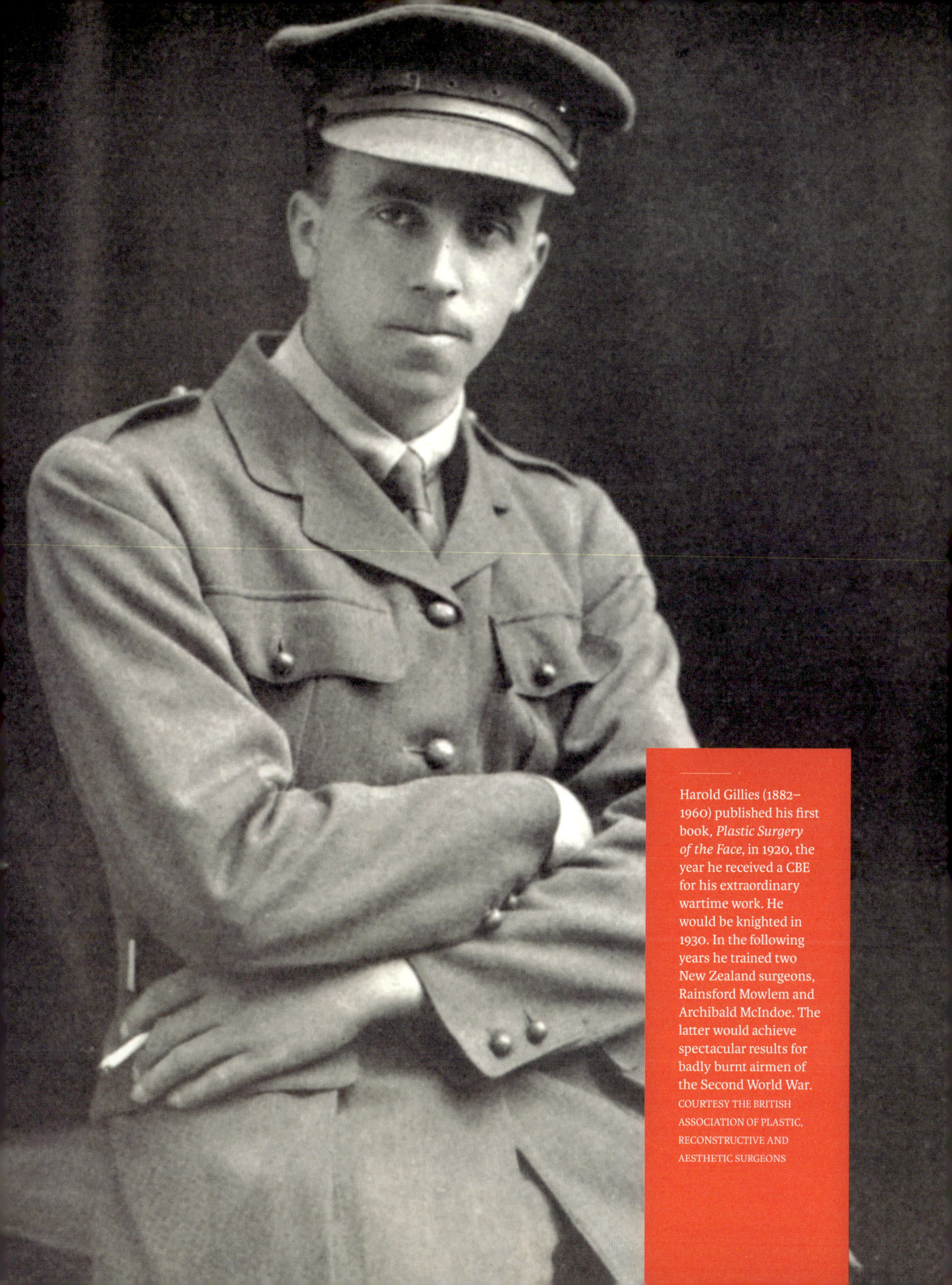

Harold Gillies (1882–1960) published his first book, *Plastic Surgery of the Face*, in 1920, the year he received a CBE for his extraordinary wartime work. He would be knighted in 1930. In the following years he trained two New Zealand surgeons, Rainsford Mowlem and Archibald McIndoe. The latter would achieve spectacular results for badly burnt airmen of the Second World War.
COURTESY THE BRITISH ASSOCIATION OF PLASTIC, RECONSTRUCTIVE AND AESTHETIC SURGEONS

Aldershot would be unable to cope with the growing numbers of facial injuries. In 1917 a new, purpose-built 1000-bed hospital was erected in the grounds of Frognal House at Sidcup in Kent. Because the patients needed months of convalescence, the enviable range of facilities included a chapel, a cinema and a canteen. Sidcup also had 'a fully equipped re-education side, where men in search of technical training or a new trade, can go on with it while their surgical treatment is running through its necessary prolonged course'.[95] Under Gillies as clinical director, separate British, Canadian, New Zealand and Australian surgical teams performed extraordinary pioneering surgery. From its opening on 18 August 1917 until 1925, the Queen's Hospital at Sidcup, and its associated hospitals, would treat some 5000 Allied soldiers and perform over 11,500 operations.[96]

The staff Gillies assembled was more than purely medical. As well as facial surgeons, dentists, radiologists and anaesthetists, there were artists to depict the faces before and after surgery. An amateur artist himself, Gillies often did his own pre-operative sketches. The best known of the Sidcup artists were Henry Tonks from London's Slade School of Fine Art and Australia's Daryl Lindsay, but former marine artist Herbert Cole, who was serving with the NZMC, was also involved. 'His work,' wrote William Parkes after a visit to Sidcup in March 1918, 'is quite satisfactory and will prove a valuable acquisition to the Medical Section of the War Museum in New Zealand.'[97] On the team, too, were sculptors, including Antarctic explorer Robert Falcon Scott's widow Kathleen, who, among other tasks, fashioned the plaster casts on which Gillies and his colleagues worked out operation procedures.

A lively, engaging and idiosyncratic man, 'who called everyone, man or woman, "my dear" or "honey"',[98] Gillies was keen not simply to mend wounds but to improve appearances. He would show his patients photographs of handsome young men and ask them to choose the chin or nose they might like. 'Broken and septic teeth were removed, dentures fitted, broken bones reset and skin-grafting carried out to reconstruct noses and jaws.'[99] Eye sockets were filled, too, and ears replaced. Gillies and his team also salvaged poorly treated cases, where terrible wounds had been closed by stitching without the lost tissue being replaced. Originally Gillies followed the established method of using a pedicle flap, where a piece of healthy skin, usually from the chest, was sutured to the wounded area to provide new grafted skin. The other end remained attached to the source, thereby providing a blood supply. These pedicles, particularly the longer ones, tended to curl inwards, like paper.

It was his inspiration to realise that 'If I stitched the edges of those flaps together, might I not create a tube of living tissue which would increase the blood supply to grafts, close them to infection, and be far less liable to contract or degenerate as the older methods were?' The insight came during an operation in October 1917, and Gillies immediately stitched the curling flaps into what he called 'tubed pedicles'.[100] As his biographer records, these were soon 'seen sprouting from scores of patients, carrying the promise of magical recovery to increasingly distant parts of the body. Beautifully fashioned from spare abdominal flesh, they were like slender pink orchidaceous stalks growing on to foreheads, cheeks, ears, noses and lips.'[101]

When the whole lower jaw had been blown away, depriving a man of the ability to eat and drink, or speak, milk and eggnog were popular forms of nourishment, the latter using the products of chickens on the hospital farm. After 35-year-old Horace Ellen, who had already received both the MM and the MC, was wounded in early November 1918 'by a bullet carrying away part of his lower jaw and another cutting a severe wound in one of his arms', he was taken to the Sir John Ellerman Hospital for Disabled Officers in London's Regent's Park, which was affiliated to Sidcup. 'My food is all liquid. Twelve glasses a day, and am getting an adept at drinking milk . . . but to be fed means a glass, a bib, a piece of cottonwool, and a sister to hold my head and jaw — some performance.'[102]

The treatment was neither easy nor rapid. Men often had to endure several operations — in one case, 50[103] — and the results, though mostly astonishing, were not always completely successful. Some men, at a certain point, refused further surgery. 'Tin faces', or at least partial prostheses, were sometimes still needed when full reconstruction proved impossible or a patient had had enough. Nursing those with what the French called *les gueules cassées* (broken faces) required both courage and sensitivity, lest an unguarded flinch or a glance away betrayed to the patient the awfulness of their appearance. Mirrors were banned in the Sidcup wards, but desperate men found ways to circumvent this. Appearing in public was hard. Although patients were encouraged to walk outside, 'some of the benches along the road from the Queen's Hospital to Sidcup, were painted blue for wounded soldiers only so that local residents would know that the occupant . . . was likely to have some hideous injury'.[104]

The New Zealand section at Sidcup was established on 9 January 1918 when Major Henry Pickerill, 29 patients and one dental mechanic were transferred from Walton-on-Thames. Major John Rishworth of the New Zealand Dental Corps arrived the same day, as the section's dental officer.[105] British-born Pickerill, who had become the first director of the Otago University Dental School in September 1907, took leave in 1916 and was seconded to the NZMC when he arrived in Britain early the following year. General Richardson had specifically asked for him because too many men returning to New Zealand 'were evidently improperly treated in the early stages and have suffered damage which can never be repaired'.[106] At the beginning of April 1917 Pickerill set up a unit at Walton for the treatment of facial and jaw injuries; it was this that later went to Sidcup. Despite having both medical and dental qualifications, Pickerill had no formal surgical training. He would nevertheless establish 'a considerable reputation as a plastic and reconstructive surgeon'. His background gave him 'a better appreciation of orthodontic principles than some of his surgical colleagues'.[107]

When Pickerill arrived at Walton, his 50-bed ward, as he told *Kai Tiaki*, 'did not contain one single jaw case', and he had 'no workroom and only a visiting mechanic, who knew nothing of any kind of metal or splint work'. After two months of hard work, he had a 'ward nearly full of jaw cases (forty), a workroom built and equipped, and a competent mechanic for the making of splints, etc.'. At that stage most of the cases were men who had been inadequately treated elsewhere, leaving, for example, a healed fracture but so much scar tissue, sometimes still containing minute pieces of shrapnel, that the jaw was virtually immobile. The 'fresh cases' that reached Pickerill were always very septic. 'Usually there is a piece of shrapnel somewhere

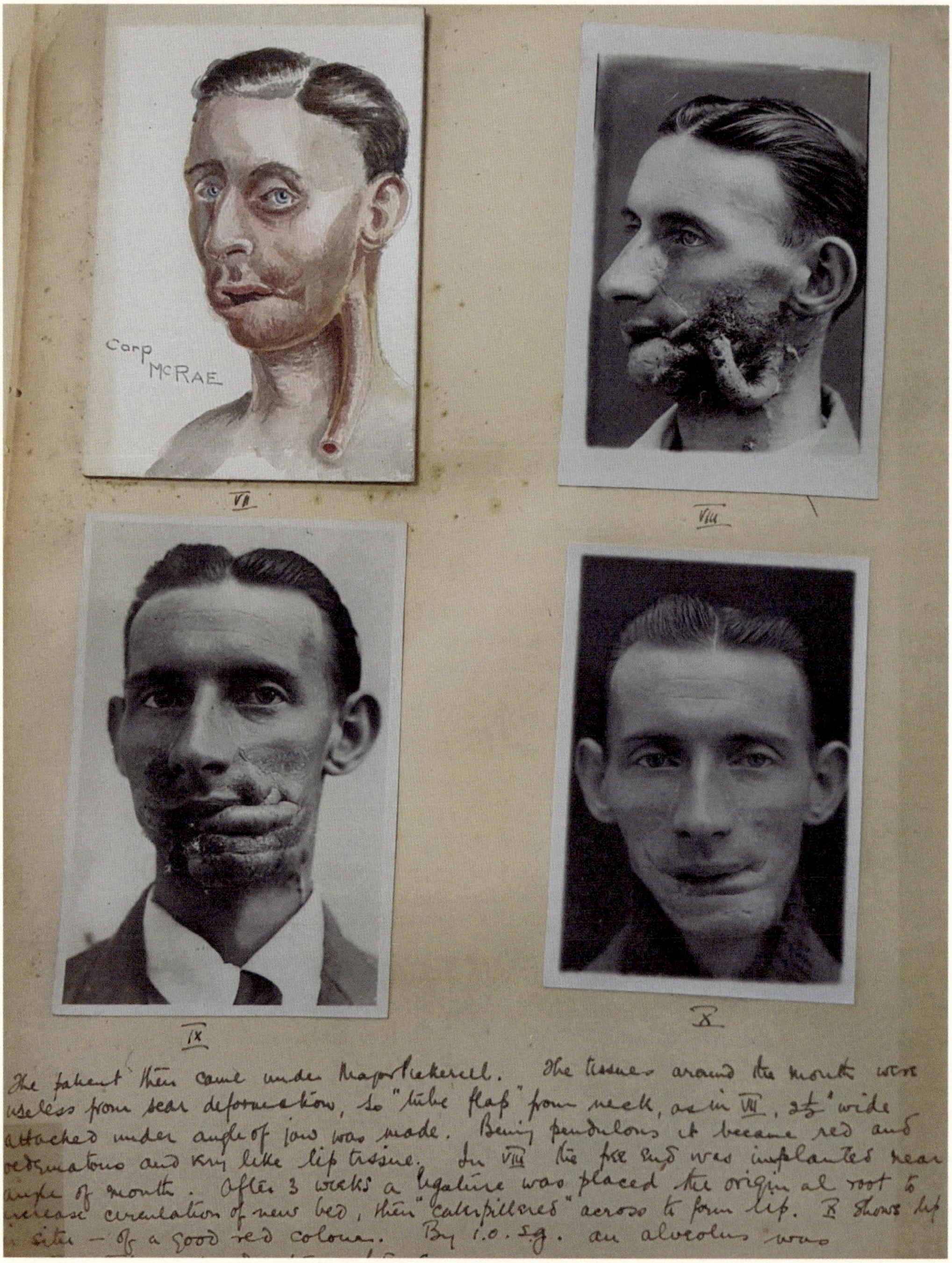

Sydney Rhind, who worked with Henry Pickerill at Sidcup, kept an album of before and after photos of patients who benefited from the pioneering surgery performed at Queen's Hospital. The revolutionary tubed pedicle introduced by Harold Gillies is clearly illustrated. ROYAL NEW ZEALAND ARMY MEDICAL CORPS HISTORY COLLECTION embedded in the tissues which has to be removed, and it is wonderful how easily one can miss these. Although the X-rays shows them quite plainly, they have, I find, a habit of moving about.'[108] There were aesthetic considerations too, such as taking skin for the upper lip from the scalp so the patient could grow a moustache. Pickerill also discovered that 'the deep scars which at first marred the face gradually disappeared', especially after the patients left the hospital, because 'the organs then received more exercise, such as talking and laughing'.[109]

Although Horace Ellen was not a patient at Sidcup itself, 'they cannot do anything to me without the sanction of a New Zealand doctor, Major Pickerill, who used to be a professor at the Dunedin University, so we ought to be well looked after'. On 19 November, 'They . . . put in my splints for the jaw, so I woke up with a mouthful.'

> To put things plainly, having anything wrong with the jaw is hell, and the pain hellish. With anything else you can clench your hands and set your teeth and bear it, but this business is the limit, but by next Sunday the first stage should be passed, and we then sit down and wait. By what I can make out, the jaw will be kept in position, and given a chance to heal itself and then if it does not heal, to graft a piece of my leg bone in and also there will be the scar to take out of the face, so there is a little to go through before I get back my ancient beauty again.[110]

On 4 December Ellen described 'the gadget I have to wear' for two months. 'Inside, on the bottom jaw, the teeth are capped on each side, and the pieces held in position by a bar. Underneath the chin is a plate and between the two are three wires with screws that tighten up underneath the plate. The wires are very thick and hollow, and the whole is gilt over with gold, so you can imagine the effect, but it means I can use my jaw a little, and get something to eat.' Once the bone was grafted in, there would be 'another operation to take out the scar in the cheek, give me sound teeth, and finish up with electrical treatment, to get the nerves right, for at present my chin is stiff, and I can back myself as a first-class dribbler, and it is very uncomfortable'. The following day Ellen was given 'another gadget', which allowed him to 'dispense with a feeder and get back to a cup again . . . though when we eat, we need a lot of loud music, as we have to suck our food in'.[111]

Pickerill and his staff carried out 113 'plastic operations' at Sidcup between 11 February and 14 July 1918. Queen Alexandra, the widow of King Edward VII, was among the visitors impressed with the New Zealanders' work; Godley was another.[112] At the beginning of May, Captain Sydney Rhind MC of the NZMC, who had been gassed twice in France, became Pickerill's assistant. He soon proved himself 'a very useful & efficient officer'.[113] Pickerill had been reluctant to move his team to Sidcup, and two days after arriving suggested to Allen that, as planned, he should return to Otago. Because 'the second or reparative stage — bone grafting etc.' could be undertaken only many months or even two years after the original wound had healed, it made more sense for such cases to be sent home, where Pickerill would treat them at Dunedin Hospital, 'which I cd. quite well do without interfering with my University duties'.[114] But Pickerill's 'intense sense of responsibility' won out, and he became deeply involved in Sidcup.[115] He did not come home until May 1919, to run a special section for returned soldiers

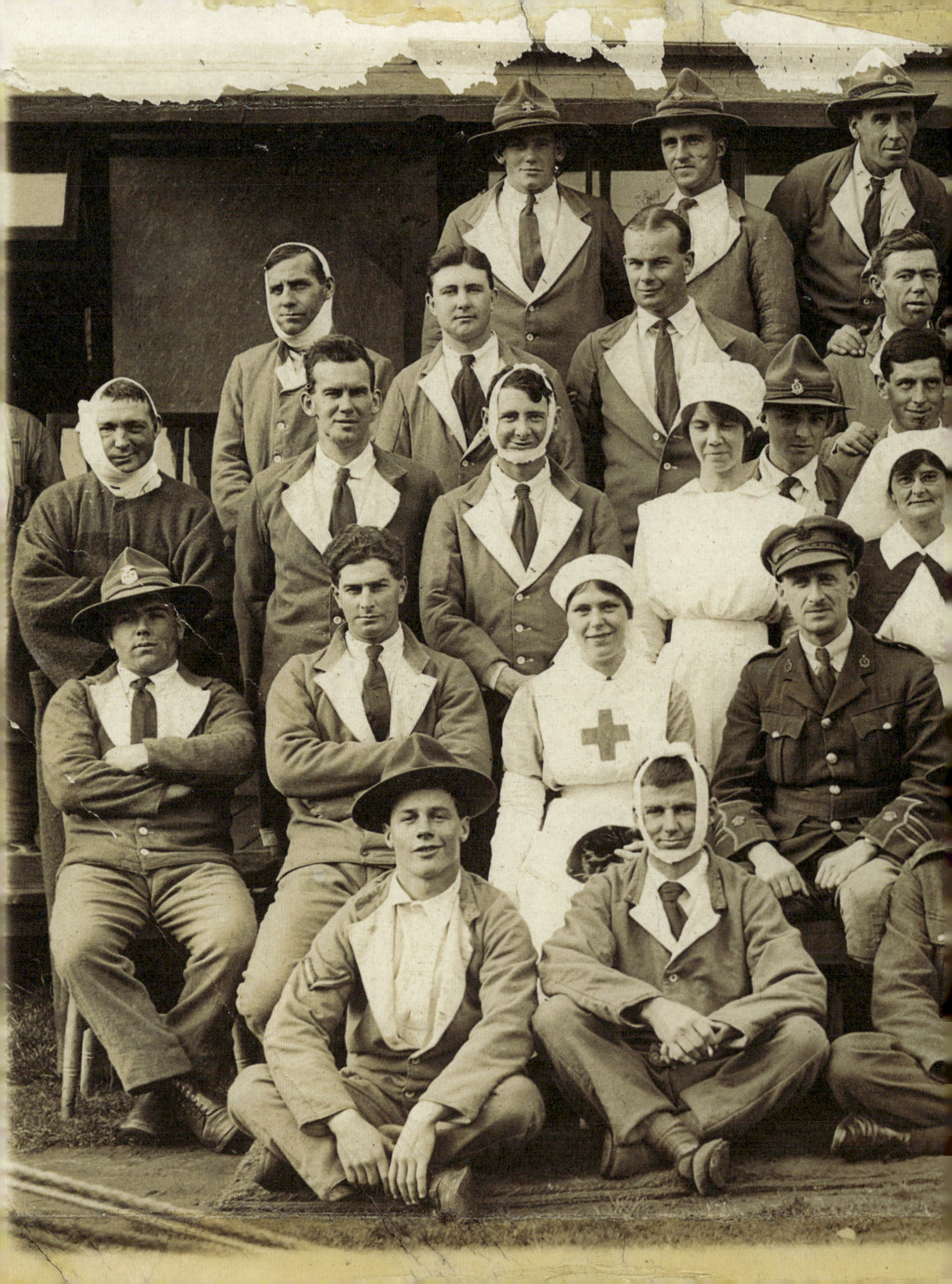

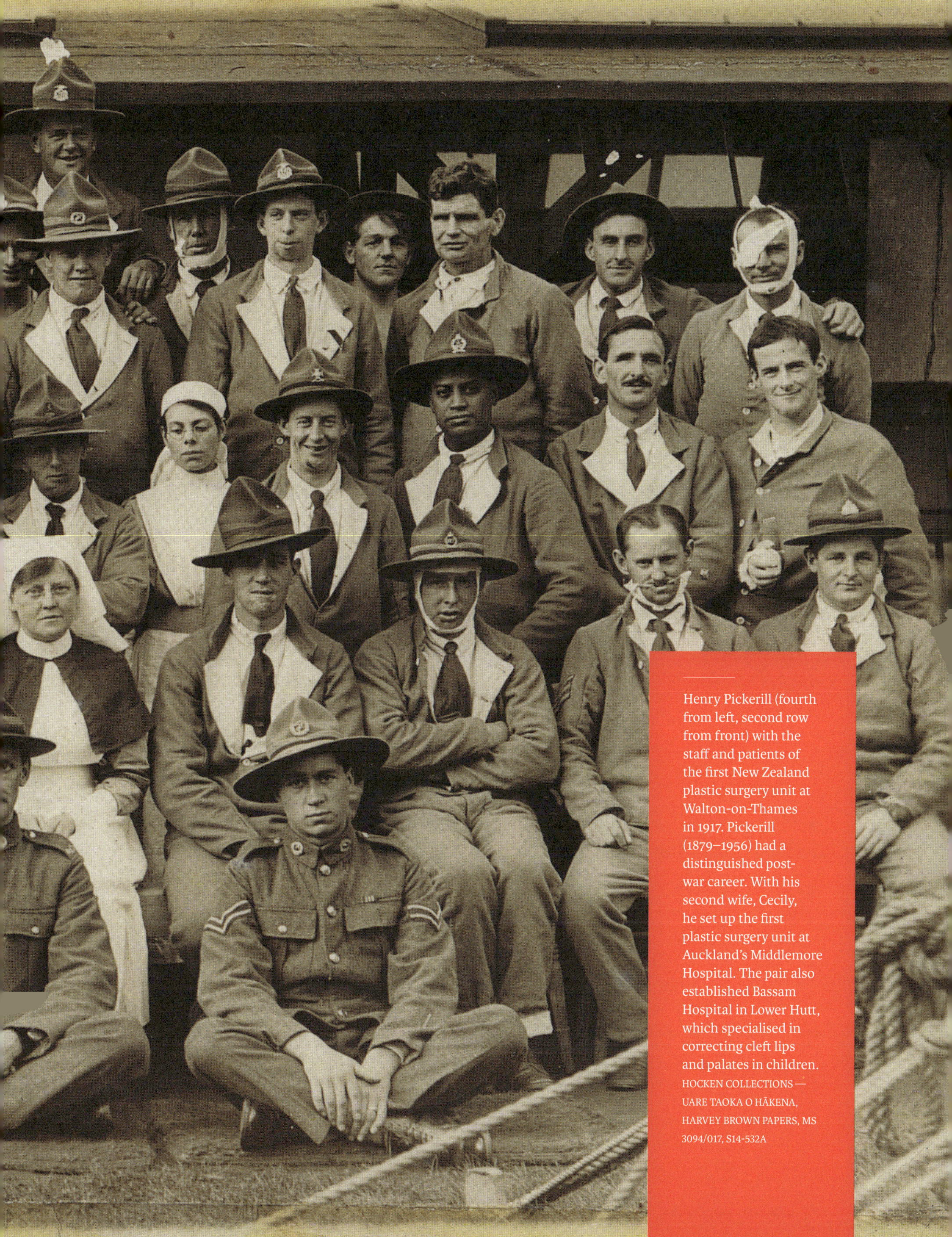

Henry Pickerill (fourth from left, second row from front) with the staff and patients of the first New Zealand plastic surgery unit at Walton-on-Thames in 1917. Pickerill (1879–1956) had a distinguished post-war career. With his second wife, Cecily, he set up the first plastic surgery unit at Auckland's Middlemore Hospital. The pair also established Bassam Hospital in Lower Hutt, which specialised in correcting cleft lips and palates in children.
HOCKEN COLLECTIONS — UARE TAOKA O HĀKENA, HARVEY BROWN PAPERS, MS 3094/017, S14-532A

with jaw and facial injuries while also resuming his Dental School role. The operative part of the work was carried out in a special ward at Dunedin Hospital, while Woodside, a mansion in north Dunedin that had been rented, renovated and furnished by the Red Cross Society, housed patients unable to undergo immediate surgery.[116]

One afternoon in November 1919, heeding James Allen's recent suggestion that this 'remarkable work . . . should be made more widely known', an *Evening Star* reporter spent an hour with Lieutenant-Colonel Pickerill in his office. The purple prose flowed freely. '[T]rue it is that Madame Tussaud's galleries never contained a more ghastly record of human mutilation than is emblazoned in the wax models (tinted with horrid particularity) hanging in this room.' Side by side with these, however, were 'the models of the same faces made anew or restored'. The reporter also admired the 'wonderful mechanical appliances' invented by the unit, and the 'extraordinarily minute record, pictorial and literary, which is kept of each case'. The expert staff who had been 'transported en bloc from Sidcup' included anaesthetist Angus Marshall, dental surgeon William Seed, artist Herbert Cole and Sisters Alice Finlayson and Mary McBeth. 'It would be possible to lengthen this brief account . . . with much detail of the work done at Sidcup and Walton . . . But we need go no further abroad than our own streets for testimony of the beneficent wonders of the new surgery. Si monumentum requiris, circumspice! [If you seek a monument, look around you!]'[117]

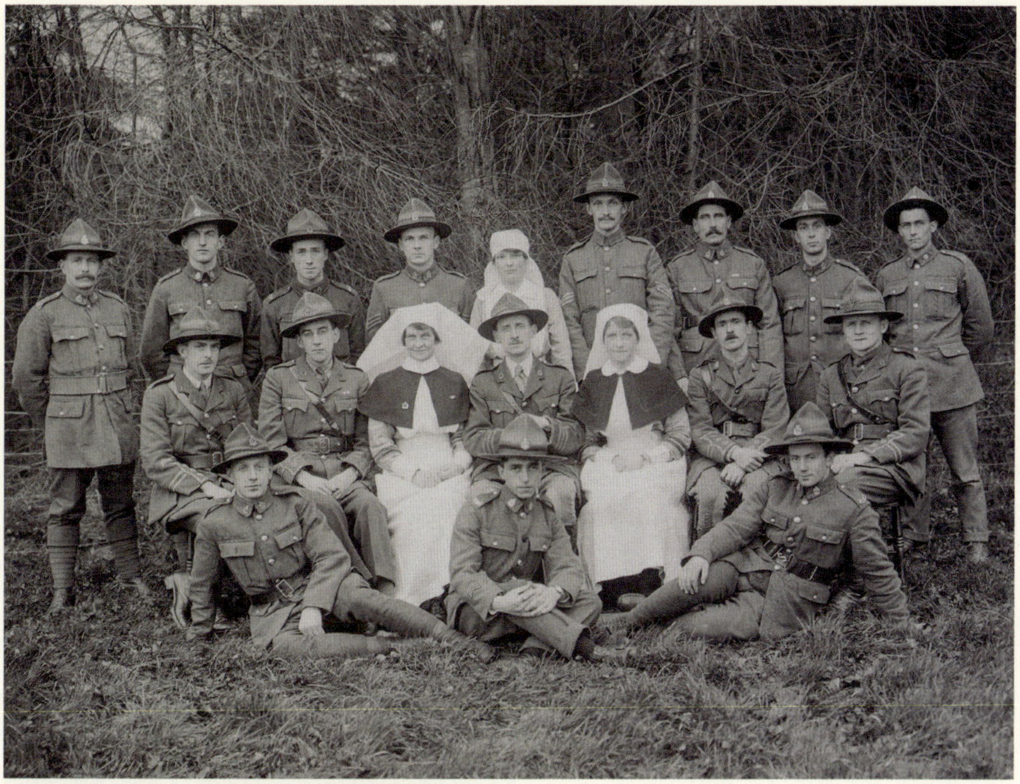

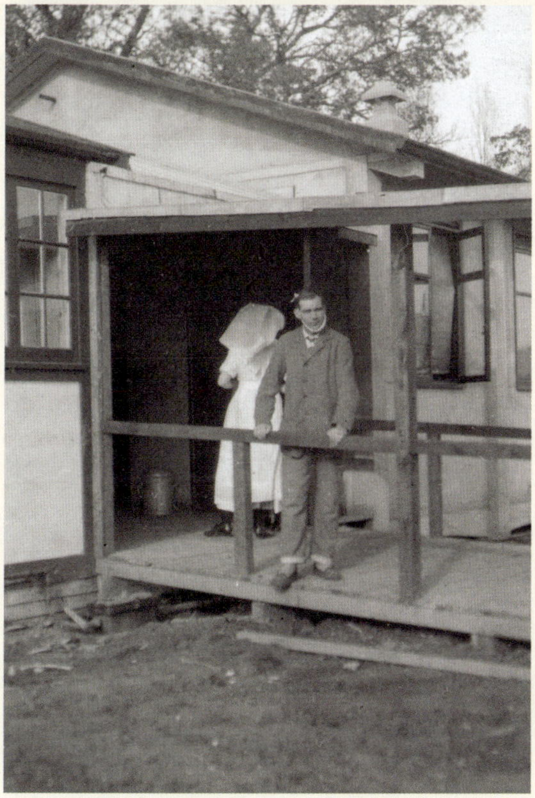

left In late 1918 NZMC man George Thomson photographed bandaged mate Laurie Reid outside a ward at Sidcup. Reid, a Linotype operator before the war, had been severely wounded in the head, back and abdomen in July that year. He also suffered a fractured jaw. After returning to New Zealand on the *Tainui* in March 1919, Reid became an inpatient at Dunedin Hospital, where he was treated by Pickerill and his staff. AUCKLAND WAR MEMORIAL MUSEUM, PH-2003-1-55

above The staff of the New Zealand unit at Sidcup. Major Henry Pickerill, in the centre, is flanked by Sisters Mary McBeth (on his right) and Alice Finlayson. The officers in that row, from left to right, are Captains Turner, Sydney Rhind, Angus Marshall and William Seed. AUCKLAND WAR MEMORIAL MUSEUM, PH-2003-1-74A

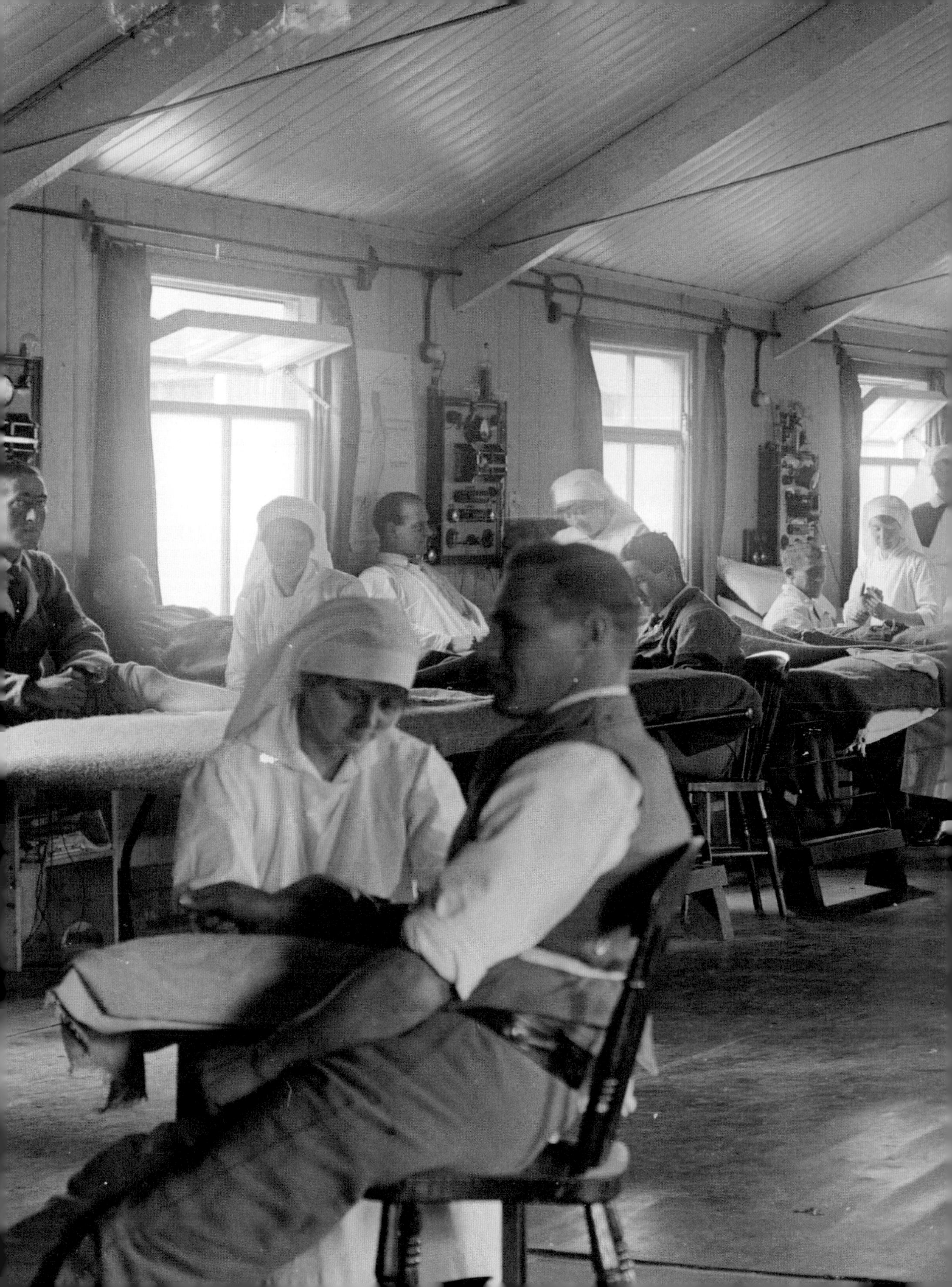

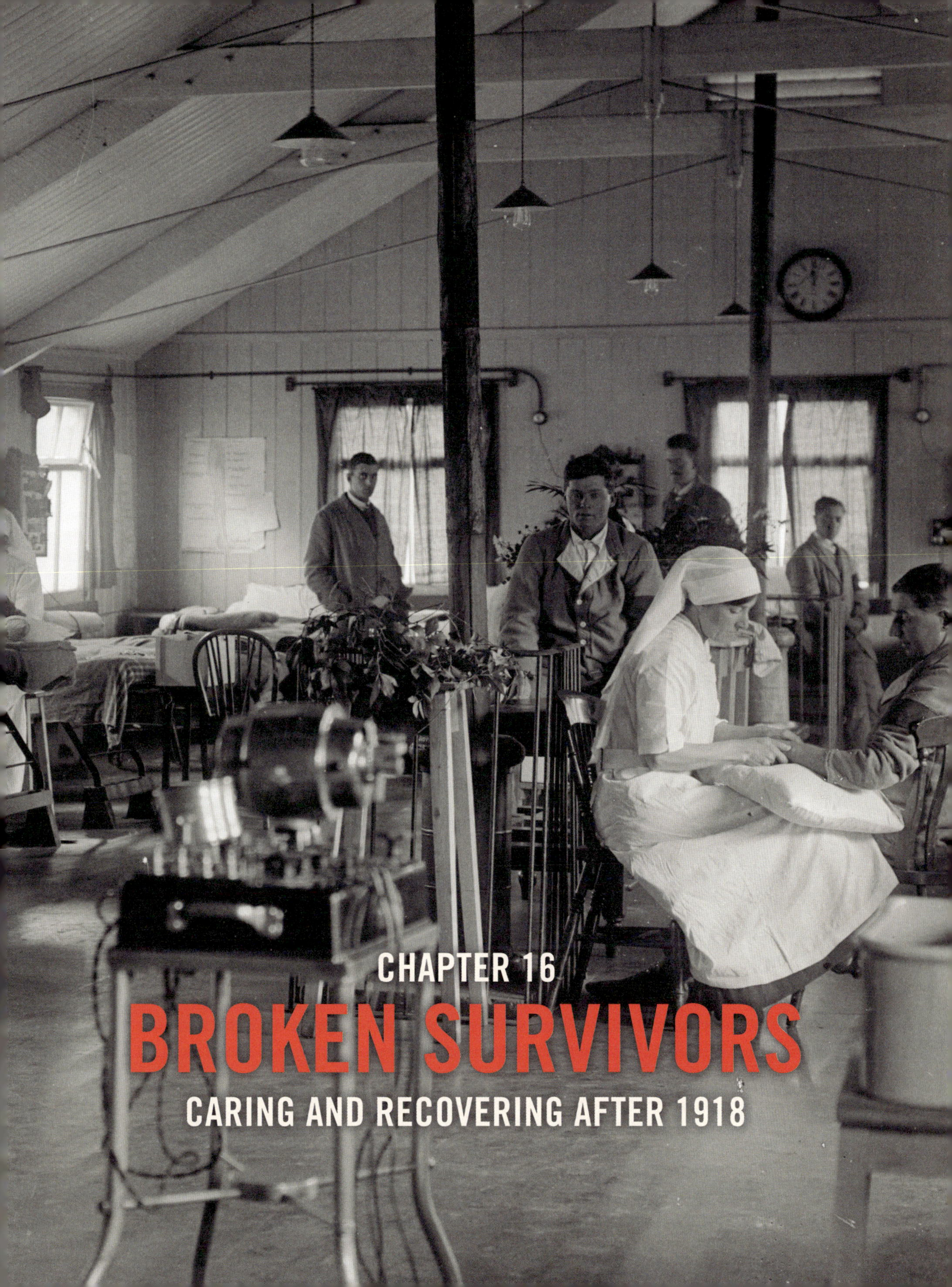

CHAPTER 16

BROKEN SURVIVORS

CARING AND RECOVERING AFTER 1918

Previous pages
As it had at Hornchurch, where this photo was taken, massage continued to play a vital role in the rehabilitation of wounded men back home in New Zealand after the war. ALEXANDER TURNBULL LIBRARY, 1/2-013999-G

> [W]ork . . . will be needed to care for the poor broken survivors . . . there will not be the excitement of preparing for a convoy of wounded, or of passing through a casualty clearing station the large numbers of recently wounded. There will not be the interest of foreign service or the tension of the submarine danger on transport or hospital ships, but . . . there will be the daily care, week in and week out, of the helpless, injured, incurable ones, the phthisical cases so hard to manage, and to bear with, the nerve cases so fractious and despondent.
>
> — *Kai Tiaki*, 1 January 1918

About 3 p.m. on 20 January 1919, a mild, sunny day with passing clouds and a south-west breeze, the former New Zealand Shipping Company vessel *Ruahine* berthed at Queen's Wharf in Auckland. She was carrying 585 invalided officers, nurses, VADs, NCOs and men. Among the patients were 94 labelled CPDI (chronic pulmonary disease intermediate) and 56 amputees. Most of the rest were surgical cases requiring dressings or massage. In the third-class saloon was an isolation hospital for 'skin affections etc' that included a VD section. The 18 cots in the smoking room turned hospital had been occupied throughout the voyage, but there were now only six bed-ridden cases.[1]

The *Ruahine* was just one of several vessels that brought sick and wounded New Zealand soldiers home from the war, along with the medical staff who had cared for them.[2] Some of the wounds were obvious — mutilated faces, missing limbs, bandaged heads — but many more, in patients and carers alike, were hidden: the cumulative effects of years of inconceivable stress, fear and horror, added to apprehension about what lay ahead.

And there had been another, more recent crisis. Although one man had died of pneumonia on the *Ruahine*, the *Herald* reporter was keen to make it clear that 'the health of the troops on arrival at Auckland was excellent'.[3] This emphasis was telling. Only weeks before, in November 1918, the country had been swept by an influenza pandemic that killed somewhere between 50 and 100 million people worldwide. Some 9000 New Zealanders had lost their lives, more than half the number who had been killed during the war.[4]

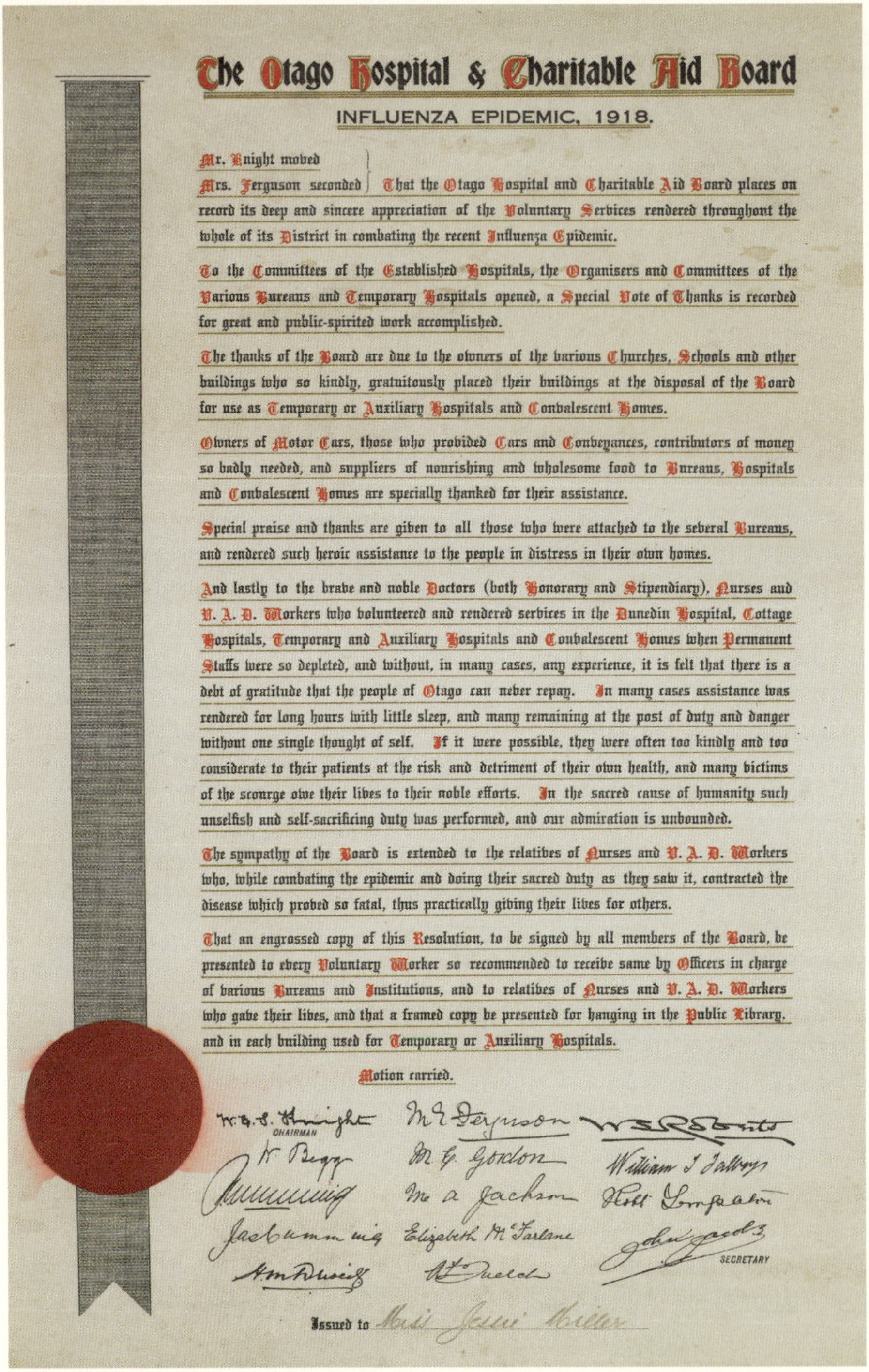

The Otago Hospital & Charitable Aid Board

INFLUENZA EPIDEMIC, 1918.

Mr. Knight moved
Mrs. Ferguson seconded } That the Otago Hospital and Charitable Aid Board places on record its deep and sincere appreciation of the Voluntary Services rendered throughout the whole of its District in combating the recent Influenza Epidemic.

To the Committees of the Established Hospitals, the Organisers and Committees of the Various Bureaus and Temporary Hospitals opened, a Special Vote of Thanks is recorded for great and public-spirited work accomplished.

The thanks of the Board are due to the owners of the various Churches, Schools and other buildings who so kindly, gratuitously placed their buildings at the disposal of the Board for use as Temporary or Auxiliary Hospitals and Convalescent Homes.

Owners of Motor Cars, those who provided Cars and Conveyances, contributors of money so badly needed, and suppliers of nourishing and wholesome food to Bureaus, Hospitals and Convalescent Homes are specially thanked for their assistance.

Special praise and thanks are given to all those who were attached to the several Bureaus, and rendered such heroic assistance to the people in distress in their own homes.

And lastly to the brave and noble Doctors (both Honorary and Stipendiary), Nurses and V. A. D. Workers who volunteered and rendered services in the Dunedin Hospital, Cottage Hospitals, Temporary and Auxiliary Hospitals and Convalescent Homes when Permanent Staffs were so depleted, and without, in many cases, any experience, it is felt that there is a debt of gratitude that the people of Otago can never repay. In many cases assistance was rendered for long hours with little sleep, and many remaining at the post of duty and danger without one single thought of self. If it were possible, they were often too kindly and too considerate to their patients at the risk and detriment of their own health, and many victims of the scourge owe their lives to their noble efforts. In the sacred cause of humanity such unselfish and self-sacrificing duty was performed, and our admiration is unbounded.

The sympathy of the Board is extended to the relatives of Nurses and V. A. D. Workers who, while combating the epidemic and doing their sacred duty as they saw it, contracted the disease which proved so fatal, thus practically giving their lives for others.

That an engrossed copy of this Resolution, to be signed by all members of the Board, be presented to every Voluntary Worker so recommended to receive same by Officers in charge of various Bureaus and Institutions, and to relatives of Nurses and V. A. D. Workers who gave their lives, and that a framed copy be presented for hanging in the Public Library, and in each building used for Temporary or Auxiliary Hospitals.

Motion carried.

CHAIRMAN

SECRETARY

Issued to Miss Jessie Miller

'Brave and noble' doctors, nurses and VADs are among those thanked on this certificate of appreciation issued by the Otago Hospital and Charitable Aid Board in 1918 after the influenza epidemic. TE PAPA, GH012027

On 22 August 1918 the troopship *Tahiti*, carrying the Fortieth Reinforcements from New Zealand to Britain, called at Freetown in Sierra Leone. The second wave of the virulent influenza was raging in the port,[5] and although no troops or crew were permitted to go ashore, locals came on board to coal the vessel. The damage was done. By the time the ship reached Plymouth, hundreds of men had reported sick and almost 80 had died. Another nine, including 31-year-old nurse Esther Tubman, who had enlisted in June after working at Featherston camp, where she 'had endeared herself greatly to the staff',[6] lost their lives soon afterwards. They were the first New Zealand deaths in the pandemic.

On 27 August, the day after the *Tahiti* left Freetown, Rifleman Marcus Hansen noted in his diary, 'An epidemic of influenza seems to have broken out on board.' By the following day, 'The sickness is going around the ship very rapidly and every available bit of floor space is being converted into a hospital . . . [T]o see big strong men just bowled over and hardly able to walk . . . is quite pitiful.' On the 29th there were 200 or 300 more on sick parade, 'and the nurses and doctors have their hands full'.[7] The former, led by Bessie Maxfield, immediately 'set to and did all we possibly could. Unfortunately for us, our P.M.O. was one of the first to go down. Next morning we sisters had to attend the sick parade and help get through the companies of sick men.' A second MO soon collapsed, though both later recovered. Nurses, too, became ill. About seven days after the outbreak, 'our cases began to suddenly grow worse and die'.

> They responded to no treatment whatever — stimulate and nourish them as we would — they went downhill rapidly, and this was the worst time of all. To see the poor boys die on our hands, one after the other . . . It was hard for us to see them go, but harder, I think, for their mates. Such a number of them were quite lads, [aged] about twenty. Having no lights on the decks made it twenty times harder for us, and one night almost every way we turned we found men, who a few moments before had seemed fairly well lying in a collapsed condition, dying about an hour later.

After being quarantined on arrival in Plymouth, the nurses were sent to the Brighton rest home, then to various hospitals, where they were soon caring for more influenza patients. As Hester Maclean proudly reported, the women were 'mentioned in despatches in terms of the highest commendation for their splendid work and devotion to duty under the most trying circumstances'.[8]

The first, milder wave of the pandemic, originating in the United States in late 1917 and early 1918 and taken to Europe by American troops, had largely abated by June. But then came what historian Geoffrey Rice has described as 'a highly infectious flu, with sudden onset and an alarming propensity for pneumonic complications'.[9] By mid-August, this was roaring through France. In September New Zealand nurse Bertha Taylor, at the NZSH in Wisques, noted the recent arrival of French soldiers suffering from a 'malignant' influenza. Some had died 'and nothing seemed able to save them'. Eva Brooke, too, reported many deaths among German and other patients later in the year from an influenza that was 'rampant and a very dreadful type with a very high mortality, owing, chiefly, to lung complications'.[10] In mid-December, Ira

Robinson, convalescing at Hornchurch, told his sister Lizzie of the 'thousands & thousands of people ill in England and Europe . . . They do not seem to be able to stamp it out here at all.'[11] In Taylor's words, 'After four years of hard work it is the saddest part of all, boys who had faced death hundreds of time in battle went "west" with "Flu". Some things are past understanding.'[12] The Middle East was not immune. On top of the malaria that devastated the New Zealanders in the Jordan Valley, 'there has been an epidemic of Spanish influenza, resulting in chest complications in many cases'.[13]

By the time Matron Mary Early was writing from the Aotea Convalescent Home at the beginning of March 1919, she and many others still serving overseas had heard what was happening at home. '[J]udging from the sad news in . . . papers coming to hand New Zealand has been a sadly unhealthy country lately. What a dreadful scourge influenza has been in our fair land! We are only now getting full details of the terrible time you must have gone through.'[14] As 'N.Z.M.C.' would write in the *New Zealand Herald* in February 1920, 'our boys were appalled when the casualty lists from New Zealand reached them in letters from home, and they could hardly believe that the infection was identical in the two countries'.[15] Too often, the loved ones they had been forced to leave behind, and had dreamt of seeing again, had died.

The war not only contributed to the pandemic via infected returning troops, but also reduced New Zealand's ability to fight the flu because so many medical personnel were still away. A nurse at the New Zealand Discharge Depot in Torquay wrote on 4 March 1919: 'What a dreadful time you have had . . . It made us all feel very sad and long to help, especially as at that time we were not at all busy over here.'[16] Those nurses who had come back lent a willing and expert hand, and the NZMC offered personnel from the military camps, along with useful organisational advice. It was their recommendation, for instance, that Auckland be divided into 22 districts, each with a depot or bureau where locals could report severe flu cases or request assistance.[17] Alfred Hollows, who had enlisted in October 1918, was one of 20 NZMC men sent to Wellington, 'which was having a very torrid time'. He worked in an emergency hospital set up in a hall 'hastily fitted with beds . . . By about 18 or 19 November, our death rate was quite appalling, something like a dozen a day.' Hollows paid tribute to the work of Dr Henry Hardwick-Smith, who had been on the third charter of the *Marama* and returned to New Zealand in May 1918. He was 'truly a wonderful man. The only sleep he got was catnaps in the back of the motor car as he was driven from case to case.'[18]

Other doctors who had served overseas also contributed. With the help of a nurse, Elizabeth Gunn organised a medical centre in the Soldiers' Club on Wellington's Sydney Street in Thorndon; in Dunedin, Louis Barnett operated on some surgical cases at a private hospital, because four of the five public hospital house surgeons were ill; at Christchurch Hospital, where half the nursing staff had influenza, along with the medical superintendent and the matron, Colonel David Wylie, who had just arrived to establish the new Chalmers orthopaedic unit, brought much-needed help: 'His experience in busy army hospitals overseas was soon put to good use.' In Temuka, desperately short of doctors, the arrival of Captain Frank Ulrich, NZMC, on 18 November, on his way from Timaru to Christchurch, seemed an 'answer to a prayer'. The town clerk immediately asked the authorities if he could stay on.[19]

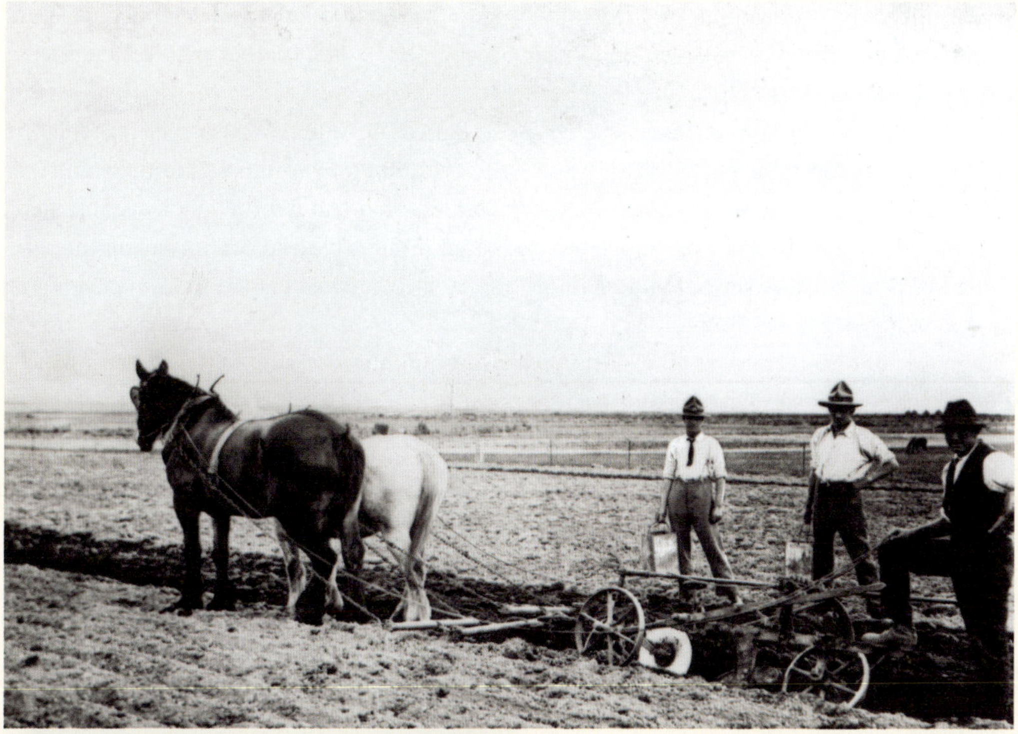

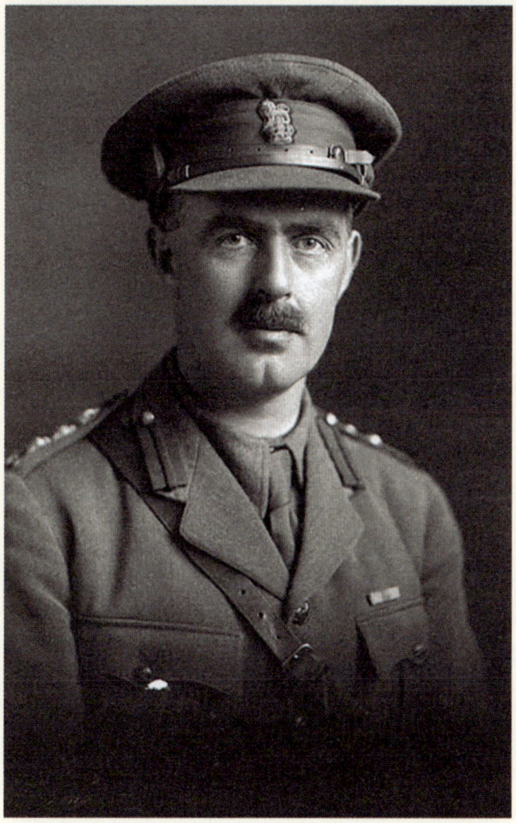

left When he died of influenza in 1919, surgeon Charles Mackie Begg CB CMG was the most decorated member of the New Zealand Medical Corps. He was mentioned in despatches three times and received the highest order of the Croix de Guerre. He began the war as the head of the New Zealand Field Ambulance and ended it as director of medical services. ARCHIVES NEW ZEALAND TE RUA MAHARA O TE KĀWANATANGA, AALZ 25044 BOX 3 F1211 15

above Tuberculosis was a widespread problem for returned servicemen. Some of those fit enough to learn lighter farming work were sent to one of the Repatriation Department's state training farms, such as this one at Tauherenikau in Wairarapa. ALEXANDER TURNBULL LIBRARY, PACOLL-8550-30

Ulrich, who had come home on the *Ionic* in August, later became sick himself but recovered, as did William Will, who was working at Christchurch Hospital.[20] Other medical men were not so fortunate. On 15 November 1918, 28-year-old Major Aubrey Short, who had served overseas and been mentioned in despatches and awarded the Military Cross, died of influenza in Christchurch Hospital. For Winifred Muff, halfway through her nurse's training, Short was 'a favourite house surgeon'.[21] Colonel Mathew Holmes, who had led the medical contingent to Samoa in August 1914, served in Egypt and France and become ADMS in Wellington, had battled ill-health before returning home in February 1918. He lost his life to influenza in the capital on 15 November.

As Rice has observed, their concentrations of large numbers of men in the susceptible 25–45-year age range made New Zealand's military camps 'among the most dangerous places to be during November 1918'. More than 280 died there. Carbery had only admiration for the NZMC personnel, 'depleted by sickness and death in their own ranks, [who] wrought unceasingly with splendid devotion', and for the 'quiet heroism' of the combatant volunteers 'in their unwonted terrible and dangerous work'.[22] Captain Allan Christie, who had been with the RAMC, then joined the NZMC as a surgeon, had suffered numerous health problems during the war, including pleurisy and tuberculosis. This history cannot have helped him when he went to Featherston in July 1918; he died in Greytown Hospital on 9 November.

After training at Awapuni, Major John Sale was to have sailed with the Forty-third Reinforcements, but when their departure was delayed by the pandemic he was posted to Trentham. He would die there of influenza at 5 a.m. on Armistice Day.[23] A retired NZMC man, 67-year-old Lieutenant-Colonel William Bey, did not let his age deter him from 'daily attending the sick men in Papawai Camp at the time of the epidemic'; he died on 14 November. Among some 14 ORs of the NZMC to lose their lives was 32-year-old Bertram Boock, who died at the Racecourse Hospital, Featherston, on 10 November, from 'bronchopneumonia following influenza'. His gravestone in Wellington's Karori Cemetery has inscriptions in both Hebrew and English.[24] Ten days later, 24-year-old Frederick Atyeo from Christchurch died of influenza and pneumonia at Trentham Military Hospital. A member of the Mounted Field Ambulance, he had been invalided home in November 1915 and discharged the following year because of 'dysentery resulting in debility', but re-enlisted and was posted to Trentham in June 1918.[25]

Not all the fatalities were male. On 10 November, 34-year-old Sister Mabel Whishaw died of influenza at Featherston. She had been on the military hospital staff for three years as night sister, and 'was a most capable and devoted nurse'. Her mother, Catherine, had lost two sons in the war: Harry was killed at the Somme in 1916 and Bernard died of pneumonia only a month before his sister.[26] On 25 November, 26-year-old VAD Corale Lumley died, also at Featherston.

New Zealand doctors died overseas, too. Colonel Charles Begg, promoted on 30 November 1918 to succeed William Parkes as DMS, had but a brief period in his new London-based role. After contracting influenza, then acute pneumonia, he died at Twickenham on 2 February 1919 and was buried at Walton-on-Thames three days later. He was 39 years old. Only three years his senior was Captain William Paterson from Dunedin, who had left New Zealand on the *Marama* on 1 June 1918 and been posted to Walton, then Hornchurch. After his death at Hornchurch on 14 November, a letter from the New Zealand Record Office revealed the grim practicalities of burials. '[O]wing to the recent epidemic of influenza, the Government Contractor is unable to carry out the arrangements for the funeral [at Brookwood Cemetery in Surrey] . . . Please arrange for the coffin to be supplied locally.' Enclosed was a railway warrant 'for the conveyance of the body by Ambulance from your hospital to the Necropolis Station'. (Brookwood is also known as the London Necropolis.)[27]

The Armistice on 11 November 1918 did not rule a neat line between conflict and peace. As Fanny Speedy put it, 'The whole thing seems too big to realise and too sad to understand.' Nurse Louisa Higginson 'did not know whether to laugh, shout or cry . . . there seems a short distance between laughter & tears'.[28] Hundreds of men were still wounded, sick and dying, the New Zealand hospitals in Britain had not closed, and ahead lay the enormous logistical task of getting everyone safely home. Then there was the challenge of providing the right kind of care, in convalescent homes and hospitals, for all those affected physically and psychologically. Like the soldiers, the medical personnel also faced the prospect of negotiating a much altered post-war world.[29]

Until the Defence Department took sole responsibility for the treatment of returned men in March 1918, joint Health/Defence control had been, in Carbery's words, 'cumbersome, [and] uneconomical, led to considerable delay in execution and was not productive of military efficiency'.[30] To fill the gaps left by overcrowded public hospitals and the inadequate provision of military hospitals, patriotic associations had, with government encouragement, established a number of small soldiers' hospitals and convalescent homes, many in buildings offered by wealthy citizens, but their 'scattered distribution' had defeated efficient administration and control.[31] After Defence took over, most of them eventually closed, but they had fulfilled an important role, providing vitally needed rest and peace. On warm days, during his few weeks convalescing at Taumaru, attorney-general Francis Dillon Bell's sheltered and lovely home at Lowry Bay, Wellington, a badly wounded and traumatised Clifford Collingwood 'used to lie on the little wharf and boat-house, and read my volume of Shakespeare, or take photos'.[32]

Rotorua already had a sanatorium, but the King George V Hospital had been opened in January 1916. For one patient, the 'beautiful new building situated on Pukeroa Hill, overlooking Lake Rotorua, and just above the Maori village of Ohinemutu . . . could not be more suitably situated', and the food was 'very good' — there was even trout for breakfast, as well as porridge and tea.[33] Hospital head Dr A. S. Herbert and his team created a number of 'clever contrivances', such as ambulatory splints, which allowed men once 'obliged to lie helpless' to walk about, and a glove with attached elastic bands 'to do the work of sinews' in a paralysed hand.[34] Hanmer Springs in North Canterbury, which had opened as a convalescent home in 1915, was reborn as the Queen Mary Military Hospital, in a building designed to be identical to Rotorua's, in June 1916.[35] Under the new Defence-run system, King George V and Queen Mary hospitals, along with all convalescent homes that had been overseen by the Public Health Department, became military institutions.[36]

There had been complaints about the struggling public hospitals, where returned men had been forced to wait for crucial dressings and massage, but these also had positive medical outcomes. In April 1917, for example, the Auckland Hospital Board could instance 'some very successful operations on wounded soldiers', such as 'the uniting of certain nerves which had been severed by bullet or shrapnel, and the correction of various deformities'. At the hospital's Military Annexe in the Domain, '310 returned men had been treated with the happiest results, though five passed beyond human aid as the direct result of wounds'.[37] Frederick Foote benefited from 'the gracious care, and generous service' of the nursing staff there and never lost his 'feeling of good will towards them'.[38] By July 1919, the annexe, rechristened the Auckland Military Hospital, had, among other new facilities, an 'up-to-date operating theatre', X-ray and developing rooms, and a 'suite . . . devoted to the electrical bath treatment'.[39]

Under the Defence-run system, men went from their ships to Trentham, where their medical needs were assessed before they were dispatched to the appropriate institution for treatment. An orthopaedic case, for example, would be sent to the 'special massage and electrical department' in Christchurch's recently opened Chalmers Military Hospital (which boasted 'all the latest improvements of baths, plaster departments, and everything used in the re-education of muscles and limbs injured in the war' and offered 'really up-to-date teaching in the latest methods' of massage),[40] to an enlarged Trentham Hospital, to Rotorua's King George V Hospital (which was extended to become, by 1920, a 300-bed orthopaedic hospital),[41] or to Dunedin Public Hospital.

Tuberculosis patients were treated in the sometimes too invigorating hilltop air at Christchurch's Cashmere Sanatorium or the Pukeora Sanatorium near Waipukurau, opened in September 1919. Heart problems meant a stay at Featherston or Auckland's Narrow Neck hospital. Pickerill continued his reconstructive surgery in Dunedin after returning to New Zealand, and Hanmer flourished as the specialist centre for men with neurological and psychological problems. 'What more lifting place,' asked the *Sun*, 'for the nerve-shattered . . . warrior to recover his lost vitality?'[42] The permanently incapacitated men designated as 'incurables' found their way to convalescent homes: Evelyn Firth in Auckland, Rannerdale in Christchurch and Montecillo in Dunedin.

The dedicated voluntary work of aid societies and patriotic groups was important. The Red Cross helped to provide, in hospitals and convalescent homes, much-needed and appreciated recreation rooms, and supplied copious comforts, including cigarettes. Just as it had overseas, the YMCA made sure that, where possible, there were picture theatres, facilities especially welcomed by those condemned to lengthy treatments or multiple surgeries. Always on hand, too, was the Salvation Army. After arriving home on the *Marama* in August 1917, Clifford Collingwood was taken to the Victoria Military Ward of Wellington Hospital. 'Salvation Army ladies . . . visited us every week and issued to each of us a copy of the "War Cry", a bag of lollies, fruit and a handkerchief — they are good & kindly women.' He was also called on by YMCA and RSA representatives.[43]

VD remained a focus of opprobrium. In mid-1916 the director of military hospitals had assured the press that 'the number of cases of venereal disease had been very greatly exaggerated', that the percentage among the returned soldiers was 'remarkably low' and, moreover, that 'as a result of modern science, no diseases of this character are now regarded as incurable'.[44] But infected men did return to New Zealand, and they were condemned to compulsory isolation and treatment, on Otago Harbour's Quarantine Island (Kamau Taurua) and later in Featherston camp's hospital. There were other punishments: docked pay, a ban on wearing uniform, refusal of railway passes for leave.[45]

Post-war medical treatment could be a lengthy and wearying business; many returned men continued to be public hospital outpatients for years.[46] Some could not face completing their prescribed treatments. After Len Coley arrived on the *Rimutaka* and caught the train home to Palmerston North, he reported, as ordered, to the military ward of the public hospital and spent the next nine weeks there. Despite struggling with his breathing after being gassed, and feeling the concussive effects of shelling 'almost every day', he jibbed at the prospect of 11 weeks of reporting as an outpatient. He asked for his discharge and made use of his free 28 days of railway travel.[47]

When Frederick Foote got home, the open wound in his right elbow, 'as large as a big saucer', was dressed daily in a big room where five or six nurses worked. Eating was a challenge. 'My left arm had dropped wrist and most of my hand was dead as far as feeling went, and my right hand was completely out of action being bound up in a sling. By grasping the great wooden handle of fork or spoon in my left hand and persisting I got some sort of meal.' Some months later, having admired the dexterity of a fellow patient who 'quickly and very neatly' put on a shirt, studded collar and tie with one hand, Foote practised every day for six months until he could do the same 'as quickly as the average man'.[48]

Clifford Collingwood still had a long, hard and painful medical journey ahead of him after his time in the Victoria Ward and at Lowry Bay. About April 1918 he had the plaster cut off his leg and a Thomas splint fitted, with a hole bored through the heel of his shoe so he could lock the end to make walking safer. He spent most of 1920 in Trentham Military Hospital, having his leg reset. Having refused a further operation, and 'in a hell of a pain', early in 1921 he visited a civilian doctor, who prescribed bismuth and opium, which Collingwood took for the next decade. Only about 1930 was he fitted with an appropriate boot that enabled him to walk in more comfort with his splint.[49]

Early death was not uncommon. Men came home with unhealed wounds that later proved fatal or heightened the risk of death in subsequent operations and from cardiovascular disease. The likelihood of suicide was greatly increased for those suffering from serious mental and physical disability, disfigurement and chronic pain.[50] Often overlooked, too, both then and since, was what historian Marina Larsson has called the 'family fallout' from physical and psychological disability. With the longed-for reunion at the quayside, where wives, sweethearts, parents and siblings suddenly confronted the reality of their loved one's impairments — blindness, loss of hearing, inability to speak clearly or to walk, the vacant stare of a sadly changed personality — an unanticipated new era of hardship began.[51]

Tuberculosis, then incurable, often fatal and greatly feared, also cast a long shadow over the lives of a number of veterans and their families.[52] Many men had unwittingly carried the symptoms of tuberculosis with them to war, and the cramped and often unsanitary conditions of trench warfare, overcrowded troopships and packed military hospitals 'undoubtedly facilitated the transmission of the bacilli, awakened "old tubercules" in soldiers' lungs, and accelerated the progression of TB to the active stage'.[53] Returned men with tuberculosis were separated from their families by being sent to a sanatorium, or, if living at home, had to sleep alone, use separate cutlery and, worst of all, avoid intimacy with their wives and children, for fear of transmitting the disease. Tuberculosis also caused difficulties with getting pensions, because of uncertainty over whether it was contracted during the war, and men's ability to work.

Rehabilitation had been a large part of the treatment at the New Zealand hospitals in Britain, and classes for sick and wounded men were held during the voyages home. On the *Ruahine*, English, mathematics, economics, commercial law, bookkeeping, shorthand and motor engineering had been on offer, along with lectures on poultry keeping.[54] This mixture of occupational therapy and vocational training remained a significant part of recovery at home, as James Allen explained in September 1918. What he called 'functional treatment' — 'basket work, leather work, wood carving and so on' — was 'fairly well developed' in the hospitals. There was 'a certain amount of gardening work in some places', and Rotorua was 'establishing workshops for wood-turning, metal turning, electrical work, motor engineering, plaster-casting, splint-making, etc.'.[55] Less taxing farming jobs such as beekeeping and poultry farming were taught to veterans with TB or chest problems at a state training farm set up on the site of the former Tauherenikau camp between 1919 and 1923.[56] There were other such farms, also run by the Repatriation Department.

Many returned men with significant injuries managed to make a living against severe odds. When farmer Frank Fougere, shot in both forearms on Gallipoli, got home in 1916, he was sent to Rotorua for months of massage treatment, then 'just knocked about the country', living on a mess allowance paid by the army and going into 'whatever hospital was handy when an abscess would form upon my [right] arm'. Once he was finally discharged, he took up a bush-covered rehab property that, over 30 years, he cleared and turned into 'a real good farm'. 'I managed quite well.'[57] The Repatriation Department

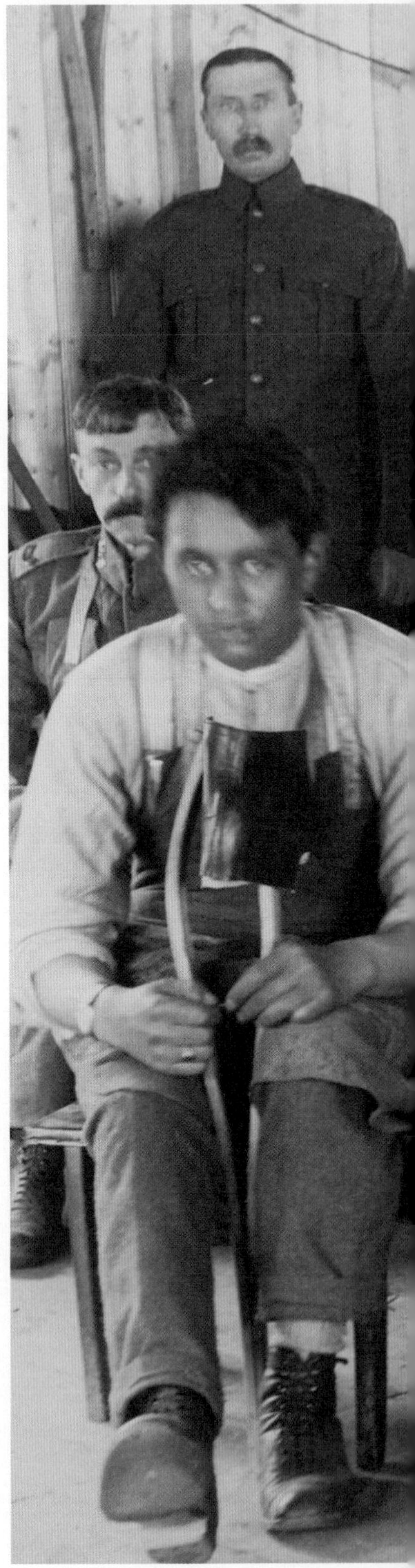

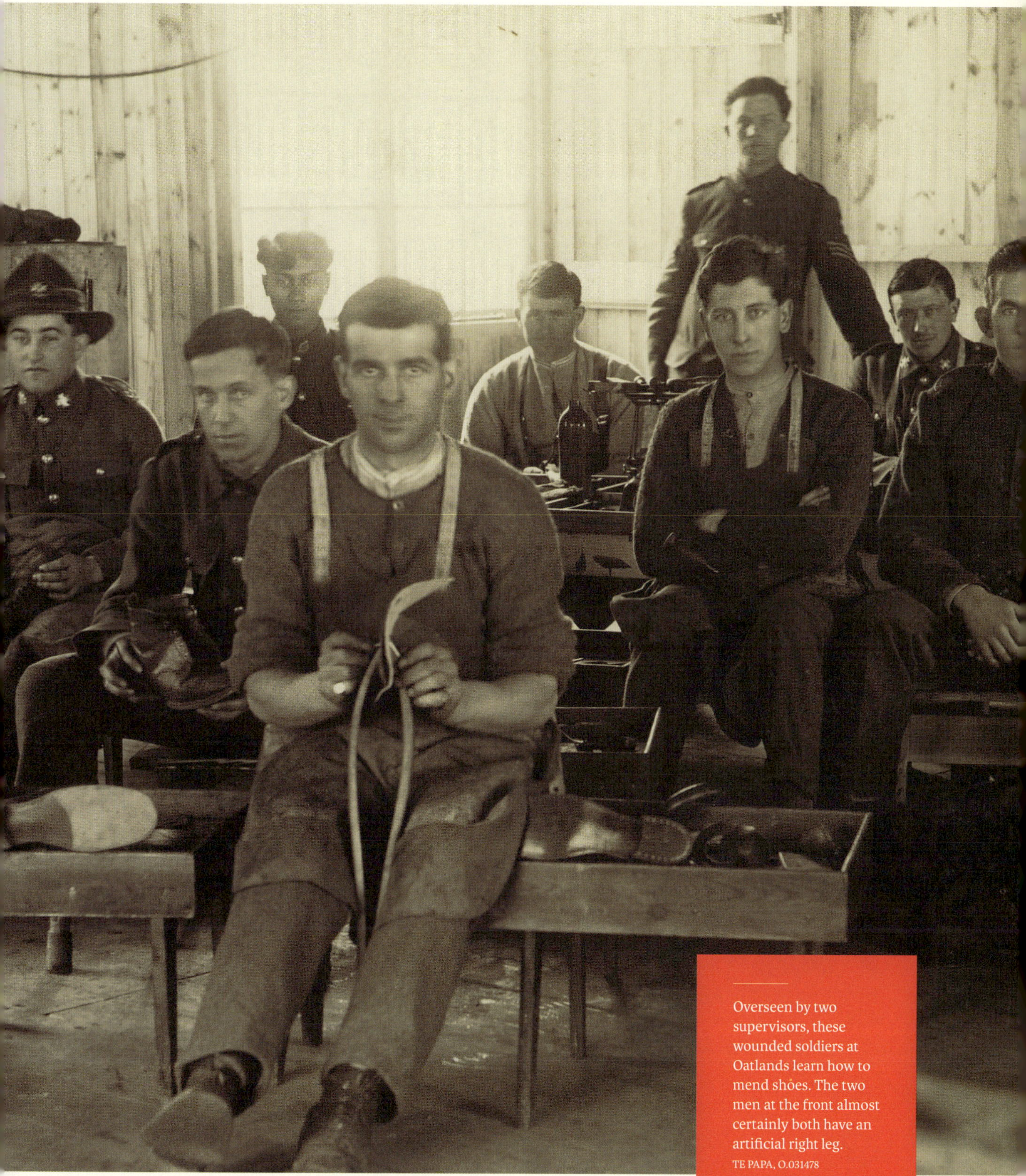

Overseen by two supervisors, these wounded soldiers at Oatlands learn how to mend shoes. The two men at the front almost certainly both have an artificial right leg.
TE PAPA, O.031478

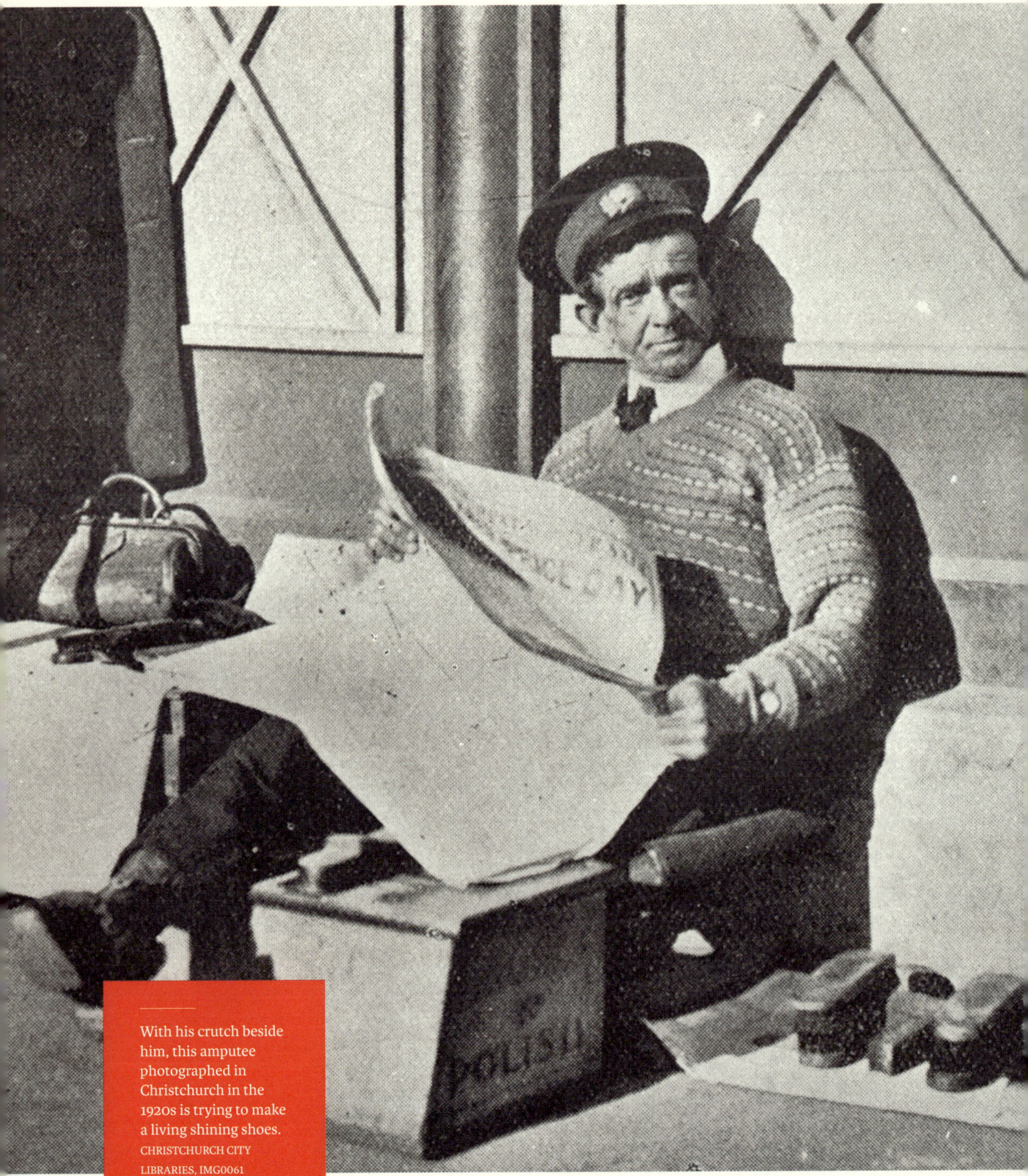

With his crutch beside him, this amputee photographed in Christchurch in the 1920s is trying to make a living shining shoes.
CHRISTCHURCH CITY LIBRARIES, IMG0061

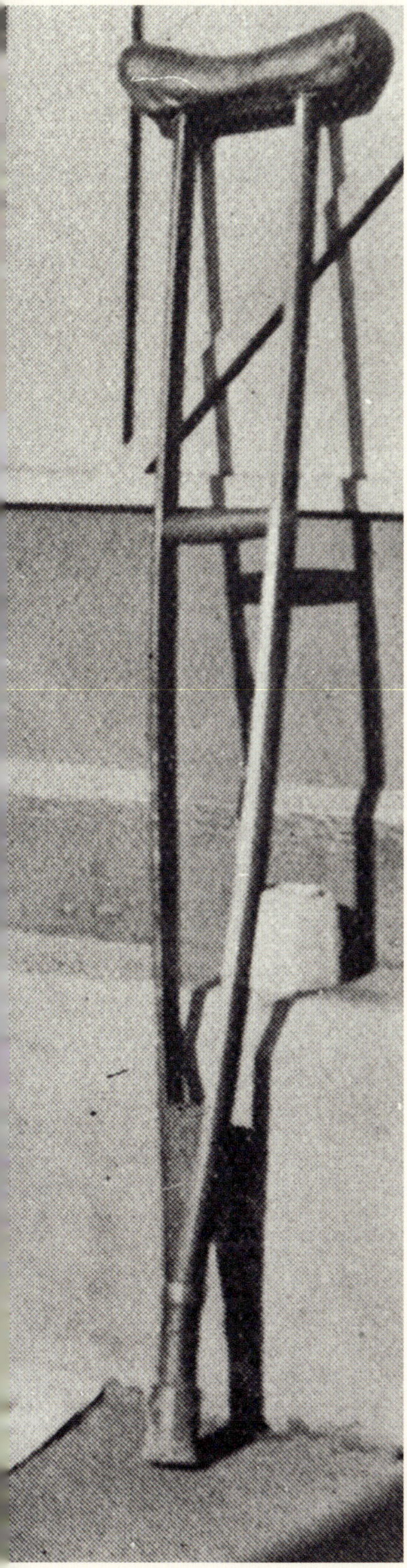

subsidised wages so that employers were more willing to take on partly trained returned men who were not yet able to work at full strength. Men keen to set up small businesses could take advantage of cheap loans.[58]

Sick and wounded returned men needed medical treatment, which was free, and then financial support in the form of a pension and assistance with finding suitable employment. This process, however, was frequently neither smooth nor problem-free, despite the fact that war disability was 'perceived as a more terrible and heroic experience' than its civilian counterpart, and therefore more deserving of expert medical treatment.[59] Reliant on pensions that were sometimes difficult to acquire, and often unable to work, such men struggled even more — and were less regarded as special cases — when economic depression hit the country from the 1920s.

As they had during the war, medical board doctors decided, before the troops left their ships, whether they required further treatment as hospital in- or outpatients, and how bad and lasting their wound or wounds were, in order to recommend a pension rate. Those who did need more medical attention had to appear regularly before the pensions board 'until their disability either healed or stabilised and a permanent pension was granted'.[60] The War Pensions Act 1915 allowed NZEF members or their dependants to receive a pension 'if the soldier had been disabled or had died as a result of service in the current war'.[61] War pensions boards decided on pension claims and the rate to be paid, which was tied to a soldier's rank and degree of seniority. Further legislation in 1917 increased the maximum disablement and war widows' pensions and, in an attempt at standardisation, introduced a schedule of disabilities that assigned pensions on a percentage basis.[62]

At the 100 per cent level were losses — of two limbs, of limb and eye, of both hands, of all fingers and thumbs, of both feet, of hand and foot — blindness, complete paralysis, lunacy, permanent confinement to bed, wounds or injuries to the head or another organ involving total permanent disabling effects, advanced incurable disease and very serious facial disfigurement. The sad catalogue of harm to the human body continued, from 85 per cent for such injuries as amputation of the right arm through the shoulder-joint and loss of speech, down to 20 per cent for the loss of an index finger on either hand.[63] There were variations to the prescribed list. Roland Bremner, who had his left arm amputated following a gunshot wound at the Somme, and who also suffered shell wounds to his penis and scrotum, 'with injury to the urethra', was judged to have 90 per cent disability.[64] An independent War Pensions Medical Appeal Board established in 1920 lasted only two years, suspended after the Returned Soldiers' Association roundly criticised its 'narrow and ungenerous approach'. The onus of proof was on the applicant, and there could be disagreements between civilian doctors and military medics.[65]

As Sydney Stanfield recalled, 'The medical boards you went before were almost hostile. You had to be proof-positive, so to speak, or you didn't get anything.' He suspected doctors were chosen to suit the circumstances. 'They wouldn't want to be too sympathetic or it would cost the country too much.'[66] The capriciousness of boards was well illustrated in a July 1917 story in Dunedin's *Evening Star*. A man the paper called Brown had served on Gallipoli and then in France, where he was seriously wounded. After hospitalisation in England, he reached New Zealand on 12 May and, after three weeks' leave, was thoroughly examined by a medical board and discharged on 9 June. Eight days later that decision was rescinded and he was reboarded cursorily on the 19th, by the same two doctors he had previously seen, who proclaimed the bullet in his chest to be 'Just a scratch'. Brown ended up in the Twenty-eighth Reinforcements, awaiting a return to the front. As the *Star*'s informant said, 'Brown is quite willing to go to the war a second time if he is physically fit; but he does not feel at all fit, the bullet in his chest giving him trouble, which occasionally becomes acute, and he does not know what would happen to him under stress.'[67]

Nurses, too, had trouble with boards. Edith Austen was discharged in April 1919, when all she had wanted was two months' sick leave to 'rest quietly' before returning to work. 'I am only suffering from war strain and am really a very strong person.' When *Marquette* survivor Mary Grigor was boarded on 30 May 1919, she was not examined 'in any way' but asked whether she wanted to be discharged and then marked fit for duty. Although she felt 'quite well', a medical board in England had decreed that she would be unwise to nurse for a minimum of a year. 'I do not in the least mind working again if it is safe to do so, but I would very much like to first of all be overhauled by . . . someone who knows something of Chest troubles.'[68] Hester Maclean fought hard for the women to be 'treated in the same way as soldiers of similar rank', finally, in August, convincing the authorities to send her all nurses' medical board proceedings.

The wartime ambivalence towards shell-shock cases, and the pressure on doctors dealing with the physically wounded, meant that many men suffering from psychological damage did not even report themselves as ill. With some medical boards reluctant to ascribe the condition of returned servicemen to their war experiences, seeking a pension for a non-physical complaint was 'doubly difficult and many were probably discouraged from applying'.[69] The Pensions Department faced a huge challenge. As historian Tim Shoebridge has noted, 'The volume of applications exploded . . . By 1920 [the department] had received nearly 55,000 applications, mainly in the previous two years, all of which had to be investigated.' At that point, over 34,500 pensions were being paid out, more than two-thirds of them temporary payments for men recovering from injury or illness. It was little wonder that there were complaints about delays.[70]

The final paragraphs of Andrew Carbery's First World War medical service history leave the reader with two main impressions: first, that the personnel's return to civilian life was generally untroubled and positive, and, second, that no nurses had been involved. Many NZMC officers, he writes, returned to private practice, or worked in such government organisations as the Pensions and the Public Health departments. A number joined the staffs of the public hospitals, where they 'continue[d] to supervise the after care of disabled soldiers' in the 1920s. The 'special knowledge or skill' brought back by each 'trained medical officer of the N.Z.E.F. . . . was of immediate avail to the civil population and so the profitable lessons taught by the war became a powerful uplift to the civilian medical organisations of the Dominion'. Carbery briefly mentions the rank and file, who 'also played an important part in the after war medical reorganisation, as radiographers, laboratory assistants, male nurses, masseurs, and as employees of the civil hospitals or the state departments engaged in medical work', but his final flourish entirely ignores the nurses: 'whatever praise the New Zealand Medical Services may have won in the Great War was, in greater part, earned by the soldierly conduct of the non-commissioned officers and the men of our Corps.'[71]

At the end of 1919, many nurses were 'still retained in the service and their posts' at military hospitals and convalescent homes. At Trentham, for example, Samoa veteran Vida MacLean had a staff of 63 NZANS nurses; Bertha Nurse, the matron at Rotorua's King George V Hospital, was managing eight. Isabella McRae, in charge at Christchurch's Chalmers block, oversaw 24 women. Eva Brooke, who had served first in Samoa, then on the *Maheno* and the *Marama* and in military hospitals overseas, was matron of the Military Convalescent Hospital at Narrow Neck in Auckland.[72] In 1921, the year after she was demobilised, this remarkable woman, the only New Zealand nurse awarded the Royal Red Cross and bar, became matron of Christchurch's Rannerdale Home for disabled veterans.

Coming home was often no easier for the doctors, nurses, vets, stretcher-bearers, orderlies and ambulance men than it was for their former patients. Lieutenant-Colonel Charles Thomas did not return to New Zealand, but he had been worried about the future. 'How I am going to make a living when I come back I don't know,' he wrote to his wife Milly from Gallipoli only three weeks before he was killed.

> This life entirely unfits you for general practice. Besides I am getting too old to start and build up a practice again. Mine will have practically speaking left me. I don't think there is much chance of my getting a military appointment in the medical branch of the service because I was never a Territorial. Besides there are others after the jobs who are senior to me because they were Territorials. None of them have anything like the service that I have got. In any case I don't suppose the appointment would be worth very much.[73]

Some NZMC men never recovered physically from their war service and died too young. Private George Knox, who had been wounded in France in May 1917, died on 16 November 1920 of 'Pneumonia — Accelerated by Gas poisoning'. He was 34, as was former Dunedin Hospital house surgeon Cyril Baigent OBE, wounded on Gallipoli, when he died of kidney disease in 1923. After establishing a large practice in Ashburton, Baigent 'found that he had not escaped unscathed from the privations of the war, and about six months ago he was able to diagnose a trouble caused in the first instance by a severe chill or exposure'. Despite knowing that the condition was incurable, 'he nevertheless decided to carry right on, which he did, and he successfully performed a serious operation on the morning of his collapse'.[74] Thirty-year-old NZMC Private George Black, who served on the first charter of the *Marama*, died later in 1916 of intestinal obstruction, toxaemia and peritonitis — 'Death due to War Service'. He had been sent home with debility following appendicitis. *Marquette* survivor David Fitzgibbon, who had been affected by gas at Hazebrouck and was invalided home with pleurisy, took charge of an auxiliary hospital in Whangarei during the influenza epidemic, despite his 'indifferent health'. Before his death, at 41, in October 1919, he suffered frequent heart attacks 'following the original chest trouble'.[75] Two nurses died as a direct result of their war work: Margaret Thompson was the victim of tuberculosis in 1921 while nursing chronically ill soldiers in a Wellington rest home, and Mary Edge, formerly Ellis, died a year after her retirement from war work in October 1918.[76]

Alcohol caused significant problems for returned men. In late May 1918 the Medical Committee of the New Zealand Returned Soldiers' Association 'viewed with grave regret . . . the ravages that alcoholism is making', describing drink as 'the sheerest poison' in shell-shock and neurasthenic cases.[77] Medical personnel were vulnerable too. When vet Thomas Lilico died in Christchurch on 5 April 1917, a year after returning to New Zealand, an inquest named alcoholism as the cause of death. William Smith of the New Zealand Veterinary Corps died of alcoholic poisoning, delirium tremens and heart failure in May 1920, aged only 46. On 1 July 1916 he had been court-martialled for being drunk in Heliopolis, severely reprimanded, sent home and discharged. At the hearing he had attributed his position to 'the hot weather' and insisted that he had consumed only two whiskies. Veterinarian Charles Neale OBE died of delirium tremens in February 1928.[78]

Major Charles Maguire, the SMO on the *Ulimaroa* when she brought sick and wounded men home in April 1916, was forced to inform the DMS that one of his staff, courageous William McAra from Gallipoli, had suffered 'several attacks of mania' which he attributed 'to alcohol with abuse of drugs supperadded. Latterly Capt. [actually Major] McAra has been in the habit of inhaling chloroform. He became so bad that I deemed it advisable to relieve him of his duties.' He believed that McAra should never again be 'placed in medical charge of troops, as I consider that, when he is under the influence of drugs, he is dangerous to himself and others'.[79] McAra died in 1934 of lymph adenoma, a condition affected by alcohol. Ironically, he had noted in his diary for 8 August 1915 the return to New Zealand of dentist Captain Peter Hume: 'Sorry for him but D.T.s. No place for him here or for anybody who drinks.'[80] Hume, who had left New Zealand with the Second Reinforcements and been appointed dental surgeon to Lady Godley's Convalescent Home, was diagnosed as an alcoholic by two medical boards when he got home. He also had tuberculosis, from which he died in Nelson in 1916, aged 34.[81]

Returning to civilian life was often hard, too, for the nurses and VADs. 'I missed the companionship that nursing carries with it, but I had to settle down, as many duties fell to my

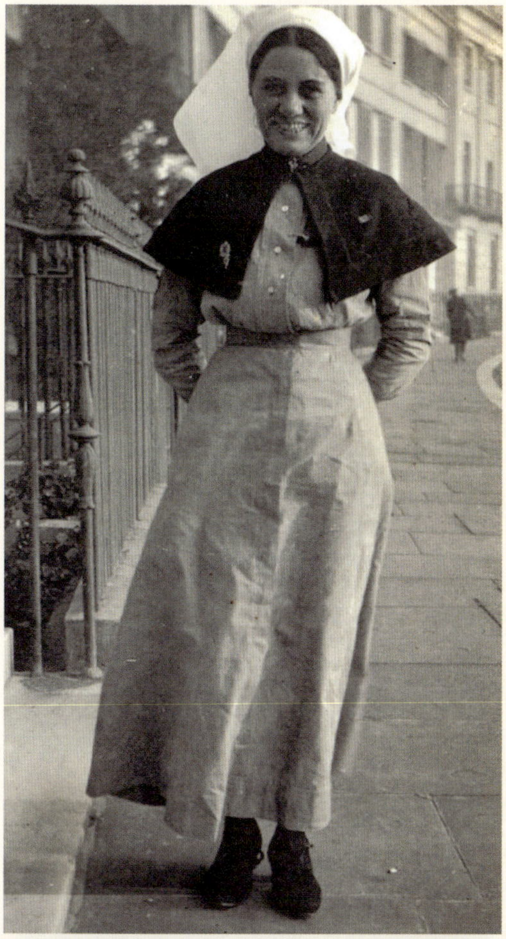

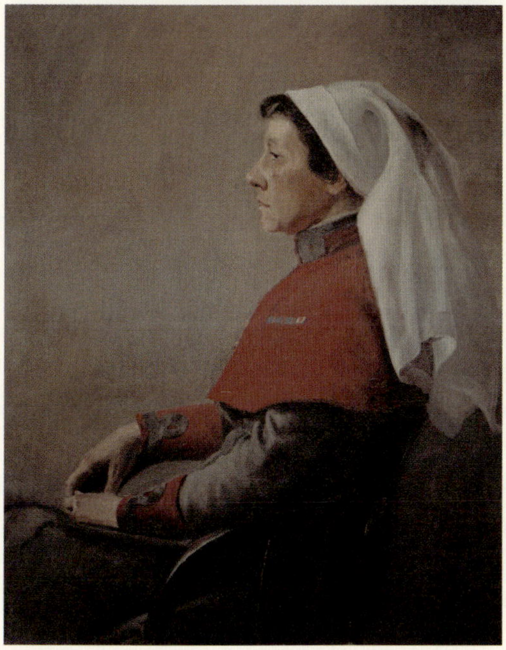

above Usually known as Eva, Evelyn Mary Brooke (1879–1962) served from 1914, when she went to Samoa, until the end of the war in a variety of highly responsible roles both overseas and in New Zealand. From 1921 until her marriage in 1925 she was matron of Christchurch's Rannerdale Home for disabled veterans. NATIONAL ARMY MUSEUM, 1990.223.1

below Mabel Thurston (1869–1960) had already received the Royal Red Cross, first class, in 1917 and would be appointed CBE two years later for her sterling and taxing work as matron-in-chief of the NZEF in Britain. Her considerable and lauded contribution did not, however, prevent the Christchurch Hospital board from insisting on her post-war resignation. NATIONAL COLLECTION OF WAR ART, AAAC 898 NCWA 522 share after my fathers death, and the frailty of my Mother who became my responsibility.'[82] VAD Gladys Luxford's sad and stoic words echoed the experience of many women forced to exchange the adventure and high emotion of wartime service for the yoke of family expectation or the much duller routine of non-military nursing. Physical exhaustion was common — 'quite a number were war-worn and not really fit for duty'.[83] For example, when Cora Anderson, mentioned in despatches and holder of the Royal Red Cross, was boarded on 10 May 1919, the diagnosis was debility caused by the 'stress and strain' of active service, which had resulted in weakness and brachycardia (slow heart rate).[84]

As had been the case with doctors, the loss of so many nurses to overseas service had caused a severe shortage of experienced senior staff in hospitals. A number who had been on leave returned to their pre-war posts, but former Christchurch Hospital 'lady superintendent' Mabel Thurston was not among them. She had been granted leave of absence for the duration of the war, initially to become matron at Walton-on-Thames on little more than half her Christchurch salary, and publicly lauded for her patriotism. Her devoted work in the challenging NZEF matron-in-chief role, which involved supervising the NZANS nurses on active duty in England, France and Egypt and organising the supply of nurses and VADs to New Zealand's military hospitals in England, earned her both the Royal Red Cross and a CBE. At the end of August 1918, however, the North Canterbury Hospital and Charitable Aid Board wrote to say that her long absence had 'adversely affected the hospital' and forced the acting matron to turn down job offers. Thurston's appointment was terminated.[85]

The board was not swayed by her eloquent protests and explanations, which were backed up by letters of support from Brigadier-General George Richardson and William Parkes, among others, and by a meeting of angry locals. Thurston had to resign. She became matron at King George V Military Hospital at Rotorua in January 1920 before assuming the same role at Hanmer, and, between 1923 and 1927, at Pukeora. Replying to Godley's hope, expressed in July 1920, that nurses and matrons would be 'treated well in the future', James Allen said, 'You need have no fear about this, except perhaps in the case of Miss Thurston. The Christchurch Hospital Board does not appear to have treated her quite well.'[86]

Other nurses opted for private nursing, sometimes joining forces to set themselves up in business. Some, as we have seen, established massage practices; Sister May Chalmer opened a private hospital in Ngaruawahia in 1920 and later one in Feilding; Vida MacLean and Fanny Wilson, both former matrons of New Zealand military hospitals in Britain, took over a small private hospital in Wellington's Willis Street. Some women, though, might 'be glad to take up some clerical work, or work on the land, such as gardening or poultry-farming', and they should be 'eligible as soldiers to receive assistance in settling on the land'.[87]

Nurses were officially included in the land settlement scheme aimed at putting returned soldiers on farms of their own, but only after a legislative change.[88] Ellen Schaw was one of just a half-dozen or so nurses who seem to have applied. According to a newspaper report, she was 'the first woman in the Wellington district, and probably in the Dominion', to obtain land under the Discharged Soldiers Settlement Act.[89] After being invalided for some months on coming home, she 'got the very section she wanted', 4 acres at Cloverlea near Palmerston

North, in a soldiers' land ballot. She began with 'one cow, horse and trap, three chickens, three cats, one dog'. A few months later — as soon as the fowlhouse could be built — she was planning to start a 'little poultry farm with more fowls, and also getting more cows. Fruit trees are also to be planted.'[90] In 1925 *Marquette* survivor Edith McLeod applied for a 105-acre block at the Hikutaia settlement near Opotiki that had been abandoned by its returned soldier owner and turned it into a profitable concern, fulfilling the prophecy of a member of the Land Board in Gisborne, who considered that 'the lady would make a very capable farmer'.[91] A few nurses, including Annie Buckley, who had left on the *Rotorua* in 1915, learnt beekeeping and horticulture at the Ruakura Government Farm and were given a small living allowance.

There could be a lack of appreciation and understanding when medical personnel came home. On 11 March 1919 the *New Zealand Herald* published a letter headed 'AMBULANCE MAN'S COMPLAINT' and signed 'Stretcher-Bearer. N.Z. Medical Corps, Rotorua'. Since reporting to the hospital a few days before, 'after considerable service in the field', the correspondent had been 'surprised and not a little disgusted to observe the attitude taken by people in this town towards men of the N.Z.M.C.'.

> Is it possible that people can have such a small conception of what work in the Medical Corps really amounts to? . . . Do they consider the heart-breaking toil of stretcher-bearing for two, three or four days and nights in all weathers and in most cases back and forwards through shell-fire, exposed to all that comes from the German guns? Can they imagine what it means to carry out a badly wounded man, on a pitch black night when German gas is thick and one has to wear a mask, stumbling along blindly, your only thought and aim, to get that man 'out.'

Now, 'given a job for awhile before he is discharged', he had been insulted — more than once. 'There are men in the Medical Corps drawing 5s per day, when they might be drawing three or four times as much outside. Are they to be blamed because they are sent here for duty?' He regarded this as the 'most unfair treatment' he had ever received, and through him it was extended to 'men who have been out since 1914'.[92]

The men and women of the medical services were, however, widely praised and recognised with many awards. At the Battle of Messines alone, New Zealand's doctors and ambulance men received a DSO, four Military Crosses, 15 Military Medals and three Military Service Medals; three were mentioned in despatches.[93] The nurses, too, were honoured during the war, with 14 Royal Red Crosses, more than 70 associate or second-class RRCs and almost 50 mentions in despatches. In 1920 Hester Maclean received the rarely bestowed Florence Nightingale Medal. VADs, too, were given several MBEs and MIDs, among other decorations.[94]

But many medical lives were lost. Of the more than 3600 men who served overseas, 662 — 56 officers and 606 other ranks — were killed or died of wounds, disease or accident. Over 450 men were wounded, several more than once.[95] Sixteen nurses died, 13 while serving with the NZANS, and three while working for other organisations: Ella Cooke, who nursed with the French Flag Nursing Corps and the QAIMNS, was killed in an accident in Egypt; Elise Kemp lost her life on the Western Front while serving with the Territorial Forces Nursing Service; Lily Lind, also with the French corps, died of consumption while returning to New Zealand in 1916. The number of VADs who died is uncertain. The known names are those of Wilmet Bennett and Corale Lumley, who died of illness, and Winifred Starling, a VAD at No. 2 New Zealand General Hospital, who was drowned when RMS *Leinster* was torpedoed in the Irish Sea on 10 October 1918.[96]

Words such as heroism and sacrifice are used too frequently and too easily, especially about the First World War. There was no glory here. As medical historian Leo van Bergen has written, 'War is about everything, but above all it is about killing and being killed.'[97] It is, too, about being wounded, often horribly or repeatedly, and about debilitating illness, disfigurement and psychological trauma. But war is also about courage — the courage to continue working, in appalling, perilous conditions and for inhumanly long hours, to save lives — and it is about compassion. Even for trained personnel, this was a terrible new world. Doctors used to treating patients in comfortable rooms, and surgeons accustomed to operating in sterile, well-organised theatres, found themselves in trenches and dug-outs, often under fire. Men who had been clerks or shop assistants or students or farmers found themselves staggering through deep mud carrying stretchers while trying to dodge snipers' bullets. Nurses who had staffed calm, organised wards found themselves in crowded tent hospitals full of severely hurt and dying men with stinking wounds and shattered limbs. As soldier poet Siegfried Sassoon rightly said, it was hell, and the brave, skilled and caring New Zealand medical personnel who went through it with the troops must, like them, never be forgotten.

MAPS

NEW ZEALAND HOSPITALS IN ENGLAND

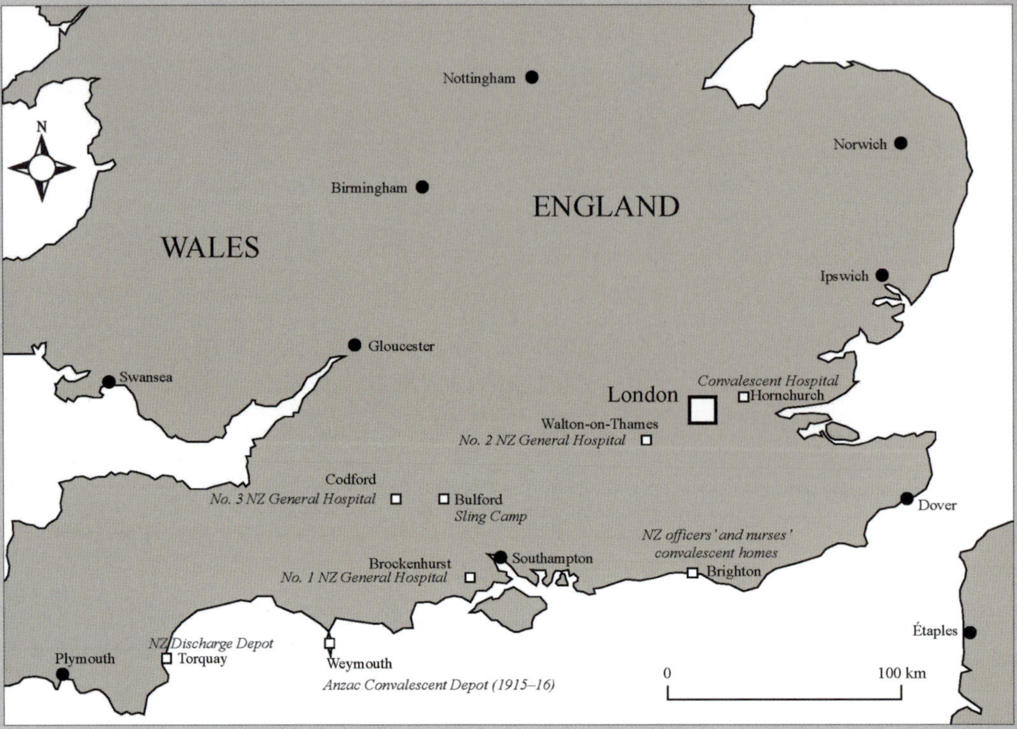

THE WESTERN FRONT

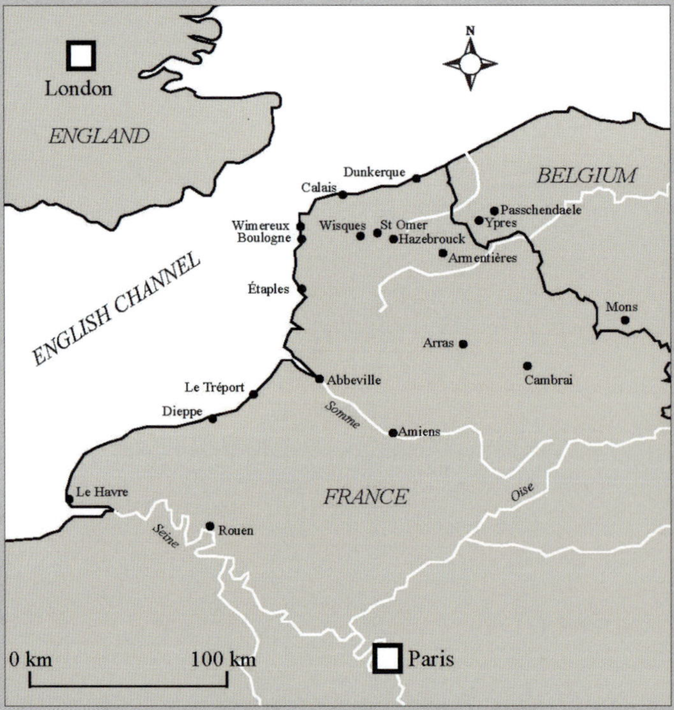

NEW ZEALANDERS IN EGYPT

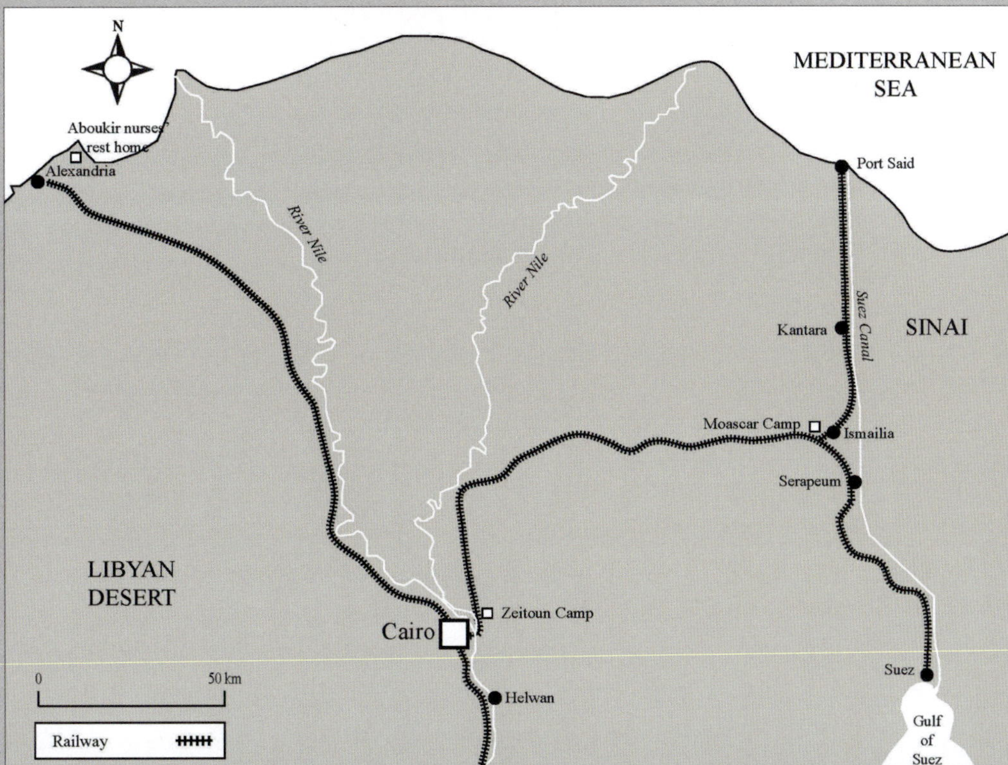

Page 410, above: New Zealand's wartime general hospitals, No. 1 at Brockenhurst, No. 2 at Walton-on-Thames and No. 3 at Codford, and the convalescent hospital at Hornchurch, were essential to the care and treatment of ill and wounded New Zealanders. They also gave a welcome and restorative taste of home. The convalescent homes for nurses and officers in Brighton were also vital.

Page 410, below: New Zealand's busy hospital in France moved twice during the war, from Amiens to Hazebrouck and then, following an air attack, to Wisques near St Omer.

This page: Port Said, Cairo and Alexandria were the significant places in the arrival, departure and treatment of sick and wounded New Zealand soldiers, particularly after Gallipoli and during the Sinai–Palestine campaign.

ABBREVIATIONS, NOTES, BIBLIOGRAPHY, ACKNOWLEDGEMENTS, ABOUT THE AUTHOR, INDEX

ABBREVIATIONS

ADMS	assistant director of medical services
ADS	advanced dressing station
ADVS	assistant director of veterinary services
AGH	Australian General Hospital
ANZAC	Australian and New Zealand Army Corps
ASC	Army Service Corps
BIPP	bismuth iodoform paraffin paste
CBE	Commander of the Most Excellent Order of the British Empire
CCS	casualty clearing station
CO	commanding officer
CSM	cerebro-spinal meningitis
DAH	disordered action of the heart
DCM	Distinguished Conduct Medal
DDMS	deputy director of medical services
DDS	director of dental services
DMS	director of medical services
DRS	divisional rest station
DSO	Distinguished Service Order
FA	field ambulance
GHQ	General Headquarters
HE	high explosive
ICC	Imperial Camel Corps
ISTM	Incorporated Society of Trained Masseuses
MBE	Member of the Most Excellent Order of the British Empire
MC	Military Cross
MDS	main dressing station
MEF	Mediterranean Expeditionary Force
MFA	Mounted Field Ambulance
MM	Military Medal
MO	medical officer
NCO	non-commissioned officer
NZANS	New Zealand Army Nursing Service
NZEF	New Zealand Expeditionary Force
NZFA	New Zealand Field Artillery
NZGH	New Zealand General Hospital
NZMC	New Zealand Medical Corps
NZSH	New Zealand Stationary Hospital
NZVC	New Zealand Veterinary Corps

OBE	Officer of the Most Excellent Order of the British Empire
OC	officer commanding
ORs	other ranks
PMO	principal medical officer
PUO	pyrexia of unknown origin
PVO	principal veterinary officer
QAIMNS	Queen Alexandra's Imperial Military Nursing Service
QM	quartermaster
RAMC	Royal Army Medical Corps
RAP	regimental aid post
RMO	regimental medical officer
SMO	senior medical officer
SRF	Serbian Relief Fund
SWH	Scottish Women's Hospitals for Foreign Service
TV	typhoid vaccine
VAD	Voluntary Aid Detachment
VC	Victoria Cross
WCA	New Zealand War Contingent Association
YMCA	Young Men's Christian Association

NOTES

ABBREVIATIONS

AJHR	*Appendix to the Journals of the House of Representatives*
ANZ	Archives New Zealand
ATL	Alexander Turnbull Library
AWM	Australian War Memorial
AWMM	Auckland War Memorial Museum
NAM	National Army Museum

INTRODUCTION

1 Letter 23 August 1918, John Keith Moloney, War diary, MS-Papers-1194, ATL.

2 Damien Fenton, with Caroline Lord, Gavin McLean and Tim Shoebridge, *New Zealand and the First World War 1914–1919* (Auckland: Penguin in association with the Ministry for Culture and Heritage, 2013), p. 80.

3 As Kevin Brown has noticed, the intimate relationship between health, medicine and war is reflected linguistically: 'We speak of the battle against infection, we wage war on bacteria and patients fight for life.' Kevin Brown, *Fighting Fit: Health, Medicine and War in the Twentieth Century* (Stroud: The History Press, 2008), p. 9.

4 Georg Friedrich Nicolai, *Aufruf an die Europäer: Manifesto to the Europeans*, quoted Leo van Bergen, *Before My Helpless Sight: Suffering, Dying and Military Medicine on the Western Front, 1914–1918* (Surrey: Ashgate, 2009), p. 357.

5 'Was World War I Good for Medicine?', http://www.nato.int/docu/review/2014/war-medicine/WWI-WW1-Health-care-medicine/EN/index.htm, accessed 1 May 2017. In the view of Mark Harrison, without this development of forward treatment it was 'unlikely that the British and other combatant nations would have been able to continue the war for so long', 'War, Health and Medicine: The Medical Lessons of World War I', Professor Mark Harrison, Gresham College, 6 May 1915, YouTube, accessed 1 August 2017.

6 Bergen, *Helpless Sight*, pp. 408–9, 411.

7 *He Rau Mahara: To Remember the Journey of our Ngāi Tahu Soldiers from the Pā to the Battlefields of the Great War* (Christchurch: Te Rūnanga o Ngāi Tahu, 2017), p. 25; Moloney, War Diary.

8 As a medical officer told the *Dominion*, 'The one thing about a stationary hospital is that it is not stationary.' It 'follows the line and its first essential is mobility'. *Dominion*, 15 April 1915, p. 3.

9 This corps, established in 1898, had originated with a few surgeons who attached themselves to groups of volunteers set up from the early 1860s. For a summary of the history of the medical corps in New Zealand, see Ian McGibbon (ed.), *The Oxford Companion to New Zealand Military History* (Auckland: Oxford University Press, 2000), pp. 313–15.

10 Ibid., p. 313.

11 *Hastings Standard*, 9 December 1913, p. 2.

12 A. D. Carbery, *The New Zealand Medical Service in the Great War, 1914–1918* (Auckland: Whitcombe & Tombs, 1924), pp. 11–12.

13 Ibid., p. 19. Other South Africa veterans who served overseas or in New Zealand during the war were Eugene O'Neill, Walter Pearless and Charles Thomas.

14 Ibid., p. 69.

15 Tim Shoebridge, 'Manawatu's First World War Camps, 1915–1919', *Manawatu Journal of History*, no. 9, 2013, pp. 11–21.

16 Ormond Edward Burton, Autobiography — A Rich Old Man (unpublished), MS-Papers-0438-059, ATL. I am indebted to Ray Grover for showing me this material.

17 31 October 1915, W. H. Parkes, OC, NZGH Egypt to DMS Wellington, Medical — Staff (Medical) Egypt, AD1 970 49/213, ANZ.

18 12 May 1915, Thomas Russell Ritchie, Papers, MS-Papers-3705-1, ATL. Ritchie gave no first name, but the orderly was possibly 6/1649 Peter McCann, from Millerton.

19 Godley to Allen, 28 February and 13 March 1915, [Correspondence between] General Sir Alexander Godley [Commander New Zealand Expeditionary Force] and Colonel Hon. Sir James Allen, Minister of Defence, 2 April–19 December 1915, WA 252 1 [2], ANZ.

20 Allen to Godley, 19 April 1915, Ministerial Files — Correspondence with General Godley, Allen 1 1 M1/15 1, ANZ.

21 *Dominion*, 17 January 1916, p. 7.

22 Ibid.; Randolph Norman Gray, Papers relating to World War One, MS-Papers-4134, ATL, folder 1.

23 *Dominion*, 14 February 1916, p. 6.

24 *New Zealand Herald*, 29 January 1916, p. 8.

25 *Dominion*, 14 January 1916, p. 7.

26 4 November 1916, Gray papers, folder 2.

27 *Dominion*, 17 January 1916, p. 7.

28 *Press*, 11 January 1917, p. 6.

29 Reports — Reports progress — Ambulance Reinforcements for Egypt, AD1/881 39/145, ANZ.

30 Gray papers, folder 1.

31 *Dominion*, 14 June 1917, p. 6.

32 Carbery, *Medical Service*, p. xii; Pat Clarkson Medical Practitioner Research Project, list of First World War doctors serving overseas, pers. comm., October 2016.

33 I am indebted to John Crawford for this information. See also Glyn Harper, with Christine Clement and Rebecca Johns, *For King and Other Countries: The Untold Story of the New Zealanders Who Served in Other Countries' Services in the First World War* (Auckland: Massey University Press, 2019).

34 Derek Dow, 'Springs of Charity? The Development of the New Zealand Hospital System, 1876–1919', in Linda Bryder (ed.), *A Healthy Country: Essays on the Social History of Medicine in New Zealand* (Wellington: Bridget Williams Books, 1991), pp. 60–1.

35 *Evening Post*, 3 September 1914, p. 3.

36 *Press*, 10 June 1915, p. 8.

37 Letter to Thomas Mackenzie, 22 June 1915, Louis Edward Barnett file, N/N, ANZ.

38 *Auckland Star*, 8 July 1915, p. 9.

39 *Southland Times*, 4 October 1918, p. 5.

40 William McAra file, 3/529, ANZ.

41 C. T. Hand-Newton, DSO, *A Physician in Peace and War* (Christchurch: N. M. Peryer, 1967), pp. 19–20.

42 *Nelson Evening Mail*, 10 August 1914, p. 8.

43 *New Zealand Herald*, 17 January 1916, p. 7.

44 *Press*, 16 July 1917, p. 10.

45 Rex Carrington Brewster file, 3/2147, ANZ.

46 William Barclay Memoirs, 2000.980, NAM, p. 104.

47 *Free Lance*, 3 March 1916, p. 4.

48 Lieutenant-Colonel W. S. Austin, *The Official History of the New Zealand Rifle Brigade* (Wellington: L. T. Watkins Ltd, 1924), p. 543. 22/280 Ada Florence Kilgour would later serve on the *Maheno*.

49 Pat Cotter, 'A Tribute: The Contribution of the Otago University Medical School and its Students in

World War 1', *New Zealand Medical Journal*, 5 April 2005, vol. 118, no. 1213, http://www.nzma.org.nz/journal/118-1213/1406/, accessed 4 January 2017. Along with Aitken, Milne and Withers, the others were Ivan Blaubaum, John Connor, Selwyn Haslett, Philip Jory, Kenneth MacCormick, David MacKay, Angus Marshall, George Redpath, Oswald Reid, William Reid, Thomas Ritchie, William Scannell, George Sharp, Aubrey Short, Wilfred Wallis, Ernest Webb, Noel Whitton and William Will.

50 War Memoirs by Dr. W. Aitken, M.C., MD, F.R.A.C.P., 1st New Zealand Field Ambulance, Australian War Memorial, 392L 2422, p. 1. Aitken and the other students were not registered, however. Pat Cotter suggests that they had probably not completed their obstetrics and gynaecology training.

51 *Otago Daily Times*, 31 July 1915, p. 8.

52 On 2 August, John Thomson of No. 1 Field Ambulance noted that 'The 4th & 5th year meds, including Glasgow, Will, Spencer and Denniston went away to return to N.Z. on Wednesday', John H. Thomson, 3/453 No. 1 N.Z. Fd. Amb., Diary from 13 April 1915 to Jan 21st 1916, PC-0316, Hocken. Several students, including Kitchen, were aboard the *Tahiti* when she returned to New Zealand in mid-March 1916.

53 *Star*, 28 July 1916, p. 2. For more detail on the OTC training, see *Evening Star*, 28 August 1916, p. 7.

54 Carbery, *Medical Service*, pp. 27–8.

55 M. W. Wilson, C. Marquand and H. J. McCann, 'Official History of the Royal New Zealand Nursing Corps', 1978, pp. 4, 5.

56 Nurses for Expeditionary Forces — Offers of by the New Zealand Government, AD 49/34, ANZ.

57 Ibid., Allen to Duff, 3 September 1914.

58 Ibid.

59 Public Health and Hospitals and Charitable Aid: Report Thereon by the Inspector-General of Hospitals and Charitable Institutions and Chief Health Officer, *AJHR*, 1915 Session I, H-31, p. 6. Allen had also checked with Godley, on 18 January 1915. He told him about the deputation and added, 'I should be glad [to] know if there are plenty of trained women nurses, and if there is any need for more being sent.' He also solicited Godley's opinion about sickness on ships 'because the question has been raised more than once, whether it would not be better for us to send female nurses with the transports'. A few days later Allen asked, 'If female trained nurses are really required for our troops and there are not sufficient in Egypt, we should be glad to send some.' Ministerial files — correspondence with General Godley, Allen 1 1, M1/15, ANZ.

60 Jan Rodgers, '"A Paradox of Power and Marginality": New Zealand Nurses' Professional Campaign During War, 1900–1920', PhD thesis, History, Massey University, 1994, p. 105.

61 Diary 5, 8 April 1915, Collection — Sister Mabel Crook — WW1, 2016.280.1, NAM.

62 *Kai Tiaki*, January 1916, p. 23.

63 Letter to Ethel, 28 March 1917, Wilfred Collinson Smith, Correspondence, MS-Papers-2352, ATL, folder 1.

64 C. H. Weston, *Three Years With the New Zealanders* (London: Skeffington & Son, 1918), Chapter XIII.

65 Nurses for Expeditionary Forces — Offers of by the New Zealand Government, AD 49/34, ANZ.

66 Edna Pengelly, *Nursing in Peace and War* (Wellington: Wingfield Press, 1956), p. 51.

67 Ibid., p. 65, 6 November 1916.

68 New Zealand Army Nursing Service — NZANS overseas records, correspondence — Matron-in-chief, AD78 23 67/3/1A, ANZ.

69 Pengelly, *Nursing*, p. 75.

70 Lyn Macdonald, *The Roses of No Man's Land* (Harmondsworth, UK: Penguin Books, 1980), p. 155.

71 Pengelly, *Nursing*, p. 62.

72 Weston, *Three Years*, Chapter XIII.

73 Letters 3, 6 and 29 January, 28 February 1915, 26 May, 16 July 1916, Carruthers family: Extracts from letters to Carruthers family/Walter [Carruthers], MS-Papers-4107, ATL.

74 A. L. Logan, Dental Service with the First New Zealand Expeditionary Force, MS-2004-66, AWMM, p. 102.

75 10 November 1915, Diary of William McAra, Gallipoli, June–December 1915, MS-2943/002, Hocken.

76 *Kai Tiaki*, January 1918, p. 9.

77 *Kai Tiaki*, January 1919, p. 45.

78 Thomson diary, Hocken.

79 Godley to Allen, 24 March 1916, [Correspondence between] General Sir Alexander Godley [Commander New Zealand Expeditionary Force] and Colonel Hon. Sir James Allen, Minister of Defence, 4 January–29 December 1916, WA 252 1 [3], ANZ. Godley would continue to criticise Fenwick. It is very possible that the latter had post-Gallipoli psychological problems: on 1 November 1916, when Fenwick was in charge of Codford, Godley feared he would 'not last again. They tell me he has begun to get nervy and excitable, though not at the front.'

80 Godley to Colonel J. J. Esson, Treasury, Wellington, 8 June 1916, Semi-personal letters by General Officer Commanding, 5 September 1914–31 October 1916, WA 252 3 [6], ANZ.

81 Godley to Allen, 18 August 1916, WA 252 1 [3], ANZ.

82 William Mandeno Smallfield, War Letters, Diaries and Papers, MS 2007/37, AWMM; Wilfred Collinson Smith, Correspondence, MS-Papers-2352, ATL, folder 3.

83 *Kai Tiaki*, January 1916, p. 28, letter 10 November 1915.

84 Allan Marriott, *Mud Beneath My Boots: A Poignant Memoir of the Effects of War on a Young New Zealander* (Auckland: HarperCollins, 2005), p. 53.

85 Glyn Harper (ed.), *Letters from the Battlefield: New Zealand Soldiers Write Home 1914–1918* (Auckland: HarperCollins, 2001), p. 54, 3 July 1916; 26 July 1915, McAra diary.

86 Letters: Ronald Watson (*Letters from a Padre: A Record of the War Service of Ronald S. Watson. M.C.*, edited by Nigel M. Watson, privately printed, Melbourne), 1998.2491, NAM, p. 23, 14 November 1917.

87 *Sun*, 13 December 1915, p. 10.

88 5 October 1915, McAra diary.

CHAPTER 1: CROSSING THE SEA

1 *Press*, 11 August 1914, p. 8; *Evening Star*, 17 August 1914, p. 8.

2 Among them were Dr Henry Monk from Auckland and Wellington surgeon Arnold Izard, who both served there in 1915. When Major Monk returned to New Zealand early in 1919, the *Observer*'s 'Pars About People' column, on 1 February, recalled him in Apia, 'feeling pulses and prescribing Epsoms for the hard-bitten crowd of Enzedders then camped under the palms. He was always a popular "quack" with the boys.'

3 A. D. Carbery, *The New Zealand Medical Service in the Great War 1914–1918* (Auckland: Whitcombe & Tombs, 1924), p. 15.

4 *Kai Tiaki*, October 1914, p. 157.

5 L. Ida G. Willis, *A Nurse Remembers: The Life Story of L. Ida G. Willis O.B.E., A.R.R.C., E.D.* (Lower Hutt: A. K. Wilson Ltd, n.d.), p. 231.

6 Stephen Smith, *The Samoa (N.Z.) Expeditionary Force 1914–1915* (Wellington: Ferguson & Osborn Ltd, 1924), pp. 37–8.

7 Smith, *Samoa*, p. 112; *Kai Tiaki*, October 1914, p. 169.

8 Smith, *Samoa*, p. 77.

9 The incidence of dysentery and dengue fever had decreased by the beginning of 1915. Holmes put the reduction in the latter down to 'universal use of mosquito curtains, and the prompt removal of cases to hospital'. PMO Samoa Expeditionary Force — War Diary — 18 December 1914–14 January 1915, WA213 215 [231f], ANZ; Smith, *Samoa*, p. 114.

10 *Kai Tiaki*, January 1915, p. 35.

11 *Samoanische Zeitung*, 28 November 1914, p. 7; Smith, *Samoa*, p. 130.

12 AD 1 49/65, Nurses — Samoa Correspondence re, ANZ; *Kai Tiaki*, January 1915, p. 35.

13 *Free Lance*, 30 April 1915, p. 22; Allen to Godley, 22 March 1915, Ministerial files — correspondence with General Godley, Allen 1 1, M1/15, ANZ.

14 The origin and composition of the medical force is outlined by Carbery, *Medical Service*, pp. 18–19.

15 Carbery, *Medical Service*, p. 19. The horses should have been on the same vessel as the field ambulance. This mistake caused 'some inconvenience' on arrival in Egypt, as the ambulance 'had to encamp without tents or cooking appliances'. Carbery felt that 'in transport, both as regards ambulance and general service waggons, the 4th Australian Field Ambulance was much better equipped than ours', *Medical Service*, pp. 21, 29. Captain Alexander Trotter of the New Zealand Mounted Rifles Field Ambulance was not impressed when, on 6 September, '15 vehicles of various sorts' arrived in Wellington: 'Some of the wagons would make excellent firewood.' Diaries of A. M. Trotter/transcribed by A. A. S. Trotter, MS-3397/004, Hocken.

16 O. E. Burton, *The Silent Division: New Zealanders at the Front, 1914–1919* (Sydney: Angus & Robertson, 1935), p. 5.

17 Carbery, *Medical Service*, p. 19; Cecil Malthus, letter to Hazel, on board transport ship, 25 October 1914, Cecil Malthus: World War I Papers, Christchurch City Libraries; William Malone, Diary, 3 November 1914, Jock Phillips, Nicholas Boyack and E. P. Malone (eds), *The Great Adventure: New Zealand Soldiers Describe the First World War* (Wellington: Allen & Unwin/Port Nicholson Press, 1988), pp. 24, 28.

18 Carbery, *Medical Service*, p. 20; Andrew Gilmore Carnachan, Letters Relating to Gallipoli, MS 2006/34, AWMM, p. 2.

19 William Taylor, *The Twilight Hour: A Personal Account of World War I* (Morrinsville: Sutherland, 1978), p. 24.

20 Clifford Collingwood, 'My Diary from 24 August 1915 to 14 July 1917', Diary and Scrapbook: New Zealand, Egypt & Western Front — WW1, 2007.139, NAM; Letters: Ronald Watson (*Letters From a Padre: A Record of the War Service of Ronald S. Watson. M.C.*, edited by Nigel M. Watson, privately printed, Melbourne), 1998.2491, NAM, p. 2.

21 Although the terms inoculation and vaccination are, and were, used almost interchangeably, they have different meanings. Vaccination originally referred to injection with cowpox serum to prevent smallpox. Inoculation referred to being injected with live smallpox serum taken from a patient who had largely recovered from the disease. Today 'vaccination' generally refers to preventative injections, while inoculation includes both preventative shots and post-infection treatments, such as anti-toxin given after a snakebite.

22 Diary of Private P. M. Thompson, 4th Battalion Otago Regiment, Suez & Gallipoli 3 August 1914–15 September 1915, 1999.803, NAM; John Crawford (ed.), *The Devil's Own War: The First World War Diary of Brigadier-General Herbert Hart* (Auckland and Wollombi: Exisle Publishing, 2008), p. 32.

23 10 November 1915, Trotter diaries.

24 C. H. Weston, *Three Years With the New Zealanders* (London: Skeffington & Son, 1918), Chapter V.

25 William Mandeno Smallfield, War letters, diaries and papers, MS 2007/37, AWMM; letter to Tot and Willie, 13 November 1916, Margaret and William Cook: Letters from Stewart Callaghan, MS-Papers-5004, ATL.

26 'The Right to Refuse: Compulsory Vaccination in the New Zealand Expeditionary Force During World War 1, 1914–1918', paper presented by Lea Doughty, 27 June 2017 (History of Medicine lectures, University of Otago), pp. 3–4, 24.

27 Malone, letter to wife, 24 November 1914, John Crawford (ed.) with Peter Cooke, *No Better Death: The Great War Diaries and Letters of William G. Malone* (Auckland: Reed, 2005), p. 81.

28 Benjamin Clyde Colbran, Diaries, MS-Papers-1431, ATL. For the British battle on this subject, see Anne Hardy, '"Straight Back to Barbarism": Antityphoid Inoculation and the Great War, 1914', *Bulletin of Historical Medicine*, vol. 74, 2000, pp. 265–90, discovery.ucl.ac.uk, accessed 9 October 2016.

29 Godley to Allen, 16 December 1914; Allen to Godley, 12 February 1915, Ministerial files — correspondence with General Godley, Allen 1 1, M1/15, ANZ.

30 Letter 26 October 1915, Randolph Norman Gray: Papers relating to World War One, MS-Papers-4134-1, ATL.

31 *Dominion*, 10 February 1915, p. 6.

32 Allan Marriott, *Mud Beneath My Boots: A Poignant Memoir of the Effects of War on a Young New Zealander* (Auckland: HarperCollins, 2005), pp. 83–4.

33 A. L. Logan, Dental Service with the First New Zealand Expeditionary Force, MS-2004-66, AWMM, p. 17.

34 Thomas E. Catchpole, Letters, Egypt & Gallipoli — WWI, 2000.316, NAM, p. 9.

35 Carbery, *Medical Service*, p. 21.

36 Trotter diaries.

37 Jack Gilchrist file, 3/323, ANZ.

38 Diary Trooper William Rupert Pyle 9/76 Otago Mounted Rifles, 1996.292, NAM; Thompson diary, NAM.

39 12 November 1914, Charles Ernest Thomas, Letters, 2015/106, South Canterbury Museum.

40 Trotter diaries; Carbery, *Medical Service*, p. 21.

41 Catchpole letters, p. 16.

42 *Dominion*, 10 February 1915, p. 6.

43 Colbran Diaries, folder 1. When Godley wrote to Allen on 17 December 1914, 119 men were in hospital, 84 at Abbassia — 'unclassified; mostly influenza, with a few cases of Egyptian Fever; Nothing serious', Ministerial files — correspondence with General Godley, Allen 1 1, M1/15, ANZ.

44 Godley memo, Semi-personal letters by General Officer Commanding, 5 September 1914–31 October 1916, WA 252 3 [6], ANZ.

45 Malone, diary 11 December 1914, Crawford (ed.), *No Better Death*, p. 98.

46 1st New Zealand Field Ambulance — War Diary, 11 August 1914–18 February 1919, WA 119 173 [119r], ANZ; also ibid., Appendix II.

47 Letters 2 and 6 January 1915, Carruthers family: Extracts from letters to Carruthers family/Walter [Carruthers], MS-Papers-4107, ATL; Diary of Gordon Clive Breen (1/131) Ambulance Corps, 1999.96, NAM.

48 Malone, diary 15 February 1915, Crawford (ed.), *No Better Death*, p. 125.

49 Norman Edgar Hassell, Memories of 1914, Bottom of Form, MS-Papers 2295, ATL. Len Coley was given castor oil: Marriott, *Mud Beneath My Boots*, p. 83.

50 Letter 22 November 1915, Gray papers, folder 1; *Oamaru Mail*, 24 February 1916, p. 4.

51 Letter 13 March 1915, Malthus papers; Thompson diary.

52 George Barclay, James Jeffery's transcripts of war letters, diaries and related material, MS-2934/002, Hocken.

53 *New Zealand Herald*, 25 March 1915 p. 8; Frederick James Foote, 'Yesteryears', Reminiscences, MS 2007/9, NAM, p. 252.

54 Collingwood diary.

55 *Ohinemuri Gazette*, 22 April 1916, p. 2; Crawford (ed.), *Devil's Own War*, p. 37.

56 Robin Hyde, *Passport to Hell*, edited and introduced by D. I. B. Smith (Auckland: Auckland University Press 2015, 1st pub. 1936), p. 91.

57 Foote, 'Yesteryears', p. 228. Cholera belts were standard issue for the troops. Generally made of red flannel or knitted wool, they were wound around the abdomen several times under the shirt, in the belief that they would prevent not only cholera, but also other illnesses thought to be caused by chilling.

58 1 March 1915, Thomas diary.

59 Carbery, *Medical Service*, p. 26; Adrian Wilmot Delamore, War Diaries, MS 2007/40, AWMM, p. 25.

60 *Dominion*, 2 October 1915, p. 6.

61 William Barclay Memoirs, 2000.980, NAM.

62 *New Zealand Herald*, 16 August 1915, p. 9.

63 *Press*, 13 December 1915, p. 7.

64 Carbery, *Medical Service*, p. 26.

65 Godley to Allen, 8 February 1915, Ministerial files — correspondence with General Godley, Allen 1 1, M1/15, ANZ.

66 As Bronwyn Dalley points out, 'When it became evident that soldiers were contracting venereal disease even before they departed for overseas, attention turned to their sexual partners. Rather than acknowledge that the men may have made the conscious decision to visit brothels, military authorities, women's groups and the general public blamed women — and alcohol — for leading men astray.' Dalley, '"Come Back with Honour": Prostitution and the New Zealand Soldier at Home and Abroad', in John Crawford and Ian McGibbon (eds), *New Zealand's Great War: New Zealand, the Allies and the First World War* (Auckland: Exisle, 2007), pp. 367–8.

67 Godley to Liverpool 14 December 1914; Godley to Allen, 10 December 1914, Ministerial Files — Correspondence with General Godley, Allen1 1 M1/15 1, ANZ.

68 Imelda Bargas and Tim Shoebridge, *New Zealand's First World War Heritage* (Auckland and Wollombi: Exisle, 2015), p. 72.

69 On 9 March 1915 Allen relayed to Godley a recommendation from a recent medical conference: 'That each soldier found to be suffering from any of the venereal diseases be isolated at an isolation hospital at Trentham under strict military discipline, and that no soldier be granted his discharge either at Home in New Zealand or abroad until he is declared to be free from danger of transmitting such diseases.' Ministerial Files — Correspondence with General Godley, Allen 1 1 M1/15 1, ANZ.

70 Philip J. Fleming, '"Shadow over New Zealand": The Response to Venereal Disease in New Zealand 1910–1945', PhD thesis, History, Massey University, 1989, p. 28.

71 Dalley, 'Come Back with Honour', p. 367. See Glyn Harper, *Johnny Enzed: The New Zealand Soldier in the First World War* (Auckland and Wollombi: Exisle, 2015), pp. 157–61 for a discussion of rates of VD infection among New Zealand troops.

72 P. S. O'Connor, 'Venus and the Lonely Kiwi: The War Effort of Miss Ettie A. Rout', *NZ Journal of History*, 1967, vol. 1, no. 1, pp. 11–32; Peter J. Lineham, 'Pettit, William Haddow', from the Dictionary of New Zealand Biography. Te Ara — the Encyclopedia of New Zealand, updated 7-Jan-2014, http://www.TeAra.govt.nz/en/biographies/3p24/pettit-william-haddow, accessed 11 October 2016.

73 *Observer*, 16 March 1918, p. 4.

74 26 August 1918, Gray papers; *Manawatu Times*, 15 August 1917, p. 4.

75 Allen to Godley, 28 January 1915, Ministerial files — correspondence with General Godley, Allen 1 1, M1/15, ANZ.

76 Thompson diary.

77 O. E. Burton, *The Silent Division: New Zealanders at the Front: 1914–1919 & Concerning One Man's War*, ed. John H. Gray (Christchurch: John Douglas Publishing, 2014), *Silent Division*, p. 41. Burton (p. 42) was unusual in his understanding of the reasons for the ubiquitous prostitution: 'It resulted from religious conceptions that made woman to be without a soul; from economic conditions that denied her right to labour; and from a social system that held no place for her other than daughter, wife or harlot.'

78 John A. Lee, *Civilian into Soldier* (Auckland: Vital Books, 1963), p. 66; 21 November 1915, John Keith Moloney, War diary, MS-Papers-1194, ATL.

79 Malone, 29 December 1914, Crawford (ed.), *No Better Death*, p. 107.

80 Unofficial letter, Fenwick to Allen, 10 October 1915, Minister of Defence — Contagious diseases, treatment of, Allen 1 8, D4/65, ANZ; Fenwick's daytime encounter plan had in fact been tried in December 1914, as Godley told Allen on the 26th: '[Officers] tell me that the march which we did in Cairo the other day, going back, as we did, through the worst slums . . . has had a good effect, as a great many of the men were horrified at seeing in daylight what the women were really like with whom they had been going at night,' Ministerial files — correspondence with General Godley, Allen 1 1, M1/15, ANZ; Malone, 29 December 1914; Crawford (ed.), *No Better Death*, p. 107.

81 Godley to Allen, 17 January 1915, 15 February 1915, Ministerial files — correspondence with General Godley, Allen 1 1, M1/15, ANZ.

82 Unofficial letter, Fenwick to Allen, 10 October 1915, Minister of Defence — Contagious diseases, treatment of Allen 1 8, D4/65, ANZ.

83 Carbery, *Medical Service*, pp. 27, 28, 29.

CHAPTER 2: GETTING IT WRONG

1 Fred Waite, Liddle Collection, Brotherton Library, University of Leeds, p. 3, courtesy Glyn Harper.

2 Gallipoli was not the only medically ill-prepared campaign of the war. As Leo van Bergen notes, in Belgium 'medical services were poorly organised' and there were problems at Mons. Leo van Bergen, *Before My Helpless Sight: Suffering, Dying and Military Medicine on the Western Front, 1914–1918* (Surrey: Ashgate, 2009), pp. 47–8, 58.

3 Kevin Fewster (ed.), *Frontline Gallipoli: C. E. W. Bean's Diary from the Trenches* (Sydney: Allen & Unwin, 1990), p. 99. On 17 May Christchurch surgeon Lieutenant-Colonel Percival Fenwick cursed 'the arrant stupidity' of the whole campaign: 'I am curtly reminded, if I speak, that I am simply a doctor and don't understand military tactics. Thank Heaven, I don't. As a mere doctor I do understand that a man foolishly exposed to fire not only is lost to our defences but fills a hospital bed for weeks and costs our Government some hundreds of pounds for nothing . . . If a thousandth part of this carelessness of human life was done in civil life, the Government would foam with indignation.' Lieutenant-Colonel Dr Percival Fenwick, *Gallipoli Diary* (Auckland: David Ling in association with Auckland War Memorial Museum, c.2000), p. 49.

4 Mark Harrison, *The Medical War: British Military Medicine in the First World War* (Oxford: Oxford University Press, 2010), p. 173; 'War, Health and Medicine: The Medical Lessons of World War I', Professor Mark Harrison, Gresham College, 6 May 1915, YouTube, accessed 1 August 2017.

5 Godley did not, however, 'feel disposed to interfere in the matter . . . I don't feel, from this distance, that I can intervene', Godley to Esson, 2 July 1915, Semi-personal letters by General Officer Commanding, 5 September 1914–31 October 1916, WA 252 3 [6], ANZ. When Hester Maclean returned to New Zealand after taking the first 50 NZANS nurses to Egypt, her report to the government suggested 'the establishment of a hospital nearer Gallipoli, so as to avoid a long journey for seriously wounded men', *Star*, 8 November 1915, p. 8. Manders had noted in his diary on 22 April that Birdwood agreed Mudros made sense, 'but it was a general Headquarters job and too late to change now', Medical Corps Memoranda — Walton on Thames, WA10 18 10/6/9, ANZ.

6 Fenwick, too, considered that Lemnos would have been 'an ideal spot for a 10,000 bed open-air hospital. I was present when Col. Manders made this suggestion, a most valuable one. It would have saved our wounded men two or four days' ship journey. Damn all the red tape, I say, when wounded are concerned,' Fenwick, *Gallipoli Diary*, 20 May 1914, p. 58.

7 A. D. Carbery, *The New Zealand Medical Service in the Great War, 1914–1918* (Auckland: Whitcombe & Tombs, 1924), p. 31.

8 Ibid., p. 33.

9 Ibid.

10 Medical Corps Memoranda — Gallipoli April — 1915 — Medical arrangements for evacuation of wounded of Australian and New Zealand Army Corps, WA10 20 10/6/11, ANZ.

11 Carbery, *Medical Service*, p. 35.

12 Christopher Pugsley, *Gallipoli: The New Zealand Story* (Libro International and Pen & Sword Books, 5th edn, 2014, 1st pub. 1984), p. 147.

13 Carbery, *Medical Service*, pp. 25, 29. Unable to communicate with anyone in charge, the *Hindu*, carrying sorely needed medical staff, remained at sea off Cape Helles until 5 p.m. on the 29th, when she was finally ordered to go to Gaba Tepe. The next day hospital members were sent to various transports.

14 Diary of Sergeant Gordon Clive Breen (1/131) Ambulance Corps, 1999.96, NAM.

15 Fenwick, *Gallipoli Diary*, p. 9.

16 Fred Glover Diary, Documents K96/1764, Imperial War Museum, courtesy Glyn Harper.

17 *Dominion*, 16 July 1915, p. 6.

18 Fenwick, *Gallipoli Diary*, p. 8.

19 Diary of William Henry Winter WW1 1915, horowhenua.kete.net.nz, accessed 25 August 2016.

20 Fenwick, *Gallipoli Diary*, p. 9.

21 *Star*, 22 April 1916, p. 6; Fenwick, *Gallipoli Diary*, 5 May 1915, p. 17.

22 Carbery, *Medical Service*, p. 38. Two New Zealand field ambulance units served on the peninsula: No. 1 New Zealand Field Ambulance as part of the NZMC, and the New Zealand Mounted Rifles Field Ambulance attached to the New Zealand Mounted Rifles Brigade. 'New Zealand Medical Corps', https://nzhistory.govt.nz/war/medical-units/new-zealand-medical-corps (Ministry for Culture and Heritage), updated 22-Mar-2017.

23 Medical Corps Memoranda — Gallipoli April — 1915 — Medical arrangements for the evacuation of wounded of Australian and New Zealand Army Corps, WA 10 20, 10/6/11, ANZ.

24 Glover diary.

25 *Otago Witness*, 4 August 1915, p. 8. The strain took its toll: Lindsay was evacuated from the peninsula at the beginning of June with 'nervous debility', Alexander Edward Lindsay file, 3/303, ANZ. As Norman Hassell recalled, the Indians on Gallipoli were 'invaluable' as stretcher-bearers, being able to 'manage their stretchers well over the roughest of country', Memories of Norman E. Hassell, Window into WW1, Palmerston North City Library, http://ww1.pncc.govt.nz/blog/2015/11/18/object-memories-of-1914-norman-e-hassell.

26 Fenwick, *Gallipoli Diary*, 5 May, p. 17.

27 *Wanganui Herald*, 14 July 1915, p. 8.

28 Medical Corps Memoranda — Gallipoli April — 1915 — Medical arrangements for the evacuation of wounded of Australian and New Zealand Army Corps, WA 10 20, 10/6/11, ANZ.

29 Godley to Allen, 6 June 1915, also Godley to Colonel R. A. Chaffey, CO Canty District, 6 September 1915, [Correspondence between] General Sir Alexander Godley [Commander New Zealand Expeditionary Force] and Colonel Hon. Sir James Allen, Minister of Defence, 2 April–19 December 1915, WA 252 1 [2], ANZ.

30 Jane Tolerton, *An Awfully Big Adventure: New Zealand World War One Veterans Tell Their Stories* (Auckland: Penguin, 2013), p. 60.

31 John Crawford (ed.), *The Devil's Own War: The First World War Diary of Brigadier-General Herbert Hart* (Auckland and Wollombi: Exisle Publishing, 2008), p. 61.

32 Glover diary.

33 Colonel C. M. Begg, statement to Dardanelles Commission, CAB 19/28, National Archives (UK), quoted Harrison, *The Medical War*, p. 180.

34 Non-medical men were called on to help even before they reached Gallipoli. Walter Carruthers, on his way to the peninsula in early May with the Wellington Infantry Battalion, 'was helping the Doctor take the sick parade. We have one every morning and night and I am becoming quite an expert among the drugs and bandages . . . I was told by an Australian Doctor one day that I put in some very good work.' Letter 17 May 1915, Carruthers family: Extracts from letters to Carruthers family/Walter [Carruthers], MS-Papers-4107, ATL.

35 Fenwick, *Gallipoli Diary*, pp. 9–10.

36 J. B. Condliffe, *Te Rangi Hiroa: The Life of Sir Peter Buck* (Christchurch: Whitcombe & Tombs, 1971), p. 133.

37 *Otago Witness*, 4 August 1915, p. 8.

38 Fenwick, *Gallipoli Diary*, pp. 14–15.

39 A. G. Butler, R. M. Downes, F. A. Maguire and R. W. Cilento, *The Australian Army Medical Services in the War of 1914–1918*, vol. I, *Gallipoli, Palestine and New Guinea* (Melbourne: Australian War Memorial, 2nd edn, 1938), p. 165.

40 On the night of the landing, NZMC doctors Thomas Ritchie and William Abbot, on the transport *Seeang Bee*, had received a message from the *Lutzow* asking for a medical officer. Ritchie was ready to go but the captain refused to lower a boat because he had no instructions from the admiral. The two men sent a message asking the *Lutzow* to dispatch a boat, but none came. Later Ritchie found out that the message never arrived. Thomas Russell Ritchie, Papers, MS-Papers-3705-1, ATL.

41 O. E. Burton, *The Silent Division: New Zealanders at the Front: 1914–1919 & Concerning One Man's War*, ed. John H. Gray (Christchurch: John Douglas Publishing, 2014), *One Man's War*, p. 268.

42 A.D.M.S. New Zealand & Australian Division M.E.F. ANZAC Interview with Col. Walton, 16th July 1919, Medical Corps Memoranda — Walton on Thames, WA10 18 10/6/9, ANZ; Fenwick, *Gallipoli Diary*, 21 May 1915, p. 61; 22 August 1915, Diaries of A. M. Trotter/transcribed by A. A. S. Trotter, MS-3397/004, Hocken.

43 Burton, *One Man's War*, p. 269.

44 Burton, *Silent Division*, p. 63.

45 *Auckland Star*, 29 June 1915, p. 4.

46 Crawford, *The Devil's Own War*, p. 61.

47 *Kai Tiaki*, January 1916, p. 28.

48 Breen diary, p. 44; Fenwick, *Gallipoli Diary*, p. 88.

49 *Auckland Star*, 29 June 1915, p. 4.

50 Benjamin Clyde Colbran, Diaries, Top of Form MS-Papers-1431, ATL.

51 C. T. Hand-Newton, DSO, *A Physician in Peace and War* (Christchurch: N. M. Peryer, 1967), pp. 22, 24.

52 *Auckland Star*, 7 July 1919, p. 7.

53 4 and 5 May 1915, John H. Thomson, 3/453 No. 1 N.Z. Fd. Amb., Diary from 13 April 1915 to Jan 21st 1916, PC-0316, Hocken.

54 Loftus diary, Medical Corps memoranda — Extracts from diary of 3/172 Sergeant Loftus NZMC, 1 January–9 December 1915 — Narrative of Captain R.D. Barron NZMC, attack on Abraham's Heights morning of 4 October 1917 — No. 2 Australian Casualty Clearing Station 1915–1917 — New Zealand Dental Corps — Venereal statistics, 4 January 1918, WA10 16 10/6/21, ANZ.

55 23 July 1915, Thomson diary.

56 Carbery, *Medical Service*, pp. 521–5, 531. In his 'Nominal Roll of Wounded in N.Z.M.C.' he was often unable to supply a date and place for wounding. Field ambulance man Norman Gray recalled 24 deaths in his unit on Gallipoli, Diary 22 September 1916, Randolph Norman Gray, Papers relating to World War One, MS-Papers-4134, ATL, folder 2.

57 Fenwick, *Gallipoli Diary*, 5 May 1915, p. 15.

58 *Auckland Star*, 14 August 1915, p. 6.

59 https://ww100.govt.nz/bearing-the-wounded, accessed 14 August 2017.

60 Christopher Pugsley and Charles Ferrall (eds), *Remembering Gallipoli: Interviews with New Zealand Gallipoli Veterans* (Wellington: Victoria University Press, 2015), p. 231; *Evening Star*, 31 January 1917, p. 2. Ross does not give the man's name in his 26 November 1916 report, and I have been unable to find it.

61 *Otago Witness*, 4 August 1915, p. 8.

62 *Star*, 27 July 1915, p. 8.

63 Medical Corps memoranda, WA10 16 10/6/21, ANZ, pp. 39, 41, 42.

64 Fenwick, *Gallipoli Diary*, 19 May 1915, p. 57.

65 24 October 1915, Diary of William McAra, Gallipoli, June–December 1915, MS-2943/002, Hocken.

66 'The Evolution of an R.A.P.', Medical Corps Memoranda — Gallipoli & Egypt, April 1916–2 March 1919, WA10 17 10/6/8, ANZ.

67 Trotter diaries.

68 Medical Corps Memoranda, WA10 17 10/6/8, ANZ.

69 Carbery, *Medical Service*, p. 57.

70 Begg article, 'Field Ambulance Work at Anzac' for *British Medical Journal*, 4 December 1915, Medical Corps Memoranda, WA10 17 10/6/8, ANZ.

71 Fenwick, *Gallipoli Diary*, 3 June 1915, p. 87.

72 Penetrating abdominal wounds were those that reached the peritoneum, the serous membrane lining the cavity of the abdomen and covering the abdominal organs.

73 Begg, 'Field Ambulance Work at Anzac'.

74 Breen diary; Carbery, *Medical Service*, p. 57. Other dressing stations were forced to move. While William McAra was with an Australian field ambulance, the death of a patient after three afternoons of shelling compelled a shift to 'what we were told is an absolutely safe place'. Shrapnel wounded three men the afternoon they arrived. 6 October 1915, McAra diary.

75 9 November 1915, McAra diary.

76 Begg, 'Field Ambulance Work at Anzac'; Godley to Allen, 23 July 1915, [Correspondence between] General Sir Alexander Godley [Commander New Zealand Expeditionary Force] and Colonel Hon. Sir James Allen, Minister of Defence, 2 April–19 December 1915, WA 252 1 [2], ANZ.

77 Fenwick, *Gallipoli Diary*, 30 May 1915, p. 86, 14 May 1915, p. 36.

78 Ibid., 16 May 1915, p. 45.

79 Michael Tyquin, *Gallipoli: An Australian Medical Perspective* (Canberra: Army History Unit, 2012), p. 46.

80 Letter Roy W. O. Dalrymple — Gallipoli — WW1, 2009.1196, NAM.

81 Pugsley, *Gallipoli*, p. 307.

82 Condliffe, *Te Rangi Hiroa*, pp. 131–3.

83 Carbery, *Medical Service*, p. 86.

84 Burton, *Silent Division*, p. 65.

85 Tyquin, *Gallipoli*, p. 49.

86 Waite, Liddle Collection.

87 Burton, *Silent Division*, p. 95.

88 Dalrymple letter.

89 Letter William John Rusden Hill, 1990.163, NAM.

90 Dalrymple letter.

91 Tyquin, *Gallipoli*, p. 81.

92 Hill letter.

93 Michael Fitzgerald and Claire Regnault, *Berry Boys: Portraits of First World War Soldiers and Families* (Wellington: Te Papa Press), 2014, p. 146.

94 Condliffe, *Te Rangi Hiroa*, p. 135.

95 Baigent, Medical Corps Memoranda, WA10 17 10/6/8, ANZ; Pugsley, *Gallipoli*, p. 308. Manders, who was replaced by Begg, died on the same day as William Malone; Sergeant Loftus wrote: 'Rough day: Col. Manders killed — every regiment cut up,' Medical Corps Memoranda, WA10 16 10/6/21, ANZ.

96 'Extracts from Diary R.M.O. Canterbury Mounted Rifles, August 1915, Capt. Guthrie N.Z.M.C.', Medical Corps Memoranda, WA10 17 10/6/8, ANZ.

97 Extract from message, Major Newton to ADMS, Medical Corps Memoranda, WA10 17 10/6/8, ANZ.

98 24 September 1915, McAra diary; George William Thomson, Papers, MS-2003-72, AWMM.

99 Carbery, *Medical Service*, pp. 48–9.

100 Butler et al., *Australian Army Medical Services*, vol. 1, pp. 32, 33, 35.

101 Carbery, *Medical Service*, pp. 39–43.

102 Ibid., pp. 50–1.

103 Quoted ibid., p. 541.

104 Ibid.

105 19[?] May 1915, Trotter diaries.

106 Fenwick, *Gallipoli Diary*, 26 May 1915, p. 74.

107 Quoted Peter Liddle, *Men of Gallipoli: The Dardanelles and Gallipoli Experience, August 1914 to January 1916* (London: Allen Lane, 1976), p. 278.

108 Harrison, *The Medical War*, p. 201.

109 *AJHR*, 1916 I, H-19b, p. 3.

110 Harrison, 'War, Health and Medicine'.

111 Quoted Tyquin, *Gallipoli*, p. 51.

CHAPTER 3: SICK AND TIRED

1 *Evening Post*, 3 September 1914, p. 4.

2 There had, however, been illness among the troops at Lemnos en route to Gallipoli. Peter Thompson reported 'a number' down with pneumonia and pleurisy, and cases of measles. 'Cases continue to leave for the Hospital daily.' Diary of Pte P. M. Thompson 4th Bn Otago Regt Suez & Gallipoli 3 August 1914–15 September 1915, 1999.803, NAM.

3 A. D. Carbery, *The New Zealand Medical Service in the Great War, 1914–1918* (Auckland: Whitcombe & Tombs, 1924), pp. 57, 59; Medical Corps Memoranda — Walton on Thames WA10 18 10/6/9, ANZ; C. T. Hand-Newton, DSO, *A Physician in Peace and War* (Christchurch: N. M. Peryer, 1967), p. 24.

4 *Dominion*, 16 August 1915, p. 6.

5 James Foster Rudd letter, Liddle Collection, Brotherton Library, University of Leeds, courtesy Glyn Harper.

6 Carbery, *Medical Service*, p. 108.

7 'A Note on Typhoid and Paratyphoid Fever in the Gallipoli Campaign (1915)', by Adam Patrick, M.D., F.R.C.P., Professor of Medicine, University of St. Andrews, *Journal of the Royal Army Medical Corps*, 1938, vol. 71, pp. 182–4, http://jramc.bmj.com/, accessed 24 October 2016.

8 Memories of Norman E. Hassell, Window into WW1, Palmerston North City Library, http://ww1.pncc.govt.nz/blog/2015/11/18/object-memories-of-1914-norman-e-hassell.

9 Section of Epidemiology and Medicine. President — Dr. G. S. Buchanan. (December 7, 1917.) President's Address. 'Epidemics of the Eastern Campaigns'. By G. S. Buchanan, M.D., Hon. Lieutenant-Colonel R.A.M.C. http://journals.sagepub.com/doi/pdf/10.1177/003591571801101301, accessed 24 June 2017; Carbery, *Medical Service*, p. 117.

10 New Zealand Expeditionary Force. Report of Lieut.-Colonel the Hon. R. Heaton Rhodes, T.D., M.P. Commanding the Canterbury Mounted Rifles Brigade, On his Mission to the New Zealand Expeditionary Force in Malta, Mudros, Gallipoli, and Egypt, as the Representative of the Government, *AJHR*, 1916, H-19b, p. 10.

11 O. E. Burton, *The Silent Division: New Zealanders at the Front: 1914–1919 & Concerning One Man's War*, ed. John H. Gray (Christchurch: John Douglas Publishing, 2014), *One Man's War*, p. 279.

12 Thompson diary, NAM; 25 August 1915, Diaries of A. M. Trotter/transcribed by A. A. S. Trotter, MS-3397/004, Hocken.

13 17 July 1915, Charles Wallace Saunders, World War I diary, Misc-MS-0267, Hocken.

14 Burton, *One Man's War*, p. 279.

15 Nick Wilson, Nhung Nghiem, Jennifer A. Summers, Mary-Ann Carter and Glyn Harper, 'A Nutritional Analysis of New Zealand Military Food Rations at Gallipoli in 1915: Likely Contribution to Scurvy and other Nutrient Deficiency Disorders', *New Zealand Medical Journal*, vol. 126, no. 1373, 19 April 2013, pp. 12–29; Buchanan, 'Epidemics of the Eastern Campaigns', p. 26: 'There was no doubt that the dietary in many cases had produced bad nutrition and in not a few cases this was associated with pronounced cardiac weakness.'

16 Frederick James Foote, 'Yesteryears', Reminiscences, MS 2007/9, NAM.

17 As Peter Stanley points out, for religious reasons, the Indian troops on Gallipoli ate fresh goat and sheep meat, although their standard rations were 'heavy on protein and carbohydrate and long reliance on them fostered scurvy': http://www.indiansongallipoli.com/indians-and-gallipoli/hill-60/, accessed 8 March 2017.

18 John Macbeth Russell Reminiscences, MS-Papers-1696, ATL.

19 Robin Hyde, *Passport to Hell*, edited and introduced by D. I. B. Smith (Auckland: Auckland University Press 2015, 1st pub. 1936), pp. 108–9.

20 1 May 1915, 13 June 1915, John H. Thomson, 3/453 No. 1 N.Z. Fd. Amb., Diary from 13 April 1915 to Jan 21st 1916, PC-0316, Hocken.

21 Allan Marriott, *Mud Beneath My Boots: A Poignant Memoir of the Effects of War on a Young New Zealander* (Auckland: HarperCollins, 2005), p. 83; Memories of Norman E. Hassell.

22 *Timaru Herald*, 5 August 1915, p. 4.

23 Russell Reminiscences, p. 42.

24 Carbery, *Medical Service*, p. 62.

25 Letter: Louis Hamilton Browne — WW1, 2002.330.1, NAM.

26 Reprinted *Taranaki Herald*, 14 August 1915, p. 3; James Jeffery's transcripts of war letters, diaries and related material, MS-2934/002, Hocken.

27 See Otago Mounted Rifles (OMR) — War Diary, 1–26 July 1915, WA44, 55/[440], ANZ. I am indebted to Ian McGibbon for this reference. On 27 July ambulance man John Thomson reported, 'Rations now include 1/8 tin of milk every second day instead of jam. We also get ½ lb of bread occasionally,' Thomson diary.

28 *Feilding Star*, 18 November 1915, p. 4.

29 Quoted Carbery, *Medical Service*, p. 115.

30 Burton, *Silent Division*, p. 82; George Barclay, James Jeffery's transcripts of war letters, diaries and related material, MS-2934/002, Hocken. The 2013 Gallipoli diet study suggests that 'modest amounts' of vegetables and fruits could have been added with only a small increase in cost, though transport would have been a consideration. Wilson et al., 'New Zealand Military Food Rations at Gallipoli'.

31 Pugsley, *Gallipoli*, p. 255; Godley to Liverpool, 13 September 1915, WA 252 2 [8] Letters to and from His Excellency the Earl of Liverpool and General Sir Alexander Godley [Commander New Zealand Expeditionary Force], 15 October 1915–5 October 1918, ANZ.

32 Letters: Thomas E. Catchpole — Egypt & Gallipoli — WW1, 2000.316, NAM, p. 32; Eric Arnold Burnett, Diary and letters, MS-Group-1701, ATL, letter 4 March 1916.

33 Thomson diary, Hocken.

34 Burnett, ATL, letter 15 October 1915.

35 Diary of William McAra, Gallipoli, June–December 1915, MS-2943/002, Hocken.

36 Cody letter, AD78 27 G15/25, History of the War (Gallipoli — Medical —1915), ANZ.

37 Carbery, *Medical Service*, p. 114.

38 Michael Tyquin, *Gallipoli: An Australian Medical Perspective* (Canberra: Army History Unit, 2012), p. 12.

39 Carbery, *Medical Service*, p. 116.

40 Glyn Harper (ed.), *Letters from the Battlefield: New Zealand Soldiers Write Home 1914–1918* (Auckland: HarperCollins, 2001), p. 29. The water shortage also meant that wounds sometimes had to be dressed using salt water, Tyquin, *Gallipoli*, p. 126.

41 John Crawford (ed.) with Peter Cooke, *No Better Death: The Great War Diaries and Letters of William G. Malone* (Auckland: Reed, 2005), p. 231.

42 Hyde, *Passport*, p. 108; Russell Reminiscences, ATL, p. 17.

43 Thomson diary, Hocken, 13 June 1917.

44 Thomas Russell Ritchie, Papers, MS-Papers-3705-1, ATL.

45 Carbery, *Medical Service*, p. 64.

46 Ibid., pp. 110, 111.

47 Frank Woolmer Parker, Liddle Collection, Brotherton Library, University of Leeds, courtesy Glyn Harper; Lieutenant-Colonel Dr Percival Fenwick, *Gallipoli Diary* (Auckland: David Ling in association with Auckland War Memorial Museum, c.2000), 9 May 1915, p. 25.

48 Crawford, *No Better Death*, pp. 217, 231.

49 1st New Zealand Field Ambulance — War Diary, 11 Aug 14–18 Feb 19, WA 119 173[119r], ANZ.

50 Russell Reminiscences, ATL, p. 44.

51 Christopher Pugsley, *Gallipoli: The New Zealand Story* (Libro International and Pen & Sword Books, 5th edn, 2014, 1st pub. 1984), pp. 251–2.

52 Fenwick, *Gallipoli Diary*, p. 94.

53 Burton, *Silent Division*, p. 81.

54 John Crawford (ed.), *The Devil's Own War: The First World War Diary of Brigadier-General Herbert Hart* (Auckland and Wollombi: Exisle Publishing, 2008), p. 74.

55 Leonard Hart, letter January 1916, Letters of Leonard and Adrian Mitchell Hart, MS-Papers-2157, ATL, folder 4; Cody letter, History of the War (Gallipoli — Medical —1915) AD78 27, G15/25, ANZ.

56 Carbery, *Medical Service*, p. 59; Ritchie papers.

57 8 September 1915, Trotter diaries.

58 13 June 1915, Thomson diary.

59 Fenwick, *Gallipoli Diary*, 5 May 1915, p. 17.

60 Memories of Norman E. Hassell.

61 Christopher Pugsley and Charles Ferrall (eds), *Remembering Gallipoli: Interviews with New Zealand Gallipoli Veterans* (Wellington: Victoria University Press, 2015), pp. 151, 153, 154.

62 Joseph George Gasparich, Liddle Collection, Brotherton Library, University of Leeds, courtesy Glyn Harper.

63 Ibid.

64 Memories of Norman E. Hassell.

65 Diary — Henry M. Clark — NZ Hospital — England — WW1, 1993.1000, NAM.

66 *Kai Tiaki*, April 1917, p. 74.

67 25 September 1915, McAra diary.

68 Fenwick, *Gallipoli Diary*, pp. 94, 100.

69 Thomson diary.

70 23 September, 19 October and 8 November 1915, McAra diary.

71 Burton, *One Man's War*, p. 293.

72 Carbery, *Medical Service*, p. 117.

73 Burton, *Silent Division*, p. 80.

74 Russell Reminiscences, p. 44.

75 Fenwick, *Gallipoli Diary*, pp. 20, 93, 94.

76 Godley to Allen, 8 July 1915, [Correspondence between] General Sir Alexander Godley [Commander New Zealand Expeditionary Force] and Colonel Hon. Sir James Allen, Minister of Defence, 2 April–19 December 1915, WA 252 1 [2], ANZ; *Wanganui Herald*, 14 October 1915. p. 8; diary 21 June 1915, Ritchie papers; 2 January 1916, Thomson diary.

77 25 July 1915, Trotter diaries.

78 Hand-Newton, *Physician*, p. 26.

79 Carbery, *Medical Service*, pp. 108, 110.

80 Crawford (ed.), *Devil's Own War*, pp. 73–4.

81 Fenwick, *Gallipoli Diary*, p. 74.

82 Pugsley, *Gallipoli*, p. 226.

83 Thomson diary.

84 *Hawera & Normanby Star*, 20 October 1915, p. 8. Warwood was one of 15 employees of Christchurch firm W. Strange who volunteered: one was killed in action, Warwood died of disease, one was reported wounded and missing, and two were wounded, *Press*, 30 October 1915, p. 2.

85 Cecil Malthus, *Anzac: A Retrospect* (Auckland: Reed, 2000, 1st pub. 1965), p. 41; Crawford, *No Better Death*, 23 April 1915, p. 160; Jane Tolerton, *An Awfully Big Adventure: New Zealand World War One Veterans Tell Their Stories* (Auckland: Penguin, 2013), p. 54.

86 Kate Hunter and Kirstie Ross, *Holding On to Home: New Zealand Stories and Objects of the First World War* (Wellington: Te Papa Press, 2014), p. 51, quoting Gordon Harper to mother 10 July 1915, MS-Papers-1444-4, ATL; Charles Saunders Wallace: World War I diary, Misc-MS-0267, Hocken.

87 12 November 1915, McAra diary.

88 Hand-Newton, *Physician*, pp. 28–9.

89 Carbery, *Medical Service*, p. 130.

90 Letter 2 December 1915, Carruthers family: Extracts from letters to Carruthers family/Walter [Carruthers], MS-Papers-4107, ATL.

91 Hand-Newton, *Physician*, p. 30.

92 Carbery, *Medical Service*, p. 132.

93 Hand-Newton, *Physician*, pp. 32–3.

94 Ibid., p. 33.

95 Carbery, *Medical Service*, p. 133.

96 Crawford (ed.), *Devil's Own War*, p. 90.

97 'The Gallipoli campaign', https://nzhistory.govt.nz/war/the-gallipoli-campaign/introduction, (Ministry for Culture and Heritage), updated 17-May-2017.

98 Letter 16 December 1915, Carruthers letters.

CHAPTER 4: FROM DESERT TO DISASTER

1 *Press*, 20 July 1915, p. 8.

2 Godley to Allen, 9 April 1915, [Correspondence between] General Sir Alexander Godley [Commander New Zealand Expeditionary Force] and Colonel Hon. Sir James Allen, Minister of Defence, 2 April–19 December 1915, WA 252 1 [2], ANZ. Allen had told Godley on 12 February: 'I wish to goodness you could stifle some of the grumbles that are continually coming from Egypt. Unfortunately there are some papers here who pick out all the grumbling correspondence for political purposes and to try and irritate the public mind.' Ministerial files — correspondence with General Godley, Allen 1 1, M1/15, ANZ. Allen would later admit that he had 'received private letters which had raised grave doubts as to the treatment of the sick and wounded', *New Zealand Herald*, 7 July 1915, p. 9.

3 *Kai Tiaki*, 1 January 1916, pp. 24, 25.

4 *Dominion*, 20 May 1915, p. 3.

5 *Press*, 22 June 1915, p. 8.

6 Reported 5 August 1915 to John H. Thomson, 3/453 No. 1 N.Z. Fd. Amb., Diary from 13 April 1915 to Jan 21st 1916, PC-0316, Hocken.

7 *Press*, 14 June 1915, p. 9.

8 Report for Colonel Valintine, Director of Military Hospitals, New Zealand Hospitals in Egypt, 14 October 1915, Reports — Reports Hospitals in Egypt — Matron in Chief, AD 1 887 39/180, ANZ.

9 *New Zealand Herald*, 7 July 1915, p. 9.

10 A. D. Carbery, *The New Zealand Medical Service in the Great War, 1914–1918* (Auckland: Whitcombe & Tombs, 1924), p. 72.

11 One of the first New Zealand nurses to care for Gallipoli casualties was an unnamed Christchurch woman who had followed her soldier husband overseas — he was killed on Gallipoli — and joined the QAIMNS in Britain before going to Egypt. She was working at Ras-el-Tin Hospital when 'the first batch of wounded [was] brought there after the historic landing, [including] a great number of Australians and two or three dozen New Zealanders', *Press*, 20 July 1915, p. 8.

12 *New Zealand Herald*, 18 June 1915, p. 4.

13 Letter: Louis Hamilton Browne — WW1, 2002.330.1, NAM; Jane Tolerton, *An Awfully Big Adventure: New Zealand World War One Veterans Tell Their Stories* (Auckland: Penguin, 2013), p. 66.

14 Godley to Allen, 15 February 1915, Ministerial files — correspondence with General Godley, Allen 1 1, M1/15, ANZ.

15 A. G. Butler, R. M. Downes, F. A. Maguire and R. W. Cilento, *The Australian Army Medical Services in the War of 1914–1918*, vol. I, *Gallipoli, Palestine and New Guinea* (Melbourne: Australian War Memorial, 1938, 2nd edn), pp. 203–4.

16 Letters 1, 2 and 18 December 1915, Randolph Norman Gray: Papers relating to World War One, MS-Papers-4134, ATL, folder 1.

17 Diary and later account, Collection — Sister Mabel Crook — WW1, 2016.280.1, NAM.

18 *Wanganui Herald*, 14 October 1915, p. 8.

19 Edna Pengelly, *Nursing in Peace and War* (Wellington: Wingfield Press, 1956), p. 29; *Press*, 12 December 1916, p. 5.

20 Kevin Clunie (comp.) and Ron Austin (ed.), *From Gallipoli to Palestine: The War Writings of Sergeant GT Clunie of the Wellington Mounted Rifles, 1914–1919* (McCrae, Victoria: Slouch Hat Publications, 2009), p. 88; *New Zealand Herald*, 19 August 1915, p. 8.

21 Pengelly, *Nursing*, pp. 28, 30.

22 Fanny Helena Speedy, Diaries, MS-Papers-1703, ATL.

23 Pengelly, *Nursing*, p. 49.

24 New Zealand Army Nursing Service — NZANS overseas records, correspondence — Matron-in-chief, AD78 23 67/3/1A, ANZ.

25 *Kai Tiaki*, October 1915, p. 170.

26 *Star*, 12 July 1915, p. 4.

27 *Kai Tiaki*, January 1916, p. 24.

28 Ibid., p. 22.

29 *Kai Tiaki*, October 1915, p. 170.

30 *Dominion*, 13 November 1915, p. 10.

31 *Northern Advocate*, 15 July 1915, p. 1.

32 Carbery, *Medical Service*, p. 73.

33 Hester Maclean's report to Valintine, 14 October 1915, Reports — Report Hospital in Egypt — Matron in Chief, AD1 887 39/180, ANZ.

34 *Wanganui Chronicle*, 11 September 1915, p. 3.

35 *Taranaki Daily News*, 28 September 1915, p. 3.

36 *Evening Post*, 19 May 1915, p. 8.

37 Tolerton, *Awfully Big Adventure*, p. 83.

38 *Press*, 13 September 1915, p. 2.

39 Joseph George Gasparich, Liddle Collection, Brotherton Library, University of Leeds, courtesy Glyn Harper.

40 Tolerton, *Awfully Big Adventure*, p. 85.

41 *Press*, 13 September 1915, p. 2.

42 *Dominion*, 22 October 1915, p. 7; *Observer*, 22 January 1916, p. 4.

43 *Dominion*, 2 October 1915, p. 6.

44 Ibid.

45 As Armitage explained in a report, Britain, Australia and New Zealand all faced the 'impossibility of obtaining adequate Bacteriological equipment in Egypt', so arranged with the Egyptian government for dysentery and enteric specimens to be examined at the Public Health Department on behalf of various military hospitals. This 'enabled very thorough examination' and meant that the ordinary lab work at the New Zealand hospital could be 'more satisfactorily carried out'. Report of Bacteriological Laboratory — 1st Novr. 1915 to 31st May 1916, Medical Corps memoranda — Walton on Thames, WA10 18 10/6/9, ANZ.

46 *Kai Tiaki*, January 1916, p. 26.

47 *Southland Times*, 18 February 1916, p. 2.

48 14 November 1915, Diary of William McAra, Gallipoli, June–December 1915, MS-2943/002, Hocken.

49 Letters 17 January and 2 February 1916, Medical — Staff (Medical) Egypt, AD1 970 49/213, ANZ.

50 *Press*, 23 May 1916, p. 3.

51 Godley to Allen, 13 March 1915, Ministerial files — correspondence with General Godley, Allen 1 1, M1/15, ANZ.

52 Reports — Report — Hospital in Egypt, AD1 881, 39/140, ANZ.

53 Godley to Allen, 10 April 1915, Ministerial files — correspondence with General Godley, Allen 1 1, M1/15, ANZ.

54 *Sun*, 8 June 1915, p. 4; Godley to Allen, 2 April 1915, [Correspondence between] General Sir Alexander Godley [Commander New Zealand Expeditionary Force] and Colonel Hon. Sir James Allen, Minister of Defence, 2 April–19 December 1915, WA 252 1 [2], ANZ.

55 Godley to Allen, 29 May 1915, WA 252 1 [2], ANZ.

56 *Wanganui Chronicle*, 30 July 1915, p. 3.

57 Medical Corps Memoranda — Gallipoli & Egypt, April 1916–2 March 1919, WA10 17 10/6/8, ANZ.

58 Godley to Allen, 19 February 1916, [Correspondence between] General Sir Alexander Godley [Commander New Zealand Expeditionary Force] and Colonel Hon. Sir James Allen, Minister of Defence, 4 January–29 December 1916, WA 252 1 [3], ANZ.

59 *Wanganui Chronicle*, 30 July 1915, p. 3.

60 Godley to Allen, 3 June 1916, Ministerial Files — Correspondence with General Godley, Allen 1 2, M1/15, ANZ.

61 *Wanganui Chronicle*, 31 July 1915, p. 4.

62 *Kai Tiaki*, April 1919, p. 60.

63 *Wanganui Chronicle*, 15 January 1916, p. 7.

64 Letter 11 December 1915, Eric Arnold Burnett, Diary and letters, MS-Papers 2091, ATL, folder 1.

65 *Wanganui Chronicle*, 22 February 1916, p. 6; 9 January 1918, p. 7.

66 *Kai Tiaki*, April 1919, p. 60.

67 *Observer*, 20 July 1918, p. 4.

68 Clunie (comp.), *From Gallipoli to Palestine*, pp. 95–6.

69 Letters 22 January and 13 February 1916, Burnett, Diary and letters, folder 2.

70 *Dominion*, 18 November 1915, p. 7.

71 *Press*, 24 November 1915, p. 6.

72 *Marlborough Express*, 29 December 1915, p. 6.

73 *New Zealand Herald*, 17 December 1915, p. 9.

74 *Marlborough Express*, 29 December 1915, p. 6.

75 *Colonist*, 16 January 1916, p. 7. Melville Mirfin, better known as Paddy, had served in Samoa before joining No. 1 NZSH. As the *Free Lance* noted in its 'Palmerston Doings' column on 24 March 1916, 'Always a quiet, unassuming sort of fellow, [he] was not looking for lime-light, and news of his gallantry is just coming to us through indirect channels.'

76 *Timaru Herald*, 1 January 1916, p. 11.

77 *Marlborough Express*, 29 December 1915, p. 6.

78 *Kai Tiaki*, January 1916, p. 10.

79 Edith Wilkin, letter to mother, 7 November 1915, Nurses' Memorial Chapel, Christchurch.

80 'New Zealand nurses lost in Marquette sinking', https://nzhistory.govt.nz/page/new-zealand-nurses-lost-in-marquette-sinking, (Ministry for Culture and Heritage), updated 20-Jan-2017.

81 It has been suggested that the British hospital ship *Grantully Castle* was in Alexandria at the same time as the *Marquette* and had room for the New Zealand medical staff, but as Peter Rees points out in *The Other Anzacs: Nurses at War, 1914–18* (Crows Nest, NSW: Allen & Unwin, 2008), p. 145, the diary of Australian nursing sister Kath King makes it clear that this was not the case.

82 *Hawera & Normanby Star*, 21 December 1915; David Fitzgibbon letter, *Northern Advocate*, 17 January 1916, pp. 1, 4.

83 *West Coast Times*, 21 January 1916, p. 2.

84 *Kai Tiaki*, January 1916, p. 12.

85 *Poverty Bay Herald*, 1 March 1916, p. 6. After seven months in Salonika, Leahy, who had 'a wide experience of bacteriological work', was invalided home to New Zealand, where he became the PMO at Trentham camp, *Observer*, 27 October 1917, p. 4.

86 *New Zealand Herald*, 7 January 1916, p. 4.

87 *Press*, 14 January 1916, p. 5.

88 *Auckland Star*, 13 April 1916, p. 4.

89 *Manawatu Times*, 13 March 1916, p. 3.

90 *Marlborough Express*, 13 March 1916, p. 2.

91 Ibid.

92 *Manawatu Times*, 13 March 1916, p. 3.

93 Carbery, *Medical Service*, p. 146.

94 Medical — Staff (Medical) Egypt, AD1 970 49/213, ANZ. No. 2 NZSH converted to general hospital, Routine Orders 10 January 1916.

CHAPTER 5: SURVIVING IN THE SAND

1 *Evening Post*, 12 February 1918, p. 6.

2 Terry Kinloch, *Devils on Horses: In the Words of the Anzacs of the Middle East* (Auckland: Exisle Publishing, 2007), p. 21; 'Sinai campaign', https://nzhistory.govt.nz/war/sinai-campaign, (Ministry for Culture and Heritage), updated 3-Nov-2017.

3 *Otago Daily Times*, 25 July 1916, p. 6.

4 Lindsay Baly, *Horseman, Pass By: The Australian Light Horse in World War I* (Staplehurst, Kent: Spellmount Ltd, 2004, 1st pub. 2003), p. 16.

5 *Auckland Star*, 5 December 1917, p. 7; *N.Z. Truth*, 2 March 1918, p. 6; Diary Charles Malone Sinai & Palestine — WW1, 1990.1620, NAM.

6 *Press*, 29 December 1917, p. 9; Diary Trooper Leslie Angus McInnes, 6th Reinforcements, Auckland Regiment 13/2054, 2008.269, NAM.

7 Frederick James Foote, 'Yesteryears', Reminiscences, MS 2007/9, AWMM, p. 255; Baly, *Horseman*, p. 34.

8 The Diary of Cervantes Jason Bell, Service in Mesopotamia December 1916 to May 1918, transcribed by Jane Hall, née Bell, courtesy of Glyn Harper.

9 Jane Tolerton, *An Awfully Big Adventure: New Zealand World War One Veterans Tell Their Stories* (Auckland: Penguin, 2013), p. 242.

10 Letter to mother, Palestine, 1 January 1918, Hubert Hatrick, Liddle Collection, Brotherton Library, University of Leeds, courtesy Glyn Harper; Foote, 'Yesteryears'.

11 *Auckland Star*, 17 October 1916, p. 7; *Evening Post*, 12 February 1918, p. 6.

12 *North Otago Times*, 3 March 1917, p. 2.

13 A. H. Wilkie, *Official War History of the Wellington Mounted Rifles Regiment 1914–1919* (Auckland: Whitcombe & Tombs, 1924), p. 107.

14 Letter to 'Dear Tell', 18 November 1916, Letters Pte F. A. Crum — WW1, 2008.25, NAM.

15 C. T. Hand-Newton, DSO, *A Physician in Peace and War* (Christchurch: N. M. Peryer, 1967), p. 39.

16 A. D. Carbery, *The New Zealand Medical Service in the Great War, 1914–1918* (Auckland: Whitcombe & Tombs, 1924), pp. 451, 471.

17 A. G. Butler, R. M. Downes, F. A. Maguire and R. W. Cilento, *The Australian Army Medical Services in the War of 1914–1918*, vol. I, *Gallipoli, Palestine and New Guinea* (Melbourne: Australian War Memorial, 1938, 2nd edn), p. 565; *Dominion*, 24 August 1918, p. 8.

18 Wilkie, *Mounted Rifles*, p. 107.

19 Trooper Arthur Ames, evacuated with enteric, appears to have been the exception. 'The first fifteen miles we had to do on camels, two men on each side slung in a kind of stretcher. It was a bit rough at first, but after a time you seem to get used to the motion; in fact, I had a sleep on the journey.' *Dominion*, 23 July 1918, p. 7.

20 Butler et al., *Australian Army Medical Services*, p. 563.

21 Ibid., p. 564.

22 Foote, 'Yesteryears', p. 262.

23 *Dominion*, 24 August 1918, p. 8.

24 Wilkie, *Mounted Rifles*, p. 107.

25 John Robertson, *With the Cameliers in Palestine* (Wellington: A. H. & A. W. Reed, 1938), p. 168.

26 Foote, 'Yesteryears', p. 262.

27 Kinloch, *Devils*, pp. 108–9.

28 *Press*, 29 December 1917, p. 9.

29 Letter 16 August 1916, Kevin Clunie (comp.) and Ron Austin (ed.), *From Gallipoli to Palestine: The War Writings of Sergeant GT Clunie of the Wellington Mounted Rifles, 1914–1919* (McCrae, Victoria: Slouch Hat Publications, 2009), pp. 88–9.

30 Tolerton, *Awfully Big Adventure*, p. 154.

31 Foote, 'Yesteryears', pp. 291–3.

32 Ibid., p. 294.

33 Diary C. L. Sommerville — Sinai & Palestine — WW1, 1997.255, NAM.

34 Carbery, *Medical Service*, p. 451.

35 *North Otago Times*, 3 March 1917, p. 2.

36 Crum letters.

37 Butler et al., *Australian Army Medical Services*, p. 561; Carbery, *Medical Service*, p. 451–2.

38 Carbery, *Medical Service*, pp. 452, 471.

39 Ibid., pp. 473–4.

40 Ibid., pp. 454–5.

41 John Kirkup, 'Fracture Care of Friend and Foe During World War 1', *ANZ Journal of Surgery*, vol. 73, no. 6, June 2003, pp. 453–9.

42 Carbery, *Medical Service*, p. 453.

43 Ibid., p. 466.

44 Ibid., p. 457.

45 Crum letters.

46 *North Otago Times*, 3 March 1917, p. 2.

47 Wilkie, *Mounted Rifles*, p. 129; Robertson, *Cameliers*, p. 166.

48 John Graham Gow file, 3/3394, ANZ.

49 Carbery, *Medical Service*, p. 477.

50 Colonel C. G. Powles, *The History of the Canterbury Mounted Rifles 1914–1919* (Auckland: Whitcombe & Tombs, 1928), p. 134.

51 Carbery, *Medical Service*, p. 455.

52 Powles, *Canterbury Mounted Rifles*, p. 118.

53 Dennis Shanks, 'Formation of Medical Units in Response to Epidemics in the Australian Imperial Force in Palestine 1918', *Journal of Military and Veterans' Health*, vol. 22, no. 2, June 2014, pp. 14–19.

54 Carbery, *Medical Service*, p. 470. NCI stood for 96% naphthalene, 2% creosote, 2% iodoform.

55 Robertson, *Cameliers*, p. 147.

56 Powles, *Canterbury Mounted Rifles*, p. 225.

57 *Dominion*, 24 August 1918, p. 8.

58 Bayly, *Horseman*, p. 222; *Press*, 29 December 1917, p. 9.

59 *Dominion*, 24 August 1918, p. 8; *Auckland Star*, 17 October 1916, p. 7.

60 Foote, 'Yesteryears', p. 281.

61 Malone diary, 1917.

62 Bayly, *Horseman*, p. 222.

63 *Kai Tiaki*, January 1917, p. 9.

64 *Dominion*, 23 July 1918, p. 7.

65 Quoted Powles, *Canterbury Mounted Rifles*, p. 239.

66 Carbery, *Medical Service*, p. 481.

67 A. Briscoe Moore, *The Mounted Riflemen in Sinai and Palestine: The Story of New Zealand's Crusaders* (Auckland: Whitcombe & Tombs, n.d.), p. 142.

68 *Kai Tiaki*, April 1919, pp. 60–1.

69 Carbery, *Medical Service*, p. 481.

70 *New Zealand Herald*, 11 January 1918, p. 6.

71 Moore, *Mounted Riflemen*, pp. 142–3.

72 *Dominion*, 23 July 1918, p. 7.

73 Roy David McCormack 13/1075, Diary: Egypt & Sinai/Palestine WW1, 1999.2619, NAM; Roy David McCormack file, 13/107, ANZ.

74 Moore, *Mounted Riflemen*, p. 144.

75 Collection of 3/2643 Private Eric Sidney Bardell, Diary of the First trip of the 5th Charter of H.M.N.Z.S. "Maheno" July 6th to October 22nd 1918, 1996.1682.1, NAM.

76 Crum letters; Fred Albert Crum file, 3/240, ANZ.

CHAPTER 6: MEDICS IN THE MUD

1 Letters 22 November and 31 December 1915, Randolph Norman Gray, Papers relating to World War One, MS-Papers- 4134, ATL, folder 1.

2 A. D. Carbery, *The New Zealand Medical Service in the Great War, 1914–1918* (Auckland: Whitcombe & Tombs, 1924), p. 160; Letter 17 April 1916, Gray papers, folder 3; War Memoirs by Dr. W. Aitken, M.C., MD,

FRACP. 1st N.Z. Field Ambulance, 3DRL/2422, Australian War Memorial, pp. 9–10.

3 Carbery, *Medical Service*, p. 160. The transport and animals for the field ambulance had arrived on 19 April: 52 horses and mules, six GS wagons, four limbered GS wagons, three water carts and a Maltese cart. The two water-testing cases per ambulance were designed to estimate the amount of chlorination required in a given water supply.

4 12 May 1916, John Keith Moloney, War diary, MS-Papers-1194, ATL.

5 William Roy Robson, Documents 16812, Imperial War Museum, courtesy Glyn Harper.

6 Diary 16 November 1916, Gray Papers, folder 2.

7 *Star*, 4 July 1917, p. 7.

8 Diary 4 May 1918, Vincent Jervis, MS-Papers-2241, ATL; Moloney diary, early 1917.

9 William Kingston Wilson, Diary, 1994.2314, NAM, pp. 109–10. My thanks to Ray Grover for alerting me to this material.

10 Clifford Collingwood, Diary and Scrapbook: New Zealand, Egypt & Western Front — WW1, 2007.139, NAM. Men often resented being ill. When Henry Clark reached Southampton in August 1915 on the *Maunganui*, he wrote that 'I mean to throw off my sickness at the earliest possible', 26 August 1915, Diary — Henry M. Clark — NZ Hospital — England — WW1, 1993.1000, NAM. When Vincent Jervis, with a temperature of 101°F, was marked for the base in March 1918, he noted, 'Ye Gods if I get down there Claude & Co will put me down as an out & out lead swinger', 17 March 1918, Jervis diary.

11 Margaret and William Cook: Letters from Stewart Callaghan, MS-Papers-5004, ATL. The note also says, 'Mustard Gas was the cause of his troubles', but there is nothing on Callaghan's file to suggest this. He became ill before this weapon was used by the Germans.

12 Rachel Hird, *Good bye Bill Massey No more Khaki: Reg Hird's Letters from the Great War* (Miramar, Wellington: author, 2015), p. 47.

13 Ian McGibbon, *New Zealand's Western Front Campaign* (Auckland: David Bateman, 2016), p. 210.

14 Mark Harrison, *The Medical War: British Military Medicine in the First World War* (Oxford: Oxford University Press, 2010), pp. 157–8.

15 I am indebted to Ian McGibbon for this information.

16 John A. Lee, *Civilian into Soldier* (Auckland: Vital Books, 1963, 1st pub. London), p. 57.

17 Carbery, *Medical Service*, pp. 176–7.

18 Ibid., p. 263; Brendan O'Carroll, *Khaki Angels: Kiwi Stretcher-bearers in the First and Second World Wars* (Wellington: Ngaio Press, 2009), p. 24. The long research required to 'prove that the real cause [of trench fever] lay in the scratching-in of louse excreta' included 'a trial involving elderly volunteers who submitted to having four hundred lice crawling over them and biting them', Nick Bosanquet, 'Health Systems in Khaki: The British and American Medical Experience', in Hugh Cecil and Peter Liddle (eds), *Facing Armageddon: The First World War Experienced* (Barnsley, UK: Pen & Sword, 2003, 1st pub. 1996), p. 458.

19 Diary 14 October 1916, Gray papers, folder 2; Carbery, *Medical Service*, p. 176.

20 Wilson diary, pp. 149–50.

21 New Zealand Sanitary Section — War Diary, 7 February 1916–25 February 1919, WA182 196 [182a], ANZ.

22 Edward Morris Dillon Diary (Stephen Clarke), courtesy Glyn Harper. As Alec Hutton wrote to his mother on 9 June 1918, 'The French are an admirable race in many ways but they don't seem to have studied the science of sanitation,' Letters to the Hutton family from Alexander Louis Hutton, MS-Papers-3906, ATL, folder 2.

23 Diary of Events April 11th to 30th 1916, Medical Corps Memoranda — Precis of events in France, 11 April 1916–10 June 1917, WA10 19, 10/6/10 28/6, ANZ.

24 Leo van Bergen, *Before My Helpless Sight: Suffering, Dying and Military Medicine on the Western Front, 1914–1918* (Surrey: Ashgate, 2009), pp. 132, 139; Memories of Norman E. Hassell, Window into WW1, Palmerston North City Library, http://ww1.pncc.govt.nz/blog/2015/11/18/object-memories-of-1914-norman-e-hassell.

25 Bergen, *Helpless Sight*, p. 148.

26 Roy David McCormack file, 13/1075, ANZ.

27 Ian McGibbon (ed.), *The Oxford Companion to New Zealand Military History* (Auckland: Oxford University Press, 2000), p. 314; 'War, Health and Medicine: The Medical Lessons of World War I', Professor Mark Harrison, Gresham College, 6 May 1915, YouTube, accessed 1 August 2017.

28 Arthur Anderson Martin, *A Surgeon in Khaki: Through France and Flanders in World War I* (Lincoln and London: University of Nebraska Press, 2011, 1st pub. 1915), p. 137; William Mandeno Smallfield, War Letters, Diaries and Papers, MS 2007/37, AWMM.

29 *Manawatu Standard*, 13 September 1916, p. 5.

30 Jane Tolerton, *An Awfully Big Adventure: New Zealand World War One Veterans Tell Their Stories* (Auckland: Penguin, 2013), p. 171.

31 'Sydney Stanfield remembers Passchendaele', https://nzhistory.govt.nz/media/sound/sidney-stanfield-remembers-passchendaele, (Ministry for Culture and Heritage), updated 11-Jul-2017.

32 Allan Marriott, *Mud Beneath My Boots: A Poignant Memoir of the Effects of War on a Young New Zealander* (Auckland: HarperCollins, 2005), pp. 36, 44.

33 C. H. Weston, *Three Years With the New Zealanders* (London: Skeffington & Son, 1918), Chapter XIII.

34 O. E. Burton, *The Silent Division: New Zealanders at the Front: 1914–1919 & Concerning One Man's War*, ed. John H. Gray (Christchurch: John Douglas Publishing, 2014), *One Man's War*, p. 401; Carbery, *Medical Service*, p. 312.

35 John Kirkup, 'Fracture Care of Friend and Foe During World War 1', *ANZ Journal of Surgery*, vol. 73, no. 6, June 2003, 453–9, p. 454.

36 'New Zealand Medical Corps', https://nzhistory.govt.nz/war/medical-units/new-zealand-medical-corps, (Ministry for Culture and Heritage), updated 22-Mar-2017. A field ambulance was divided into three sections, A, B, and C, each made up of a bearer subdivision and a tent subdivision. The former carried the stretchers, collected the wounded and administered first aid from a surgical haversack carried by the leader of the squad, before going to the RAP and dressing stations. The tent division was responsible for setting up and running the dressing stations. See Carbery, *Medical Service*, p. xix, for a detailed summary of the medical arrangements for the New Zealand Division in France.

37 John Kirkup, 'Fracture Care of Friend and Foe During World War 1', *ANZ Journal of Surgery*, vol. 73, no. 6, June 2003, pp. 453–9.

38 Harry Baverstock, quoted Lyn Macdonald, *1914–1918: Voices and Images of the Great War* (London: Michael Joseph, 1988), p. 170.

39 For example, Ploegsteert, March 1917, Medical Corps memoranda — Precis of events in France, 11 April 1916–10 June 1917, WA10 19 10/6/10, ANZ; Diary 11 May 1916, Gray papers, folder 2.

40 Red signalled a bad case, white a less alarming one. Early in October 1917, ADMS McGavin ordered that a blue cross on a bandage would indicate that a man did not require further dressing at an ADS; the letter M in indelible pencil on a forehead would denote 'Morphia Given', Carbery, *Medical Service*, p. 164; 'Medical Instructions in the Event of an Offensive', Medical Corps Memoranda — Precis of Events in France, 10 June–31 December 1917, WA10 20, 10/6/12, ANZ.

41 Burton, *One Man's War*, p. 326.

42 William Taylor, *The Twilight Hour: A Personal Account of World War I* (Morrinsville: Sutherland, 1978), p. 70; Collingwood diary.

43 *Wanganui Chronicle* (supplement), 21 July 1919, p. 7.

44 Medical Corps Memoranda — Precis of Events in France, 10 June–31 December 1917, WA10 20, 10/6/12, ANZ.

45 'Medical Units of the NZEF', https://nzhistory.govt.nz/war/medical-units, (Ministry for Culture and Heritage), updated 22-Mar-2017.

46 Tom Scotland, 'War Surgery, 1914–18, National Army Museum', 11 January 2003, YouTube, accessed 1 August 2017.

47 Gray papers, folder 2.

48 'To check acidosis, the depletion of the alkaline reserve (bicarbonate content) in the blood and body tissues, sodium bicarbonate was administered and very small doses of morphine; an intravenous transfusion of gum acacia raised the blood pressure. Before blood transfusion became common, infusions of saline or of "Bayliss' gummy solution" — a colloid preparation of gum arabic (from the sap of the Acacia tree) were used to treat shock from blood loss.' http://www.kumc.edu/wwi/essays-on-first-world-war-medicine/index-of-essays/medicine/blood-transfusion.html, accessed 19 January 2017.

49 Carbery, *Medical Service*, p. 361. At the MDS set up near Le Quesnoy in 1918, No. 3 Field Ambulance had special heating arrangements: 'each case, whilst being treated, was placed over a blanketed frame heated by oil stoves', Lieutenant-Colonel W. S. Austin, *The Official History of the New Zealand Rifle Brigade* (Wellington: L. T. Watkins Ltd, 1924), p. 566.

50 Bergen, *Helpless Sight*, p. 333.

51 Medical Corps Memoranda — Precis of events in France, 11 April 1916–10 June 1917, WA10 19, 10/6/10, ANZ.

52 *Dominion*, 23 August 1916, p. 6.

53 Carbery, *Medical Service*, p. 172.

54 *North Otago Times*, 25 September 1916, p. 7.

55 Austin, *Rifle Brigade*, p. 550.

56 *Kai Tiaki*, July 1918, p. 144.

57 Kevin Brown, *Fighting Fit: Health, Medicine and War in the Twentieth Century* (Stroud, UK: The History Press, 2008), p. 43.

58 *Kai Tiaki*, July 1918, pp. 138–9.

59 *Manawatu Standard*, 13 September 1916, p. 5.

60 *Taranaki Herald*, 1 September 1917, p. 4; diary 20 March 1918, Jervis papers; *Thames Star*, 2 December 1916, p. 4; Burton, *One Man's War*, p. 377.

61 Iain Gordon, *Lifeline: A British Casualty Clearing Station on the Western Front, 1918* (Stroud, UK: The History Press, 2013), p. 29.

62 *Kai Tiaki*, January 1917, p. 12.

63 *New Zealand Herald*, 23 August 1916, p. 8.

64 'Resume of Division Medical Arrangements', Medical Corps Memoranda — Precis of events in France, 11 April 1916–10 June 1917, WA10 19, 10/6/10, ANZ.

65 Letter 23 April 1918, Callaghan; William Fleming, Reminiscences, Misc-MS-1908, Hocken.

66 Carbery, *Medical Service*, p. xix. Also part of the ambulance system were 'men on motor-cycles' attached to the field ambulances, who went around the dressing stations to ascertain how many men 'needed to be moved by motor', so the right number of cars went to the right places, Surgeon-General Robert Henderson lecture, *Dominion*, 4 August 1917, p. 8; 1st New Zealand Field Ambulance — War Diary, 11 August 1914–18 February 1919, WA 119 173 [119r], ANZ; Carbery, *Medical Service*, p. 163.

67 'Indeed, use of motorised ambulances, well-trained stretcher-bearers, and improvements in fracture/wound management by medical services have been described as factors reducing the case fatality level among the wounded in later stages of the war,' Nick Wilson, Jennifer A. Summers, Michael G. Baker, George Thomson and Glyn Harper, 'Fatal Injury Epidemiology among New Zealand Military Forces in the First World War', *New Zealand Medical Journal*, vol. 126, no. 1385, 1 November 2013, p. 23; Surgeon-General Henderson also suggested that they saved wounded men from being taken prisoner, *Dominion*, 4 August 1917, p. 8.

68 Collingwood diary; Wilson diary.

69 *Dominion*, 23 August 1916, p. 6.

70 Tolerton, *Awfully Big Adventure*, p. 144.

71 *Dominion*, 8 February 1917, p. 6; 'At the big bases the motor ambulances convey the wounded from

the train to the Base Hospitals or to the ships' sides at the quays', *Manawatu Standard*, 13 September 1916, p. 5.

72 3rd New Zealand Field Ambulance — War Diary, 1 April 1916–4 February 1919, WA 121 176 [121a], ANZ.

73 Henderson, *Dominion*, 4 August 1917, p. 8.

74 *Evening Post*, 16 January 1917, p. 2; 18 May 1917, p. 8.

75 Allen to Godley, 12 February 1915, Ministerial files — correspondence with General Godley, Allen 1 1, M1/15, ANZ.

76 Minister of Defence — Motor ambulances, offers overseas, Allen 1 7, D1/17 2480, ANZ.

77 Modris Eksteins, *Rites of Spring: The Great War and the Birth of the Modern Age* (London: Black Swan, 1989), p. 223.

78 In crises orderlies often found themselves working as stretcher-bearers. At the Somme, William Robson of No. 2 Field Ambulance had already been working for 20 hours when he and several others volunteered to 'go out and pick up some men', Robson, documents.

79 *Timaru Herald*, 1 January 1917, p. 3.

80 Christine E. Hallett, *Veiled Warriors: Allied Nurses of the First World War* (Oxford: Oxford University Press, 2014), p. 79.

81 Aitken, Memoirs, p. 11.

82 Carbery, *Medical Service*, p. 253.

83 Ibid., p. 311–12. The Novita apparatus was also used by the tunnellers.

84 Medical Corps Memoranda — Precis of Events in France, 10 June–31 December 1917, WA10 20, 10/6/12, ANZ.

85 simonjoneshistorian.com, accessed 10 January 2017; Rachel Hird, *Good bye Bill Massey*, p. 67; Medical Corps Memoranda — Precis of Events in France, 10 June–31 December 1917, WA10 20, 10/6/12, ANZ.

86 Juliet Nicolson, *The Great Silence 1918–1920: Living in the Shadow of the Great War* (London: John Murray, 2009), p. 25.

87 Gordon, *Lifeline*, pp. 57, 58; Medical Corps Memoranda — Precis of Events in France, 10 June–31 December 1917, WA10 20, 10/6/12, ANZ.

88 Ibid.

89 *Evening Post*, 18 January 1918, p. 8.

90 Glyn Harper (ed.), *Letters from the Battlefield: New Zealand Soldiers Write Home 1914–1918* (Auckland: HarperCollins, 2001), pp. 120–30; Edwin Farrell file, 6/1838, ANZ.

91 3rd New Zealand Field Ambulance — War Diary, 1 April 1916–4 February 1919, WA 121 176 [121a], ANZ.

92 Carbery, *Medical Service*, p. 168; Memories of Norman E. Hassell.

93 *Evening Star*, 21 December 1916, p. 5.

94 Medical Corps Memoranda — Precis of Events in France, 10 June–31 December 1917, WA10 20, 10/6/12, ANZ.

95 *Hawera & Normanby Star*, 21 February 1917, p. 5.

96 *Timaru Herald*, 1 January 1917, p. 3.

97 Bergen, *Helpless Sight*, p. 299.

98 Weston, *Three Years*, Chapter XIII.

99 Austin, *Rifle Brigade*, p. 564.

100 *Dominion*, 23 August 1916, p. 6.

101 *Dominion*, 8 February 1917, p. 6.

102 *Timaru Herald*, 1 January 1917, p. 3.

103 PH stood for phenate hexamine, which offered protection against chlorine and phosgene gas.

104 Carbery, *Medical Service*, p. 297.

105 Wilson diary, pp. 66–7.

106 Weston, *Three Years*, Chapter XIII. There was another aspect to the German bearer assistance, as the New Zealand Rifle Brigade 'repeatedly observed': 'many German prisoners came back with brand-new brassards, the badges of the medical service, upon their arm . . . When the German medical officer was asked why the men donned them . . . when our troops were close up to them, he stated that everyone in the German army went through various courses of training, and that when a man had completed a course in first-aid he was entitled to wear a Red Cross brassard. Many of the Germans evidently treasured these as a safeguard to be used as a last resort.' Austin, *Rifle Brigade*, pp. 560–1.

107 *Dominion*, 8 February 1917, p. 6.

108 Robson documents.

109 Tolerton, *Awfully Big Adventure*, p. 119.

110 Figures courtesy Glyn Harper, pers. comm., 19 March 2018.

111 McGibbon (ed.), *Oxford Companion*, p. 55.

112 Burton, *One Man's War*, p. 377; Bergen, *Helpless Sight*, p. 92.

113 Moloney diary.

114 During October, 3140 sick men from the New Zealand Division were evacuated to CCSs. 'The principal diseases were Local Septic conditions and Skin Disease, Myalgia, Diseases of the Respiratory and Digestive Systems. P.I.O. and Diarrhoea were very prevalent and there was a marked incidence of Diseases of the Nervous Syst. . . . Generally, the sickness wastage was considerably higher than at the Somme in 1916.' Medical Corps Memoranda — Precis of Events in France, 10 June–31 December 1917, WA10 20, 10/6/12, ANZ.

115 Night of 11/12 October 1917, Medical Corps Memoranda — Precis of Events in France, 10 June–31 December 1917, WA 10 20, 10/6/12, ANZ.

116 Moloney diary; 'Sydney Stanfield remembers Passchendaele'.

117 Report from Captain McGhie to Major McCormick, 14 October 1917, Medical Corps Memoranda — Precis of Events in France, 10 June–31 December 1917, WA 10 20, 10/6/12, ANZ.

118 Col. Begg DDMS, II Anzac Corps Report on Medical Aspect of Operations 1–18 October 1917, Medical Corps Memoranda — Precis of Events in France, 10 June–31 December 1917, WA 10 20, 10/6/12, ANZ.

119 Estimate of Wastage New Zealand Division, Medical Corps Memoranda — Precis of Events in France, 10 June–31 December 1917, WA 10 20, 10/6/12, ANZ; Carbery, *Medical Service*, p. 363.

120 Godley to Allen, 16 October 1917, [Correspondence between] General Sir Alexander Godley [Commander New Zealand Expeditionary Force] and Colonel Hon. Sir James Allen, Minister of Defence, 6 January–28 December 1917, WA 252 1 [4], ANZ; Medical Corps Memoranda — Precis of Events in France, 10 June–31 December 1917, WA 10 20, 10/6/12, ANZ.

121 Carbery, *Medical Service*, pp. 521–5.

122 Diary 22 September 1916, Gray papers, folder 2.

123 *North Otago Times*, 25 September 1916, p. 7. Martin wrote an important pamphlet to this effect after serving at Béthune in 1914–15, Ian McGibbon, pers. comm., 23 October 2017.

124 *Dominion*, 8 February 1917, p. 6.

125 Austin, *Rifle Brigade*, p. 544; *Manawatu Standard*, 15 July 1916, p. 5.

126 *Dominion*, 11 July 1918, p. 4.

127 James Ayson Marshall file, 3/1120, ANZ.

128 As Kevin Brown points out, there could be another side to doctor heroism. Gallant acts 'could deprive a whole unit of medical aid, leading to calls for medical officers to be forbidden to expose themselves too recklessly, but heroes continued to be heroes', Brown, *Fighting Fit*, p. 42.

129 Confidential report October 1917, Samuel Llewellyn Serpell file, 3/2874, ANZ.

130 Austin, *Rifle Brigade*, p. 561.

131 A. L. Logan, Dental Service with the First New Zealand Expeditionary Force, MS-2004, AWMM.

132 Quoted John McGhie file, 3/2123, ANZ; diary 4 November 1916, Gray papers, folder 2.

133 *London Gazette*, 17 December 1917, p. 13201.

134 Glyn Harper and Colin Richardson, *Acts of Valour: The History of the Victoria Cross in New Zealand* (Auckland: HarperCollins, 2016), pp. 166–7.

135 Letter 21 December 1917, Carruthers family: Extracts from letters to Carruthers family/Walter [Carruthers], MS-Papers-4107, ATL.

136 Thomas Parsons file, 3/1184, ANZ.

137 *Manawatu Standard*, 24 July 1917, p. 5.

CHAPTER 7: NOT FAR FROM THE FIGHTING

1 Ian McGibbon, *New Zealand's Western Front Campaign* (Auckland: David Bateman, 2016), pp. 207–8.

2 Ned O'Neill, letter to Bertha Taylor, 22 June 1918, Bertha Emily Taylor, Letters and journal, MS-Papers-1291, ATL. Le Tréport was the British hospital for infectious diseases on the coast. As one New Zealand nurse who worked there reported, 'The hospital is right up on a cliff overlooking the sea, and as the M.O. remarked, "it would be a pretty tough old germ that could hang on while these gales are blowing",' *Kai Tiaki*, July 1917, p. 139.

3 Herbert H. Farrant, Elizabeth Morey and Delysse Storey (eds), *A Strong Sense of Duty: The First World War Letters of Chaplain the Reverend Clive Mortimer Jones 1917–1920* (Auckland: New Zealand Military Historical Society, 2013), p. 65.

4 When McGavin was appointed ADMS in October 1916, he was replaced as head of No. 1 NZSH by E. J. O'Neill.

5 A. D. Carbery, *The New Zealand Medical Service in the Great War, 1914–1918* (Auckland: Whitcombe & Tombs, 1924), p. 190; *Kai Tiaki*, October 1916, p. 201.

6 Carbery, *Medical Service*, p. 190.

7 *Evening Post*, 2 February 1917, p. 2.

8 *Kai Tiaki*, October 1916, p. 196.

9 Ibid., p. 189.

10 L. Ida G. Willis, *A Nurse Remembers: The Life Story of L. Ida G. Willis O.B.E., A.R.R.C., E.D.* (Lower Hutt: A. K. Wilson Ltd, n.d.), pp. 38–9.

11 *Evening Post*, 2 February 1917, p. 2; Carbery, *Medical Service*, p. 191. That month the NZSH admitted 1297 sick and 97 wounded.

12 *Evening Post*, 2 February 1917, p. 2.

13 *Kai Tiaki*, April 1917, p. 75.

14 Quoted Lyn Macdonald, *The Roses of No Man's Land* (Harmondsworth, UK: Penguin Books, 1993, 1st pub. 1980), p. 11; American nurse Ellen La Motte, quoted Leo van Bergen, *Before My Helpless Sight: Suffering, Dying and Military Medicine on the Western Front, 1914–1918* (Surrey: Ashgate, 2009), p. 337.

15 *Kai Tiaki*, October 1916, p. 196.

16 McGibbon, *Western Front*, p. 209.

17 *Kai Tiaki*, January 1917, p. 11.

18 *Kai Tiaki*, July 1917, p. 142.

19 Elsie Prudentia Grey, Diary, MS-Papers-5994, ATL.

20 Rachel Hird, *Good bye Bill Massey No more Khaki: Reg Hird's Letters from the Great War* (Miramar, Wellington: author, 2015), p. 54.

21 *Kai Tiaki*, July 1918, pp. 138–9.

22 *Kai Tiaki*, October 1919, pp. 181, 183.

23 Ibid., p. 183.

24 Ibid.

25 Ibid., p. 185.

26 Letters: Ronald Watson (*Letters From a Padre: A Record of the War Service of Ronald S. Watson. M.C.*, edited by Nigel M. Watson, privately printed, Melbourne), 1998.2491, NAM, pp. 15

27 Thurston to Hester Maclean, 27 July 1917, New Zealand Army Nursing Service — NZANS overseas records, correspondence — Matron-in-chief, AD78 23 67/3/1A, ANZ.

28 *Kai Tiaki*, July 1918, p. 136. The unnamed writer was almost certainly Ida Willis.

29 Carbery, *Medical Service*, p. 302.

30 McGibbon, *Western Front*, p. 224. Cushing 'was to impress observers with his use of a magnet to extract metal fragments from the brains of the injured after X-rays had located them . . . In an attempt to speed things up, he began to use a catheter to suck our depressed bone fragments . . . and operated using a local anaesthetic, talking to the conscious soldier as he performed brain surgery on him.' Kevin Brown, *Fighting Fit: Health, Medicine and War in the Twentieth Century* (Stroud, UK: The History Press, 2008), p. 45.

31 Grey diary.

32 Watson, *Letters from a Padre*, pp. 17, 18.

33 Grey diary.

34 Ibid.

35 *Kai Tiaki*, July 1918, p. 137; McGibbon, *Western Front*, p. 225.

36 Watson, *Letters from a Padre*, p. 18

37 *Kai Tiaki*, April 1919, pp. 65, 66, 67.

38 John Keith Moloney, War diary, MS-Papers-1194, ATL.

39 Willis, *A Nurse Remembers*, p. 44.

40 Carbery, *Medical Service*, p. 497.

41 *Kai Tiaki*, October 1918, p. 171.

42 Taylor, letters and journal.

43 *Taranaki Daily News*, 28 May 1918, p. 7.

44 Glyn Harper (ed.), *Letters From the Battlefield: New Zealand Soldiers Write Home 1914–1918* (Auckland: HarperCollins, 2001), p. 121.

45 Mary Reidy interview with James McNeish, 1969, Sound Archives/Nga Taonga Korero Ref T1327.

46 Harper, *Letters From the Battlefield*, p. 122.

47 C. T. Hand-Newton, DSO, *A Physician in Peace and War* (Christchurch: N. M. Peryer, 1967), p. 47.

48 Taylor, Letters and journal, p. 34.

49 Carbery, *Medical Service*, pp. 497–8.

50 *Kai Tiaki*, April 1919, pp. 64–7.

51 Ibid., p. 68.

52 Ibid., April 1919, pp. 64–7.

53 Letter 16 July 1916, Barbara Mildred Tilly, Papers, MS-Papers-1451, ATL; letter 31 December 1915, Ella Cooke Letters, MS 94/36, AWMM; letter 28 August 1918, Beth Sutherland, *My Dear Chick: A New Zealand Love Story 1911–1948* (Masterton: Fraser Books, 2008), p. 204; Louisa Higginson, Diaries transcribed by Mrs R. L. Wilson, MS-Papers-2477, ATL.

54 *Grey River Argus*, 15 June 1916, p. 4.

CHAPTER 8: A GOOD HOME

1 *Ohinemuri Gazette*, 21 December 1917, p. 3.

2 *Sun*, 17 September 1915, p. 3.

3 *New Zealand Herald*, 23 October 1915, p. 8; *Star*, 30 September 1915, p. 1.

4 *Otago Daily Times*, 5 November 1915, p. 6.

5 *Evening Post*, 29 February 1916, p. 8.

6 Some of the funds for the hospital had come from the 'substantial amount in hand' left over from fitting out the *Maheno*; the governor 'considered himself justified in forwarding the sum to this kindred object'. *Dominion*, 6 October 1915, p. 6.

7 *Press*, 11 September 1915, p. 16; *Press*, 2 October 1915, p. 2.

8 2 New Zealand General Hospital — War Diary, 1 August 1915–31 December 1917, WA141 178 [141a], ANZ.

9 *Press*, 2 October 1915, p. 2.

10 *New Zealand Herald*, 15 September 1915, p. 11.

11 *N.Z. Truth*, 16 September 1916, p. 2.

12 2 New Zealand General Hospital — War Diary, WA141 178 [141a], ANZ. In winter the hospital's location would prove too damp for some tubercular patients.

13 George William Nuttall, Liddle Collection, Brotherton Library, University of Leeds, courtesy Glyn Harper.

14 William Taylor, *The Twilight Hour: A Personal Account of World War I* (Morrinsville: Sutherland, 1978), p. 73.

15 John A. Lee, *Soldier* (Wellington: A. H. & A. W. Reed, 1976), pp. 94, 96; Edna Pengelly, *Nursing in Peace and War* (Wellington: Wingfield Press, 1956), p. 62.

16 Letter 24 November 1918, Letters to the Hutton family from Alexander Louis Hutton, MS-Papers-3906, ATL, folder 4; *Wanganui Chronicle*, 27 July 1917, p. 3. Music could exacerbate loneliness. Clifford Collingwood, lying wounded in a British hospital in Boulogne, was missing his 'old mates very keenly . . . In fact, when music was played in the Ward, more than once I had to cover my face to hide the tears which ran down my face.' Clifford Collingwood, Diary and Scrapbook: New Zealand, Egypt & Western Front — WW1, 2007.139, NAM.

17 2 New Zealand General Hospital War Diary, WA141 178 [141a], ANZ; *Press*, 12 April 1916, p. 9. The NZEF had recently established its own Military Police; William Kingston Wilson, Diary, 1994.2314, NAM, p. 68. My thanks to Ray Grover for alerting me to this material.

18 Lord Plunket, New Zealand War Contingent Association pamphlet, William Massey and Joseph Ward's visit 13 November 1916, Medical Corps Memoranda — Walton on Thames, WA10 18 10/6/9, ANZ.

19 A February 1916 comparison had shown that the much bigger Royal Victoria Military Hospital at Netley, per 300 patients, had 22 sisters, 15 nurses and 45 orderlies. For the same number of beds, excluding the matron and her assistant, and the nurses working in the massage department, Walton had nine sisters, 18 staff nurses, 23 probationers, seven Red Cross probationers and just 15 orderlies. 2 New Zealand General Hospital War Diary, WA141 178 [141a], ANZ.

20 Godley to Allen, 1 November 1916, [Correspondence between] General Sir Alexander Godley [Commander New Zealand Expeditionary Force] and Colonel Hon. Sir James Allen, Minister of Defence, 6 January–28 December 1917, WA 252 1 [4], ANZ.

21 *Press*, 3 July 1919, p. 2.

22 Godley to Allen, 30 June 1916; reply from Allen 4 July 1916, [Correspondence between] General Sir Alexander Godley [Commander New Zealand Expeditionary Force] and Colonel Hon. Sir James Allen, Minister of Defence, WA 252 1 [4], ANZ. Parkes, as DDMS, agreed. In a private letter to Allen on 25 August, he wrote: 'Walton Hospital was not handed over to us with good grace, and considerable resentment was shown . . . However the change of administration was really needed for the patients suffered from over-indulgence and were not amenable to discipline.' Ministerial Files — Correspondence with Colonel Parkes, Allen 1 3, M1/34, ANZ.

23 Parkes to Allen, Ministerial Files — Correspondence with Colonel Parkes, Allen1 3, M1/34, ANZ.

24 *Kai Tiaki*, January 1917, p. 6.

25 Wilson diary, pp. 67–8.

26 Ibid., p. 69.

27 Diary 6, 7 September 1918, Vincent Jervis, MS-Papers-2241, ATL; letter to Fannie 19 October 1918, Letters to the Hutton family from Alexander Louis Hutton, MS-Papers-3906, ATL, folder 4.

28 Letter 20 November 1918, Hutton letters, folder 4; *Evening Post*, 7 March 1917, p. 11.

29 *Kai Tiaki*, October 1917, p. 203.

30 Diary 1 July 1917, Clifford Collingwood, Diary and Scrapbook: New Zealand, Egypt & Western Front — WW1, 2007.139, NAM.

31 Edna Pengelly, *Nursing in Peace and War* (Wellington: Wingfield Press, 1956), pp. 81, 83.

32 Ibid., pp. 76–7; letter 20 November 1918, Hutton letters, folder 4.

33 *Evening Post*, 11 December 1917, p. 7.

34 *Otago Daily Times*, 19 January 1918.

35 *Evening Post*, 6 January 1916, p. 7.

36 Letter 28 October 1916; Cecil Malthus: World War I Papers, http://christchurchcitylibraries.com/Heritage/Digitised/WarsAndConflicts/WorldWarI/Malthus/Thumbnails/.

37 Letter 20 November 1918, Hutton letters, folder 4.

38 William T. Carnes, who had become an amputee after a factory accident, patented his artificial arms from 1911. In the United States they were advertised as the artificial limb 'that puts you back on the payroll'. www.freepatentsonline.com; billingsgazette.com, accessed 12 October 2017. Artificial limbs made by the English firm of Chas. A Blatchford & Sons, founded in 1890, were also popular.

39 *Otago Daily Times*, 19 January 1918.

40 *Press*, 3 March 1917, p. 7.

41 *New Zealand Herald*, 5 November 1915, p. 6.

42 Lee, *Soldier*, pp. 90–1, 125.

43 Pengelly, *Nursing*, p. 52.

44 Nicholas Boyack and Jane Tolerton, *In the Shadow of War: New Zealand Soldiers Talk About World War One and Their Lives* (Auckland: Penguin Books, 1990), pp. 100–1.

45 In fact, as Carbery pointed out, because Walton and Brockenhurst served only the New Zealand Division, 'at times in a quiet sector, at times engaged in costly fighting, the admissions were so irregular as to necessitate breathless spells of work during active operations and comparative inactivity at other times', A. D. Carbery, *The New Zealand Medical Service in the Great War, 1914–1918* (Auckland: Whitcombe & Tombs, 1924), p. 371.

46 Pengelly, *Nursing*, pp. 60, 62–3.

47 *Kai Tiaki*, January 1918, p. 12.

48 Letter 4 September 1917, William Mandeno Smallfield, War Letters, Diaries and Papers, MS 2007/37, AWMM.

49 *Dominion*, 3 February 1917, p. 10.

50 *Northern Advocate*, 16 January 1919, p. 1.

51 Letter 23 September 1918, Hutton letters, folder 4; *Kai Tiaki*, January 1918, p. 9.

52 *Northern Advocate*, 16 January 1919, p. 1.

53 Diary 4 July 1917, Collingwood diary and scrapbook.

54 Letter 8 September 1918, Hutton letters, folder 3; letter 29 November 1916, Malthus papers.

55 Carbery, *Medical Service*, p. 487.

56 Letter Barnett to Henderson 12 April 1917, William Marshall Macdonald file, 3/3305, ANZ.

57 Carbery, *Medical Service*, p. 370.

58 *Press*, 27 July 1916, p. 2.

59 New Zealand Convalescent Hospital — War Diary, 6 July 1916–28 December 1917, WA146 178/[146a], ANZ.

60 Ian McGibbon, *New Zealand's Western Front Campaign* (Auckland: David Bateman, 2016), p. 36.

61 Letters 29 November, 14 December 1916, Malthus papers.

62 Rifleman Gladstone (Gladdie) Graham, Letters: Egypt, France, England — WW1, 2005.585, NAM.

63 *Wanganui Herald*, 16 October 1916, p. 6.

64 Elsie Prudentia Grey, Diary, MS-Papers-5994, ATL.

65 Collection — Sister Mabel Crook — WW1, 2016.280.1, NAM.

66 *Kai Tiaki*, October 1917, p. 193.

67 *Press*, 10 January 1917, p. 6.

68 Bertha Emily Taylor, Letters and journal, MS-Papers-1291, ATL.

69 Beth Sutherland, *My Dear Chick: A New Zealand Love Story 1911–1948* (Masterton: Fraser Books, 2008), p. 102.

70 Grey diary; John Keith Moloney War diary, MS-Papers-1194, ATL.

71 New Zealand Convalescent Hospital — War Diary, 6 July 1916–28 December 1917, WA146 178/[146a], ANZ.

72 Carbery, *Medical Service*, p. 372.

73 Moloney diary.

74 3 New Zealand General War Diary 1 January–31 December 1918, WA142178 [142d], ANZ.

75 *Taranaki Herald*, 28 January 1919, p. 5.

76 *Hawera & Normanby Star*, 19 May 1917. Jack Johnson was the first African-American world heavyweight boxing champion, holding the title from 1908 to 1915.

77 New Zealand Convalescent Hospital — War Diary, 6 July 1916–28 December 1917, WA146 178/[146a], ANZ.

78 Ibid.

79 New Zealand Convalescent Hospital — War Diary, 1 January–31 December 1918, WA146 178 [146h], ANZ. In her 1918 article on Hornchurch, Hilda Keane noted that Aucklander Walter Hill, 'well-known before his soldiering as an especially skilled farmer', had, since recovering from illness at Hornchurch, 'become the instructor, with a success that amounts to genius, of garden work. He has revolutionised the life of the men . . . they grow all the required vegetables and crops, and their enthusiasm is one of the most infectious results of the war. He is simply invaluable to the authorities.' *New Zealand Herald*, 22 June 1918, supplement. p. 1.

80 New Zealand Officers' Convalescent Home, Brighton — War Diary, 1 January 1915–31 December 1917, WA145 178, 145a, ANZ.

81 Lieutenant-Colonel Myers, 'The New Zealand Hospitals in the United Kingdom', in H. T. B. Drew (ed.), *The War Effort of New Zealand* (Auckland: Whitcombe & Tombs, 1923), pp. 125–6.

82 Letter 16 November 1918, Letters: Ronald Watson (*Letters from a Padre: A Record of the War Service of Ronald S. Watson. M.C.*, edited by Nigel M. Watson, privately printed, Melbourne), 1998.2491, NAM.

83 Mabel Thurston to Hester Maclean, 21 September 1918, New Zealand Army Nursing Service — NZANS overseas records, correspondence — Matron-in-chief, AD78 23 67/3/1A, ANZ.

84 Pengelly, *Nursing*, p. 71.

85 Godley to Allen, 24 March 1916, [Correspondence between] General Sir Alexander Godley [Commander New Zealand Expeditionary Force] and Colonel Hon. Sir James Allen, Minister of Defence, 6 January–28 December 1917, WA 252 1 [4], ANZ.

86 Godley to Allen, 1 November 1916, /11/16, WA 252 1 [4], ANZ. Bertha Nurse's story, as revealed in her personnel file, is a sad one. She had received a RRC in Egypt and Hester Maclean defended her, but she does seem to have had problems exercising leadership. 'In a smaller sphere,' Parkes wrote to Surgeon-General Henderson on 12 July 1917, 'her work would probably be satisfactory but as matron of a General Hospital she was overweighed by the responsibility, hence the unfortunate result.' Bertha Grace Nurse file, 22/1, ANZ.

87 Cable, Mackenzie to Massey 28 August 1915, Medical — Hospital — Walton-on-Thames — General file, AD1 965 49/116, ANZ; Diary — Henry M. Clark — NZ Hospital — England — WW1, 1993.1000, NAM.

88 Edward O'Neill letter, 1 March 1918, Taylor, letters and journal. As Henry Pickerill wrote to Allen from Sidcup on 11 January 1918, 'I think our patients are quite comfortable & happy though they might not get quite as well fed & the discipline may be a little more strict.' Medical — Dental hospital — England — Sidcup (Queens Hospital), AD1 971, 49/229, ANZ.

89 Letter 15 September 1915, Kitson letters and diary.

90 Ibid.; Wilson diary; letter 13 September 1918, Hutton letters, folder 4.

91 O'Neill letter, 1 March 1918; letter 21 August 1917, Smallfield war letters, diary and papers.

92 Letter 5 October 1916, Malthus papers; *Southland Times*, 3 November 1916, p. 2; letter 19 October 1918, Hutton letters, folder 4. This had also happened on Gallipoli. Late in October 1915, at a sick parade, William McAra 'sent a man Fraser to hospital. He remembered me in Mataura where he was buyer for Borthwick & Sons.' Diary of William McAra, Gallipoli, June–December 1915, MS-2943/002, Hocken.

93 Fanny Helena Speedy diaries, MS-Papers-1703, ATL.

94 Myers, 'New Zealand Hospitals', p. 126.

95 *Kai Tiaki*, October 1919, p. 180.

96 Myers, 'New Zealand Hospitals', p. 119.

97 http://blog.tepapa.govt.nz/2011/09/05/stories-from-the-first-world-war-soldiers-commemorated-at-walton-on-thames/, accessed 12 October 2017; *Wairarapa Daily Times*, 25 November 1918, p. 4.

98 Roughly half died of wounds and half of disease, though some suffered from both. Of the 12 Māori soldiers interred here, 10 died of tuberculosis or pneumonia. Clare Church, *New Zealand Graves at Brockenhurst: 93 Soldiers Remembered from World War One* (Lymington: Elizabeth Church, 2002), pp. 37–8.

99 Collection Sydney A. Davies 4/895, 2006.1294, NAM.

CHAPTER 9: SAFE AT SEA

1 John Macbeth Russell Reminiscences, MS-Papers-1696, ATL.

2 Newspapers had reported in early May that the Admiralty had acquired the steamer *Karoola* as Australia's first hospital ship and was sending her to the Dardanelles, but she continued to function as a troop transport until fitted out for her new role in August 1915. Peter Plowman, *Coast to Coast: The Great Australian Coastal Liners* (New South Wales: Rosenberg, 2007), pp. 60–1.

3 *Wanganui Herald*, 19 May 1915, p. 7.

4 *Press*, 19 May 1915, p. 8.

5 *Ashburton Guardian*, 20 May 1915, p. 2.

6 *Poverty Bay Herald*, 5 August 1915, p. 9.

7 *Auckland Star*, 20 May 1915, p. 2.

8 *Dominion*, 21 May 1915, p. 2; *Poverty Bay Herald*, 25 May 1915, p. 3; *Wanganui Chronicle*, 25 May 1915, p. 5.

9 *Wanganui Herald*, 1 July 1918, p. 7.

10 *Evening Star*, 26 May 1915, p. 5.

11 *Ashburton Guardian*, 5 August 1915, p. 3.

12 *Evening Post*, 5 July 1915, p. 8.

13 *Kai Tiaki*, July 1915, p. 130.

14 Godley to Allen, 3 September 1915, [Correspondence between] General Sir Alexander Godley [Commander New Zealand Expeditionary Force] and Colonel Hon. Sir James Allen, Minister of Defence, 2 April–19 December 1915, WA 252 1 [2], ANZ.

15 *Evening Post*, 12 July 1915, p. 2; Uniforms, etc — Dress — NZAMC, AD 1 750 13/266, ANZ.

16 *Kai Tiaki*, October 1915, p. 171.

17 *Kai Tiaki*, April 1916, p. 84.

18 Collection of 3/2643 Private Eric Sidney Bardell, Diary of the First trip of the 5th Charter of H.M.N.Z.S. "Maheno" July 6th to October 22nd 1918, 1996.1682.1, NAM.

19 William Barclay Memoirs, 2000.980, NAM.

20 L. Ida G. Willis, *A Nurse Remembers: The Life Story of L. Ida G. Willis O.B.E., A.R.R.C., E.D.* (Lower Hutt: A. K. Wilson Ltd, n.d.), p. 25; Anon. ['Aunt Jane'], 'We go through the Red Sea, Nursing in World War I', MS-99/57, AWMM.

21 Diary of Michael O'Malley 3/799 NZMC *Maheno*, 1991.1278, NAM.

22 Private S. G. Gibb NZMC, Diary from 25.5.15 to 9.9.19; Russell Reminiscences, p. 37.

23 John D. Duder, Papers, 82/8, MS-1160, NAM.

24 O'Malley diary; *Manawatu Standard*, 14 January 1916, p. 2.

25 Extract, letter 31 August 1915, from Staff Sergeant Clarence Ernest Schofield NZMC 3/821, History of the War (Gallipoli — Medical —1915), AD78 27 G15/25, ANZ.

26 28 August 1915, O'Malley diary.

27 Quoted Norma Chick and Jan Rodgers (eds), *Looking Back, Moving Forward: Essays in the History of New Zealand Nursing and Midwifery* (Palmerston North: Department of Nursing and Midwifery, Massey University, 1997), p. 60.

28 29 August 1915, O'Malley diary.

29 *Kai Tiaki*, April 1916, p. 78.

30 *Kai Tiaki*, January 1916, pp. 18–19.

31 O'Malley diary.

32 3 September 1915, Diaries of A. M. Trotter/transcribed by A. A. S. Trotter, MS-3397/004, Hocken.

33 10 November 1915, Diary of William McAra, Gallipoli, June–December 1915, MS-2943/002, Hocken.

34 *Auckland Star*, 1 January 1916, p. 9.

35 8 December 1915, O'Malley diary.

36 *Auckland Star*, 1 January 1916, p. 9.

37 Allen to Godley, 4 January 1916, Ministerial Files — Correspondence with General Godley, Allen 1 1 M1/15 1, ANZ.

38 *Auckland Star*, 11 April 1916, p. 6. Goldien seems to have managed to work after the war: when he died in 1947 he was described as a retired farm labourer.

39 Diary 13 July 1917, Clifford Collingwood, Diary and Scrapbook: New Zealand, Egypt & Western Front — WW1, 2007.139, NAM.

40 Gavin McLean, *The White Ships: New Zealand's First World War Hospital Ships* (Wellington: New Zealand Ship & Marine Society, 2013), p. 114. That week, New Zealand nurses were also working on British hospital ships. Kate Barnitt was on the *Oxfordshire*: 'on one voyage we carried 1500 patients — all surgical. Oh! the wounds, and the bravery of the men when their wounds were being dressed, and the excitement of the men as they neared Blighty,' *Kai Tiaki*, April 1917, p. 74.

41 His Excellency the Earl of Liverpool (comp.), *The Voyages of His Majesty's New Zealand Hospital Ships 'Marama' and 'Maheno' (Second Volume)* (Auckland et al.: Whitcombe & Tombs, 1917), pp. 140–3.

42 Barclay memoirs.

43 Liverpool, *Voyages*, p. 143.

44 *Auckland Star*, 22 April 1919, p. 6.

45 *Press*, 21 September 1915, p. 6.

46 Godley to Allen, 20 September 1915, [Correspondence between] General Sir Alexander Godley [Commander New Zealand Expeditionary Force] and Colonel Hon. Sir James Allen, Minister of Defence, 2 April–19 December 1915, WA 252 1 [2], ANZ.

47 McLean, *White Ships*, pp. 100–1.

48 *Kai Tiaki*, January 1916, p. 14; Godley to Sir James Wilson, 7 June 1916, Semi-personal letters by General Officer Commanding, 5 September 1914–31 October 1916, WA 252 3 [6], ANZ.

49 *Kai Tiaki*, October 1915, p. 201; *Kai Tiaki*, July 1917, p. 133.

50 Letters before Christmas 1915, 29 January 1916, Barbara Mildred Tilly, Papers, MS-Papers-1451, ATL.

51 *Kai Tiaki*, October 1916, p. 202.

52 Ibid., p. 201.

53 *Kai Tiaki*, January 1916, p. 19.

54 Letter 12 August 1916, Tilly papers.

55 Bertha Emily Taylor, Letters and Journal, MS-Papers-1291, ATL.

56 3 May 1917, Gibb diary.

57 *Kai Tiaki*, July 1917, p. 145.

58 Collingwood, diary and scrapbook.

59 *Kai Tiaki*, October 1917, p. 201.

60 Lieutenant-Colonel J. S. Elliott, 'The New Zealand Hospital Ships', in H. T. B. Drew (ed.), *The War Effort of New Zealand* (Auckland: Whitcombe & Tombs, 1923), p. 136.

61 Bardell collection.

62 *Kai Tiaki*, October 1917, p. 201; *Evening Star*, 27 August 1917, p. 4.

63 *Dominion*, 30 April 1918, p. 6.

64 *Auckland Star*, 27 January 1919, p. 6.

65 McLean, *White Ships*, p. 6.

66 *Evening Star*, 24 December 1919, p. 8.

67 Collingwood, diary and scrapbook.

68 Of the 13 invalided men, at least three had syphilis and were discharged. At least two had neurasthenia: one was discharged and one later re-enlisted. Orien Knight, who had been sent home with a 'rheumatic heart', died in 1918, as did William Barman, who had chronic eczema.

69 Plowman, *Coast to Coast*, p. 60.

70 *New Zealand Herald*, 14 July 1915, p. 4.

71 *Evening Star*, 15 July 1915, p. 6.

72 Allen to Godley 17 July 1915, [Correspondence between] General Sir Alexander Godley [Commander New Zealand Expeditionary Force] and Colonel Hon. Sir James Allen, Minister of Defence, 2 April–19 December 1915, WA 252 1 [2], ANZ.

73 *Press*, 14 August 1915, p. 12.

74 *Evening Post*, 11 September 1915, p. 4.

75 Imelda Bargas and Tim Shoebridge, *New Zealand's First World War Heritage* (Auckland and Wollombi: Exisle, 2015), p. 135.

76 Allen to Godley, 20 September 1915, [Correspondence between] General Sir Alexander Godley [Commander New Zealand Expeditionary Force] and Colonel Hon. Sir James Allen, Minister of Defence, 2 April–19 December 1915, WA 252 1 [2], ANZ.

77 12 July 1915, McAra diary; Crowther Garside file, 6/2137, ANZ.

78 *Kai Tiaki*, April 1918, p. 67.

79 Frederick James Foote, 'Yesteryears', Reminiscences, MS 2007/9, NAM.

80 *Kai Tiaki*, April 1918, p. 67.

81 Ibid.

82 *Free Lance*, 4 February 2016, p. 14.

83 *Press*, 22 April 1916, p. 7.

84 Memories of Norman E. Hassell, Window into WW1, Palmerston North City Library, http://ww1.pncc.govt.nz/blog/2015/11/18/object-memories-of-1914-norman-e-hassell.

85 *Kai Tiaki*, April 1916, p. 79.

86 Collection — Sister Mabel Crook — WW1, 1979.5805, NAM.

87 A. D. Carbery, *The New Zealand Medical Service in the Great War, 1914–1918* (Auckland: Whitcombe & Tombs, 1924), p. 494.

88 Collingwood, diary and scrapbook.

89 *Auckland Star*, 15 July 1915, p. 2.

90 *Dominion*, 17 March 1916, p. 6.

91 *Kai Tiaki*, January 1916, pp. 49–51.

92 Collingwood, diary and scrapbook.

CHAPTER 10: TEETH TROUBLE

1 *Sun*, 17 August 1914, p. 8.

2 *Ashburton Guardian*, 13 August 1914, p. 6.

3 *Marlborough Express*, 17 August 1914, p. 2; Christopher Pugsley, *Gallipoli: The New Zealand Story* (Libro International and Pen & Sword Books, 5th edn, 2014, 1st pub. 1984), p. 48.

4 Charles Wallace Saunders: World War I diary, Misc-MS-0267, Hocken. Saunders also failed to mention the loose cartilage in his right knee caused by a sporting injury. He was later forced to put this back into place himself.

5 *Hastings Standard*, 21 July 1911, p. 11.

6 *Maoriland Worker*, 5 August 1914, p. 8.

7 Geoffrey Victor Wild, Diary and Letters Relating to War Service (compiled Dorothy Wakelin), MS 2004/59, AWMM.

8 *Wanganui Chronicle*, 7 August 1914, p. 4.

9 *Akaroa Mail & Banks Peninsula Advertiser*, 11 August 1914, p. 3.

10 Frederick James Foote, 'Yesteryears', Reminiscences, MS 2007/9, AWMM.

11 *Press*, 7 September 1914, p. 9.

12 Lieutenant-Colonel T. A. Hunter, 'New Zealand Dental Corps' in H. T. B. Drew (ed.), *The War Effort of New Zealand* (Auckland: Whitcombe & Tombs, 1923), p. 141.

13 A. L. Logan, Dental Service with the First New Zealand Expeditionary Force, MS-2004, AWMM, p. 2.

14 Hunter, 'Dental Corps', p. 141.

15 Quoted Pugsley, *Gallipoli*, p. 66. Such vigorous treatment was not unknown on the Western Front: when Vincent Jervis had three 'old stumps' yanked out, as he put it, at Hazebrouck in March 1918, 'I thought my head was coming off with the last', 1 March 1918, Vincent Jervis, MS-Papers-2241, ATL.

16 *Clutha Leader*, 17 November 1914, p. 7.

17 Logan, Dental Service, p. 4.

18 Hunter, 'Dental Corps', p. 141.

19 Christopher Pugsley and Charles Ferrall (eds), *Remembering Gallipoli: Interviews with New Zealand Gallipoli Veterans* (Wellington: Victoria University Press, 2015), p. 246.

20 Diary Captain J. A. Berry NZMC, England & Western Front — WW1, 2000.727, NAM.

21 William Kingston Wilson, Diary, 1994.2314, NAM, p. 21. My thanks to Ray Grover for alerting me to this material.

22 Logan, Dental Service, pp. 21–2.

23 Ibid., p. 27.

24 Hunter, 'Dental Corps', p. 42.

25 A. D. Carbery, *The New Zealand Medical Service in the Great War, 1914–1918* (Auckland: Whitcombe & Tombs, 1924), p. 60.

26 *Ashburton Guardian*, 18 May 1918, p. 2. McKenzie also took a turn acting as sanitary officer at Anzac Cove and, said Fenwick, 'a very excellent one he is, tremendously energetic and very outspoken'. Lieutenant-Colonel Dr Percival Fenwick, *Gallipoli Diary* (Auckland: David Ling in association with Auckland War Memorial Museum, c.2000), 23 May 1915, p. 65.

27 Hunter, 'Dental Corps', p. 142.

28 *Ashburton Guardian*, 18 May 1918, p. 2.

29 John Macbeth Russell Reminiscences, MS-Papers-1696, ATL; Ormond Burton, 'Army Biscuits', *The Anzac Book, Written and Illustrated in Gallipoli by The Men of ANZAC* (London, New York, Toronto and Melbourne: Cassell and Company Ltd, 1916), p. 61.

30 Jan Chamberlin, *Shrapnel and Semaphore: My Grandfather's Diary of Gallipoli* (Auckland: RadioWorks, 2001), pp. 14–29.

31 Ibid., p. 52.

32 Diary 19 May 1918, The Diary of Cervantes Jason Bell, Service in Mesopotamia December 1916 to May 1918, transcribed by Jane Hall, née Bell, courtesy Glyn Harper.

33 William Mandeno Smallfield, War Letters, Diaries and Papers, MS 2007/37, AWMM.

34 O. E. Burton, *The Silent Division: New Zealanders at the Front: 1914–1919 & Concerning One Man's War*, ed. John H. Gray (Christchurch: John Douglas Publishing, 2014), *One Man's War*, p. 416.

35 Foote, 'Yesteryears'.

36 25 July 1915, Ross McCandlish (compiler), 'Between the Lines: The Diary and Letters of 11/92 Trooper Roderick McCandlish, Wellington Mounted Rifles', www.nzmr.org/McCandlish.

37 Carbery, *Medical Service*, p. 127.

38 *West Coast Times*, 8 December 1915, p. 2; 1st Field Ambulance — War Diary, 11 Aug 1914–18 Feb 1919, WA119 173 [119r], ANZ.

39 24 October 1915, Diary of William McAra, Gallipoli, June–December 1915, MS-2943/002, Hocken.

40 Logan, Dental Service, pp. 69–71.

41 Medical Corps Memoranda — Gallipoli & Egypt, April 1916–2 March 1919, WA10 17 10/6/8, ANZ.

42 Carbery, *Medical Service*, p. 123.

43 *North Otago Times*, 6 December 1915, p. 3.

44 Bertram Sibbald Finn, 12/591, http://www.aucklandmuseum.com/war-memorial/online-cenotaph; Logan, Dental Service, p. 94. Finn, who also served in the Second World War, was made a CBE in 1945.

45 Letter 7 January 1916, Thomson papers.

46 Frederick Stanley Welsh file, 4/859, ANZ.

47 Hunter, 'Dental Corps', p. 138.

48 *Dominion*, 23 October 1915, p. 3.

49 Godley to Allen, 19 November 1915, [Correspondence between] General Sir Alexander Godley [Commander New Zealand Expeditionary Force] and Colonel Hon. Sir James Allen, Minister of Defence, 2 April–19 December 1915, WA 252 1 [2], ANZ.

50 *Free Lance*, 19 November 1915, p. 22.

51 Hunter, 'Dental Corps', pp. 139–40. Civilian dentists and corps dentists in the camps filled 6335 teeth, took out 5237 extractions and made 854 dentures.

52 *Sun*, 14 November 1916, p. 6; Will Lawson, *Historic Trentham, 1914–1917: The Story of a New Zealand Military Training Camp, and Some Account of the Daily Round of the Troops within its Bounds* (Wellington: Wellington Publishing Company, 1917).

53 *Observer*, 3 November 1917, p. 2.

54 *Evening Post*, 11 August 1919, p. 2.

55 Carbery, *Medical Service*, pp. 263–4.

56 *Auckland Star*, 15 May 1917, p. 7.

57 Logan, Dental Service, p. 97.

58 1st Field Ambulance — War Diary, 11 Aug 1914–18 Feb 1919, WA119 173 [119r], ANZ.

59 Carbery, *Medical Service*, p. 146.

60 2nd New Zealand Field Ambulance — War Diary, 26 March 1916–25 March 1919, WA 120 174 [120a], ANZ.

61 Diary of Events April 11th to 30th 1916 Medical Corps Memoranda — Precis of events in France, 11 April 1916–10 June 1917, WA10 19, 10/6/10, ANZ; 2nd New Zealand Field Ambulance — War Diary, 26 March 1916–25 March 1919, WA 120 174 [120a] [29/5], ANZ; also Carbery, *Medical Service*, p. 179, and Hunter, 'Dental Corps', p. 143.

62 Logan, Dental Service, p. 114.

63 Ibid., p. 119.

64 Carbery, *Medical Service*, p. 237.

65 Logan, Dental Service, p. 128.

66 Carbery, *Medical Service*, p. 238.

67 Logan, Dental Service, p. 130.

68 *Ashburton Guardian*, 18 May 1918, p. 2.

69 Russell Reminiscences, p. 168.

70 Logan, Dental Service, p. 153.

71 Ibid., pp. 132, 131, 141.

72 *Ashburton Guardian*, 18 May 1918, p. 2.

73 William Habberfield Short, War Diary, MS-2006-40, AWMM; letter 11 March 1918, Smallfield letters, diary and papers.

74 Carbery, *Medical Service*, p. 323.

75 Hunter, 'Dental Corps', p. 145.

76 Clifford Collingwood, Diary and Scrapbook: New Zealand, Egypt & Western Front — WW1, 2007.139, NAM.

77 New Zealand Section, Queen's Hospital [Sidcup] — War Diary, 12 January–9 July 1918, WA143 178, [143A], ANZ.

78 Logan, Dental Service, pp. 201, 200.

79 *Ashburton Guardian*, 18 May 1918, p. 2. The statistics were impressive. Between September 1914 and the end of January 1918, there were 57,257 extractions, 73,066 fillings, 8324 root fillings, 23,614 minor operations, 21,565 dentures and 15,212 repairs. The total number of patients treated was 114,677. Those figures, Ross pointed out, did not include the work done by the New Zealand dentists lent to the British and Australians on Gallipoli and in Egypt for eight months.

80 Arther Lunan Logan file, 11/721a, ANZ.

81 *Free Lance*, 15 June 1917, p. 4.

82 *Evening Post*, 22 November 1918, p. 8.

83 *Evening Post*, 4 December 1918, p. 2.

84 David Nathan Isaacs file, 3/72, ANZ.

85 *Wairarapa Age*, 25 January 1918, p. 5.

86 Charles Kay Ward file, 3/71, ANZ.

CHAPTER 11: CARING FOR THE ANIMALS

1 'New Zealand's First World War horses', https://nzhistory.govt.nz/war/nz-first-world-war-horses, (Ministry for Culture and Heritage), updated 8-Nov-2016.

2 This applied in all the armies of the First World War. 'Martin Gilbert calculates that in the years 1914 to 1918 more than half a million horses died violent deaths, drowned or succumbed to sickness and exhaustion. This may be a conservative estimate . . . 375,000 horses . . . died in the war on the British side alone.' Leo van Bergen, *Before My Helpless Sight: Suffering, Dying and Military Medicine on the Western Front, 1914–1918* (Surrey: Ashgate, 2009), p. 26.

3 *Dominion*, 18 April 1908, p. 12. The other PVOs were Majors John Clayton, Joseph Lyons, Charles Neale, Charles Sanderson, William Snowball and Alexander Young, and Captains Peter Edgar and Herbert Kyle. Also gazetted as officers in 1908 were Captains Alexander Brodie, Samuel Burton, John Charlton, Thomas Lilico, Henry Marsack, George Owen, Thoric Palgrave, Donald Rait, Harry Reid and Frederick Robertson. (Sanderson and Palgrave resigned their commissions in 1910.) www.nzmr.org.

4 Dr. C. J. Reakes, 'New Zealand Veterinary Corps', in H. T. B. Drew (ed.), *The War Effort of New Zealand* (Auckland: Whitcombe & Tombs, 1923), p. 151.

5 *Dominion*, 24 September 1915, p. 1; Defence Forces of New Zealand, Report of the General Officer Commanding the Forces from 26th June, 1915, to 31st May, 1916, *AJHR*, 1916 Session I, H-19, p. 14.

6 Reakes, 'Veterinary Corps', pp. 151–3. The average price paid was £17 1s 10d for riding horses and £24 10s for artillery horses.

7 *Dominion*, 10 August 1914, p. 6.

8 Reakes, 'Veterinary Corps', p. 151.

9 *Dominion*, 8 November 1916, p. 6.

10 Letter 22 December 1914, Letters: Thomas E. Catchpole — Egypt & Gallipoli — WW1, 2000.316, NAM; A. D. Carbery, *The New Zealand Medical Service in the Great War, 1914–1918* (Auckland: Whitcombe & Tombs, 1924), p. 29.

11 Following the South African War, 'most A&P shows held classes to judge horses suitable for military purposes'. Carolyn Jean Mincham, 'A Social and Cultural History of the New Zealand Horse', PhD thesis, History, Massey University, 2008, p. 164.

12 Reakes, 'Veterinary Corps', p. 153.

13 Strangles (*Streptococcus equi*) is characterised by severe inflammation of the upper respiratory tract with abscess formation of the adjacent lymph glands. It is very debilitating and can lead to pneumonia and death. It is a particular problem when horses are together. Poor feeding and cold, damp weather can also increase horses' vulnerability to the disease. Neil Bruere, pers. comm., 9 August 2016.

14 C. G. Nicol, *The Story of Two Campaigns: Official War History of the Auckland Mounted Rifles Regiment, 1914–1919* (Auckland: Wilson & Horton, 1921), pp. 6–7.

15 Terry Kinloch, *Echoes of Gallipoli: In the Words of New Zealand's Mounted Riflemen* (Auckland: Exisle Publishing, 2005), p. 35.

16 Imelda Bargas and Tim Shoebridge, *New Zealand's First World War Heritage* (Auckland and Wollombi: Exisle, 2015), p. 62.

17 Geoffrey Victor Wild, Diary and Letters Relating to War Service (compiled Dorothy Wakelin), MS 2004/59, AWMM, p. 7.

18 Bargas and Shoebridge, *Heritage*, p. 62.

19 'German Samoa', https://nzhistory.govt.nz/war/nz-first-world-war-horses/german-samoa, (Ministry for Culture and Heritage), updated 27-Aug-2014.

20 Horses, mules, etc. — Horses for Samoa — Supply of, AD1 900 40/72, ANZ.

21 Alexander Malcolm Brodie file, 3/2709, ANZ.

22 Brodie report, Horses, mules, etc. — Horses for Samoa — Supply of, AD1 900 40/72, ANZ.

23 'The end of the war', https://nzhistory.govt.nz/war/nz-first-world-war-horses/end-of-the-war, (Ministry for Culture and Heritage), updated 4-Nov-2014.

24 *Feilding Star*, 25 September 1914, p. 4.

25 Defence Forces of New Zealand. Report of the General Officer Commanding the Forces from 26th June,

1915, to 31st May, 1916. *AJHR*, 1916 Session I, H-19, p. 14.

26 Reakes, 'Veterinary Corps', pp. 153–4, 155. According to one newspaper report, experts had 'generally considered that at least 10 per cent of the horses would die on such a lengthy voyage', *Evening Post*, 14 January 1915, p. 2.

27 A. L. Logan, Dental Service with the First New Zealand Expeditionary Force, MS-2004, AWMM, pp. 4–5, 6.

28 Lieutenant-Colonel Dr Percival Fenwick, *Gallipoli Diary* (Auckland: David Ling in association with Auckland War Memorial Museum, c.2000), pp. 22, 98.

29 Nicol, *Two Campaigns*, pp. 14, 17.

30 Logan, Dental Service.

31 Diary Trooper William Rupert Pyle 9/76 Otago Mounted Rifles, 1996.292, NAM.

32 Logan, Dental Service.

33 *New Zealand Herald*, 28 September 1914, p. 7.

34 3 March 1916, report from Captain John Danskin NZVC on *Waihora*, AD1 881 39/140 Reports — Report — Hospital in Egypt, ANZ.

35 Trooper Ben Gainfort, Jane Tolerton, *An Awfully Big Adventure: New Zealand World War One Veterans Tell Their Stories* (Auckland: Penguin, 2013), p. 150.

36 11 November 1914, Diaries of A. M. Trotter/transcribed by A. A. S. Trotter, MS-3397/004, Hocken; Remembering Gallipoli p. 50.

37 Memories of Norman E. Hassell, Window into WW1, Palmerston North City Library, http://ww1.pncc.govt.nz/blog/2015/11/18/object-memories-of-1914-norman-e-hassell.

38 Ibid.

39 27 June 1915, Diary of William McAra, Gallipoli, June–December 1915, MS-2943/002, Hocken.

40 *Te Puke Times*, 13 July 1915, p. 2.

41 Memories of Norman E. Hassell.

42 Nicol, *Two Campaigns*, p. 20; Pyle diary.

43 4 December 1915, Trotter diaries; Justin Aylmer Westenra, Liddle Collection, Brotherton Library, University of Leeds, courtesy Glyn Harper; Kinloch, *Echoes*, p. 75.

44 Reakes, 'Veterinary Corps', p. 155.

45 Catchpole letters, pp. 15–16.

46 *Observer*, 27 February 1915, p. 16; *Southland Times*, 5 April 1916, p. 2.

47 Tolerton, *Awfully Big Adventure*, p. 152; Major J. Stafford, Senior Veterinary Officer, Monthly Report of the New Zealand Veterinary Services (Egypt) for August 1917 and NZMR for month of July 1917 (horses killed in action/died and destroyed), WA10 12, ZMR 10/1/1, ANZ.

48 Frederick James Foote, 'Yesteryears', Reminiscences, MS 2007/9, AWMM, pp. 286–7. Founder or laminitis is a painful inflammation of horses' feet.

49 Kevin Clunie (comp.) and Ron Austin (ed.), *From Gallipoli to Palestine: The War Writings of Sergeant GT Clunie of the Wellington Mounted Rifles, 1914–1919* (McCrae, Victoria: Slouch Hat Publications, 2009), p. 191.

50 Foote, 'Yesteryears', pp. 286–7; letter 20 October 1916, Hubert Hatrick, Liddle Collection, Brotherton Library, University of Leeds, courtesy Glyn Harper.

51 Reakes, 'Veterinary Corps', p. 155; Kinloch, *Echoes*, p. 35.

52 Reakes, 'Veterinary Corps', p. 155; www.nzmr.org.

53 John Crawford (ed.), *The Devil's Own War: The First World War Diary of Brigadier-General Herbert Hart* (Auckland and Wollombi: Exisle in association with the New Zealand Defence Force, 2008), p. 55.

54 'Egypt and Gallipoli', https://nzhistory.govt.nz/war/nz-first-world-war-horses/egypt-gallipoli, (Ministry for Culture and Heritage), updated 29-Jul-2014, accessed 17 February 2017.

55 Pyle diary; 5 May 1915, Trotter diaries: '[W]e are to leave in a few days as infantry. It is very satisfactory to be getting away but there is naturally a lot of dissatisfaction . . . that we should go dismounted.'

56 Diary Vol. 1, 6 May 1915, Thomas Russell Ritchie, Papers, MS-Papers-3705, ATL, folder 1.

57 'Egypt and Gallipoli', https://nzhistory.govt.nz/war/nz-first-world-war-horses/egypt-gallipoli, (Ministry for Culture and Heritage), updated 29-Jul-2014, accessed 17 February 2017.

58 Crawford, *Devil's Own War*, p. 88.

59 Reakes, 'Veterinary Corps', pp. 155–6.

60 Alfred Thomas Stratton, First World War 1916–1918 in France after Gallipoli, MS-Papers-3823, ATL.

61 Catchpole letters, p. 15; *Otago Daily Times*, 2 March 1915, p. 6.

62 Peter Stanley, *Die in Battle, Do Not Despair: The Indians on Gallipoli, 1915* (Solihull, UK: Helion & Co. in association with the United Service Institution of India, 2015), pp. 78, 80, 105; http://i.stuff.co.nz/national/last-post-first-light/79254250/Indian-army-contributed-valiantly-at-Gallipoli, accessed 10 March 2017.

63 Stanley, *Die in Battle*, p. 80. As Australian war correspondent Charles Bean recorded, the mules could be trained to be silent, which added to their value on nocturnal missions. Ibid., p. 275.

64 Letter William John Rusden Hill, 1990.163, NAM.

65 Fenwick, *Gallipoli Diary*, p. 25.

66 Stanley, *Die in Battle*, p. 244.

67 4 May 1915, John H. Thomson, 3/453 No. 1 N.Z. Fd. Amb., Diary from 13 April 1915 to Jan 21st 1916, PC-0316, Hocken; letter 18 June 1915, published in *New Zealand Medical Journal*, vol. 12, no. 45, 1915, republished *New Zealand Medical Journal*, vol. 128, no. 1412, 17 April 2015.

68 Foote, 'Yesteryears', pp. 239–40.

69 27 January 1916, Godley to Lieutenant-Colonel J. E. Watson, 8th Southland Regiment, Invercargill, Semi-personal letters by General Officer Commanding, 5 September 1914–31 October 1916, WA 252 3 [6], ANZ.

70 Reakes, 'Veterinary Corps', p. 156.

71 Foote, 'Yesteryears', p. 239.

72 Ibid., p. 24. Because, unlike cows or sheep, horses nibble with their lips, sand consumption was all too easy. Neil Bruere, pers. comm., 9 August 2016.

73 *Dominion*, 13 March 1916, p. 7; Tolerton, *Awfully Big Adventure*, p. 259; Reakes, 'Veterinary Corps', p. 156.

74 Letters 17 May 1916, 26 June 1944, James Foster Rudd, Liddle Collection, Brotherton Library, University of Leeds, courtesy Glyn Harper.

75 'Taini', 'Work of "Mobile Vets.", *Kia Ora Coo-ee: The Magazine for the Anzacs in the Middle East, 1918*, Second Series, no. 2 (Sydney: Cornstalk Publishing, 1981), 15 August 1918, p. 9; Tolerton, *Awfully Big Adventure*, p. 153; Reakes, 'Veterinary Corps', p. 156.

76 Bell diary.

77 Diary Charles Malone Sinai & Palestine — WW1, 1990.1620, NAM.

78 Reakes, 'Veterinary Corps', p. 157.

79 Interview with veteran of the New Zealand MR, 1964, Sound Archives, Nga Taonga, 158670.

80 Tolerton, *Awfully Big Adventure*, p. 126.

81 'Cameliers and camels at war', https://nzhistory.govt.nz/war/camel-corps/camels-and-cameliers, (Ministry for Culture and Heritage), updated 2-Sep-2014.

82 Letter 20 October 1916, Hatrick.

83 John Robertson, *With the Cameliers in Palestine* (Wellington: A. H. & A. W. Reed, 1938), p. 31.

84 William Kingston Wilson, Diary, 1994.2314, NAM, p. 61.

85 'Western Front', https://nzhistory.govt.nz/war/nz-first-world-war-horses/western-front, (Ministry for Culture and Heritage), updated 15-Apr-2016; Ian M. Parsonson, *Vets at War: A History of the Australian Army Veterinary Corps 1909–1946* (Canberra: Australian Military History Publications, 2005), p. 91.

86 Parsonson, *Vets at War*, p. 91.

87 2nd New Zealand Field Ambulance — War Diary, 26 March 1916–25 March 1919, WA 120 174 [120a], ANZ.

88 Crawford, *Devil's Own War*, p. 210.

89 Beth Sutherland, *My Dear Chick: A New Zealand Love Story 1911–1948* (Masterton: Fraser Books, 2008), p. 191.

90 Letter 18 September 1916, Harold Ernest Kretschmar, War Letters and Diaries, MS 2007/36, AWMM.

91 New Zealand Sanitary Section — War Diary, 7 February 1916–25 February 1919 WA182 196 [182a], ANZ. Efficient disposal of horse manure was also a challenge. It was supposed to be collected and stacked, but this did not always happen as it should have: 'Given a spell of hot weather with the continuance of the present slovenly methods . . . there will be a serious plague of flies.' Diary of Events April 11th to 30th 1916 Medical Corps Memoranda — Precis of events in France, 11 April 1916–10 June 1917, WA10 19, ANZ.

92 Eric Wilson Hames, 'How I Won the Great War', MS 2013/1, AWMM, p. 40; Crawford, *Devil's Own War*, p. 259; Tolerton, *Awfully Big Adventure*, p. 254.

93 Geoffrey Victor Wild, Diary and Letters Relating to War Service (compiled Dorothy Wakelin), MS 2004/59, AWMM, p. 66; Russell diary, p. 116.

94 1st New Zealand Field Ambulance — War Diary, 11 August 1914–18 February 1919, WA119 173 [119r], ANZ.

95 Headquarters New Zealand and Australian Division — New Zealand Division — Assistant Director of Veterinary Services (ADVS) — War Diary, 1 July–31 July 1917, WA27 36 [27m], ANZ.

96 Alexander Wilson, Liddle Collection, Brotherton Library, University of Leeds, courtesy Glyn Harper; 27 September 1916, Clarence Albany Hankins, Diary, MS-Papers-1439, ATL.

97 Memories of Norman E. Hassell, Window into WW1, Palmerston North City Library, http://ww1.pncc.govt.nz/blog/2015/11/18/object-memories-of-1914-norman-e-hassell.

98 26 December 1917, Russell diary, p. 106.

99 Mange in horses is caused by microscopic mites, mainly *Sarcoptes scabiei*, which burrow into the skin and lay many eggs that hatch into nymphs and cause acute irritation. Because the life cycle is quick, about seven to 14 days, animals become infested very rapidly. In the war, congregation of horses, poor husbandry and cold, damp weather all contributed to its spread, and it was very difficult to treat as no effective acaricides were available. The troops did their best to contain the disease by washing the horses in lime sulphur solutions.

100 1st New Zealand Field Ambulance — War Diary, 11 August 1914–18 February 1919, WA119 173 [119r], ANZ; *Observer*, 4 May 1918, p. 18; Crawford, *Devil's Own War*, p. 205.

101 L. P. Leary Q.C., *Not Entirely Legal* (Christchurch: Whitcoulls, 1977) pp. 54–5; L. P. Leary, 'For King and Country', Spectrum 420, Nga Taonga 21534. Another consideration was how much precious food a wounded horse would consume while recovering.

102 Hankins diary; Parsonson, *Vets at War*, p. 94.

103 Ibid., p. 98.

104 Headquarters New Zealand and Australian Division — New Zealand Division — Assistant Director of Veterinary Services (ADVS) — War Diary, 1 April–30 April 1917, WA27 36 [27j], ANZ.

105 Memories of Norman E. Hassell.

106 Reakes, 'Veterinary Corps', p. 161; Parsonson, *Vets at War*, p. 94.

107 *Dominion*, 12 January 1918, p. 8.

108 The Royal Army Veterinary Corps had a number of hospitals on the Western Front, usually in groups comprising a reception hospital, a mange hospital and a general hospital; there were different wards for different cases, such as chest complaints. Some had isolation lines and a contagious diseases yard for infectious illnesses; some even had their own abattoir. http://www.westernfrontassociation.com/education/universities/dissertations-post-graduate/the-care-development-and-importance-of-the-british-horse-on-the-western-front-in-world-war-one.html#, accessed 25 February 2017.

109 Reakes, 'Veterinary Corps', p. 161.

110 Ibid., pp. 159–60.

111 History of No. 4 New Zealand Veterinary Hospital from Formation until the Armistice, WA10 12, ZMR 10/4/1, ANZ.

112 *Dominion*, 25 April 1919, p. 4.

113 'Western Front', https://nzhistory.govt.nz/war/nz-first-world-war-horses/western-front, (Ministry for Culture and Heritage), updated 15-Apr-2016; 'The end of the war', https://nzhistory.govt.nz/war/nz-first-world-war-horses/end-of-the-war, (Ministry for Culture and Heritage), updated 4-Nov-2014.

114 Reakes, 'Veterinary Corps', p. 159.

115 Jean Bou, 'They shot the horses — didn't they?', *Wartime*, no. 44, 2008, pp. 54–7, www.awm.gov.au/wartime/44/page54_bou; Reakes, 'Veterinary Corps', p. 159.

116 Tolerton, *Awfully Big Adventure*, p. 262.

117 'The end of the war', https://nzhistory.govt.nz/war/nz-first-world-war-horses/end-of-the-war (Ministry for Culture and Heritage), updated 4-Nov-2014.

118 Letter, NZMR 130GE, in the Field, Xmas Eve [1916], courtesy Susanna Norris.

119 In the view of Nigel Allsopp, the New Zealand Brigade in Egypt owed more to the farriers, and to Stafford, 'than can ever be told'. Nigel Allsopp, *A Centenary of Australian Animals at War* (Australia: InHouse Publishing, n.d.), p. 206.

120 *Dominion*, 11 November 1916, p. 6.

121 Machattie is remembered on the Ellesmere County War Memorial in the main street of Leeston, Canterbury, where he was living before the war.

122 George Noel Waugh file, 10/86, ANZ.

123 Headquarters New Zealand and Australian Division — New Zealand Division — Assistant Director of Veterinary Services (ADVS) — War Diary, 1 May–31 May 1917, WA27 36 [27k], ANZ.

124 *Northern Advocate*, 6 September 1917, p. 1.

125 'Otago Mounted Rifles Regiment', https://nzhistory.govt.nz/war/otago-mounted-rifles (Ministry for Culture and Heritage), updated 21-Apr-2017.

126 *Dominion*, 25 April 1919, p. 4.

CHAPTER 12: HOLY MEN AND HEALING HANDS

1 John A. Lee, *Soldier* (Wellington: A. H. & A. W. Reed, 1976), p. 79.

2 Zane Kidd, 'God is on Our Side: Chaplain Colonel (William) John Aldred Luxford', in John Crawford, David Littlewood and James Watson (eds), *Experience of a Lifetime: People, Personalities and Leaders in the First World War* (Auckland: Massey University Press, 2016), p. 269.

3 Chaplains were represented 'according to the percentage of adherents of each denomination to the total New Zealand population'. Ibid., footnote 4.

4 Gavin McLean, *The White Ships: New Zealand's First World War Hospital Ships* (Wellington: New Zealand Ship & Marine Society, 2013), p. 116.

5 Excerpt from Luxford's report to the Reverend S. J. Serpell, former president NZ Methodist Conference, Kidd, 'God is on Our Side', pp. 283–4.

6 Chris Pugsley, *Te Hokowhitu a Tu: The Maori Pioneer Battalion in the First World War* (Auckland: Reed, 1995), pp. 44, 67.

7 *Press*, 8 December 1917, p. 8.

8 Kidd, 'God is on Our Side', p. 289.

9 *Southland Times*, 19 August 1916, p. 3.

10 Letters: Ronald Watson (*Letters from a Padre: A Record of the War Service of Ronald S. Watson. M.C.*, edited by Nigel M. Watson, privately printed, Melbourne), 1998.2491, NAM.

11 Letter 9 June 1918, Herbert H. Farrant, Elizabeth Morey and Delysse Storey (eds), *A Strong Sense of Duty:*

The First World War Letters of Chaplain the Reverend Clive Mortimer Jones 1917–1920 (Auckland: New Zealand Military Historical Society, 2013), pp. 80–1.

12 Letter 25 November 1918, ibid., p. 88.

13 Clement Houchen file, 18/12, ANZ; Kidd, 'God is on Our Side', p. 269.

14 *Grey River Argus*, 17 December 1917, p. 8.

15 *Southland Times*, 20 April 1918, p. 5.

16 *Poverty Bay Herald*, 6 September 1915, p. 3.

17 A. L. Logan, Dental Service with the First New Zealand Expeditionary Force, MS-2004, WMM, p. 17.

18 C. G. Nicol, *The Story of Two Campaigns: Official War History of the Auckland Mounted Rifles Regiment, 1914–1919* (Auckland: Wilson & Horton, 1921), p. 84.

19 Roger Lang and Dr Jennifer Batham-Lang, *Chaplains of Anzac: New Zealand's Fallen Chaplains of the Great War* (New Zealand: Lang Book Publishing, 2015), p. 48.

20 *Evening Post*, 19 July 1918, p. 7.

21 Watson, *Letters from a Padre*, p. 29.

22 Quoted *Kai Tiaki*, April 1915, p. 76.

23 https://otago150years.wordpress.com/2016/02/29/the-massage-school/, accessed 3 April 1917. As Hester Maclean would write in *Kai Tiaki* in April 1918 (p. 59), for many years massage had 'been held in disrepute, owing as much to its abuse for evil purposes as to the lack of a proper standard of training and qualification'.

24 *New Zealand Times*, 17 January 1916, p. 9.

25 *Kai Tiaki*, July 1913, p. 114; https://otago150years.wordpress.com/2016/02/29/the-massage-school/, accessed 3 April 1917. In 1915, 'apparently to the relief of the university', responsibility for administering the massage school passed to the Otago Hospital Board.

26 *Kai Tiaki*, July 1915, p. 144.

27 The *New Zealand Herald* reported on 7 May 1915 that Hawke's Bay's Mrs A. E. Westall, an ISTM member, joined the corps and worked at the No. 3 Military Hospital in Wandsworth. When the *Willochra* brought home more wounded in September 1916, with them came New Zealander Nurse Edwards, who had been working at a French and then several British hospitals. 'She was wearing dark blue, with a cloak, and a veiled bonnet . . . On a red badge were the letters "A.P.M.C," the official uniform and badge of the Almeric Paget Massage Corps', *Evening Post*, 30 September 1916, p. 7.

28 Letters 6 October 1915, 28 December 1915, Henry Kitson, Letters and diary, MS-Papers-4540, ATL.

29 Letter 27 January 1916, Kitson, Letters and diary; letter 24 November 1918, Letters to the Hutton family from Alexander Louis Hutton, MS-Papers-3906, ATL, folder 4.

30 'The Story of Hobart and Ruby Tennent From October 4th 1883 to September 14th 1978', collated by Patrick Tennent in 2002, 2003.644, NAM, p. 32.

31 *Evening Star*, 22 November 1916, p. 6.

32 *New Zealand Herald*, 20 June 1916, p. 9.

33 *Star*, 24 January 1916, p. 8.

34 Jane Tolerton, *Ettie: A Life of Ettie Rout* (Auckland: Penguin Books, 1992), p. 142.

35 H. Maclean, 'New Zealand Army Nurses', in H. T. B. Drew (ed.), *The War Effort of New Zealand* (Auckland: Whitcombe & Tombs, 1923), pp. 103–4.

36 'Story of Hobart and Ruby Tennent'.

37 *New Zealand Herald*, 15 May 1918, p. 6.

38 *New Zealand Herald*, 30 January 1917, p. 8; A. D. Carbery, *The New Zealand Medical Service in the Great War, 1914–1918* (Auckland: Whitcombe & Tombs, 1924), p. 371.

39 New Zealand Army Nursing Service — NZANS overseas records, correspondence — Matron-in-chief, AD78 23 67/3/1A, ANZ. There was a shortage in New Zealand too. On 3 September 1917 Thurston sent

Maclean the address of a woman applying for a masseuse position: 'As I know you are short handed I think you would be wise to take her, it is most annoying the length of time we are kept waiting for those who should arrive from New Zealand.' New Zealand Army Nursing Service — NZANS [New Zealand Army Nursing Service] overseas records, correspondence re VADs, Brocklehurst, AD78 23 67/5/1A, ANZ.

40 *Kai Tiaki*, April 1918, p. 62.

41 Dorothy McKenzie and Lindsay Malcolm (eds), *Boots, Belts, Rifle & Pack: A New Zealand Soldier at War 1917–1919* (Dunedin: L. M. Malcolm, 1992), pp. 133–4.

42 *Taranaki Herald*, 28 January 1919, p. 5.

43 Thurston to Maclean, 15 November 1917, 21 February 1918, New Zealand Army Nursing Service — NZANS overseas records, correspondence — Matron-in-chief, AD78 23 67/3/1A, ANZ. Brandon later dropped out of the massage course.

44 *Kai Tiaki*, January 1919, p. 43.

45 Thurston to Maclean, 9 January 1918, New Zealand Army Nursing Service — NZANS overseas records, correspondence — Matron-in-chief, AD78 23 67/3/1A, ANZ.

46 *Kai Tiaki*, October 1918, pp. 213, 215.

47 *Kai Tiaki*, April 1918, p. 59.

48 *Kai Tiaki*, October 1918, p. 196.

49 New Zealand Army Nursing Service — NZANS overseas records, AD78 23 67/3/1, ANZ. Hester Maclean was not alone in her call for more trained masseurs: see letter 'Massage Treatment', *Evening Post*, 13 April 1918, p. 12.

50 *Kai Tiaki*, July 1920, p. 153.

51 Letter 4 October 1915, Cecil Malthus: World War I Papers, http://christchurchcitylibraries.com/Heritage/Digitised/WarsAndConflicts/WorldWarI/Malthus/Thumbnails/; Randolph Norman Gray, Papers relating to World War One, MS-Papers- 4134, ATL, folder 1; letter 14 May 1916, Harry Hall, Diary and letters 1915–1917 (compiled Christopher S. (Kit) Withers), MS 2002/72, AWMM. Gray also observed an interesting chiropodial technique in Colombo on 5 November 1915: 'One man set himself up — or rather down — as corn extractor . . . The chappie cut around the corn until he got it well exposed and then made two small incisions down into the root. He then put a small rubber sucker — just like a finger stall for the little finger — on the corn and sucked at it until he got the root out.'

52 Medical — Chiropodists — Appointment of — General file, AD1 973 49/250, ANZ.

53 Medical Corps Memoranda — Walton on Thames 1915–19, WA10 18, 10/6/9, ANZ.

54 *Dominion*, 29 September 1915, p. 7.

55 Medical — Chiropodists — Appointment of — General file, AD1 973 49/250, ANZ.

56 Medical — Chiropodists — Trentham Camp — return of work done, AD1 972 49/235, ANZ.

57 *Dominion*, 3 February 1917, p. 7.

58 Tim Shoebridge, *Featherston Military Training Camp and the First World War* (Wellington: Manatū Taonga/Ministry for Culture & Heritage, 2012, 1st pub. April 2011), p. 29.

59 Carbery, *Medical Service*, p. 179.

60 Ibid., p. 246; *Dominion*, 6 March 1917, p. 6.

61 William Mandeno Smallfield, War Letters, Diaries and Papers, MS 2007/37, AWMM. As Carbery pointed out, the number of men in a division 'with the necessary goodwill, education and ability to make efficient chiropodists' was probably very limited, and this may have accounted for the 'small proportion' of successful candidates. Carbery, *Medical Service*, p. 247.

62 Diary 12 June 1916, James Currie, letters and diary, in the possession of David Sewell, Wanganui, courtesy Glyn Harper; O. E. Burton, *The Silent Division: New Zealanders at the Front: 1914–1919 & Concerning One Man's War*, ed. John H. Gray (Christchurch: John Douglas Publishing, 2014), *One Man's War*, p. 393.

63 Leo van Bergen, *Before My Helpless Sight: Suffering, Dying and Military Medicine on the Western Front, 1914–1918* (Surrey: Ashgate, 2009), p. 145.

64 C. H. Weston, *Three Years With the New Zealanders* (London: Skeffington & Co., 1918), Chapter VIII.

65 Diary 14 October 1916, Gray papers, folder 2; Jane Tolerton, *An Awfully Big Adventure: New Zealand World War One Veterans Tell Their Stories* (Auckland: Penguin, 2013), p. 180.

66 Carbery, *Medical Service*, p. 362.

67 Medical Corps memoranda — Precis of events in France, 11 April 1916–10 June 1917, WA10 19 10/6/10, ANZ.

68 *Evening Post*, 26 August 1916, p. 10; quoted Carbery, *Medical Service*, pp. 362–3.

69 Carbery, *Medical Service*, p. 247.

70 A. H. Wilkie, *Official War History of the Wellington Mounted Rifles Regiment 1914–1919* (Auckland: Whitcombe & Tombs, 1924), pp. 170–1.

71 *Press*, 3 August 1917, p. 4.

72 A roll of honour published by the Pharmacy Board of New Zealand in 1919 identified 89 members of the Pharmaceutical Society (registered pharmacists) who served in the First World War; nine of them had died. Another 186 soldiers entered 'chemist' as their trade or calling on their enlistment attestation form, as recorded on the Auckland War Memorial Museum Cenotaph database; 13 put 'dispenser'. Sixteen more who entered 'chemist' or chemist assistant' have been identified from other sources. There are probably more. I thank Euan Galloway, who has done considerable work in this area, for this total.

73 Reg Combes, *Pharmacy in New Zealand: Aspects and Reminiscences* (Auckland: Ray Richards for the Pharmaceutical Society of New Zealand, 1981), p. 188. Thanks to Euan Galloway for this reference.

74 *Dominion*, 5 June 1916, p. 8. The newspaper misspelt his name as 'Bronley Hall'. To be a registered pharmaceutical chemist under the 1908 Pharmacy Act, a person had to be at least 21, have passed examinations in such subjects as 'materia medica, botany, chemistry, practical chemistry, pharmacy, and practical pharmacy', and have served 'for at least three years under articles of apprenticeship as the apprentice of a registered chemist, or chemist and druggist, or homoeopathic chemist'. Euan Galloway, who kindly supplied this information, also suggests that several of the men who enlisted giving their profession as chemist still had to complete their apprenticeships or pass the required exams, or were not yet 21. Others might have been employed as assistants in chemist shops with no intention to qualify.

75 *Dominion*, 4 August 1915, p. 11. 'Fair Play' subsequently claimed that the young dispenser on the *Maheno* had 'failed to pass in his chemist's examinations', *Dominion*, 12 August 1915, p. 6.

76 *Dominion*, 5 June 1916, p. 8.

77 Lea Doughty, pers. comm., 15 August 2017.

78 *Evening Post*, 5 February 1916, p. 3.

79 Jonathan Chilton-Towle, 'Pharmacists Front and Centre in New Study on WW1', *Pharmacy Today*, 21 June 1917.

80 http://www.slideshare.net/WW1C/medical-services-world-war-i, accessed 18 January 2017.

81 Robin Hyde, *Passport to Hell*, edited and introduced by D. I. B. Smith (Auckland: Auckland University Press 2015, 1st pub. 1936), p. 113.

82 *Dominion*, 2 September 1916, p. 3.

83 Doughty, pers. comm., 15 August 2017; Chilton-Towle, 'Pharmacists'.

84 *Ashburton Guardian*, 2 November 1915, p. 4.

85 *Marlborough Express*, 8 December 1915, p. 5; George Everett Hards file, 3/1322, ANZ.

86 Douglas McKenzie file, 3/2109, ANZ.

87 James Ernest Watson file, 3/3164, ANZ; Frederick Horace Dolphin file, 3/2055, ANZ. Watson was registered in 1909, Dolphin after the war.

88 *Dominion*, 10 July 1915, p. 6.

89 *Manawatu Standard*, 25 June 1923, p. 5.

90 Adolph Duncan McLennan file, 3/1062; letter 28 October 1915, Gray Papers, folder 1.

91 *Free Lance*, 16 July 1915, p. 16. Lea Doughty notes that in Australia, dispensers were also responsible for

sterilising surgical instruments and overseeing the medical stores. But in times of crisis there was no strict division of labour. Lea Doughty, pers. comm., 15 August 2015.

92 *Evening Post*, 27 September 1918, p. 3; *Sun*, 12 December 1918, p. 5.

93 *Dominion*, 20 July 1915, p. 6.

94 *Free Lance*, 6 September 1915, p. 21.

95 *He Rau Mahara: To Remember the Journey of our Ngāi Tahu Soldiers from the Pā to the Battlefields of the Great War* (Christchurch: Te Rūnanga o Ngāi Tahu, 2017), p. 47.

96 *Southland Times*, 29 September 1915, p. 5.

97 *Auckland Star*, 31 December 1915, p. 6.

98 *Auckland Star*, 11 April 1916, p. 6.

99 *Otago Witness*, 24 November 1915, p. 28.

100 *Press*, 5 October 1915, p. 4.

101 PharmacyToday.co.nz/in-print/2015/march-2015/april-2015/retired-chief-pharmacist-embarks-on-Anzac-research, accessed 18 April 2017; Cyril James McHardie file, 3/700, ANZ.

102 *Taranaki Herald*, 23 December 1916, p. 3; Richard Egbert Compere Dowling file, 3/128, ANZ.

103 Another NZMC man lost on the *Marquette*, John Ross, had been working at Dunedin's Friendly Societies Dispensary before the war. *Star*, 4 November 1915, p. 5.

104 William Ingle, who had been a self-employed qualified chemist and dispenser in Marton, was a member of the NZMC. He died in France on 28 July 1918 while serving with No. 2 New Zealand Field Ambulance, but whether he was a dispenser is unknown. Registered pharmacist Douglas Goddard, from Woodville, served with No. 1 Field Ambulance on Gallipoli, in what capacity is uncertain. He transferred to the infantry on 5 November 1916 and was killed in action near Armentières three weeks later. Euan Galloway, 'Members of the Pharmaceutical Society of New Zealand Killed in World War 1', 6 December 2017, pers. comm.

105 Hospital pharmacy was acceptable early as a job for women, but an apprenticeship in a retail pharmacy was considered too physically demanding and would also entail the discussion of such sensitive subjects as venereal disease. Lea Doughty, pers. comm., 15 August 2017.

106 Her New Zealand Defence Force record describes her as 'Dispensing Chemist, New Zealand Red Cross', AABK, 22525, W5725, 1/, B.R. 37/99B, ANZ. Since Edith Rayner and William Porteous married in London, it is likely that she had a British qualification. More British women managed to do wartime dispensing work, among them future crime queen Agatha Christie, whose experience at a military hospital pharmacy gave her a useful authorial knowledge of poisons, Kevin Brown, *Fighting Fit: Health, Medicine and War in the Twentieth Century* (Stroud, UK: The History Press, 2008), p. 74.

107 *Timaru Herald*, 18 November 1916, p. 2. Although the article concerned his wife, it was headed 'Dr W. J. Porteous in a Dug-Out' and did not give her first name.

108 *New Zealand Times*, 1 April 1916, p. 5.

CHAPTER 13: WOMEN AT WAR

1 *Free Lance*, 7 April 1916, p. 5; Godley to Parkes, 22 August 1916, Semi-personal letters by General Officer Commanding, 5 September 1914–31 October 1916, WA 252 3 [6], ANZ. Accommodation was a problem. At Brockenhurst nurses and VADs lived in rented houses until purpose-built quarters were erected. From September 1917 DMS Parkes was asking for more VAD accommodation, in the form of a large hut, as the women were sleeping in Ward 20, which was needed for an expected influx of casualties. Delays in finding a solution led to VADs resigning or refusing to renew their contracts. Buildings — Accommodation nurses and VADs — Brockenhurst 24 September 1917–7 August 1918, WA1 13, 5/19, ANZ.

2 Anne Powell, *Women in the War Zone: Hospital Service in the First World War* (Stroud, UK: The History Press, 2013, 1st pub. 2009), p. 21.

3 7 May 1915, Diaries of A. M. Trotter/transcribed by A. A. S. Trotter, MS-3397/004, Hocken.

4 Letter 30 October 1915, Eric Arnold Burnett, Diary and letters, MS-Papers-2901, ATL, folder 1.

5 New Zealand Army Nursing Service — NZANS overseas records, correspondence re VADs, Brocklehurst, AD78 23 67/5/1A, ANZ. Nurses could misbehave too. In a letter of 8 February 1917 Thurston reported to Maclean that a staff nurse on a recent voyage of the *Tofua* 'is often indiscreet in her attitude towards men, and is too eager for their company'. Thurston sent her home and asked Maclean to keep her in New Zealand. New Zealand Army Nursing Service — NZANS overseas records, correspondence — Matron-in-chief, AD78 23 67/3/1A, ANZ.

6 Ibid.

7 Jan Rodgers, '"A Paradox of Power and Marginality": New Zealand Nurses' Professional Campaign During War, 1900–1920', PhD thesis, History, Massey University, 1994, p. 205.

8 *Kai Tiaki*, October 1915, p. 160.

9 *Kai Tiaki*, April 1915, p. 84.

10 Bertha Emily Taylor, Letters and journal, MS-Papers-1291, ATL; Edna Pengelly, *Nursing in Peace and War* (Wellington: Wingfield Press, 1956), p. 61.

11 'It is important to maintain a sufficient reserve in France to replace wastage and I am expecting to rely largely upon V.A.D. assistance in Base Hospitals in place of orderlies.' Parkes to Allen, 25 August 1916, Ministerial Files — Correspondence with Colonel Parkes, Allen1 3, M1/34 , ANZ.

12 *Kai Tiaki*, October 2016, pp. 206, 211.

13 Thurston to Maclean, 30 January 1917, New Zealand Army Nursing Service — NZANS overseas records, correspondence — Matron-in-chief, AD78 23 67/3/1A, ANZ. On 30 April 1917 the DDMS had told the DGMS that 'A large number of New Zealand ladies are working as V.A.Ds in the various hospitals and giving complete satisfaction', Cora Beattie Anderson file, 22/12, ANZ.

14 Thurston to Maclean, 4 January 1918 (in response to enquiry from Henderson), New Zealand Army Nursing Service — NZANS overseas records, correspondence — Matron-in-chief, AD78 23 67/3/1A, ANZ.

15 New Zealand Army Nursing Service — NZANS overseas records, correspondence re VADs, Brocklehurst, AD78 23 67/5/1A, ANZ.

16 Ethel Marion Gould MBE, JP née Hirst, biographical note, Gladys Violet Luxford, 'How I came to be interested in war and why I went to World war One', MS94/36, AWMM.

17 Luxford, 'How I came to be interested in war'; letter 8 December 1916.

18 Pengelly, *Nursing*, 26 July 1916, p. 57.

19 *Evening Post*, 21 September 1916, p. 9 (report based on letters from masseuse Christine Smith at Brockenhurst). Bell later worked for the Women's Army Auxiliary Corps as a clerk in Rouen. For more on Pearce and Bell, and other ambulance drivers, see Jane Tolerton, *Make Her Praises Heard Afar: New Zealand Women Overseas in World War One* (Wellington: Booklovers Books, 2017).

20 Pengelly, *Nursing*, pp. 57, 72.

21 RNZ Spectrum, 'One Woman, One Ambulance', 5 June 2015, http://www.radionz.co.nz/national/programmes/spectrum/audio/201757875/one-woman,-one-ambulance,-wwi.

22 Deborah Pitts Taylor, Diary and letters, MS-2000-20, AWMM.

23 Jane Tolerton tells more of Gladys Henning's remarkable story in *Make Her Praises*, pp. 276–8, 340–1; *New Zealand Herald*, 21 January 1919, p. 6.

24 *Kai Tiaki*, January 1918, p. 15. The CBE, OBE and MBE were created in 1917 by King George V to recognise the 'service of all classes of men and women during the war'.

25 *Kai Tiaki*, April 1918, p. 70.

26 *Kai Tiaki*, July 1920, p. 109.

27 For coverage of marriage for NZANS nurses, see Sherayl McNabb, *100 Years New Zealand Military Nursing: New Zealand Army Nursing Service — Royal New Zealand Nursing Corps 1915–2015* (Wairoa: author, 2015).

28 *Kai Tiaki*, April 1918, p. 107; *Evening Post*, 18 January 1917, p. 9.

29 See Tolerton, *Make Her Praises.* The doctors who served included Jessie Maddison from Christchurch, who worked as a surgeon in Sheffield's Wharncliffe Hospital, and New Zealand's first female medical graduate doctor, Emily Seideberg, who also served in Sheffield, at the Royal Infirmary.

30 M.-F. Weiner, 'The Scottish Women's Hospital at Royaumont, France 1914–1919', *Journal of the Royal College of Physicians of Edinburgh*, 2014, no. 44, pp. 328–36, http://dx.doi.org/10.4997/JRCPE.2014.418.

31 A typical contemporary attitude was expressed by the dean of the medical faculty at Otago University in March 1916 in response to a request from the surgeon-general for more junior doctors. Of the five students who had recently passed the requisite exams, 'The three boys were immediately placed as house surgeons and I suppose the girls would hardly meet your requirements.' Letter to Henderson from Dean of Medical Faculty at Otago University, 23 March 1916, Medical — Medical Corps for NZEF — General File 1916–1921 AD 1 967 49/148 Pt 2, ANZ.

32 The great women of anaesthesia: Mary Alice Blair by Monica Cronin, Curator | Dec 19, 2016, http://www.geoffreykayemuseum.org.au/the-great-women-of-anaesthesia-mary-alice-blair/, accessed 11 May 2017.

33 A brief January 1915 report from London said that 'Dr. Mary Blair (late of Wellington) has been over at a hospital in Boulogne for a few weeks. She hopes to return there again later.' *Evening Post*, 9 March 1915, p. 3. The Women's Hospital Corps, founded by British doctors Louisa Garrett Anderson and Flora Murray, had established a hospital in a Paris hotel in September 1914; a second at Wimereux, just north of Boulogne, opened on 6 November. Blair may have worked there for a while. Leah Leneman, 'Medical Women at War, 1914–1918', *Medical History*, 1994, vol. 388, no. 2, April 1994, pp. 160–77.

34 scottishwomenshospitals.co.uk, accessed 11 May 2017.

35 *Dominion*, 13 September 1916, p. 2.

36 Cronin, 'Great women'.

37 *Oamaru Mail*, 3 July 1915, p. 4.

38 *Star*, 9 July 1915, p. 6.

39 Fiona Ward, 'Scott, Jessie Ann', from the Dictionary of New Zealand Biography. Te Ara — the Encyclopedia of New Zealand, http://www.TeAra.govt.nz/en/biographies/3s7/scott-jessie-ann, accessed 15 May 2017.

40 *Auckland Star*, 26 February 1916, p. 8.

41 Ibid.

42 *Otago Witness*, 17 May 1916, p. 52.

43 *Press*, 23 April 1917, p. 4.

44 Barbara Brookes, 'A Corresponding Community: Dr Agnes Bennett and her Friends from the Edinburgh Medical College for Women of the 1890s', *Medical History*, April 2008, vol. 52, no. 2, pp. 237–56.

45 Beryl Hughes, 'Bennett, Agnes Elizabeth Lloyd', from the Dictionary of New Zealand Biography. Te Ara — the Encyclopedia of New Zealand, http://www.TeAra.govt.nz/en/biographies/3b28/bennett-agnes-elizabeth-lloyd, accessed 15 May 2017.

46 Letter 22 September 1932, reply from office of Adjutant and QMG, Military HQ, Wgtn. S. H. Crump to New Zealand Women's Medical Association query, Elizabeth Catherine Gunn file 3/2062, ANZ.

47 Tolerton, *Make Her Praises*, p. 69.

48 *Dominion*, 13 November 1915, p. 10.

49 *New Zealand Herald*, 21 July 1916, p. 9.

50 *Kai Tiaki*, January 1917, p. 21.

51 *Press*, 17 April 1919, p. 2; Medical — Health — Troops on transports — Returning with invalids, AD1 982 49/467 [a], ANZ.

52 Brookes, 'Corresponding Community'; *Dominion*, 7 July 1913, p. 2.

53 Medical — Health — Troops on transports — Returning with invalids, AD1 982 49/467 [a], ANZ.

54 This and all following quotes from Elizabeth Catherine Gunn file, 3/2062, ANZ.

55 Margaret Tennant, 'Gunn, Elizabeth Catherine', from the Dictionary of New Zealand Biography. Te Ara

— the Encyclopedia of New Zealand, http://www.TeAra.govt.nz/en/biographies/3g24/gunn-elizabeth-catherine, accessed 18 May 2017.

56 *Evening Post*, 29 September 1916, p. 9.

57 *Star*, 24 July 1917 p. 4.

58 *Star*, 24 July 1917, p. 4.

59 *Evening Post*, 28 July 1917, p. 9.

60 *Kai Tiaki*, April 1918, p. 74.

61 The initiative followed a British army order of 3 November 1917. Only volunteers were selected, and references from an OC and a matron were required. The women who did the course and were posted to hospitals and CCSs 'also gained considerable clinical experience in the nursing and resuscitation of wounded soldiers together with the use of intravenous infusions including blood.' R. E. Rawstron, *A Unique Nursing Group: New Zealand Army Nurse Anaesthetists of WWI* (Christchurch: Rawstron Publishing Co., 2005), p. 1.

62 *Kai Tiaki*, January 1919, pp. 5–6.

63 *Kai Tiaki*, July 1919, pp. 117–18.

64 *Kai Tiaki*, January 1919, pp. 5–6.

65 Rodgers, 'Paradox', footnote, Chapter 8; *Kai Tiaki*, 1 July 1919, pp. 117–18.

66 As Jane Tolerton notes, Rout chose the minimum age of 30 specifically to avoid the charges of naivety and youthfulness that were sometimes hurled at VADs, *Ettie: A Life of Ettie Rout* (Auckland: Penguin Books, 1992), p. 105.

67 *Sun*, 5 July 1917, p. 11.

68 *Press*, 20 July 1915, p. 8.

69 Tolerton, *Ettie*, pp. 106, 107, 108.

70 Diary 27 February 1916, John Keith Moloney, War diary, MS-Papers-1194, ATL.

71 *Colonist*, 16 September 1916, p. 2.

72 *New Zealand Times*, 20 October 1915, p. 9; Godley to Allen, 30 June 1916, [Correspondence between] General Sir Alexander Godley [Commander New Zealand Expeditionary Force] and Colonel Hon. Sir James Allen, Minister of Defence, 4 January–29 December 1916, WA 252 1 [3], ANZ.

73 *Sun*, 8 December 1916, p. 4.

74 *Wanganui Chronicle*, 27 July 1917, p. 3.

75 Jane Tolerton, 'Rout, Ettie Annie', Dictionary of New Zealand Biography, first published in 1996. Te Ara — the Encyclopedia of New Zealand, https://teara.govt.nz/en/biographies/3r31/rout-ettie-annie, accessed 26 January 2018.

76 *Taranaki Daily News*, 15 October 1919, p. 5.

77 *Free Lance*, 6 February 1919, p. 4.

78 *Observer*, 20 December 1919, p. 10.

CHAPTER 14: VISIBLE AND INVISIBLE

1 *Kai Tiaki*, January 1915, p. 50.

2 O. E. Burton, *The Silent Division: New Zealanders at the Front: 1914–1919 & Concerning One Man's War*, ed. John H. Gray (Christchurch: John Douglas Publishing, 2014), *One Man's War*, p. 374.

3 A. D. Carbery, *The New Zealand Medical Service in the Great War, 1914–1918* (Auckland: Whitcombe & Tombs, 1924), p. 25.

4 Robin Hyde, *Passport to Hell*, edited and introduced by D. I. B. Smith (Auckland: Auckland University Press 2015, 1st pub. 1936), p. 105.

5 Leo Van Bergen, *Before My Helpless Sight: Suffering, Dying and Military Medicine on the Western Front, 1914–1918* (Surrey: Ashgate, 2009), pp. 168–9.

6 *Timaru Herald*, 5 August 1915, p. 4; *Star*, 15 July 1915, p. 4.

7 Bergen, *Helpless Sight*, p. 170.

8 18 June 1917, Clifford Collingwood, Diary and Scrapbook: New Zealand, Egypt & Western Front — WW1, 2007.139, NAM.

9 Bergen, *Helpless Sight*, p. 171.

10 Brendan O'Carroll, *Khaki Angels: Kiwi Stretcher-bearers in the First and Second World Wars* (Wellington: Ngaio Press, 2009), pp. 18–19.

11 1 May 1915, John H. Thomson, 3/453 No. 1 N.Z. Fd. Amb., Diary from 13 April 1915 to Jan 21st 1916, PC-0316, Hocken; 21 July 1915, Charles Wallace Saunders: World War I diary, Misc-MS-0267, Hocken.

12 John A. Lee, *Civilian into Soldier* (Auckland: Vital Books, 1963), p. 91.

13 *Dominion*, 23 August 1916, p. 6.

14 John A. Lee, *Soldier* (Wellington: A. H. & A. W. Reed, 1976), pp. 85, 87.

15 William Taylor, *The Twilight Hour: A Personal Account of World War I* (Morrinsville: Sutherland, 1978), p. 71.

16 O'Carroll, *Khaki*, pp. 18–19.

17 *Star*, 17 November 1915, p. 5. Named after the heavyweight champion boxer, a 'Jack Johnson' was the British nickname for the Germans' largest artillery shell, which could create a crater 20ft deep; William Anderson, 'Great Grandfather's Tales', p. 72, courtesy Bill Anderson.

18 Frederick James Foote, 'Yesteryears', Reminiscences, MS 2007/9, AWMM.

19 *Otago Witness*, 4 August 1915, p. 8.

20 Lee, *Soldier*, p. 72.

21 *Dominion*, 27 October 1915, p. 7; Glyn Harper (ed.), *Letters from the Battlefield: New Zealand Soldiers Write Home 1914–1918* (Auckland: HarperCollins, 2001), p. 71.

22 Bergen, *Helpless Sight*, p. 168.

23 *Dominion*, 16 July 1915, p. 6.

24 *Star*, 15 July 1915, p. 4.

25 Taylor, *Twilight*, p. 102; Harper, *Letters*, p. 113.

26 Diary of William Henry Winter WW1 1915, horowhenua.kete.net.nz, accessed 25 August 2016.

27 Medical Corps Memoranda — Gallipoli & Egypt, April 1916–2 March 1919, WA10 17 10/6/8, ANZ; Hyde, *Passport*, pp. 122–3.

28 Michael Tyquin, *Gallipoli: An Australian Medical Perspective* (Canberra: Army History Unit, 2012), p. 67.

29 Martin Boswell, Imperial War Museum, quoted https://eandt.theiet.org/content/articles/2014/06/ww1-combat-helmet-technology-the-brodie-steel-helmet/, accessed 26 May 2017.

30 5 June 1916, William Kingston Wilson, Diary, 1994.2314, NAM.

31 On 30 September 1917, Major Robert Adams 'was out when shells were falling about, and suddenly found himself on his back; two fragments of shell had struck his steel helmet and driven it in on his head, making a scalp wound. He says that these helmets undoubtedly save thousands of lives. He was sent to the base hospital, and after nine days' rest rejoined his battery.' *Southland Times*, 26 December 1917, p. 5.

32 War Memoirs by Dr. W. Aitken, M.C., MD, F.R.A.C.P., 1st New Zealand Field Ambulance, Australian War Memorial, 392L 2422, pp. 11–12.

33 Marina Larsson, *Shattered Anzacs: Living With the Scars of War* (Sydney: University of New South Wales Press, 2009), p. 46.

34 *Wanganui Herald*, 14 July 1915, p. 5; *New Zealand Herald*, 14 July 1915, p. 4; *Evening Star*, 14 October 1915, p. 3.

35 *Wanganui Herald*, 14 October 1915, p. 8.

36 *Dominion*, 16 July 1915, p. 6.

37 *Wanganui Chronicle*, 9 November 1916, p. 4.

38 Letter 13 September 1918, Letters to the Hutton family from Alexander Louis Hutton, MS-Papers-3906, ATL.

39 Extract from letter, Joseph Frederick Cody, History of the War (Gallipoli — Medical —1915), AD78 27, G15/25, ANZ.

40 *Dominion*, 16 July 1915, p. 6.

41 Cyril Vernon Wallace file, 12/1823, ANZ.

42 Medical Corps Memoranda — Gallipoli & Egypt, April 1916–2 March 1919, WA10 17 10/6/8, ANZ.

43 Letter Roy W. O. Dalrymple — Gallipoli — WW1, 2009.1196, NAM, p. 8.

44 Ibid.

45 Howard Karl Kippenberger — World War One Diary, MS-Papers-8181-147, ATL.

46 Beth Sutherland, *My Dear Chick: A New Zealand Love Story 1911–1948* (Masterton: Fraser Books, 2008), p. 109.

47 Claude Weston, *Three Years With the New Zealanders* (London: Skeffington & Son, 1918), Chapter XIII.

48 20 June 1917, Collingwood diary.

49 Weston, *Three Years*, Chapter XIII; letter 4 October 1918, Hutton letters, folder 3.

50 Weston, *Three Years*, Chapter XIII.

51 Lee, *Soldier*, pp. 72–3, 74.

52 Burton, *One Man's War*, p. 388. Burton's treatment of the wound was interesting. 'I did not report to the R.A.P. officially, as we had a new doctor whose reactions might have been unpredictable.' He and a friend 'fomented [the wound] and bandaged it up' (p. 389). With rest, Burton recovered completely.

53 2 August 1915, Malone diary.

54 John Crawford (ed.), *The Devil's Own War: The First World War Diary of Brigadier-General Herbert Hart* (Auckland and Wollombi: Exisle in association with New Zealand Defence Force, 2008), p. 116.

55 Christopher Pugsley, *On the Fringe of Hell: New Zealanders and Military Discipline in the First World War* (Auckland: Hodder & Stoughton, 1991), pp. 73–4.

56 Allan Marriott, *Mud Beneath My Boots: A Poignant Memoir of the Effects of War on a Young New Zealander* (Auckland: HarperCollins, 2005), p. 161.

57 Section 18 of the 'Notes for R.M.Os. of the New Zealand Division' written by ADMS Colonel Donald McGavin and published in August 1917, in Carbery, *Medical Service*.

58 Ashley Ekins and Elizabeth Stewart (eds), *War Wounds: Medicine and the Trauma of Conflict* (Auckland and Wollombi: Exisle Publishing, 2011), p. 42.

59 Hyde, *Passport*, p. 139.

60 Ekins and Stewart, *War Wounds*, p. 42.

61 29 August 1915, Diary of William McAra, Gallipoli, June–December 1915, MS-2943/002, Hocken.

62 Lee, *Civilian into Soldier*, p. 243.

63 23 September 1915, McAra diary.

64 Medical Corps Memoranda — Gallipoli & Egypt, April 1916–2 March 1919, WA10 17 10/6/8, ANZ; letter 17 May 1915, Malone.

65 Kippenberger Diary, p. 84.

66 28 and 30 June 1917, Collingwood diary.

67 Nigel Murphy, 'It Was Hell, Merrilyn, It Was Just Hell', in Nathalie Philippe (ed.), with Christopher Pugsley, John Crawford and Matthias Strohn, *The Great Adventure Ends: New Zealand and France on the Western Front* (Christchurch: John Douglas Publishing, 2013), p. 131.

68 Medical Corps Memoranda — Gallipoli & Egypt, April 1916–2 March 1919, WA10 17 10/6/8, ANZ.

69 Carbery, *Medical Service*, p. 109.

70 Medical Corps Propaganda — Gallipoli and Egypt, April 1916–2 March 1919, WA10 17, 10/6/8, ANZ.

71 *Dominion*, 16 July 1915, p. 6; 17 August 1915, Diaries of A. M. Trotter/transcribed by A. A. S. Trotter, MS-3397/004, Hocken.

72 A. G. Butler, *The Australian Army Medical Services in the War of 1914–1918*, vol. III, *Special Problems and Services* (Canberra: Australian War Memorial, 1943), p. 81.

73 Denise J. Poynter, '"The Report on her Transfer was Shell Shock", A Study of the Psychological Disorders of Nurses and Female Voluntary Aid Detachments who Served Alongside the British and Allied Expeditionary Forces During the First World War, 1914–1918', PhD thesis, University of Northampton, 2008, p. 95. Some of the gaits and physical manifestations of shell shock can be seen in a remarkable piece of film, 'War Neuroses, Netley, 1917, Seal Hayne Military Hospital, 1918', www.youtube.com/watch?v=IWHbF5jGJYO.

74 'A Contribution to the Study of Shell Shock. Being an Account of Three Cases of Loss of Memory, Vision, Smell, and Taste, Admitted into the Duchess of Westminster's War Hospital, Le Touquet', *Lancet*, vol. 185, no. 4772, 13 February 1915, pp. 316–20; Kevin Brown, *Fighting Fit: Health, Medicine and War in the Twentieth Century* (Stroud, UK: The History Press, 2008), p. 61.

75 Russell Clarke, '"Not Mad, But Very Ill": The Treatment of New Zealand's Shellshocked Soldiers 1914 to 1939', MA thesis, University of Auckland, 1991, p. 5.

76 C. S. Myers, *Shell Shock in France 1914–1918*, Cambridge, 1940, pp. 25–9, quoted Ben Shephard, *A War of Nerves: Soldiers and Psychiatrists in the Twentieth Century* (Harvard: Harvard University Press, 2003), p. 31.

77 Gwen Parsons, 'The Construction of Shell Shock in New Zealand, 1919–1939: A Reassessment', *Social History of Medicine*, vol. 26, no. 1, February 2013, p. 60. Because diagnosis was difficult, numbers were also hard to quantify. As Parsons has identified (p. 61), the only available relevant statistics show that fewer than 6.4 per cent of NZEF evacuations from the front line between May 1916 and December 1918, and under 1 per cent of British hospital admissions for the period July 1917–June 1918, were attributed to shell shock. (Reports of the Statistics Department July 1918–February 1919, War Archives Box 5, AD1, 1/4/7, ANZ)

78 Letter 12 June 1915, Henry Kitson, Letters and diary, MS-Papers-4540, ATL.

79 William Kingston Wilson, Diary, 1994.2314, NAM, p. 47. As psychiatrist Dr Sandy Macleod notes, the fact that the 'clinical consequences were rather different to WW II and Vietnam but similar to Iraq and Afghanistan suggests that maybe the blast effects were of some relevance'. Pers. comm., 6 November 2017.

80 *Evening Star*, 23 October 1916, p. 7.

81 c. 29 September 1916, 14–16 March 1917, 10 May 1917, Cyril Coxhead, MSX-7829, ATL. Coxhead's brother Edd was admitted to hospital twice for shell shock in 1917 and died on 17 January 1922 of 'Acute Mania & Heart Failure due to Shell Shock'.

82 Harry Luckman file, 46051, ANZ.

83 Memories of Norman Hassell; Sutherland, *My Dear Chick*, pp. 215–16.

84 Lee, *Civilian*, p. 202; *Wanganui Chronicle*, 13 September 1916, p. 4.

85 Charles E. Carrington, interview, Liddle Collection, Brotherton Library, Leeds, courtesy Glyn Harper.

86 Leary, *Spectrum* interview.

87 Mental Hospitals of the Dominion (report on) for 1918. By Frank Hay, The Inspector-General of Mental Defectives, presented by Sir Francis Bell, the Minister in Charge of the Department for the Care of Mental Defectives. Appendix II. A Note on the Work of the Department with respect to Soldier Patients from the Beginning of the War to the 4th August, 1919, *AJHR*, 1919, H-7, p. 27.

88 Report from Godley, 15 February 1915, Ministerial files — correspondence with General Godley, Allen 1 1, M1/15, ANZ; Baigent letter, Dan Bardsley file, 8/1186, ANZ.

89 Letter 22 March 1915, Charles Ernest Thomas, Letters, 2015/106, South Canterbury Museum.

90 Horace Maitland Haycock file, 11/59, ANZ.

91 Shephard, *War of Nerves*, p. 28. I am indebted to Dr Sandy Macleod for this insight, pers. comm., 6 November 2017.

92 Shephard, *War of Nerves*, p. 28; Jay Winter, 'Shell-Shock and the Cultural History of the Great War', *Journal of Contemporary History*, vol. 35, no. 1, Special Issue: Shell-Shock, January 2000, pp. 7–11, http://www.jstor.org/stable/261177 Accessed: 08-09-2017.

93 Shephard, *War of Nerves*, p. 25; Gwen Parsons, 'The Construction of Shell Shock', p. 59.

94 *Waikato Independent*, 8 February 1917, p. 2.

95 Bergen, *Helpless Sight*, p. 403.

96 Carrington interview.

97 Medical Corps Propaganda, Precis of Events in France, 11 April 1916–10 June 1917, WA10 19 10/6/10, ANZ.

98 Carbery, *Medical Service*, p. 296.

99 Medical Corps Memoranda — Precis of Events in France, 10 June–31 December 1917, WA10 20, 10/6/12, ANZ. In July came a further refinement: all NYDN cases were to go to a special receiving CCS, where a final decision on hospital treatment would be made, Carbery, *Medical Service*, p. 320.

100 McGavin, 'Notes for R.M.O.s'.

101 Bergen, *Helpless Sight*, p. 236.

102 Carbery, *Medical Service*, p. 319. Interestingly, Carbery himself seems to have suffered while on Gallipoli. On 26 October 1915, MO William McAra reported that he was seen to be 'getting fearfully nervous — ducks & runs at sound of every bullet'. At least two officers thought he might have 'a severe nervous breakdown', but Carbery stayed on the peninsula. McAra diary.

103 *New Zealand Herald*, 4 November 1916, p. 11. In Boyd's opinion, 'colonials were not so liable to shell shock as the British soldiers . . . due to the more open-air life which was possible in the colonies, and to the fact that life was not lived at so great a pressure'.

104 Richard Dowling file, 3/128, ANZ.

105 *Wairarapa Age*, 9 June 1916, p. 3; Frank Leyland file, 4/619, ANZ.

106 Parkes to Godley, 1 April 1918, Medical Report — Parkes to G.O.C., WA 1/3/10/30, ANZ.

107 Officers were often sent to special hospitals. These included Craiglockhart, outside Edinburgh, which found fame through its remarkable doctor, William Rivers, and his equally remarkable 'patient', the poet Siegfried Sassoon, a relationship fictionally immortalised by Pat Barker in her *Regeneration Trilogy*.

108 Godley to Allen, 30 June 1916, [Correspondence between] General Sir Alexander Godley [Commander New Zealand Expeditionary Force] and Colonel Hon. Sir James Allen, Minister of Defence, 4 January–29 December 1916, WA 252 1 [3], ANZ.

109 Elsie Prudentia Grey, Diary, MS-Papers-5994, ATL.

110 New Zealand Army Nursing Service — NZANS overseas records, correspondence — Matron-in-chief, AD78 23 67/3/1A, ANZ.

111 Arthur Owen Evans file, 3/2930, ANZ.

112 Angus McPhee Marshall file, 3/1284, ANZ.

113 *Southland Times*, 29 December 1916, p. 3.

114 Reginald William Napier file, 3/274, ANZ.

115 George Sandham file, 3/81, ANZ.

116 Frederick James Foote, 'Yesteryears', Reminiscences, MS 2007/9, AWMM, pp. 306–8.

CHAPTER 15: MAKING IT BETTER?

1 27 November 1915, Diary of William McAra, Gallipoli, June–December 1915, MS-2943/002, Hocken.

2 Letter 16 September 1917, William Mandeno Smallfield, War Letters, Diaries and Papers, MS 2007/37, AWMM.

3 Michael Tyquin, *Gallipoli: An Australian Medical Perspective* (Canberra: Army History Unit, 2012),

p. 65; Frederick James Foote, 'Yesteryears', Reminiscences, MS 2007/9, AWMM, p. 295; George Tierney, Glyn Harper (ed.), *Letters from the Battlefield: New Zealand Soldiers Write Home 1914–1918* (Auckland: HarperCollins, 2001), p. 120.

4 *Wanganui Chronicle*, 30 June 1915, p. 5. Turnbull, who also served in the Second World War, received the MC and a DSO and was mentioned in despatches three times.

5 William Kingston Wilson, Diary, 1994.2314, NAM, p. 67.

6 8 September 1915, Diaries of A. M. Trotter/transcribed by A. A. S. Trotter, MS-3397/004, Hocken.

7 A. D. Carbery, *The New Zealand Medical Service in the Great War, 1914–1918* (Auckland: Whitcombe & Tombs, 1924), p. 118.

8 31 August 1917, Smallfield letters, diaries and papers.

9 Carbery, *Medical Service*, p. 400.

10 Christopher Pugsley and Charles Ferrall (eds), *Remembering Gallipoli: Interviews with New Zealand Gallipoli Veterans* (Wellington: Victoria University Press, 2015), p. 226.

11 *Kai Tiaki*, October 1917, pp. 216–17.

12 *Star*, 29 August 1916, p. 2 (quoting *Chicago Tribune*).

13 T. Duncan M. Stout, *War Surgery and Medicine* (The Official History of New Zealand in the Second World War 1939–1945) (Wellington: Department of Internal Affairs, 1954), p. 3.

14 *Star*, 29 August 1916, p. 2 (quoting *Chicago Tribune*).

15 Clifford Collingwood, Diary and Scrapbook: New Zealand, Egypt & Western Front — WW1, 2007.139, NAM.

16 Kevin Brown, *Fighting Fit: Health, Medicine and War in the Twentieth Century* (Stroud, UK: The History Press, 2008), p. 44; *Kai Tiaki*, October 1917, pp. 216–17.

17 Robin Hyde, *Passport to Hell*, edited and introduced by D. I. B. Smith (Auckland: Auckland University Press 2015, 1st pub. 1936), p. 275. Morison described the use of BIPP in a 12 August 1916 *Lancet* article and wrote a book, *BIPP Treatment of War Wounds*, published in 1918. In the preface he said of his system, 'it is so simple that a clever surgeon is unnecessary for the achievement of the best results, though a careful one is essential'.

18 *Kai Tiaki*, October 1918, pp. 193–5; *Kai Tiaki*, January 1918, p. 9.

19 *Kai Tiaki*, April 1918, p. 82. As surgeon Duncan Stout, who served in both world wars, pointed out, after 1918, debridement, Carrel-Dakin treatment and BIPP 'were all utilised in civilian practice, especially in the treatment of serious accidental injuries'. Stout, *War Surgery*, p. 3.

20 Foote, 'Yesteryears', p. 296.

21 Tyquin, *Gallipoli*, p. 56; Lieutenant-Colonel W. S. Austin, *The Official History of the New Zealand Rifle Brigade* (Wellington: L. T. Watkins Ltd, 1924), p. 548.

22 *Kai Tiaki*, April 1915, p. 105. Plaster of Paris had, in Jones's words, proved 'a filthy method' for compound fractures, absorbing any 'suppuration' from the wound 'like blotting-paper' and becoming 'horribly offensive, adding to the infection'.

23 Medical Corps Memoranda — Precis of events in France, 11 April 1916–10 June 1917, WA10 19, 10/6/10, ANZ; Carbery, *Medical Service*, p. 311.

24 Collingwood diary.

25 http://livesonline.rcseng.ac.uk/biogs/E004298b.htm, Royal College of Surgeons, Plarr's Lives of the Fellows Online, accessed 24 July 2017.

26 *Kai Tiaki*, January 1916, p. 30. Hester Maclean added a note to Cherry's letter: 'Sister Cherry has, for about six months, had the position of charge of the surgical ward she mentions above. We may feel proud that one of our New Zealand sisters has been entrusted with such a responsible position.'

27 Carbery, *Medical Service*, p. 304.

28 24 October 1915, McAra diary.

29 Tyquin, *Gallipoli*, pp. 63, 65.

30 Richard Dowling file, 3/128, ANZ.

31 Jane Tolerton, *An Awfully Big Adventure: New Zealand World War One Veterans Tell Their Stories* (Auckland: Penguin, 2013), p. 67.

32 John Crawford (ed.) with Peter Cooke, *No Better Death: The Great War Diaries and Letters of William G. Malone* (Auckland: Reed in association with New Zealand Defence Force, 2005), p. 161.

33 Hyde, *Passport*, pp. 241, 243.

34 Carbery, *Medical Service*, p. 284; Hyde, *Passport*, pp. 122–3.

35 John A. Lee, *Soldier* (Wellington: A. H. & A. W. Reed, 1976), p. 74.

36 Hyde, *Passport*, pp. 243–4.

37 *Northern Advocate*, 11 June 1917, p. 2.

38 *Auckland Star*, 29 September 1915, p. 9. 'It is hoped that the X-ray apparatus which is not yet quite ready. will be installed this week. The radiographer will be Dr. Grace, son of the late Hon. Dr. Grace. M.L.C.. of New Zealand.'

39 *Evening* Star, 24 September 1915, p. 6.

40 *Kai Tiaki*, April 1918, pp. 80–1. The Scottish Women's Hospital even had a dedicated X-ray ambulance, known as the 'Ambulance Flottante', driven by 'a woman chauffeur', which boasted its own darkroom and water supply and could travel to wherever it was most needed. *New Zealand Herald*, 2 October 1915, supplement, p. 6.

41 *Press*, 25 May 1916, p. 3; *Timaru Herald*, 5 August 1915, p. 4; *Northern Advocate*, 9 November 1916, p. 4.

42 Kevin Clunie (comp.) and Ron Austin (ed.), *From Gallipoli to Palestine: The War Writings of Sergeant GT Clunie of the Wellington Mounted Rifles, 1914–1919* (McCrae, Victoria: Slouch Hat Publications, 2009), p. 35; *Manawatu Standard*, 13 April 1916, p. 7.

43 Jim Rotherham, *Hori Kaiporka: The Life and Stories of George Richard Rotherham Gallipoli Veteran* (Rotorua: Jamesfield Publishing, 2nd rev. edn, 1st pub. 2004), p. 68.

44 *Southland Times*, 7 October 1915, p. 2.

45 John Crawford (ed.), *The Devil's Own War: The First World War Diary of Brigadier-General Herbert Hart* (Auckland and Wollombi: Exisle in association with New Zealand Defence Force, 2008), pp. 62–3; Rotherham, *Hori Kaporka*, p. 92.

46 *Auckland Star*, 27 April 1916, p. 2.

47 *Evening Post*, 17 May 1918, p. 7. French X-ray expert Dr Maxime Ménard lost both his index fingers, 'having fallen victim to the mysterious rays', *New York Herald*, European edition, 10 September 1916.

48 *Star*, 13 October 1916, p. 5.

49 Foote, 'Yesteryears', p. 295.

50 Johanna McCamish and Rob Hawker, 'The Development, Impact and Use of Anaesthesia in World War One', *ACORN: The Journal of Perioperative Nursing in Australia*, vol. 28, no. 2, Winter 2015, pp. 20–3.

51 Tyquin, *Gallipoli*, p. 67.

52 Collection of 3/2643 Private Eric Sidney Bardell, Diary of the First trip of the 5th Charter of H.M.N.Z.S. "Maheno" July 6th to October 22nd 1918, 1996.1682.1, NAM.

53 Allan Marriott, *Mud Beneath My Boots: A Poignant Memoir of the Effects of War on a Young New Zealander* (Auckland: HarperCollins, 2005), pp. 167–8.

54 http://www.bbc.com/future/story/20160630-how-one-of-historys-bloodiest-wars-eventually-saved-lives, accessed 17 August 2017.

55 *Kai Tiaki*, July 1919, p. 117.

56 McCamish and Hawker, 'Anaesthesia in World War One'.

57 Foote, 'Yesteryears', p. 295.

58 Charles Weston, *Three Years with the New Zealanders* (London: Skeffington & Son, 1918), Chapter XIII.

59 *Kai Tiaki*, October 1915, p. 171.

60 William Taylor, *The Twilight Hour: A Personal Account of World War I* (Morrinsville: Sutherland, 1978), p. 71.

61 Reginald Pound, *Gillies: Surgeon Extraordinary* (London and Christchurch: Michael Joseph/Whitcombe & Tombs, 1964), p. 56.

62 New Zealand Section, Queen's Hospital [Sidcup] — War Diary, 12 January–9 July 1918, WA143 178, [143A] ANZ; *Neil Metcalfe,* 'The Effect of the First World War (1914–1918) on the Development of British Anaesthesia'*, European Journal of Anaesthesiology*, vol. 24, no. 8, 2007, pp. 649–57.

63 Diary August 1918, Vincent Jervis, MS-Papers-2241, ATL.

64 Brown, *Fighting Fit*, pp. 44–5.

65 Lyn Macdonald, *The Roses of No Man's Land* (Harmondsworth, UK: Penguin Books, 1980), p. 95.

66 Carbery, *Medical Service*, p. 400.

67 *Kai Tiaki*, October 1919, p. 185.

68 *Observer*, 17 August 1918, p. 4.

69 Michael Tyquin, *Gallipoli: The Medical War: The Australian Army Medical Services in the Dardanelles Campaign of 1915* (Sydney: University of New South Wales Press, 1993), p. 65.

70 *Kai Tiaki*, July 1918, p. 138.

71 Tyquin, *Gallipoli*, p. 57.

72 Diary of Lance-Corporal Victor Charles Middlemass, 1993.977, NAM.

73 *North Otago Times*, 21 December 1916, p. 8.

74 23 May 1915, Diaries of A. M. Trotter/transcribed by A. A. S. Trotter, MS-3397/004, Hocken.

75 26 July 1915, McAra diary.

76 Lee, *Soldier*, p. 95.

77 Medical — Health — Troops on transports — Returning with invalids, AD1 982 49/467 [a], ANZ.

78 Tyquin, *Gallipoli*, pp. 64, 67; George William Thomson, Papers, MS-2003-72, AWMM; *Kai Tiaki*, January 1916, p. 28.

79 *Otago Daily Times*, 19 January 1918, p. 11.

80 *Evening Post*, 26 June 1916, p. 3. Instead of receiving the £300 salary he later asked for, Tolhurst was dismissed in July 1918 with a £200 gratuity. Allen thanked him for his 'ungrudgingly given' work and explained that because trained men were coming from Britain, his services were no longer required. Tolhurst file Territorial Force — Gerald Tolhurst, AABK, 7291, W5614, 79/, D.2/7230, ANZ.

81 *Evening Post*, 26 January, 1918, p. 9.

82 Carbery, *Medical Service*, p. 516.

83 *New Zealand Herald*, 16 June 1917, p. 8.

84 *New Zealand Times*, 27 June 1916, p. 6.

85 *New Zealand Herald*, 16 June 1917, p. 8.

86 Wilson diary, p. 50; Memories of Norman E. Hassell, Window into WW1, Palmerston North City Library, http://ww1.pncc.govt.nz/blog/2015/11/18/object-memories-of-1914-norman-e-hassell.

87 Kerry Neale, 'Scarred by War: Medical Responses to Facially Disfigured Soldiers of the Great War', in Ashley Ekins and Elizabeth Stewart (eds), *War Wounds: Medicine and the Trauma of Conflict* (Auckland and Wollombi: Exisle Publishing, 2011), p. 63.

88 Juliet Nicolson, *The Great Silence 1918–1920: Living in the Shadow of the Great War* (London: John Murray, 2009), pp. 75–6.

89 *Evening Star*, 6 November 1919, p. 3.

90 George William Nuttall Diary, Liddle Collection, Brotherton Library, Leeds, courtesy Glyn Harper.

91 Quoted Pound, *Gillies*, p. 50.

92 For background on the fascinating Valadier, see Murray C. Meikle, *Reconstructing Faces: The Art and Wartime Surgery of Gillies, Pickerill, McIndoe and Mowlem* (Dunedin: Otago University Press, 2013,

reprint 2015), pp. 43–5.

93 In September 1915 this became a hutted hospital near Wimereux, north of Boulogne, and in May 1917 it was renamed the No. 83 (Dublin) General Hospital. On 14 October 1917 New Zealand ambulance man Norman Gray visited the 'New Face' ward at Wimereux, 'where some fifty men were growing new noses and lips. One chap had a piece of rib bone for his nose bridge and some of his forehead pulled down over it for a covering! He had had thirteen operations and had two more to go. The new nose and things were not exactly handsome, but some of the more advanced cases were really marvelous examples of modern surgery.' Randolph Norman Gray, Papers relating to World War One, MS-Papers-4134, ATL, folder 3.

94 Pound, *Gillies*, pp. 22–5. There had been experiments that sought 'to pad out fallen contours by the use of celluloid, imbedded in the tissue: but this method was commonly unsuccessful, since the tissue would not tolerate the foreign substance, which was forced to the surface'. *Evening Star*, 6 November 1919, p. 3.

95 *Press*, 18 January 1918, p. 5.

96 Andrew Bamji, 'Facial Surgery: The Patient's Experience', in Hugh Cecil and Peter Liddle (eds), *Facing Armageddon: The First World War Experienced* (Barnsley, UK: Pen & Sword, 2003, 1st pub. 1996); Nicolson, *Great Silence*, p. 88.

97 Report on Medical Services N.Z.E.F. (England) by Col. Parkes', 1 April, 1918, Medical — Dental hospital — England — Sidcup (Queens Hospital), AD1 971, 49/229, ANZ.

98 Nicolson, *Great Silence*, p. 82.

99 Brown, *Fighting Fit*, p. 59.

100 Quoted Pound, *Gillies*, p. 44.

101 Pound, *Gillies*, p. 45.

102 *Press*, 8 February 1919, p. 12.

103 Bamji, 'Facial Surgery', p. 495.

104 Ibid., p. 498.

105 New Zealand Section, Queen's Hospital [Sidcup] — War Diary, 12 January–9 July 1918, WA143 178, [143A], ANZ.

106 Allen to Godley, 12 and 19 December 1916, Ministerial Files — Correspondence with General Godley, Allen, 1 2 M1/15 3, ANZ.

107 Meikle, *Reconstructing*, pp. 78–9; Darryl Tong, 'Correction of Midfacial Fractures Using a Dentofacial Traction Appliance', *Journal of Military and Veterans' Health*, vol. 22, no. 2, June 2014.

108 *Kai Tiaki*, January 1918, pp. 35–7.

109 *Otago Daily Times*, 24 May 1919, p. 6.

110 *Press*, 8 February 1919, p. 12.

111 Ibid.

112 Godley to Allen, 4 July 1918, Ministerial Files — Correspondence with General Godley, Allen1 2, M1/15, ANZ.

113 New Zealand Section, Queen's Hospital [Sidcup] — War Diary, 12 January–9 July 1918, WA143 178, [143A], ANZ.

114 Pickerill to Allen, 11 January 1918, Medical — Dental hospital — England — Sidcup (Queens Hospital), AD1 971, 49/229, ANZ.

115 Neale, 'Scarred by War', p. 69.

116 *Otago Daily Times*, 24 May 1919, p. 6.

117 *Evening Star*, 6 November 1919, p. 3.

CHAPTER 16: BROKEN SURVIVORS

1 *New Zealand Herald*, 21 January 1919, p. 6; Medical — Health — Troops on transports — Returning with invalids, AD1 982 49/467 [a], ANZ.

2 For a full account of the embarkation arrangements and the vessels involved, see A. D. Carbery, *The New Zealand Medical Service in the Great War, 1914–1918* (Auckland: Whitcombe & Tombs, 1924), pp. 494ff.

3 *New Zealand Herald*, 21 January 1919, p. 6.

4 'The 1918 flu pandemic', https://nzhistory.govt.nz/culture/influenza-pandemic-1918 (Ministry for Culture and Heritage), updated 26-Jan-2018.

5 Laura Spinney, *Pale Rider: The Spanish Flu of 1918 and How it Changed the World* (London: Jonathan Cape, 2017), p. 4. Note that Marcus Hansen called it yellow fever on 23 August, and on the 29th, 'African fever of some sort', 'A Soldier's Diary', Pvt. Marcus Christian Hansen (Rifleman), Regt. No. 74744, Company: SPEC, 40th Reinforcements 1918/19, Transcribed by John W. Hansen (grandson), http://www.aucklandmuseum.com/war-memorial/online-cenotaph/record, accessed 7 February 2018.

6 *Kai Tiaki*, October 1918, p. 209. Tubman's brother Reynold had been killed at Passchendaele.

7 Hansen, 'A Soldier's Diary'.

8 *Kai Tiaki*, January 1919, pp. 15–17.

9 Geoffrey W. Rice, *Black November: The 1918 Influenza Pandemic in New Zealand* (Christchurch: Canterbury University Press, 2005, rev. edn, 1st pub. 1988), p. 57.

10 Bertha Emily Taylor, Letters and journal, MS-Papers-1291, ATL, p. 29; *Kai Tiaki*, January 1919, pp. 4, 8.

11 Chrissie Ward (ed.), *Dear Lizzie: A New Zealand Soldier Writes From the Battlefields of World War One* (Auckland: HarperCollins, 2000), p. 133. As Geoffrey Rice notes, 'Though there were many more hospital beds than in peacetime, military hospitals were geared to treating wounds rather than infectious diseases. For example, it was difficult to isolate cases in the overcrowded and desperately busy hospitals in France.' *Black November*, p. 43.

12 Taylor letters and journal, p. 34.

13 *Kai Tiaki*, January 1919, p. 7.

14 *Kai Tiaki*, April 1919, p. 61.

15 *New Zealand Herald*, 7 February 1920, supplement, p. 1.

16 *Kai Tiaki*, April 1919, p. 63.

17 Rice, *Black November*, p. 71.

18 Ibid., p. 96.

19 Ibid., pp. 95, 122, 123, 147.

20 Ibid., pp. 135, 149.

21 Ibid., p. 135.

22 Ibid., p. 211; Carbery, *Medical Service*, p. 507. Rice puts the death toll at 281, Carbery at 287.

23 Allan Leslie Christie file, 3/2915, ANZ; John Bonwell Sale file, 3/4316, ANZ.

24 Letter from Featherston Camp CO, 23 January 1919, William Bey file, N/N, ANZ; Bertram Boock file, 3/2344, ANZ.

25 Frederick George Atyeo file, 3/130a, ANZ.

26 *Kai Tiaki*, January 1919, pp. 10, 45.

27 William Fergus Paterson file, 3/4277, ANZ.

28 11 November 1918, Fanny Helena Speedy diaries, MS-Papers-1703, ATL; Louisa Higginson, Diaries transcribed by Mrs R. L. Wilson, MS-Papers-2477, ATL, Book 2, p. 12.

29 Carbery, *Medical Service*, p. 514. For the NZMC and the NZANS, final demobilisation had largely been achieved by the end of April 1920, but that year the medical personnel retained by the Defence Department were transferred to a newly created New Zealand Army Medical Department (and paid at the same rate). Almost all the 40 medical officers in the NZAMD, and almost half the 459 NCOs and men, had served overseas. There were also 210 nurses still working.

30 Carbery, *Medical Service*, p. 503; Imelda Bargas and Tim Shoebridge, *New Zealand's First World War Heritage* (Auckland and Wollombi: Exisle, 2015), pp. 200–1.

31 Carbery, *Medical Service*, p. 509.

32 Clifford Collingwood, Diary and Scrapbook: New Zealand, Egypt & Western Front — WW1, 2007.139, NAM.

33 *Evening Post*, 13 April 1916, p. 7.

34 *New Zealand Herald*, 6 October 1916, p. 9.

35 Bargas and Shoebridge, *First World War Heritage*, p. 200; Carbery, *Medical Service*, pp. 510–11.

36 Carbery, *Medical Service*, p. 505.

37 *New Zealand Herald*, 18 April 1917, p. 8.

38 Frederick James Foote, 'Yesteryears', Reminiscences, MS 2007/9, NAM, p. 301.

39 *New Zealand Herald*, 14 July 1919, p. 4.

40 *Kai Tiaki*, January 1919, p. 43.

41 Carbery, *Medical Service*, p. 511. The extended hospital took all the patients from the Military Annexe at Auckland.

42 *Sun*, 3 June 1916, p. 3.

43 Collingwood diary.

44 *Evening Post*, 26 June 1916, p. 3.

45 Bargas and Shoebridge, *First World War Heritage*, p. 206.

46 Tim Shoebridge, 'Repatriation of Returned Servicemen', https://nzhistory.govt.nz/files/documents/public-service-at-war-articles-footnoted.pdf, p. 77, accessed 29 November 2017. Although most of the sick and injured had been discharged from the military hospital system by 1921, and the hospitals were reassigned to the Health Department in 1921 and 1922, soldiers continued to be treated 'in their capacity as private citizens'.

47 Allan Marriott, *Mud Beneath My Boots: A Poignant Memoir of the Effects of War on a Young New Zealander* (Auckland: HarperCollins, 2005), pp. 196–8.

48 Foote, 'Yesteryears', p. 302.

49 Collingwood diary.

50 Nick Wilson, Jennifer A. Summers, Michael G. Baker, George Thomson and Glyn Harper, 'Fatal Injury Epidemiology Among New Zealand Military Forces in the First World War', *New Zealand Medical Journal*, 1 November 2013, vol. 126, no. 1385, p. 21.

51 Marina Larsson, *Shattered Anzacs: Living With the Scars of War* (Sydney: University of New South Wales Press, 2009), pp. 22, 24, 72–3.

52 Coralie Clarkson, 'The Reality of Return: Exploring the Experiences of World War One Soldiers After Their Return to New Zealand', MA thesis, History, Victoria University of Wellington, 2011, p. 189. Clarkson speaks of the added burden, for sufferers, of phthisiophobia — the fear of tuberculosis.

53 Larsson, *Shattered Anzacs*, p. 183.

54 *New Zealand Herald*, 21 January 1919, p. 6.

55 Allen to Parkes, 10 September 1918, Ministerial Files — Correspondence with Colonel Parkes, Allen 1, 3 M1/34, ANZ.

56 http://www.wairarapa100.co.nz/tauherenikau-military-camp#more-414, accessed 29 November 2017.

57 Jane Tolerton, *An Awfully Big Adventure: New Zealand World War One Veterans Tell Their Stories* (Auckland: Penguin, 2013), p. 270.

58 Tim Shoebridge, 'Repatriation of Returned Servicemen', https://nzhistory.govt.nz/files/documents/public-service-at-war-articles-footnoted.pdf, p. 77, accessed 29 November 2017.

59 Elizabeth Anne Walker, '"The Living Death": The Repatriation Experience of New Zealand's Disabled Great War Servicemen', MA thesis, History, Victoria University of Wellington, 2013, pp. 8–9, 34–5.

60 Ibid., p. 47.

61 Social Assistance Chronology 1844–2013: A historical summary of social security benefits, war pensions, retirement pensions, taxation measures, family assistance, housing, student support and labour market

programmes (as at May 2013), http://www.msd.govt.nz/documents/about-msd-and-our-work/about-msd/history/social-assistance-chronology-1844-2013.pdf, accessed 15 November 2017.

62 Ibid.

63 War Pensions Amendment Act, Third Schedule. Pensions Payable for Specific Injuries.

64 Roland Scott Bremner file, 23476, ANZ.

65 Social Assistance Chronology; Walker, 'Living Death', p. 50.

66 Tolerton, *Awfully Big Adventure*, p. 273.

67 *Evening Star*, 3 July 1917, p. 7.

68 Letter Edith J. Austen to Hester Maclean, 20 April 1919, letter Mary Grigor to Hester Maclean, 30 May 1919, Boarding & Treatment of Nurses, AD 1 48/858, ANZ.

69 Russell Clarke, '"Not Mad, But Very Ill": The Treatment of New Zealand's Shellshocked Soldiers 1914 to 1939', MA thesis, University of Auckland, 1991, pp. 36–7.

70 Shoebridge, 'Repatriation of Returned Servicemen', https://nzhistory.govt.nz/files/documents/public-service-at-war-articles-footnoted.pdf, p. 80, accessed 29 November 2017.

71 Carbery, *Medical Service*, p. 517.

72 *Kai Tiaki*, 1 January 1920, p. 17.

73 Letter 7 August 1915, Charles Ernest Thomas, Letters, 2015/106, South Canterbury Museum.

74 *Press*, 11 January 1923, p. 7.

75 *Northern Advocate*, 11 October 1919, p. 4.

76 Jan Rodgers, '"A Paradox of Power and Marginality": New Zealand Nurses' Professional Campaign During War, 1900–1920', PhD thesis, History, Massey University, 1994, Chapter 10.

77 *New Zealand Herald*, 29 May 1918, p. 8.

78 *Star*, 7 May 1917, p. 6; William George Charles Smith file, 17/248, ANZ; Charles Raymond Neale file, 17/294, ANZ.

79 William McAra file, 3/529, ANZ.

80 8 August 1915, Diary of William McAra, Gallipoli, June–December 1915, MS-2943/002, Hocken.

81 Peter Gulland Hume file, 3/446a, ANZ.

82 Gladys Violet Luxford, 'How I came to be interested in war and why I went to World War One', MS 94/6, AWMM, p. 6.

83 After six months of consecutive duty in a hospital or on a transport or hospital ship, they were eligible, like the soldiers, for three weeks' leave and a railway pass that gave them free travel, Orders (Standing) Nursing Service, AD 1 51/34, ANZ; Hester Maclean, *Nursing in New Zealand: History and Reminiscences* (Wellington: Tolan Printing Company, 1932), p. 232.

84 Cora Beattie Anderson file, 22/12, ANZ.

85 Jan Rodgers, 'Thurston, Mabel', Dictionary of New Zealand Biography, first published in 1996. Te Ara — the Encyclopedia of New Zealand, https://teara.govt.nz/en/biographies/3t36/thurston-mabel, accessed 13 December 2017.

86 Allen to Godley, 10 July 1920, Ministerial Files — Correspondence with General Godley, Allen1 2, M1/15, Part 6 28/1/20, ANZ.

87 *Kai Tiaki*, January 1919, p. 11.

88 Ashley Gould, 'Soldier Settlement', in Ian McGibbon (ed.), *The Oxford Companion to New Zealand Military History* (Auckland: Oxford University Press, 2000), p. 501.

89 *Dominion*, 7 November 1919, p. 9.

90 *Kai Tiaki*, January 1920, p. 49, July 1920, p. 159.

91 Rodgers, 'Paradox', Chapter 10; *New Zealand Herald*, 15 August 1925, p. 13.

92 *New Zealand Herald*, 11 March 1919, p. 5.

93 Honours and Awards for Messines June 1917, Medical Corps Memoranda — Precis of Events in France, 11 April 1916–10 June 1917, WA10 19, 10/6/10, ANZ. A full awards list appears in Carbery, *Medical Service*, pp. 526–30.

94 For a full list see Sherayl McNabb, *100 Years New Zealand Military Nursing: New Zealand Army Nursing Service — Royal New Zealand Nursing Corps 1915–2015* (Wairoa: author, 2015), pp. 484–6.

95 Carbery, *Medical Service*, gives an NZMC honour roll on pp. 521–5.

96 McNabb, *100 Years*, p. 188.

97 Leo van Bergen, *Before My Helpless Sight: Suffering, Dying and Military Medicine on the Western Front, 1914–1918* (Surrey: Ashgate, 2009), p. 407.

BIBLIOGRAPHY

UNPUBLISHED SOURCES

Alexander Turnbull Library, Wellington

Eric Arnold Burnett, Diary and letters, MS-Papers-2901

Carruthers family: Extracts from letters to Carruthers family/Walter [Carruthers], MS-Papers-4107

Margaret and William Cook: Letters from Stewart Callaghan, MS-Papers-5004

Benjamin Clyde Colbran, Diaries, Top of Form MS-Papers-1431

Cyril Coxhead, MSX-7829

Randolph Norman Gray, Papers relating to World War One, MS-Papers-4134

Elsie Prudentia Grey, Diary, MS-Papers-5994

Clarence Albany Hankins, Diary, MS-Papers-1439

Louisa Higginson, Diaries transcribed by Mrs R. L. Wilson, MS-Papers-2477

Letters to the Hutton family from Alexander Louis Hutton, MS-Papers-3906

Vincent Jervis, MS-Papers-2241

Howard Karl Kippenberger — World War One Diary, MS-Papers-8181-147

Henry Kitson, Letters and diary, MS-Papers-4540

John Keith Moloney, War diary, MS-Papers-1194

Thomas Russell Ritchie, Papers, MS-Papers-3705-1

Wilfred Collinson Smith, Correspondence, MS-Papers-2352

Fanny Helena Speedy, Diaries, MS-Papers-1703

Alfred Thomas Stratton, First World War 1916–1918 in France after Gallipoli, MS-Papers-3823

Bertha Emily Taylor, Letters and journal, MS-Papers-1291

Barbara Mildred Tilly, Papers, MS-Papers-1451

Archives New Zealand, Wellington

AABK W5829 7738 Box 1 1 [Register of Wounded Soldiers] No. 1–10,000

AABK W5829 7738 Box 2 3 [Register of Wounded Soldiers] No. 2000,01–30,000

ABVV W4763 7295 Box 1 d, New Zealand Veterinary Corps (Draft notes of the official history)

AD1 49/34 Nurses for Expeditionary Force — Offers of by New Zealand Government

AD1 718 9/260 Expeditionary Force — Remount Branch Veterinary Corps

AD1 725 10/110 Territorial Force — Exemption — Conscientious objectors

AD1 734 10/407/3 1 Territorial Force — Conscientious objectors sent abroad

AD1 750 13/266 Uniforms, etc — Dress — NZMC

AD1 795 25/159 1 Transport of forage to Egypt — Charter SS "Waihora" (ship)

AD1 881 39/140 Reports — Report — Hospital in Egypt

AD1 881 39/145 Reports — Reports progress — Ambulance Reinforcements for Egypt

AD1 887 39/180 Reports — Report Hospitals in Egypt — Matron in chief

AD1 894 39/237 Reports — Report health of troops at Trentham

AD1 900 40/27 Horses, mules, etc. — Suggestions for alleviating sufferings — Animals in war

AD1 900 40/65 Horses, mules, etc. — Horses for NZEF [New Zealand Expeditionary Force] — Requirements for 1st year of war

AD1 900 40/69 Horses, mules, etc. — Saddlery supplies to NZEF [New Zealand Expeditionary Force] at Samoa — Complaints

AD1 900 40/72 Horses, mules, etc. — Horses for Samoa — Supply of

AD1 965 49/116 Medical — Hospital — Walton-on-Thames — General file

AD1 965 49/116/1 Medical — Hospital — Walton-on-Thames — General file

AD1 967 49/148 Part 2 Medical — Medical Corps for NZEF — General File

AD1 967 49/148 Part 3 Medical — Medical Corps for NZEF — General File

AD1 970 49/213 Medical — Staff (Medical) Egypt

AD1 971 49/229 Medical — Dental Hospital — England — Sidcup (Queens Hospital)

AD1 972 49/235 Medical — Chiropodists — Trentham Camp — return of work done

AD1 973 49/250 Medical — Chiropodists — Appointment of — General file

AD1 977 49/341 Medical — Nurses — Walton-on-Thames Hospital — General staff

AD1 982 49/467 [a] Medical — Health — Troops on transports — Returning with invalids

AD1 1005 51/727/8 Publications, instructions, etc. — Histories — Regimental — New Zealand Veterinary Corps NZEF [New Zealand Expeditionary Force]

AD1 1036 62/45 Formation of Corps — Veterinary Section — Featherston Camp

AD1 1037 62/61 Formation of Corps — Corps — New Zealand Medical Corps — Formation of

AD1 1038 63/4/1 Medical Orderlies — New Zealand Medical Corps — General File 1915

AD1 1038 63/4/2 Medical Orderlies — New Zealand Medical Corps — General File 1917

AD1 1041 64/119 Returns — NZMC — Killed, wounded or died overseas

AD1 1130 210/15/2 Training — Medical — Stretcher bearers Regiment

AD78 16 27/125 Reinforcements — Conscientious objectors — General

AD78 23 67/3/1 New Zealand Army Nursing Service — NZANS [New Zealand Army Nursing Service] overseas records

AD78 23 67/3/1A New Zealand Army Nursing Service — NZANS [New Zealand Army Nursing Service] overseas records, correspondence — Matron-in-chief

AD78 23 67/5/1A New Zealand Army Nursing Service — NZANS [New Zealand Army Nursing Service] overseas records, correspondence re VADs [Voluntary Aid Detachments], Brocklehurst

AD78 27 G15/25, History of the War (Gallipoli — Medical —1915)

ALLEN1 1 M1/15 1 Ministerial Files — Correspondence with General Godley

ALLEN1 2 M1/15 3 Ministerial Files — Correspondence with General Godley

ALLEN1 2 M1/15 5 Ministerial Files — Correspondence with General Godley

ALLEN1 2 M1/15 6 Ministerial Files — Correspondence with General Godley

ALLEN1 3 M1/34 Ministerial Files — Correspondence with Colonel Parkes

ALLEN1 7 D1/17 Minister of Defence — Motor ambulances, offers overseas

ALLEN1 7 D1/22/2 Minister of Defence — Expeditionary force medical services

ALLEN1 8 D1/41 Minister of Defence — Hospital ship, "Maheno" (ship)

ALLEN1 8 D4/65 Minister of Defence — Contagious diseases, treatment of

WA1 10 2/30 Supplies — Equipment — Stores and equipment medical — Brockenhurst Hospital [New Zealand Convalescent Hospital], 12 September 1916–25 August 1919

WA1 13 5/19 Buildings — Accommodation nurses and VAD's [Voluntary Aid Detachment] — Brockenhurst, 24 September 1917–7 August 1918

WA1 20 10/76 Health, Welfare, etc. — Reports on and disposal of conscientious objectors, 16 July 1917–27 May 1919

WA10 12 ZMR 10/1/1 Monthly Report of New Zealand Veterinary Services (Egypt) for August 1917 and NZMR Brigade [New Zealand Mounted Rifle Brigade] for month of July 1917 (horses killed in action/died and destroyed) Major J. Stafford, Senior Veterinary Officer

WA10 12 ZMR 10/1/4 New Zealand Veterinary Corps (Egypt) Monthly horse state, November 1917, by Major J. Stafford [records state of horses injured, killed, or destroyed]

WA10 12 ZMR 10/1/5 New Zealand Veterinary Corps (Egypt) Monthly horse state, March 1918, by Major J. Stafford [records state of horses injured, killed, or destroyed]

WA10 12 ZMR 10/1/6 New Zealand Veterinary Corps (Egypt) Reports of Senior Officer NZEF [New Zealand Expeditionary Force] for July–August–September 1917 [records state of horses injured, killed, or destroyed]

WA10 12 ZMR 10/4/1 History of No. 4 New Zealand Veterinary Hospital from Formation until the Armistice [two photo postcards enclosed]

WA10 16 10/6/21 Medical Corps memoranda — Extracts from diary of 3/172 Sergeant Loftus NZMC [New Zealand Medical Corps], 1 January–9 December 1915 — Narrative of Captain R.D. Barron NZMC [New Zealand Medical Corps], attack on Abraham's Heights morning of 4 October 1917 — No. 2 Australian Casualty Clearing Station 1915–1917 — New Zealand Dental Corps — Venereal statistics, 4 January 1918

WA10 17 10/6/8, Medical Corps Memoranda — Gallipoli & Egypt, April 1916–2 March 1919

WA10 18 10/6/9, Medical Corps memoranda — Walton on Thames

WA10 19 10/6/10, Medical Corps memoranda — Precis of events in France, 11 April 1916–10 June 1917

WA10 20 10/6/11, Medical Corps Memoranda — Gallipoli April — 1915 — Medical arrangements for evacuation of wounded of Australian and New Zealand Army Corps

WA10 20 10/6/12, Medical Corps Memoranda — Precis of Events in France, 10 June–31 December 1917

WA27 35 [27a–n] Headquarters New Zealand and Australian Division — New Zealand Division — Assistant Director of Veterinary Services (ADVS) — War Diaries, 1 July–31 July August 1916 to 1–31 August, 1917

WA119 173 [119r], 1st New Zealand Field Ambulance — War Diary, 11 August 1914–18 February 1919

WA120 174 [120a], 2nd New Zealand Field Ambulance — War Diary, 26 March 1916– 25 March 1919

WA121 176 [121a], 3rd New Zealand Field Ambulance — War Diary, 1 April 1916–4 February 1919

WA123 175 [123f] 1st New Zealand Mobile Veterinary Section — War Diary, 1 April–30 June 1917

WA133 [134] ZG 34/58 Conscientious objectors, 4 September 1917–26 September 1918

WA136 177 [136b] New Zealand Medical Corps Reserve Depot — War Diary, 25 September 1917–16 December 1918

WA141 178 [141a], 2 New Zealand General Hospital — War Diary, 1 August 1915–31 December 1917

WA141 178/[141b], 2 New Zealand General Hospital — War Diary, 1 January–31 December

WA142 178 [142d] 3 New Zealand General War Diary 1 January–31 December 1918, WA142178 [142d]

WA143 178 [143a] New Zealand Section, Queen's Hospital [Sidcup] — War Diary, 12 January–9 July 1918

WA145 178 [145a] New Zealand Officers' Convalescent Home, Brighton — War Diary, 1 January 1915–31 December 1917

WA146 178/[146a] New Zealand Convalescent Hospital — War Diary, 6 July 1916–28 December 1917

WA146 178 [146h] New Zealand Convalescent Hospital — War Diary, 1 January–31 December 1918

WA182 196 [182a] New Zealand Sanitary Section — War Diary, 7 February 1916–25 February 1919

WA183 196 [183a] 2nd ANZAC [Australian and New Zealand Army Corps] Medical Officer Training School — War Diary, 20–30 November 1916

WA183 196 [183b] 2nd ANZAC [Australian and New Zealand Army Corps] Medical Officer Training School — War Diary, 1–31 December 1916

WA183 196 [183c] 2nd ANZAC [Australian and New Zealand Army Corps] Medical Officer Training School — War Diary, 1–31 January 1917

WA184 196 [184a] New Zealand Section Number 4 Veterinary Hospital — War Diary, Summary, 1 March 1916–24 April 1917

WA184 196 [184c] New Zealand Section Number 4 Veterinary Hospital — War Diary, 1–28 February 1918

WA184 196 [184d] New Zealand Section Number 4 Veterinary Hospital — War Diary, 1–31 March 1918

WA200 212 [200d] New Zealand Section 15 & 16 Company Imperial Camel Corps — War Diary 16 July 1917–23 June 1918

WA213 215 [213a] Principal Medical Officer Samoa Expeditionary Force — War Diary — 23 October–25 November 1914

WA213 215 [213c] Principal Medical Officer Samoa Expeditionary Force — War Diary — 26 November–17 December 1914

WA213 215 [213f] Principal Medical Officer Samoa Expeditionary Force — War Diary — 18 December 1914–14 January 1915

WA232 2 20 Trentham Camp — Report of the Committee of Inquiry into the sanitary conditions and health of troops in Trentham Military Camp, 1916

WA 252 1 [2], [Correspondence between] General Sir Alexander Godley [Commander New Zealand Expeditionary Force] and Colonel Hon. [Honourable] Sir James Allen, Minister of Defence, 2 April–19 December 1915

WA 252 1 [3], [Correspondence between] General Sir Alexander Godley [Commander New Zealand Expeditionary Force] and Colonel Hon. [Honourable] Sir James Allen, Minister of Defence, 4 January–29 December 1916

WA 252 1 [4], [Correspondence between] General Sir Alexander Godley [Commander New Zealand Expeditionary Force] and Colonel Hon. [Honourable] Sir James Allen, Minister of Defence, 6 January–28 December 1917

WA 252 2 [8] Letters to and from His Excellency the Earl of Liverpool and General Sir Alexander Godley [Commander New Zealand Expeditionary Force], 15 October 1915–5 October 1918

WA 252 3 [6], Semi-personal letters by General Officer Commanding, 5 September 1914–31 October 1916

Auckland War Memorial Museum

Anon. ['Aunt Jane'], 'We go through the Red Sea, Nursing in World War I', MS-99/57

Walter Arnold, Papers, MS-2016-9

John Budge, Letters, MS-98-67

Andrew Gilmore Carnahan, Letters Relating to Gallipoli, MS 2006/34

Ella Cooke, Letters, MS 94/36

Adrian Wilmot Delamore, War Diaries, MS 2007/40

John D. Duder, Papers, 82/8, MS-1160

Frederick James Foote, 'Yesteryears', Reminiscences, MS 2007/9

Harry Hall, Diary and letters 1915–1917 (compiled Christopher S. (Kit) Withers), MS 2002/72

Eric Wilson Hames, 'How I Won the Great War', MS 2013/1

Gilbert Martin Hames, Letters, MS 2013/2

David Alexandra Hipkins, War Diary extract, MS 2008/1

Harold Ernest Kretschmar, War Letters and Diaries, MS 2007/36

L. Logan, Dental Service with the First New Zealand Expeditionary Force, MS-2004

Gladys Violet Luxford, 'How I came to be interested in war and why I went to World War One', MS 94/6

Robert Scott, War Diary, MS-1671

William Habberfield Short, War Diary, MS-2006-40

Charles Haddon Simpkin, War Letters, MS 2007/43

William Mandeno Smallfield, War Letters, Diaries and Papers, MS 2007/37

George William Thomson, Papers, MS-2003-72

Geoffrey Victor Wild, Diary and Letters Relating to War Service (compiled Dorothy Wakelin), MS 2004/59

Christchurch City Libraries

Cecil Malthus: World War I Papers, http://christchurchcitylibraries.com/Heritage/Digitised/WarsAndConflicts/WorldWarI/Malthus/Thumbnails/

Hocken Collections — Te Uare Taoka o Hākena, Dunedin

William Fleming, Reminiscences, Misc-MS-1908

James Jeffery's transcripts of war letters, diaries and related material, MS-2934/002

Diary of William McAra, Gallipoli, June–December 1915, MS-2943/002

John H. Thomson, 3/453 No. 1 N.Z. Fd. Amb., Diary from 13 April 1915 to Jan 21st 1916, PC-0316

Diaries of A. M. Trotter/transcribed by A. A. S. Trotter, MS-3397/004

National Army Museum, Waiouru

Collection Corporal Harold Allen Alexander, 2006.1295

William Barclay Memoirs, 2000.980

Collection of 3/2643 Private Eric Sidney Bardell, Diary of the First trip of the 5th Charter of H.M.N.Z.S. "Maheno" July 6th to October 22nd 1918, 1996.1682.1

Diary Captain J. A. Berry NZMC, England & Western Front — WW1, 2000.727

Diary 49141 Harry O'Donel Bourke 2nd Wellington Regiment, 2005.332

Diary of Sergeant Gordon Clive Breen (1/131) Ambulance Corps, 1999.96

Letter: Louis Hamilton Browne — WW1, 2002.330.1

Letters: Thomas E. Catchpole — Egypt & Gallipoli — WW1, 2000.316

Diary — Henry M. Clark — NZ Hospital — England — WW1, 1993.1000

Clifford Collingwood, Diary and Scrapbook: New Zealand, Egypt & Western Front — WW1, 2007.139

Collection — Sister Mabel Crook — WW1, 2016.280.1

Letters Pte F. A. Crum — WW1, 2008.25

Letter Roy W. O. Dalrymple — Gallipoli — WW1, 2009.1196

Collection Sydney A. Davies 4/895, 2006.1294

Rifleman Gladstone (Gladdie) Graham, Letters: Egypt, France, England — WW1, 2005.585

Letter William John Rusden Hill, 1990.163

Diary: Patrick J. Keegan — Western Front — WW1, 1987.2294

Roy David McCormack 13/1075, Diary: Egypt & Sinai/Palestine WW1, 1999.2619

Diary Trooper Leslie Angus McInnes, 6th Reinforcements, Auckland Regiment 13/2054, 2008.269

Diary Charles Malone Sinai & Palestine — WW1, 1990.1620

Diary of Lance-Corporal Victor Charles Middlemass, 1993.977

Diary of Michael O'Malley 3/799 NZMC *Maheno*, 1991.1278

Diary Trooper William Rupert Pyle 9/76 Otago Mounted Rifles, 1996.292

Letters: Matthew George Sheeran — Western Front — WW1, 1999.1725

Diary C. L. Sommerville — Sinai & Palestine — WW1, 1997.255

The Story of Hobert & Ruby Tennent From October 14th 1883 to September 14th 1978 Collated by Patrick Tennent March 20th 2001, 2001.644

Diary of Pte P. M. Thompson 4th Bn Otago Regt Suez & Gallipoli 3 August 1914–15 September 1915, 1999.803

Letters: Ronald Watson (*Letters from a Padre: A Record of the War Service of Ronald S. Watson. M.C.*, edited by Nigel M. Watson, privately printed, Melbourne), 1998.2491

William Kingston Wilson, Diary, 1994.2314

Diary: Robert L. Withers — Sinai & Palestine & Western Front WW1, 2013.239.1

South Canterbury Museum, Timaru

Charles Ernest Thomas, Letters, 2015/106

Privately held papers

William Anderson, 'Great Grandfather's Tales', courtesy Bill Anderson

Private S. G. Gibb NZMC, Diary from 25.5.15 to 9.9.19, courtesy the late Pat Spale

Theses

Clarke, Russell. '"Not Mad, But Very Ill": The Treatment of New Zealand's Shellshocked Soldiers 1914 to 1939', MA thesis, University of Auckland, 1991

Clarkson, Coralie. 'The Reality of Return: Exploring the Experiences of World War One Soldiers After Their Return to New Zealand', MA thesis, History, Victoria University of Wellington, 2011

Fleming, Philip J. '"Shadow Over New Zealand": The Response to Venereal Disease in New Zealand 1910–1945', PhD thesis, History, Massey University, 1989

Mincham, Carolyn Jean. 'A Social and Cultural History of the New Zealand Horse', PhD thesis, History, Massey University, 2008

Palenski, Ron. 'Malcolm Ross: A Forgotten Casualty of the Great War', MA thesis, History, University of Otago, 2007

Poynter, Denise J. '"The Report on her Transfer was Shell Shock", A Study of the Psychological Disorders of Nurses and Female Voluntary Aid Detachments Who Served Alongside the British and Allied Expeditionary Forces During the First World War, 1914–1918', PhD thesis, University of Northampton, 2008

Rodgers, Jan. '"A Paradox of Power and Marginality": New Zealand Nurses' Professional Campaign During War, 1900–1920', PhD thesis, History, Massey University, 1994

Sargison, Patricia Ann. '"Essentially a Woman's Work": A History of General Nursing in New Zealand 1830–1930', PhD thesis, University of Otago, 2001

Tong, Darryl Chan. 'An Evidence-based and Historical Review of War Surgery of the Face and Jaws', PhD thesis, University of Otago, 2013

Walker, Elizabeth Anne. '"The Living Death": The Repatriation Experience of New Zealand's Disabled Great War Servicemen', MA thesis, History, Victoria University of Wellington, 2013

Wilson, Marcus James. 'A History of New Zealand's Military Horse: The Experience of the Horse in the Anglo-Boer War and World War One', MA thesis, History, University of Canterbury, 2007

PUBLISHED SOURCES

Books

Allsopp, Nigel. *A Centenary of Australian Animals at War*. Australia: InHouse Publishing, n.d.

Anson, T. V. *The New Zealand Dental Services* (The Official History of New Zealand in the Second World War). Wellington: Department of Internal Affairs, 1960.

The Anzac Book, Written and Illustrated in Gallipoli by The Men of ANZAC For the Benefit of Patriotic Funds Connected with the A & NZAC. London, New York, Toronto and Melbourne: Cassell and Company Ltd, 1916.

Austin, Lieutenant-Colonel W. S. *The Official History of the New Zealand Rifle Brigade*. Wellington: L. T. Watkins Ltd, 1924.

Baly, Lindsay. *Horseman, Pass By: The Australian Light Horse in World War I*. Staplehurst, Kent: Spellmount Ltd, 2004 (1st pub. 2003).

Bargas, Imelda and Tim Shoebridge. *New Zealand's First World War Heritage*. Auckland and Wollombi: Exisle, 2015.

van Bergen, Leo. *Before My Helpless Sight: Suffering, Dying and Military Medicine on the Western Front, 1914–1918* (The History of Medicine in Context series). Surrey: Ashgate, 2009.

Bourke, Joanna. *Dismembering the Male: Men's Bodies, Britain and the Great War*. Chicago: University of Chicago Press, 1996.

Boyack, Nick. *Behind the Lines: The Lives of New Zealand Soldiers in the First World War*. Wellington: Allen & Unwin/Port Nicholson Press, 1989.

Brown, Kevin. *Fighting Fit: Health, Medicine and War in the Twentieth Century*. Stroud, UK: The History Press, 2008.

Burton, O. E. *The Silent Division: New Zealanders at the Front: 1914–1919 & Concerning One Man's War*, ed. John H. Gray. Christchurch: John Douglas Publishing, 2014.

Butler, A. G. *The Australian Army Medical Services in the War of 1914–1918*, vol. III, *Special Problems and Services*. Canberra: Australian War Memorial, 1943.

Butler, A. G., R. M. Downes, F. A. Maguire and R. W, Cilento, *The Australian Army Medical Services in the War of 1914*–1918, vol I, *Gallipoli, Palestine and New Guinea*. Melbourne: Australian War Memorial, 1938 (2nd edn).

Callister, Sandy. *The Face of War: New Zealand's Great War Photography*. Auckland: Auckland University Press, 2008.

Carbery, A. D. *The New Zealand Medical Service in the Great War, 1914–1918*. Auckland: Whitcombe & Tombs, 1924.

Cecil, Hugh and Peter Liddle (eds). *Facing Armageddon: The First World War Experienced*. Barnsley, UK: Pen & Sword, 2003 (1st pub. 1996).

Chamberlin, Jan. *Shrapnel and Semaphore: My Grandfather's Diary of Gallipoli*. Auckland: RadioWorks, 2001.

Church, Clare. *New Zealand Graves at Brockenhurst: 93 Soldiers Remembered from World War One*. Lymington, UK: Elizabeth Church, 2002.

Clunie, Kevin, (comp.) and Ron Austin (ed.). *From Gallipoli to Palestine: The War Writings of Sergeant GT Clunie of the Wellington Mounted Rifles, 1914–1919*. McCrae, Victoria: Slouch Hat Publications, 2009.

Condliffe, J. B. *Te Rangi Hiroa: The Life of Sir Peter Buck*. Christchurch: Whitcombe & Tombs, 1971.

Crawford, John (ed.), with Peter Cooke. *No Better Death: The Great War Diaries and Letters of William G. Malone*. Auckland: Reed in association with the New Zealand Defence Force, 2005.

Crawford, John (ed.). *The Devil's Own War: The First World War Diary of Brigadier-General Herbert Hart*. Auckland and Wollombi: Exisle in association with New Zealand Defence Force, 2008.

__________ David Littlewood and James Watson (eds), *Experience of a Lifetime: People, Personalities and Leaders in the First World War*. Auckland: Massey University Press, 2016.

Drew, H. T. B. (ed.). *The War Effort of New Zealand*. Auckland: Whitcombe & Tombs, 1923.

Ekins, Ashley, and Elizabeth Stewart (eds). *War Wounds: Medicine and the Trauma of Conflict*. Auckland and Wollombi: Exisle Publishing, 2011.

Farrant, Herbert H., Elizabeth Morey and Delysse Storey (eds). *A Strong Sense of Duty: The First World War Letters of Chaplain the Reverend Clive Mortimer Jones 1917–1920*. Auckland: New Zealand Military Historical Society, 2013.

Fenton, Damien, with Caroline Lord, Gavin McLean and Tim Shoebridge. *New Zealand and the First World War 1914–1919*. Auckland: Penguin in association with Ministry for Culture and Heritage, 2013.

Fenwick, Lieutenant-Colonel Dr Percival. *Gallipoli Diary*. Auckland: David Ling in association with Auckland War Memorial Museum, c.2000.

Fitzgerald, Michael, and Claire Regnault. *Berry Boys: Portraits of First World War Soldiers and Families*. Wellington: Te Papa Press, 2014.

Fussell, Paul. *The Great War and Modern Memory*. Oxford: Oxford University Press, 1975, 2000, 2013.

Gordon, Iain. *Lifeline: A British Casualty Clearing Station on the Western Front, 1918*. Stroud, UK: The History Press, 2013.

Hallett, Christine E. *Veiled Warriors: Allied Nurses of the First World War*. Oxford: Oxford University Press, 2014.

Hand-Newton, C. T., DSO. *A Physician in Peace and War*. Christchurch: N. M. Peryer, 1967.

Harper, Glyn. *Massacre at Passchendaele: The New Zealand Story*. Auckland: HarperCollins, 2000.

________ (ed.). *Letters from the Battlefield: New Zealand Soldiers Write Home 1914–1918*. Auckland: HarperCollins, 2001.

________ and Queen Elizabeth II Army Memorial Museum. *Images of War: World War One: A Photographic Record of New Zealanders at War 1914–1918*. Auckland: HarperCollins, 2008.

________ (ed.). *Letters from Gallipoli: New Zealand Soldiers Write Home*. Auckland: Auckland University Press, 2011.

________ *Johnny Enzed: The New Zealand Soldier in the First World War 1914–1918*. Auckland and Wollombi: Exisle, 2015.

Harrison, Mark. *The Medical War: British Military Medicine in the First World War*. Oxford: Oxford University Press, 2010.

Hird, Rachel. *Good bye Bill Massey No more Khaki: Reg Hird's Letters from the Great War*. Miramar, Wellington: author, 2015.

Hunter, Kate, and Kirstie Ross. *Holding On to Home: New Zealand Stories and Objects of the First World War*. Wellington: Te Papa Press, 2014.

Hyde, Robin. *Passport to Hell*, edited and introduced by D. I. B. Smith. Auckland: Auckland University Press, 2015 (1st pub. 1936).

In Memoriam, Chaplain-Major Wm. Grant: His Letters from the Front. Gisborne: Herald Office, 1915.

Kinloch, Terry. *Echoes of Gallipoli: In the Words of New Zealand's Mounted Riflemen*. Auckland: Exisle Publishing, 2005.

________ *Devils on Horses: In the Words of the Anzacs of the Middle East*. Auckland: Exisle Publishing, 2007.

Lang, Roger, and Dr Jennifer Batham-Lang. *Chaplains of Anzac: New Zealand's Fallen Chaplains of the Great War*. New Zealand: Lang Book Publishing, 2015.

Larsson, Marina. *Shattered Anzacs: Living with the Scars of War*. Sydney: University of New South Wales Press, 2009.

Lawson, Will. *Historic Trentham, 1914–1917: The Story of a New Zealand Military Training Camp, and Some Account of the Daily Round of the Troops Within Its Bounds*. Wellington: Wellington Publishing Company, 1917.

Lee, John A. *Civilian into Soldier*. Auckland: Vital Books, 1963 (1st pub. Mayfair Books, London).

________ *Soldier*. Wellington: A. H. & A. W Reed, 1976.

Liddle, Peter. *Men of Gallipoli: The Dardanelles and Gallipoli Experience, August 1914 to January 1916*. London: Allen Lane, 1976.

Macdonald, Lyn. *The Roses of No Man's Land*. Harmondsworth, UK: Penguin Books, 1980.

________ *1914–1918: Voices and Images of the Great War*. London: Michael Joseph, 1988.

McGibbon, Ian (ed.). *The Oxford Companion to New Zealand Military History*. Auckland: Oxford University Press, 2000.

________ *New Zealand's Western Front Campaign*. Auckland: David Bateman, 2016.

Maclean, Hester. *Nursing in New Zealand: History and Reminiscences*. Wellington: Tolan Printing Company, 1932.

McLean, Gavin. *The White Ships: New Zealand's First World War Hospital Ships*. Wellington: New Zealand Ship & Marine Society, 2013.

McNabb, Sherayl. *100 Years New Zealand Military Nursing: New Zealand Army Nursing Service — Royal New Zealand Nursing Corps 1915–2015*. Wairoa: author, 2015.

Malthus, Cecil. *Anzac: A Retrospect*. Auckland: Reed, 2000 (1st pub. 1965).

Marriott, Allan. *Mud Beneath My Boots: A Poignant Memoir of the Effects of War on a Young New Zealander*. Auckland: HarperCollins, 2005.

Martin, Arthur Anderson. *A Surgeon in Khaki: Through France and Flanders in World War I*. Lincoln and London: University of Nebraska Press, 2011 (1st pub. 1915).

Mayhew, Lucy. *Wounded: A New History of the Western Front in World War I*. Oxford: Oxford University Press, 2014 (1st pub. 2013).

Meikle, Murray C. *Reconstructing Faces: The Art and Wartime Surgery of Gillies, Pickerill, McIndoe and Mowlem*. Dunedin: Otago University Press, 2013 (reprint 2015).

Moore, A. Briscoe. *The Mounted Riflemen in Sinai and Palestine: The Story of New Zealand's Crusaders*. Auckland: Whitcombe & Tombs, n.d.

Nicol, C. G. *The Story of Two Campaigns: Official War History of the Auckland Mounted Rifles Regiment, 1914–1919*. Auckland: Wilson & Horton, 1921.

Nicolson, Juliet. *The Great Silence 1918–1920: Living in the Shadow of the Great War*. London: John Murray, 2009.

O'Carroll, Brendan. *Khaki Angels: Kiwi Stretcher-bearers in the First and Second World Wars*. Wellington: Ngaio Press, 2009.

Parsonson, Ian M. *Vets at War: A History of the Australian Army Veterinary Corps 1909–1946*. Canberra: Australian Military History Publications, 2005.

Pengelly, Edna. *Nursing in Peace and War*. Wellington: Wingfield Press, 1956.

Philippe, Nathalie (ed.), with Christopher Pugsley, John Crawford and Matthias Strohn. *The Great Adventure Ends: New Zealand and France on the Western Front*. Christchurch: John Douglas Publishing, 2013.

Pound, Reginald. *Gillies: Surgeon Extraordinary*. London and Christchurch: Michael Joseph/Whitcombe & Tombs, 1964.

Powell, Anne. *Women in the War Zone: Hospital Service in the First World War*. Stroud, UK: The History Press, 2013 (1st pub. 2009).

Pugsley, Christopher. *Gallipoli: The New Zealand Story*. Libro International and Pen & Sword Books, 5th edn, 2014 (1st pub. 1984).

________ *On the Fringe of Hell: New Zealanders and Military Discipline in the First World War*. Auckland: Hodder & Stoughton, 1991.

________ *Te Hokowhitu a Tu: The Maori Pioneer Battalion in the First World War*. Auckland: Reed, 1995.

_________ and Charles Ferrall (eds), *Remembering Gallipoli: Interviews with New Zealand Gallipoli Veterans.* Wellington: Victoria University Press, 2015.

Rattray, Joan. *Great Days in New Zealand Nursing.* Wellington: A. H. & A. W. Reed, 1961.

Rawstron, R. E. *A Unique Nursing Group: New Zealand Army Nurse Anaesthetists of WWI.* Christchurch: Rawstron Publishing Co., 2005.

Reddiex, Glenn. *Just To Let You Know I'm Alive: Postcards from New Zealanders During the First World War.* Wellington: Grantham House, 2015.

Rice, Geoffrey W. *Black November: The 1918 Influenza Pandemic in New Zealand.* Christchurch: Canterbury University Press, 2005 (rev. edn, 1st pub. 1988).

Robertson, John. *With the Cameliers in Palestine.* Wellington: A. H. & A. W. Reed, 1938.

Rogers, Anna. *While You're Away: New Zealand Nurses at War 1899–1948.* Auckland: Auckland University Press, 2003.

Rotherham, Jim. *Hori Kaiporka: The Life and Stories of George Richard Rotherham Gallipoli Veteran.* Rotorua: Jamesfield Publishing, 2nd rev. edn, 1st pub. 2004.

'Sergeant-Major, R.A.M.C.'. *With the R.A.M.C. in Egypt.* London, New York, Toronto and Melbourne: Cassell & Co., 1918.

Shephard, Ben. *A War of Nerves: Soldiers and Psychiatrists in the Twentieth Century.* Harvard: Harvard University Press, 2003.

Shoebridge, Tim. *Featherston Military Training Camp and the First World War.* Wellington: Manatū Taonga/ Ministry for Culture & Heritage, 2012 (1st pub. April 2011).

Smith, Stephen. *The Samoa (N.Z.) Expeditionary Force 1914–1915.* Wellington: Ferguson & Osborn, 1924.

Spinney, Laura. *Pale Rider: The Spanish Flu of 1918 and How It Changed the World.* London: Jonathan Cape, 2017.

Stanley, Peter. *Die in Battle, Do Not Despair: The Indians on Gallipoli, 1915.* Solihull, UK: Helion & Co. in association with United Service Institution of India, 2015.

Stout, T. Duncan M. *War Surgery and Medicine* (The Official History of New Zealand in the Second World War 1939–1945). Wellington: Department of Internal Affairs, 1954.

Sutherland, Beth. *My Dear Chick: A New Zealand Love Story 1911–1948.* Masterton: Fraser Books, 2008.

Taylor, William. *The Twilight Hour: A Personal Account of World War I.* Morrinsville: Sutherland, 1978.

Tolerton, Jane. *Ettie: A Life of Ettie Rout.* Auckland: Penguin Books, 1992.

_________ *An Awfully Big Adventure: New Zealand World War One Veterans Tell Their Stories.* Auckland: Penguin, 2013.

_________ *Make Her Praises Heard Afar: New Zealand Women Overseas in World War One.* Wellington: Booklovers Books. 2017.

Tyquin, Michael. *Gallipoli: The Medical War: The Australian Army Medical Services in the Dardanelles Campaign of 1915.* Sydney: University of New South Wales Press, 1993.

_________ *Forgotten Men: The Australian Veterinary Corps 1909–1946.* Warriewood, NSW: Big Sky Publishing, 2011.

_________ *Gallipoli: An Australian Medical Perspective.* Canberra: Army History Unit, 2012.

Ward, Chrissie (ed.). *Dear Lizzie: A New Zealand Soldier Writes From the Battlefields of World War One.* Auckland: HarperCollins, 2000.

Weaver, John C. *Sorrows of a Century: Interpreting Suicide in New Zealand, 1900–2000.* Montreal and London: McGill-Queen's University Press; Wellington: Ithaca/Bridget Williams Books, 2014.

Weston, C. H. *Three Years With the New Zealanders.* London: Skeffington & Son, 1918.

Willis, L. Ida G. *A Nurse Remembers: The Life Story of L. Ida G. Willis O.B.E., A.R.R.C., E.D.* Lower Hutt: A. K. Wilson Ltd, n.d.

Articles

Doughty, Lea, and Susan Heydon. 'Medicine Supply During the First World War: Overcoming Shortages in New Zealand, *Health and History*, vol. 17, no. 2, 2015, Special Issue: World War I, 37–51.

Doughty, Lea. 'The Right to Refuse: Compulsory Vaccination in the New Zealand Expeditionary Force During World War 1, 1914–1918', History of Medicine Lectures, University of Otago, 27 June 2017.

Fitzgerald, Gerard J., PhD. 'Chemical Warfare and Medical Response During World War I', *American Journal of Public Health*, vol. 98, no. 4, April 2008, 611–25.

Jones, Edgar, and Simon Wessely. 'Battle for the Mind: World War 1 and the Birth of Military Psychiatry', Legacy of the 1914–18 War series, *Lancet*, vol. 384, 8 November 2014, 1708–14.

Kirkup, John. 'Fracture Care of Friend and Foe During World War 1', *ANZ Journal of Surgery*, vol. 73, no. 6, June 2003, 453–9.

McCamish, Johanna, and Rob Hawker, 'The Development, Impact and Use of Anaesthesia in World War One', *ACORN: The Journal of Perioperative Nursing in Australia*, vol. 28, no. 2, Winter 2015, 20–3.

Metcalfe, Neil. 'The Effect of the First World War (1914–1918) on the Development of British Anaesthesia', *European Journal of Anaesthesiology*, vol. 24, no. 8, 2007, 649–57.

O'Connor, P. S. 'Venus and the Lonely Kiwi: The War Effort of Miss Ettie A. Rout', *New Zealand Journal of History*, vol. 1, no. 1, 1967, 11–32.

Parsons, Gwen. 'The Construction of Shell Shock in New Zealand, 1919–1939: A Reassessment', *Social History of Medicine*, vol. 26, no. 1, February 2013, 56–73,

Shoebridge, Tim. 'Manawatu's First World War Camps, 1915–1919', *Manawatu Journal of History*, no. 9, 2013, 11–21.

_________ 'Repatriation of Returned Servicemen', https://nzhistory.govt.nz/files/documents/public-service-at-war-articles-footnoted.pdf, accessed 29 November 2017.

Weaver, John, and David Wright. 'Shell Shock and the Politics of Asylum Committal in New Zealand, 1916–22', *Health and History*, vol. 7, no. 1, 2005, 17–40.

Wilson, Nick, Nhung Nghiem, Jennifer A. Summers, Mary-Ann Carter and Glyn Harper. 'A Nutritional Analysis of New Zealand Military Food Rations at Gallipoli in 1915: Likely Contribution to Scurvy and Other Nutrient Deficiency Disorders', *New Zealand Medical Journal*, vol. 126, no. 1373, 19 April 2013, 12–29.

Wilson, Nick, Jennifer A. Summers, Michael G. Baker, George Thomson and Glyn Harper. 'Fatal Injury Epidemiology among New Zealand Military Forces in the First World War', *New Zealand Medical Journal*, vol. 126, no. 1385, 1 November 2013, 13–25.

Wilson, Nick, Christine Clement, Jennifer A. Summers, John Bannister and Glyn Harper, 'Mortality of First World War Military Personnel: Comparison of Two Cohorts', *British Medical Journal*, 349, 16 December 2014.

Winter, Jay. 'Shell-Shock and the Cultural History of the Great War', *Journal of Contemporary History*, vol. 35, no. 1, 2000, Special Issue: Shell-Shock, 7–11.

Online

Memories of Norman E. Hassell, Window into WW1, Palmerston North City Library, http://ww1.pncc.govt.nz/blog/2015/11/18/object-memories-of-1914-norman-e-hassell.

McCandlish, Ross (compiler). 'Between the Lines: The Diary and Letters of 11/92 Trooper Roderick McCandlish, Wellington Mounted Rifles', www.nzmr.org/McCandlish.

http://nzans.org/Nurses Who Served/Full NZANS WW1 Roll.html

Diary of William Henry Winter WW1 1915, horowhenua.kete.net.nz, accessed 25 August 2016.

ACKNOWLEDGEMENTS

My thanks, first, to Glyn Harper, Professor of War Studies at Massey University, who oversaw this book as part of the First World War Centenary History Programme, for his support and for kindly sharing research material. Project administrator Tessa Lyons was always helpful and patient with inquiries, as was her successor, Rebecca Johns.

I am grateful to all those who offered support, advice and information: Emily Anderson, Clare Ashton, Juliet Ashton, Neill Atkinson, Imelda Bargas, Shaun Barnett, Joe Bennett, Ross Blair, Professor Giselle Byrnes, Elizabeth Caffin, Charlotte Cantley, Carolyn Carr, Anna Cottrell, Peter Cox, David Elworthy and Ros Henry, Sam Gawn, John Gordon, Ray Grover, Joe Hollander, Peter Hurly, Dr Karen Jillings, Simon Johnson, Sophie Lennon, Chris Maclean, Owen Marshall, Susanna Montgomery Norris, Joanna Orwin, Professor Katie Pickles, Geoffrey Rice and Tim Shoebridge. Pat Clarkson's database of New Zealand First World War doctors was invaluable. My cousins, Claire and Paul White, and Dr David Richards, generously provided illustrations.

My particular thanks to: Professor Neil Bruère for his enthusiastic and knowledgeable assistance with veterinary matters; New Zealand Defence Force historian John Crawford for sterling advice and for alerting me to useful archival sources; Ashley Ekins from the Australian War Memorial for his encouragement; Peter Fry for much-needed and greatly appreciated help on military aspects; Euan Galloway and Lea Doughty for their essential contributions regarding pharmacists; Dr Sandy Macleod for useful discussions on shell shock; military historian Dr Ian McGibbon for kindly reading draft chapters; Simon Moody, research curator at the Air Force Museum of New Zealand, for giving up so much of his busy time; and Dr Kerry Neale of the Australian War Memorial for good conversation and for sharing her knowledge of maxillo-facial wounds and surgery.

As always, the friendly and knowledgeable staff at various institutions were vital. I thank the Alexander Turnbull Library, the Auckland War Memorial Museum, the Australian War Memorial, the Cotter Medical History Museum, the Hocken Collections — Uare Taoka o Hākena, the South Canterbury Museum, Dolores Ho at the National Army Museum and Noel Swift at the Linton Military Camp.

The team at Massey University Press — publisher Nicola Legat, managing editor Anna Bowbyes, editorial assistant Emily Goldthorpe and designer Kate Barraclough, who made the book so handsome — have been a pleasure to work with. My thanks to Paul Lumsden for the maps, Peter Cooke for the index, and Quentin Wilson for kindly scanning images. My editor, David Green, combined excellent stylistic advice with invaluable historical knowledge.

Last, but by no means least, I thank two people without whom I could not have written this book: my dear friend, Alison Parr, and my beloved sister, Juliet Rogers. Alison has never faltered in her support, enthusiastic and knowledgeable interest or willingness to read and discuss draft material. Juliet's unwavering encouragement, love and belief in me, her superb advice, her restorative humour and her staunch loyalty have been indispensable. I am immeasurably grateful to her.

ABOUT THE AUTHOR

Anna Rogers has spent most of her working life as a book editor. She has an MA in English from Canterbury University, and has also been a bookseller and a sub-editor for the *New Zealand Listener*. Anna has edited both fiction and non-fiction for most of the major New Zealand publishers, adapted books for radio and is a book reviewer. She has edited an anthology of writing about Christchurch and written several non-fiction titles, including *While You're Away: New Zealand Nurses at War 1899–1948*, *A Lucky Landing: The Story of the Irish in New Zealand*, and illustrated histories of Canterbury and the West Coast.

INDEX

Page numbers in bold indicate illustrations

ABOUT THE FIRST WORLD WAR CENTENARY HISTORY PROGRAMME

Massey University, the Ministry for Culture and Heritage (MCH) and the New Zealand Defence Force have joined forces and committed substantial resources to produce a series of authoritative print histories on New Zealand and the First World War. Scholarly yet accessible to broad audiences, the works in this series draw on an extensive range of primary sources held in New Zealand, Britain and elsewhere, and contain high-quality maps and illustrations. Together they form the first complete and detailed account of New Zealand's First World War experience.

These print histories are complemented by digital resources published through the www.firstworldwar.govt.nz website, part of the Ministry for Culture and Heritage's NZHistory.govt.nz site. The programme's historians are also contributing to other centenary activities, including major international conferences, museum and art exhibitions, television documentaries, heritage trails and commemorative events in New Zealand and overseas.

The Centenary History Programme Governance Group is co-chaired by Gerald Hensley and Massey University Assistant Vice-Chancellor Research, Academic and Enterprise Giselle Byrnes. The group includes MCH Chief Historian Neill Atkinson, Defence Force Historian John Crawford, Massey University Professor of War Studies Glyn Harper, and other representatives of the three agencies. More information about the Centenary History series can be found at: http://ww100.govt.nz/first-world-war-centenary-print-histories.

This volume of the Centenary History would not have been possible without generous donations to the Massey University Foundation for this purpose. The Governance Group of the Centenary History Programme would like to acknowledge and thank the following organisations for their generosity: Acurity Health Group Limited, Canterbury Equine Clinic, Keelah Farm Vets, Lotteries Commission, Medical Assurance Society, New Zealand Equine Veterinary Association, New Zealand Veterinary Association, New Zealand Defence Force, Palmerston North City Council, Royal New Zealand Army Medical Corps, Society of Sheep and Beef Cattle, Wayne McIlwraith and the William & Lois Manchester Charitable Trust.

MASSEY UNIVERSITY TE KUNENGA KI PŪREHUROA UNIVERSITY OF NEW ZEALAND
New Zealand DEFENCE FORCE Te Ope Kātua O Aotearoa NAVY NZ ARMY AIR FORCE
MASSEY UNIVERSITY FOUNDATION
Manatū Taonga Ministry for Culture & Heritage
WW100 FIRST WORLD WAR CENTENARY HISTORY

MASSEY
UNIVERSITY
PRESS

First published in 2018 by Massey University Press
Private Bag 102904, North Shore Mail Centre
Auckland 0745, New Zealand
www.masseypress.ac.nz

Text copyright © Anna Rogers, 2018
Images copyright © as credited, 2018

Design by Kate Barraclough
Cover photographs: Alexander Turnbull Library and
National Army Museum

The moral right of the author has been asserted

All rights reserved. Except as provided by the Copyright Act 1994, no part of this book may be reproduced, stored in or introduced into a retrieval system or transmitted in any form or by any means (electronic, mechanical, photocopying, recording or otherwise) without the prior written permission of both the copyright owner(s) and the publisher.

A catalogue record for this book is available from the
National Library of New Zealand

Printed and bound in China by Everbest Printing
Investment Limited

ISBN: 978-0-9951001-9-0